CLINICAL DISORDERS OF BONE AND MINERAL METABOLISM

CLINICAL DISORDERS OF BONE AND MINERAL METABOLISM

Proceedings of
the Frances and Anthony D'Anna Memorial Symposium,
Detroit, MI, May 9–13, 1983

Editors:

BOY FRAME
Clinical Professor of Medicine, University of Michigan Medical School; Physician in Charge, Bone and Mineral Division, Henry Ford Hospital, Detroit, MI, USA

JOHN T. POTTS Jr
Jackson Professor of Clinical Medicine, Harvard Medical School; Chief of the General Medical Services, Massachusetts General Hospital, Boston, MA, USA

1983

EXCERPTA MEDICA, Amsterdam–Oxford–Princeton

International Congress Series No. 617

ISBN 0 444 90315 1

Library of Congress Cataloging in Publication Data
Main entry under title:

Clinical disorders of bone and mineral metabolism.
Includes indexes.
1. Bones--Diseases--Congresses. 2. Mineral metabolism--Disorders--Congresses. 3. Hyperparathyroidism--Congresses. I. Frame, Boy. II. Potts, John T.
[DNLM: 1. Bone diseases, Metabolic--Congresses.
2. Minerals--Metabolism--Congresses. W3 EX89 no. 617 /
WE 250 F815c 1983]
RC930.C55 1983 616.7′1 83-20644
ISBN 0-444-90315-1

Publisher:
Excerpta Medica
305 Keizersgracht
P.O. Box 1126
1000 BC Amsterdam

Sole Distributors for the USA and Canada:
Elsevier Science Publishing Co. Inc.
52 Vanderbilt Avenue
New York, NY 10017

Printed in The Netherlands by Casparie Amsterdam

In memory of Frances Maria D'Anna,
loving wife and mother

The Anthony D'Anna Family

CLINICAL DISORDERS OF BONE AND MINERAL METABOLISM

Steering Committee

Co-Chairmen

Boy Frame, M.D.
John T. Potts Jr, M.D.

Members

Frederic L. Coe, M.D.
Jack Coburn, M.D.
Howard Duncan, M.D.
John G. Haddad, M.D.
Michael Kleerekoper, M.D.
Stephen Krane, M.D.
Charles E. Jackson, M.D.
Conrad C. Johnston, M.D.
Donald R. Moore, M.D.
A. Michael Parfitt, M.B., B. Chir.
Sudhaker D. Rao, M.B., B.S.

PREFACE

This book contains a compilation of papers, overviews and discussions based on the Symposium entitled Clinical Disorders of Bone and Mineral Metabolism, held at the Hyatt Regency Hotel, Dearborn, Michigan, U.S.A., from May 9–13, 1983. The Symposium was sponsored by the Bone and Mineral Division, Henry Ford Hospital, Detroit, Michigan. It was made possible in part through the generous support of Mr. Anthony D'Anna and his family in memory of Mrs. Frances D'Anna, beloved wife of Mr. D'Anna. In addition, several hundred patients of the Henry Ford Hospital's Bone and Mineral Division also contributed to the Symposium Fund.

Close to 600 medical scientists and clinicians from approximately 30 countries were in attendance during the 5-Day Symposium. The purpose of the meeting was to discuss laboratory, clinical and therapeutic features of diseases that are related to disturbances in bone and mineral metabolism.

Topics for discussion included the following: clinical applications of parathyroid hormone assays, assessment of trabecular bone status, the role of vitamin D in clinical medicine, an assessment of mineral and matrix turnover, pathogenesis of hyperparathyroidism, management of hypercalcemic hyperparathyroidism, recent developments in bone physiology, secondary hyperparathyroidism, PTH-mediated bone loss, osteomalacia and nutritional bone disease, renal osteodystrophy, non-parathyroid hypercalcemia, osteoporosis, Paget's disease, idiopathic hypercalciuria and calcium disorders in childhood including pseudohypoparathyroidism.

Manuscripts were typed on special photocopy paper to speed and facilitate publication. Unless errors were detected, the manuscripts were published as received from the author(s).

Each section is preceded by an overview written by the section moderator(s) and is meant to capture the major highlights and general flavor of the related chapters which follow. Pertinent discussion following each paper or group of related papers has been included.

Three scientific poster sessions consisting of 55 to 75 posters each were an important part of the Symposium. Twelve posters from each session were chosen for further oral discussion between the moderators, authors and participants. Overviews of the poster sessions were written by the poster session moderators. An attempt was made to record the highlights and pertinent discussion following each poster session.

On the last day of the Symposium, four simultaneous oral sessions including a variety of topics in the bone and mineral field were conducted. Again the moderators, in an overview of each oral session, attempted to record pertinent new information and relevant discussion of the papers presented.

Moderator written overviews of two workshops are included. One is related to roentgenologic features of metabolic bone disease. In the other workshop, concepts of the current management of mild asymptomatic hyperparathyroidism was discussed. In addition, criteria to assess the design of a prospective, randomized clinical trial to evaluate the benefits and risks of surgical and medical management were reviewed.

Boy Frame, M.D.
John T. Potts Jr, M.D. *November, 1983*

WELCOMING ADDRESS

On behalf of the Board of Trustees of the Henry Ford Hospital, I would like to welcome you to our Third International Symposium on Clinical Disorders of Bone and Mineral Metabolism.

I have been assured by those responsible for planning the events of the next several days that this symposium is intended to provide a forum for a free exchange of ideas by the foremost medical specialists in the field. That is, by the way, the second definition of 'symposium' according to Webster's Seventh Collegiate Dictionary. Webster's first definition of 'symposium' is 'a drinking party especially following a banquet'.

With more than 250 clinical papers and exhibits to be presented over the next several days, on a range of topics, I doubt that you will find much time to engage in the spirit of the first definition of 'symposium'.

Over the last thirty years, this hospital has sponsored a variety of gatherings – like this one today – intended to bring together specialists from all over the world and from many fields. In fact, throughout my life I've watched the growth and development of this institution. And I am proud of the many contributions it has made to medical science and the needs of the community during its 68 years.

At the time this hopital was founded in 1915, the average life expectancy was only 54.5 years. Today it is 72 years. Medical science certainly has made great strides since my grandfather's first involvement in founding this hospital.

More remarkable, children being born today can expect to live for about 83 years – 10 years more than their parents, 20 years more than their grandparents and 30 years more than their great-grandparents.

Who knows what new advances in medicine will be uncovered during their lifetimes? Or, perhaps, which of the new developments you will discuss today and this week will contribute significantly to their health – and to their quality of life?

The second international bone symposium, in 1972 at this hospital, was opened by my late brother, Benson. He characterized the meeting in 1972 – and I think accurately so – as representing a 'declaration of interdependence for all the medical specialties and disciplines'. I am certain that this gathering will carry on that tradition – adding to the wealth of medical knowledge, the advances that have been made over the past 10 years in both diagnosis and treatment of bone and mineral metabolism disorders.

I am impressed that more than 500 physicians and researchers in the audience today have come from nearly every continent on the globe – from countries including Japan, China and Greece ... as well as Italy, Argentina and Holland, to name a few. I am informed that the top authorities in the field have come to share their thinking and their research.

The English philosopher Lord Bryce once wrote that medicine is 'the only profession that labors incessantly to destroy the reason for its own existence'. It is that quality that makes your profession one of the most honored. It is that quality that I see represented here today. And it is that quality that gives me the confidence that the exchange of information, during the sessions that follow, will aid in conquering the remaining medical frontiers.

I would like to acknowledge Dr. Boy Frame of Henry Ford Hospital and Dr. John Potts Jr of Massachusetts General Hospital – who, together with their distinguished steering committee, are responsible for the planning of this meeting.

Funding for the symposium is being provided in part by the Anthony and Frances D'Anna Fund, a fund established in memory of the late Mrs. D'Anna, a patient of Dr. Frame's. I understand that Mr. D'Anna is with us today. Mr. D'Anna has a long history with the Henry Ford Hospital, and he also has a history with the Ford Motor Company – as a former Ford dealer. I am told that a number of additional patients of the Bone and Mineral Division at Henry Ford Hospital also have contributed to the symposium fund.

Finally, I hope that the next several days are productive ones. I hope that you will carry home with you a feeling of accomplishment. I also would like you to take a message back to your individual states and countries. The message is that Michigan is becoming once again a center for growth and technology and scientific achievement. Your being here is testimony to that fact.

Thank you.

Henry Ford II
Chairman, Board of Trustees
Henry Ford Hospital
Detroit, Michigan, U.S.A.

REPLY TO MR. FORD'S REMARKS

Mr. Ford, distinguished members of the symposium, guests and friends: I am deeply honored to be here this morning in such fine company – the company of great men and women, whose quest for knowledge and dedication to quality patient care is responsible for our high caliber of health today.

I am proud and thankful to have had a small part in the symposium, and pray that God will enlighten your minds so that your efforts and good intentions will be realized.

If just one person is helped by the clinical information and investigative techniques exchanged at this meeting, then you have accomplished your mission.

Your courage, your wisdom, and your compassion, like that of Dr. Boy Frame and Dr. John Potts, is reflected in your faces and numbers this morning.

I will always remember Dr. Frame and the staff of Henry Ford Hospital for the many kindnesses shown my wife, Frances, while she was ill and under their care. Their presence and concern gave her dignity and made her three year struggle with bone cancer as comfortable as possible.

When she died, she left behind a legacy of love that made me realize how important it is that your research and work continue.

In closing, I would like to thank my friends at Henry Ford Hospital and the Ford family, as well, for their assistance and encouragement. They have been more than helpful to me in my many associations with them and have helped make my life a success.

God bless you for making this symposium a reality.

Anthony D'Anna

CONTENTS

III VITAMIN D IN CLINICAL MEDICINE

IV ASSESSMENT OF MINERAL AND MATRIX TURNOVER

VIII SECONDARY HYPERPARATHYROIDISM AND PTH-MEDIATED BONE LOSS

IX OSTEOMALACIA AND NUTRITIONAL BONE DISEASE

X RENAL OSTEODYSTROPHY

XI NON-PARATHYROID HYPERCALCEMIA

XII ECTOPIC CALCITRIOL PRODUCTION INCLUDING SARCOIDOSIS

XIII OSTEOPOROSIS – PATHOGENESIS, PREVENTION AND TREATMENT

XIV PAGET'S DISEASE

XV IDIOPATHIC HYPERCALCIURIA

XVI CALCIUM DISORDERS IN CHILDHOOD

XVII PSEUDOHYPOPARATHYROIDISM (PHP) AND RELATED DISORDERS

XVIII SCIENTIFIC POSTER SESSIONS

XIX ORAL SESSIONS

XX WORKSHOPS

I CLINICAL APPLICATION OF PARATHYROID HORMONE ASSAYS

SESSION I: CLINICAL APPLICATIONS OF PARATHYROID HORMONE ASSAYS

Moderator: John T. Potts, Jr.

Department of Medicine, Harvard Medical School and Massachusetts General Hospital, Boston, MA, U.S.A.

INTRODUCTION

J. POTTS: Problems seen today in interpretation of the radioimmunoassay for parathyroid hormone were not appreciated when Berson and Yalow developed, with Aurbach and me, the first radioimmunoassay for the hormone in 1963 using bovine parathyroid hormone which Aurbach had purified. In the last two decades, there has been intensive basic research on parathyroid hormone, including structural analysis and chemical synthesis of the hormone from human and other mammalian species. What has become gradually apparent is the complexity of the biosynthesis and the metabolism of the hormone that was not evident in 1963. Multiple fragment(s) and possibly even precursors of the hormone are present in blood of humans and animals. As a result of these discoveries, there has been a growth in attempts to produce immunoassays that measure specific forms of the hormone of greatest clinical significance. Investigators in this field have moved gradually from use of bovine hormone to human hormone as the immunogen as the latter has become available. Dr. Arnaud and his colleagues first introduced C-terminal assays, based on the bovine sequence, in 1970 when the large concentrations of circulating carboyl fragments was recognized. Since then there has been a gradual movement toward the use of human hormone. Drs. Mallette, Marx, and their colleagues recently showed the value of antisera that recognize the middle region of the human molecule. Dr. Segre and his colleagues this year have introduced a very sensitive amino-terminal immunoassay developed by immunization with the synthetic human 1-34 fragment.

There are many unanswered questions in this field of clinical and basic research concerning parathyroid hormone that we hope will be clarified by today's presentations and discussions. What assays should be used in different diseases associated with abnormal function of the parathyroid? What is the biological and pathophysiological meaning of the heterogeneity of circulating hormone that accounts for the multiple circulating fragments? How best are we to use and interpret the assays to arrive at sensible answers in a cost-effective manner when we evaluate patients with hypercalcemia and hypocalcemia? What types of assays are most likely to be useful in the future?

It is beyond the scope of this clinical symposium to review the basic complexity of the biosynthesis and metabolism of the hormone and the underlying problems in performance and interpretation of radioimmunoassays of various types. The reviews by Drs. Goltzman, Arnaud, Segre and their colleagues contain references to primary papers written over the last decade on the radioimmunoassay for parathyroid hormone that could be useful to interested readers.

Parathyroid hormone is composed of 84 amino acids in human, porcine, bovine and rat species; the structures are non-identical but closely homologous. Biological activity resides in the amino-terminal portion of the hormone (residues 2-25). Once it was appreciated that fragmentation of the hormone occurs both within the gland and in the periphery, due to several as yet uncharacterized enzymes present at several sites. Obvious questions were raised about what constitutes the active molecular species. It was realized that if an amino-terminal fragment was formed, it could be biologically active.

It is not known whether the fragments that enter the blood from the gland and the fragments that are produced by peripheral metabolism are necessarily the same, nor whether the same enzymes are responsible in each site. Some groups, our own, for example, have concentrated on the peripheral metabolism, and other groups have concentrated on fragmentation within the gland. There are many methodologic difficulties in these studies, including problems with artifacts, and the need to develop special techniques to examine the products produced by glandular or peripheral metabolism. Although progress has been slow, the issues raised are very intriguing.

The entire molecule of 84 amino acids is still, by conservative estimates, the most likely candidate to interact with receptors in bone and kidney, the two known principal target organs. It is also possible, however, that a biologically active amino-terminal fragment either leaves the site of cleavage and enters the blood, or is produced by cleavage at target sites to serve as an alternate or, even sole, active molecular species as suggested by the work of Slatopolsky's group, for example. We have to understand the metabolism of the hormone in order to know what we are measuring, but also to define (and measure) all molecules that are candidates to exert significant biological activity.

Fragments produced include a large fragment of 40 to 50 amino acids, extending from the region residues 30 to 40 to the carboxyl-terminus (usually referred to as C-fragments) and an amino-terminal fragment. Carboxyl fragments disappear from blood more slowly than does the intact hormone (which is taken up by tissues and cleaved); hence there is much more carboxyl fragment in blood than the intact molecule. Several groups have data that they have detected an amino-terminal fragment(s) in the blood, but there is general agreement that, if present, its concentration is very low compared to other hormonal forms; the clearance half-time of such N-fragments must be very rapid. So, at steady state, there are at least three basic molecular species to be concerned with: the intact hormone, carboxyl fragment(s), and amino-terminal fragment(s).

Fragments arising from the gland may differ from those found to re-enter the blood from peripheral sites. Also, there may be smaller fragments formed from the initial cleavage products. No one knows today just how many circulating fragments there are. We trust that as knowledge increases concerning circulating fragments, various assays can be used more effectively to help with discrimination between primary hyperparathyroidism and tumor hypercalcemia, and other related clinical issues.

Dr. Arnaud summarizes experience with assays that measure the biologically inactive molecules (carboxyl and/or mid-region fragments). Because of the high concentration of these fragments relative to that of the intact hormone (or amino-terminal fragments), the inert fragments have been measurable with many more antisera. Drs. Fischer and Slatapolsky's short contributions summarize the issue of the relative sensitivity and detection limits required for assays that measure only the amino-terminal region of the molecule. Arnaud and Slatapolsky emphasize the utility of assays that utilize antisera based on the middle region (M) or carboxyl region (C) of the molecule, emphasizing their clinical utility as an "integrative" index of normal or abnormal glandular activity both in primary hyperparathyroidism and the secondary hyperparathyroidism of renal failure. The limitation of such M-assays or C-assays for measurement of rapid changes in glandular secretory activity is also discussed.

It is not yet clear, however desirable, that any single assay can be used effectively in all clinical disease states where parathyroid status is to be assessed. Dr. Segre presents evidence suggesting possible wide utility of amino-terminal assays utilizing an antiserum with the very high affinity constant needed to detect only the intact molecule (by an exclusive amino-terminal recognition site that does not detect inert fragments).

In most of endocrinology, we apply suppression tests when we suspect overactivity and stimulation tests when we suspect underactivity of endocrine function. Until quite recently, such approaches have not been practical with parathyroid hormone because of problems with the heterogeneity of circulating hormone and varying clearance half-times of the material produced peripherally.

Dr. Segre provides data that suggests that stimulation and suppression tests are now practical. In his reports, stimulation and suppression by varying serum calcium concentration in normal subjects and those with primary hyperparathyroidism confirms *in vivo* the findings reported *in vitro* with excised glands and primary cell cultures by Habener and Brown, respectively, that there is a set point defect in primary hyperparathyroidism.

CYTOCHEMICAL BIOASSAY FOR PARATHYROID HORMONE: VALIDATION AND CLINICAL APPLICATIONS

David Goltzman, Hilary Gomolin, Marvin Wexler and Jonathan L. Meakins

Departments of Medicine and Surgery, McGill University and Royal Victoria Hospital, Montreal, Canada

The major circulating form of parathyroid hormone (PTH) consists of carboxyl and mid-region fragments, generated by peripheral metabolism (chiefly in the liver) of the major glandular form of PTH, PTH-(1-84) and released from the parathyroid gland. The fate of the corresponding amino-terminal fragment is unknown, yet this issue is of importance in that the hormonal bioactivity seems to reside within the amino-terminal end of the molecule. In order to examine the circulating biological forms of PTH in various hyperparathyroid states, we developed a sensitive bioassay, employing a previously described cytochemical technique (1).

VALIDATION STUDIES

Several studies were first performed to validate the PTH bioassay, which is based on the hormonal stimulation of the enzyme glucose-6-phosphate dehydrogenase in guinea pig kidney tubule cells (2). Thus, synthetic PTH-(1-34) was demonstrated to stimulate the assay in parallel with PTH-(1-84) and to be equipotent on a molar basis with the intact hormone. Additionally a synthetic analog of PTH-(3-34) was shown to inhibit the action of PTH-(1-84) as it does in other in vitro bioassay systems. Human plasma was reactive in the bioassay and serial dilutions stimulated in parallel with standard PTH-(1-84). Bioactivity in plasma fell after induction of hypercalcemia and after parathyroidectomy. Consequently, the appropriate behaviour of agonists and antagonists in the assay, and of the bioactivity determined in plasma, supported the use of the assay as an index of PTH bioactivity.

A variety of non-hormonal substances tested elicited either no stimulation or non-parallel stimulation at high concentrations only. Furthermore, the segregation of bioactivity levels in plasma samples from individuals with known hyper-or hypoparathyroidism or no parathyroid disease, into high, low or intermediate respectively, suggested that the major stimulating factor in plasma was indeed PTH and not other "non-specific" factors.

CLINICAL APPLICATIONS

Having validated the specificity of the bioassay and confirmed its sensitivity (detection limit of 5fg/ml), examination of the nature of the circulating molecular forms of PTH was then begun.

In initial studies (2) plasma from patients with primary hyperparathyroidism and normal renal function were fractionated by conventional gel chromatography. The results demonstrated that the majority of the bioactivity in the plasma of these patients was recovered in a pool co-eluting with PTH-(1-84) (Fig 1A). Consequently, in these patients, the major circulating bioactive moiety was similar or identical to the major glandular form of the hormone.

Similar fractionation studies were then performed with plasma from patients with chronic renal failure on maintenance hemodialysis (2). Again, a major proportion of bioactivity recovered from the gel filtration columns co-eluted with PTH-(1-84). In addition, however, a substantial component of the recovered bioactivity eluted after PTH-(1-84), in the position of a smaller molecular-weight entity (Fig. 1B). The relationship of both moieties to PTH was shown by elimination of the bioactivity through prior incubation with anti-PTH serum. The origin of the small molecular-weight entity was then explored. When parathyroid venous effluent plasma was subjected to chromatographic analysis, the majority of the bioactivity co-eluted with PTH-(1-84), and only a minor component of small molecular-weight bioactivity was identified. Consequently, the larger amounts appearing in the periphery seemed due either to reduced clearance of the relatively minor amounts of secreted material and/or due to generation of the fragment in the periphery. The disappearance rates of total bioactivity after parathyroidectomy did not seem excessively prolonged in patients with abnormal renal function, however, suggesting that peripheral production could be responsible for the small molecular-weight entity seen in uremia.

Although pseudohypoparathyroidism is functionally a form of hypoparathyroidism, we have operationally considered it a form of hyperparathyroidism in view of the high prevailing concentrations of circulating immunoreactive PTH. The disorder is believed to be due to a defect in the target tissue response to circulating PTH, associated with a reduction in the guanyl nucleotide-binding protein of the adenylate cyclase system. Others have reported a discordance of PTH bioactivity and immunoreactivity in this syndrome (4) and have suggested that the high circulating levels of immunoreactive PTH in this disorder could be bio-inactive. We have studied one such patient in whom we observed the absence of plasma bioactivity despite high circulating levels of PTH immunoreactity. Additionally, incubation of the plasma of this patient with exogenous bovine PTH-(1-84) reduced the sensitivity of the standard curve generated in the bioassay by this hormone. Consequently, in addition to a discordance in bioactivity and immunoreactivity, the patient's plasma appeared to contain PTH inhibitory activity.

Finally, we have initiated collaborative studies to examine the circulating PTH-like moiety present in the hypercalcemia-syndrome associated with malignancy which has been called "ectopic" hyperparathyroidism (3). A subset of these patients was studied who had some biochemical manifestations in common with patients with primary hyperparathyroidism, (such as increased nephrogenous cyclic AMP excretion and reduced renal phosphate threshold), and others which differed (3). Mean levels of

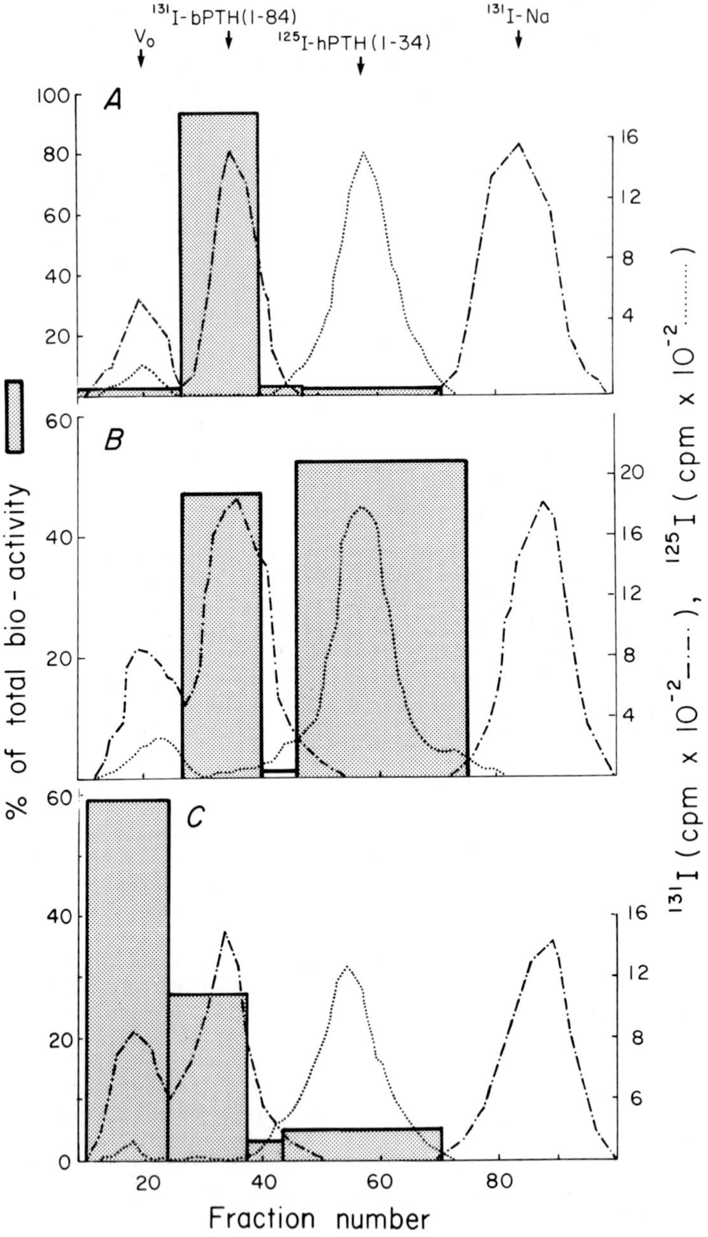

Figure 1. Gel filtration profiles of PTH bioactivity (-) after chromatography on Bio-Gel P-100 of plasma from a patient with (A) primary hyperparathyroidism (B) secondary hyperparathyroidism and chronic renal failure and (C) hypercalcemia associated with malignancy. For bioactivity, the height of the solid bars indicates the percentage of total bioactivity represented by pooled eluted fractions and the width of the bars, the size of the pools assayed. ^{131}I and ^{125}I profiles indicate the elution positions of bovine PTH-(1-84) and human PTH-(1-34) respectively.

bioactivity were elevated in these patients, and bioactivity was measurable in the medium of a resected tumor from such a patient, which was maintained in tissue culture. Analysis of plasma by gel chromatography, (Fig. 1C) revealed that the majority of the bioactivity eluted before PTH-(1-84), indicating that it differed from the major bioactive form of PTH circulating in primary hyperparathyroidism. Bioactivity extracted from tumors of these patients (5) could be detected by both renal adenylate cyclase bioassay and by cytochemical bioassay, and appeared larger than PTH-(1-84). In both bioassay systems, the synthetic analog of PTH-(3-34) inhibited bioactivity, suggesting that the bioactive moiety, could cross react with PTH receptors. The exact nature of this new entity remains to be determined.

SUMMARY AND CONCLUSIONS

Our studies have therefore employed both bioassays and immunoassays to examine the molecular nature of PTH-like substances. In primary hyperparathyroidism the major bioactive circulating moiety seems similar or identical to the major glandular form of the hormone, and hypersecretion of this entity clearly appears to be the major pathogenetic lesion. In hyperparathyroidism with chronic renal failure, higher levels of both bioactivity and immunoreactivity are generally observed and an additional small molecular-weight form of PTH was identified which seems to be generated through peripheral metabolism. In some cases of pseudohypoparathyroidism, elevated immunoreactive PTH levels may be associated with diminished bioactive levels and accompanied by PTH-inhibitory activity; an abnormal form of PTH may therefore exist in these instances. Finally, in the syndrome of hypercalcemia associated with malignancy, in a subset of patients, a discordance is again seen, however with low levels of PTH immunoreactivity and elevated levels of bioactivity. A new moiety may therefore be responsible for this syndrome which can interact with PTH receptors but which differs immuno-chemically. The use of our bioassay can therefore complement the information derived from radioimmunoassay and provide a potent tool for the exploration of the pathogenetic mechanisms of hyperparathyroid states.

REFERENCES

1. Chambers, D.J., Dunham, J., Zanelli, J.M., Parsons, J.A., Bitensky, L. and Chayen, J. (1978): Clin. Endocrinol. 9, 375.
2. Goltzman, D., Henderson, B. and Loveridge, N. (1980): J. Clin. Invest. 65, 1309.
3. Goltzman, D., Stewart, A.F., and Broadus, A.E. (1981): J. Clin. Endocrinol. Metab. 5233, 899.
4. Nagant de Deuxchaisnes, C., Fischer, J.A., Dambacher, M.A., Devogelaer, J-P., Arber, C.E., Zanelli, J.M., Parsons, J.A., Loveridge, N., Bitensky, L., and Chayen, J. (1981): J. Clin. Endocrinol. Metab. 53, 11105.
5. Stewart, A. F., Insogna, K.L., Goltzman, D. and Broadus, A.E. (1983): Proc. Natl. Acad. Sci. U.S.A. 80, 1454.

CLINICAL UTILITY OF "MID" AND "CARBOXYL" REGION SPECIFIC ASSAYS OF PARATHYROID HORMONE

Claude D. Arnaud and Linda A. Zitzner

Endocrine Unit, V.A. Medical Center and Departments of Medicine and Physiology, University of California, San Francisco, CA, U.S.A.

GENERAL COMMENTS

Our observations (1), made almost 15 years ago, concerning the extraordinary clinical utility of the parathyroid hormone (PTH) radioimmunoassay (RIA) have gradually gained broad acceptance and been recently confirmed by many laboratories. The key element in such assays appears to be the antiserum used. Not only must it have high affinity but it must also be specific for the mid (M) or carboxyl (C) regions of the native PTH molecule [PTH(1-84)] . The explanation(s) for this apparent latter requirement are not clear. In fact, this phenomenon is something of a paradox for, whereas the region of PTH(1-84) responsible for biological activity lies within the first 34 amino acid sequence, M and C fragments of PTH(1-84) have no known biological activity.

The purpose of this communication is to review our early observations concerning the clinical utility of a mid-region specific RIA of PTH (2) in relation to those made more recently by others with similar assays.

RESULTS AND DISCUSSION

Differential Diagnosis of Hypercalcemia

Our early results of M RIAs of PTH in the serum of normal subjects, patients with surgically proved primary hyperparathyroidism (1° HPT) and patients with malignancy associated hypercalcemia (MAH) are shown in Figure 1A and B. Recent studies by others using similar RIAs report almost identical results. Approximately 90% (Fig 1A) of patients with 1° HPT can be distinguished from normal subjects based on an abnormally increased serum M immunoreactive PTH (M iPTH) value alone and the majority of the remaining 10% have values that are not only in the upper range of normal but are inappropriately high for the corresponding level of serum calcium (Ca). Although not demonstrated uniformly by others, we have consistently found a significant negative correlation between the serum total Ca over the normal range and the serum M iPTH. Such a demonstration depends upon the precise and accurate measurement of the total serum Ca in fresh specimens.

Figure 1B shows that many patients with MAH can be distinguished from patients with 1° HPT on the basis of a relatively low serum M iPTH for a given serum Ca (3). This is particularly true of patients with serum Ca values > 12.5 mg/dl. Although this observation has been confirmed extensively by others, it is poorly understood, especially in the light of recent observations (4) suggesting that a large proportion of patients with MAH may have ectopic hyperparathyroidism. Coexistent 1° HPT should be suspected in patients with malignancy when serum M iPTH is increased above the normal range, however, it is clear from serum fractionation studies reported by our laboratory 10 years ago (5) that an increased serum M iPTH in some patients with MAH primarily reflects high serum concentrations of an immunoreactive species of PTH having a larger molecular size than PTH(1-84). This is in contrast to 1° HPT in which increased serum M iPTH primarily reflects an increase in circulating M and C fragments of PTH(1-84). These observations concerning differences in the molecular size of circulating M iPTH in 1° HPT and MAH have recently received considerable

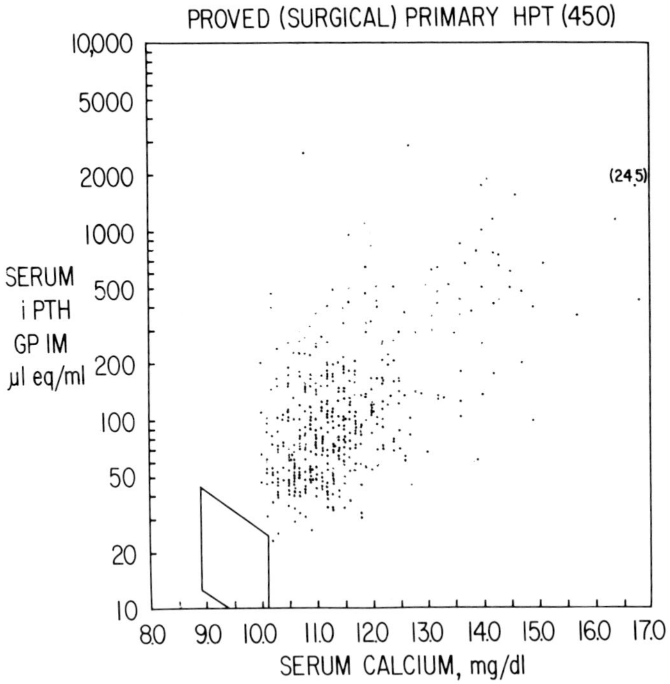

Figure 1A. Serum iPTH values in 450 patients with surgically proved primary hyperparathyroidism as a function of serum calcium concentration. The area enclosed by the solid lines represents the normal range ± 2 SD for serum iPTH and serum calcium. Note that there is a 10% overlap of serum iPTH with the normal range but that greater than 95% of normal sera and all hyperparathyroid sera have measurable iPTH. Formal discriminative analysis of serum iPTH and serum calcium separates 100% of hyperparathyroid patients from normal subjects. (From Arnaud CD, et al.: Excerpta Medica International Congress Series No. 346, Calcium Regulating Hormones, 1975, p. 19.)

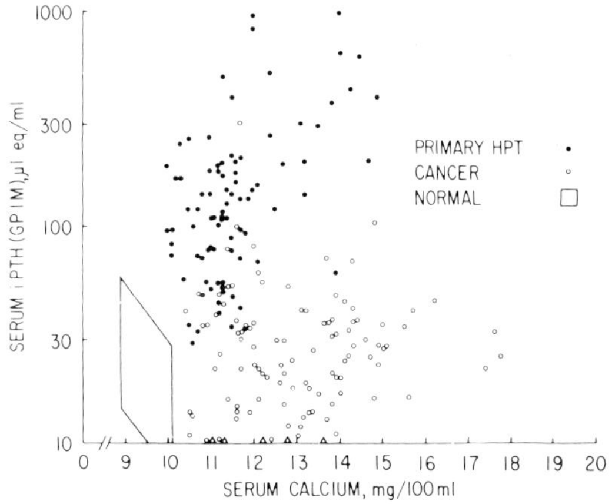

Figure 1B. Relationship between serum iPTH and serum calcium in primary hyperparathyroid patients (●) and hypercalcemic patients with cancer (0). Note that for a given serum calcium value, serum iPTH is lower in patients with cancer. Of 105 patients with cancer, 5 had undetectable serum iPTH (△). Area enclosed with solid lines indicates normal range ± 2 SD for serum iPTH and serum calcium. (From Benson RC, et al.: Am J Med 56:821, 1974.)

support from the studies of Goltzman et al. (6) using a cytochemical bioassay of PTH. These investigators showed that serum bioactive PTH fractionated on gel filtration columns similar to those we used eluted in almost identical positions as did M iPTH in our studies. Furthermore, as reported in the present volume by others and by Strewler et al. (7) of our laboratory, evidence is accumulating that a large molecular weight factor is produced by malignant cells in culture (derived from either animal models of MAH or from humans with the syndrome) which both stimulates bone resorption and binds to the PTH receptor in vitro. Paradoxically, most of such conditioned media factors have little PTH immunoreactivity (using PTH RIAs with multiple specificities) and this may explain why most sera from patients with MAH have either normal or low serum iPTH.

Although a large proportion of sera from patients with severe hypoparathyroidism contain little if any detectable M or C iPTH, many patients with hypercalcemia of non-parathyroid origin (i.e. vitamin D intoxication) contain low or even mid-range normal levels. This comprises the main drawback of M or C RIAs in the differential diagnosis of hypercalcemia. They may fail to segregate such patients from the relatively infrequent patient with occult MAH.

Differential Diagnosis of Hypocalcemia and Therapeutic Evaluation of Parathyroid Status in Chronic Renal Failure

Although history and physical examination will frequently result in the diagnosis of the underlying cause of hypocalcemia, serum M or C iPTH measurement correctly categorizes patients definitively into a group with parathyroprivic hypoparathyroidism (low or undetectable levels) or a group with either pseudohypoparathyroidism or secondary hyperparathyroidism (high values). The exception to this is in patients with severe hypomagnesemia ($<$ 1.0 mg/dl) who will have low serum M or C iPTH until this cation is replenished.

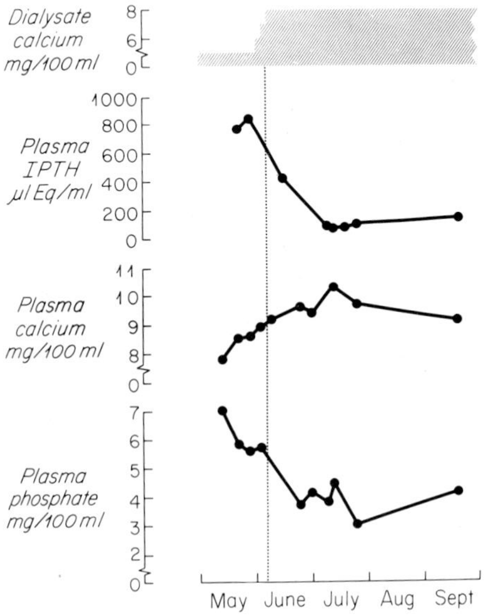

Figure 2. Serial values of plasma iPTH, calcium and phosphate during treatment of a patient with low and then high dialysate calcium. Plasma phosphate was reduced to 6 mg/dl by oral administration of aluminum hydroxide gel, after which dialysate calcium concentrations were progressively increased to 8 mg/dl. (Reproduced, with permission, from Goldsmith RS et al: Am J Med 1971;50:692).

Our general experience is that amino region (N) specific assays have the same diagnostic utility as M or C assays in assessing the hypocalcemic patient. The one exception is the patient undergoing medical treatment (i.e. phosphate restriction, Ca supplementation, vitamin D metabolite administration) for the secondary HPT associated with chronic renal failure. Such patients usually have severe parathyroid hyperplasia and, although serum N iPTH (measures largely PTH 1-84 in serum) can be rapidly (minutes) suppressed by increasing serum Ca to normal or slightly hypercalcemic values, it is very unlikely that parathyroid gland size changes appreciably with short treatment regimens. This is in contrast to serum M or C iPTH values which decrease slowly over a relatively long period of time (months) (Fig 2). Based on autopsy studies (unpublished) in successfully and unsuccessfully treated patients, we have found that serum M or C iPTH reflects the degree of parathyroid hyperplasia whereas serum N iPTH may or may not depending upon immediately antecedent therapy. These observations have great practical importance in patient management; it is easy to construe a point in time set of circumstances in a patient with severe parathyroid hyperplasia in which the value for serum N iPTH may be normal, on the one hand, correctly reflecting parathyroid secretory status, but on the other, misleading in the assessment of the potential severity of ensuing HPT if a therapeutic regimen is relaxed. These are the considerations that have led us to recommend that measurement of serum M or C iPTH be used in the long term medical management of secondary HPT in chronic renal failure. It is only fair to say that this recommendation is controversial and there are those who prefer to use N assays for this purpose. This is based on the idea that measuring the immunoreactive form of PTH likely to be bioactive will more likely reflect the presence of osteitis fibrosa cystica. Although this may be true in some cases, the fact remains that serum N assays may be normal in patients with temporarily suppressed hyperplastic parathyroid glands whereas serum M or C assays will be high, truly reflecting the need for continued intensive medical therapy.

REFERENCES

1. Arnaud, C.D., Tsao, H.S., and Littledike, T. (1971): J. Clin. Invest. 50, 21.
2. Gallagher, J.C., Riggs, B.L., Jerpbak, C. and Arnaud, C.D. (1980): J. Lab. Clin. Med. 95, 373.
3. Benson, R.C., Riggs, B.L., Pickard, B.M., and Arnaud, C.D. (1974): Am. J. Med 56, 821.
4. Stewart, A.F, Horst, R., Deftos, L., Cadman, E.C., Lang, R., and Broadus, A. (1980) N. Engl. J. Med. 303, 1377.
5. Benson, R.C., Riggs, B.L., Pickard, B.M., and Arnaud, C.D. (1974): J. Clin. Invest. 54, 175.
6. Goltzman, D., Stewart, A.F., and Broadus, A.E. (1981) J. Clin. Endocrinol Metab. 53, 899.
7. Strewler, G.J., Williams, R.D., and Nissenson, R.A. (1983) J. Clin. Invest. 71, 769.

AMINO-TERMINAL RADIOIMMUNOASSAYS FOR HUMAN PARATHYROID HORMONE

Gino V. Segre

Endocrine Unit, Department of Medicine, Massachusetts General Hospital and Harvard Medical School, Boston, MA, 02114, U.S.A.

The development of more specific quantitative techniques for measuring hormones frequently has led to rapid growth in understanding normal and disturbed hormonal function. Ideally, these assays should precisely estimate the hormone's biologic activity. However, most bioassays are difficult to perform, often imprecise, and, in general, relatively insensitive. Accordingly, an acceptable, and often preferable alternative, is to measure some specific hormonal property that correlates directly and reproducibly with the hormone's biologic activity. Because of their specificity, sensitivity and relative precision, radioimmunoassays for hormones, in general, have proved to be remarkably useful, enormously expanding our knowledge of hormonal physiology in health and pathologic states.

Radioimmunoassays for parathyroid hormone (iPTH) have served well in the differential diagnosis of hypercalcemic states and in secondary forms of hyperparathyroidism. However, the often varying results reported in the literature attest to the difficulties in performing assays for this hormone. These discrepant results (1) relate both to limitations of the specific assays employed and to previously unexpected complexities concerning the heterogeneity of circulating iPTH. In the past, most PTH radioimmunoassays have been relatively insensitive for measuring the low concentrations of circulating hormonal forms of iPTH in humans because these assays have been based on antisera raised to bovine PTH. Moreover, principally from results of studies using radioimmunoassays, it is now well recognized that intact PTH comprises only 5-25% of the total plasma iPTH. The remaining iPTH consists largely of biologically inactive middle and carboxy-terminal fragments (2). These inert fragments attain their relatively high circulating concentrations because they are cleared from plasma far more slowly ($t1/2=20-40$ min) than is intact hormone ($t1/2=$ 2-4 min). Moreover, the relative concentration of these fragments varies in normal subjects. Also, since they are cleared nearly exclusively by glomerular filtration, their concentration increases as a function of advancing age in normal humans (3), and also increases with pathologic states, such as chronic renal failure (4). Consequently, PTH radioimmunoassays based on antisera recognizing antigenic determinants in the middle and carboxy-regions of the intact molecule provide only an index of the circulating concentrations of biologically-active hormone. The accuracy of this index must be considered within the context of factors causing variability in the relative concentrations between intact hormone and these inert fragments.

Currently, no bioassay is available for the routine and precise measurement of circulating biologically-active PTH. Inasmuch as studies of structure-function relations have shown that the amino-terminal portion of the PTH sequence contains all the requisite properties responsible for the known biologic activities of the hormone, we have emphasized the development of radioimmunoassays based on antisera to synthetic human PTH-(1-34). This approach assumes that normal PTH physiology can be best defined, and distinction of normal from pathophysiologic states can be best assessed by measuring immunoreactive forms of the hormone that include the region of the molecule required for biologic activity. This proved to be a formidable undertaking because only antisera containing antibodies with extraordinarily high affinity constants would be useful for measuring the circulating concentrations of biologically-active hormone (estimated to be approximately 10^{-11}M).

CK-67, an antiserum raised in chickens immunized with synthetic human PTH-(1-34), detects 1-2 pg/tube of human PTH, recognizes intact human PTH and synthetic human PTH-(1-34) nearly equivalently on a molar basis, and gives dose-dilution curves between iPTH in plasma and the human PTH-(1-34) standard which are parallel. Using 85% of the tracer binding (antibody control) as the detection limit, 95% of normal subjects have detectable iPTH (11.9$\pm$13.2 pg/ml, mean $\pm$ 2 S.D.)(5). These estimates correlate well with those obtained using the cytochemical bioassay (6) (mean-11.3, range 2.9-29 pg/ml), suggesting that the iPTH measured in this amino-terminal radioimmunoassay accurately reflects the concentration of biologically-active hormone. This agreement should be regarded as being only approximate, however, because different standards were used in these two studies. A formal comparison is currently in progress through a collaborative study between Dr. Goltzman's laboratory and ours.

We have measured iPTH in matched samples in this amino-terminal assay and in assays with GP-1. GP-1 is a biterminal antiserum, recognizing determinants in the amino- and carboxy-terminal portions of the PTH sequence (2). However, since carboxy-terminal fragments predominate in plasma, most of the "signal" recognized by GP-1 reflects the high circulating concentrations of these inert fragments. In 93% of over 60 patients with surgically-confirmed primary hyperparathyroidism, 80% of whom had serum calcium concentrations below 12 mg/dl, iPTH was elevated in the amino-terminal assay, whereas only 65% were elevated in assays with GP-1. As expected, most patients with severe chronic renal failure undergoing hemodialysis, even though they were relatively well-managed, had elevated iPTH in the CK-67 assay, but the mean was indistinguishable from patients with primary and other forms of secondary hyperparathyroidism. By comparison, nearly all patients had elevated iPTH in assays with GP-1 and the mean value was strikingly higher; findings consistent with the measurement of high concentrations of carboxy-terminal fragments which are slowly cleared in renal failure. Moreover, in collaborative studies, quantitative bone histomorphometric parameters indicative of osteitis fibrosa in patients with chronic renal failure correlated better with results from the amino-terminal assay than with those from a carboxy-terminal assay (7).

Preliminary experience with measurements of iPTH in cancer patients with hypercalcemia shows that about half of the plasmas contain material which reduces binding of the radioligand. In nearly all of these instances, the "apparent iPTH" is within the normal range. This contrasts to our previous experience using GP-1 in which only rarely did such patients have a detectable "signal." Initial chemical experiments clearly show that the "apparent iPTH" can be distinguished from authentic PTH and its fragments, but its chemical nature and the explanation for its immunochemical properties remain unknown.

Although development of assays to better distinguish classic forms of hyperparathyroidism are our central goal, the availability of an assay which measures only the short-lived, biologically-active hormone and not the long-lived carboxy-terminal fragments has permitted us to examine PTH secretory patterns and dynamically test parathyroid gland function; studies which were difficult, if not impossible, to perform with previously available assays.

PTH secretion was found to be pulsatile in normal subjects. Fortunately, in less than 0.3% of nearly 800 measurements in 16 normal subjects did iPTH levels exceed the upper limit of normal. Pulsatile secretion also is typical of patients with primary hyperparathyroidism, but only rarely do values fall within the normal range. Hence, these pulsatile changes do not significantly interfere with the usefulness of static measurements in differential diagnosis. Whether loss or accentuation of these pulsatile patterns are significant in the pathogenesis of some forms of hyperparathyroidism, or of other diseases involving bone loss or renal calculi remain to be explored.

We are currently completing studies to define PTH secretory dynamics in response to uniform perturbations of plasma calcium concentrations in normal subjects, and also have begun comparing these responses to those observed in patients with primary hyperparathyroidism. Since the inert, carboxyl-terminal fragments whose circulating concentrations are high, and whose clearance is slow are not detected by this assay, rapid changes in hormone concentration can be detected (Fig. 1). In all normal subjects and most patients with primary hyperparathyroidism, there is a sigmoidal iPTH response to experimentally raising and lowering the plasma ionized calcium. Perturbations of less than 0.04 mM in ionized calcium result in compensatory PTH secretory responses. Most patients with primary hyperparathyroidism show evidence for both an altered "set-point" in PTH secretion (the plasma calcium concentration required to suppress plasma iPTH by 50%), as well as an increased level of non-suppressible, calcium-independent PTH secretion. However, not all patients with primary hyperparathyroidism demonstrate the same response pattern, suggesting that primary hyperparathyroidism may be associated with different pathophysiologic defects.

Clearly, measurements of iPTH using this amino-terminal radioimmunoassay have particular advantages. The assay sensitivity, and specificity provide excellent discrimination among normal subjects, patients with various forms of hyperparathyroidism, and patients with hypercalcemia associated with malignancy. Hence, a single assay can serve reliably to measure iPTH in patients with various disease states and in normal subjects regardless of age. Its application to measurements of plasma iPTH as a function of induced changes in plasma calcium through stimulation and suppression studies will allow detailed definition of normal PTH physiology. In addition, studies with this assay will contribute to defining the pathophysiologic defects in primary hyperparathyroidism, and may define subtle and relatively small aberrations in calcium or vitamin D status in elderly subjects. Furthermore, studies with this amino-terminal radioimmunoassay may demonstrate functionally significant alterations in PTH secretory patterns or small quantitative changes in the control of PTH secretion which may be present in common and chronic disorders of calcium metabolism, particularly those involving bone loss and renal calculi formation.

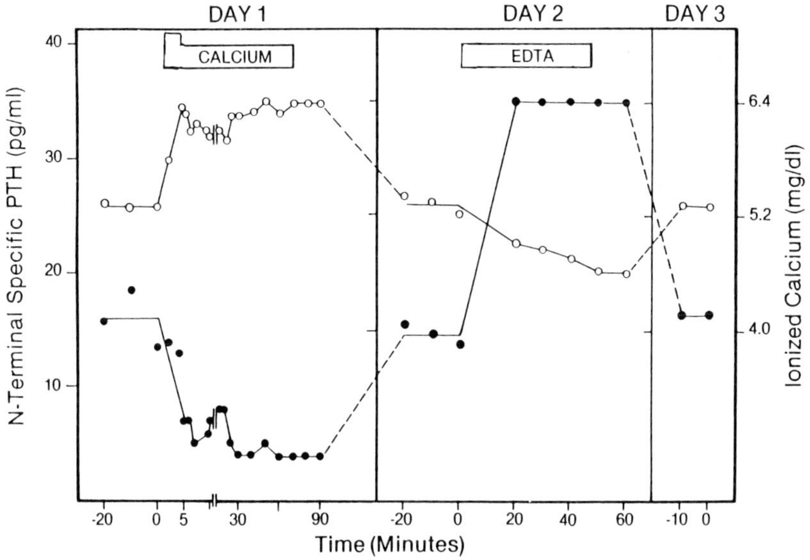

Figure 1

When iPTH is measured in a normal subject, there is a rapid fall as the blood ionized calcium is abruptly elevated (t 1/2 of iPTH < 5 min), and a rapid rise in iPTH as the blood ionized calcium is elevated by infusion of EDTA. Upon infusion of EDTA, iPTH exceeded 35 pg/ml. Unfortunately, insufficient plasma precluded precise determination of the iPTH in these samples. Blood ionized calcium (o-o) and iPTH (o-o) are plotted as a function of time.

REFERENCES

1. Raisz, L.G., Yajnik, C.H., Bockman, R.S. and Bower, B.B. (1979): Ann. Intern. Med., 91, 739.
2. Segre, G.V., Habener, J.F., Powell, D., Tregear, G.W. and Potts, J.T., Jr. (1972): J. Clin. Invest., 52, 3163.
3. Berlyne, G.M., Ben Ari, J., Kusheleusky, A., Idelman., A., Galinsky, D., Hirsch, M., Shainkin, B., Yagil, R. and Zlotnik, M. (1975): Quart. J. Med., 44, 501.
4. Freitag, J., Martin, K.J., Hruska, K.A., Anderson, C., Conrades, M., Ladenson, J., Klahr, S. and Slatopolsky, E. (1978): N. Engl. J. Med., 298, 29.
5. Segre, G.V., Harris, S.T., Tully, G. and Neer., R. (1981): Annual Meeting of the Endocrine Society (abstr).
6. Goltzman, D., Henderson, B. and Loveridge, N. (1980): J. Clin. Invest., 65, 1309.
7. Endres, D., Brickman, A., Goodman, W., Maloney, N. Sherrard, D. and Segre, G.V. (1981): Annual Meeting of the Endocrine Society (abstr).

THE CONTRIBUTION OF SYNTHETIC HUMAN PARATHYROID HORMONE AND OF ITS FRAGMENTS TO PARATHYROID HORMONE MEASUREMENTS

F.A. Tschopp, M.A. Dambacher and J.A. Fischer

Research Laboratory for Calcium Metabolism, Departments of Orthopedic Surgery and Medicine, University of Zurich, Forchstrasse 340, 8008 Zurich, Switzerland

Circulating parathyroid hormone (PTH) levels are generally measured radioimmunologically. At present, antibodies are usually raised to extracts of human parathyroid tumors or to synthetic human PTH fragments. We have extracted peptides coeluting with intact PTH-(1-84) and its fragments on HPLC and gel permeation chromatography with a yield of 1-4 mg PTH per 100 g parathyroid glands. The amount of crude extract (1-4% purity) from 100 g parathyroid tissue is sufficient for the successfull immunisation of two to four goats using previously described procedures (4). Moreover, synthetic human PTH fragments are used for immunization. Optimal sensitivity and specificity for the measurement of circulating PTH in man can be achieved with the use of radioiodinated synthetic intact human PTH-(1-84) and its fragments. As an example, antibodies have been raised in a goat to a crude extract of human parathyroid tumors and the antiserum dilution yielding 50% binding (B/F = 1) determined with various radioiodinated PTH peptides (Fig. 1A). In this particular bleeding the antibodies generated recognized synthetic [131-I]human PTH-(1-84) and -(Tyr27-48) best, followed by human PTH-(Tyr43-68), -(1-44) and -(Tyr52-84), and by bovine PTH-(1-84). Binding to human PTH-(1-34) was negligible. The polyclonal antibodies are directed to different antigenic determinants and can be further purified using affinity chromatography methodology.

In the present study we have developed a radioimmunoassay system suitable for the measurement of PTH in human serum. Since the antibodies were not recognized to any great extent by the amino-terminal PTH fragment-(1-34), they are presumably directed predominantly to recognition sites located in the middle and the carboxyl-terminal regions of intact PTH-(1-84). The antibodies were incubated with radiolabelled intact human PTH and its fragments and with intact bovine PTH in dilutions yielding 25-35% binding (B/F 0.3-0.5) and immunodilution curves were obtained with pooled serum from patients with primary hyperparathyroidism (Fig. 1B). Using [131-I]human PTH-(Tyr43-68) a 50% inhibition of the immunological reaction was obtained with 15 µl hyperparathyroid serum, whereas 50 µl were required with [131-I]human PTH-(1-84) and -(Tyr27-48). Circulating PTH was only minimally detected with radioiodinated human PTH-(Tyr52-84) and intact bovine PTH and not recognized with [131-I]human PTH-(1-44). Even though high titer antibodies were recognized by radiolabelled synthetic intact human PTH and the fragment (Tyr27-48), the RIA systems were not sensitive enough for the measurement of circulating PTH in the majority of normal subjects. Similarly, using the radioiodinated amino- and carboxyl-terminal human PTH fragments-(1-44) and -(Tyr52-84) and bovine PTH endogenous PTH has not been detected to any great extent, whereas a sensitive assay was established with [131-I]human PTH-(Tyr43-68). Radiolabelled human PTH-(44-68) has been successfully used in recently developed radioimmunoassays (1, 6).

Homologous radioimmunoassay systems can be successfully used for the measurement of PTH in the circulation of normal human subjects and hyperparathyroid patients. The discrimination, although not perfect, is usually adequate for the differentiation of raised PTH levels in hyperparathyroid

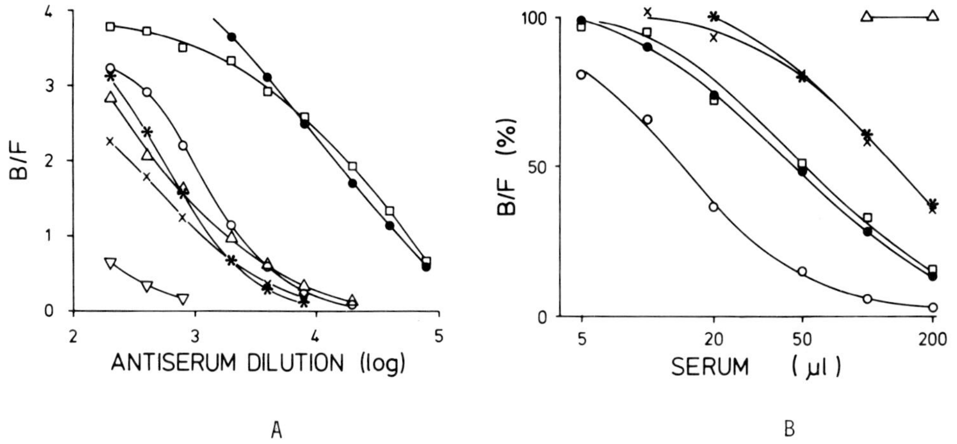

Figure 1. Quantitative and qualitative properties of antibodies to extracted human PTH. A, specific binding of [131-I] synthetic human PTH-(1-84) (Peninsula) (●), -PTH-(1-34) (courtesy of the late J. Parsons) (▽), -(1-44) (△), -(Tyr27-48) (□), -(Tyr43-68) (o) and -(Tyr52-84) (Universal Biologicals) (x) and extracted bovine PTH-(1-84) (Medical Research Council) (*). B, inhibition of specific binding (100% B/F = 0.4) of the radioactive ligands by pooled serum of patients with primary hyperparathyroidism.

patients from undetectable or normal values in normal subjects or patients with hypercalcemia unrelated to parathyroid tumors. Most radioimmunoassay systems recognize predominantly carboxyl-terminal PTH fragments in peripheral human serum besides small amounts of intact PTH-(1-84) (2-6).

Only few so-called N assays have been successfully used for the measurement of circulating PTH. The sensitivity is usually inadequate for the measurement of the rather low amounts of intact PTH (<30 pg/ml) in normal subjects (3). Basal PTH levels in unextracted normal human serum are probably largely the result of non-specific inhibition of the immunological reaction by plasma proteins and salts. Nonetheless, this type of assay has proved to be useful especially in hyperparathyroid patients for the evaluation of rapid secretory and metabolic changes of circulating PTH components (2, 5, Segre: this Symposium).

In conclusion, homologous PTH radioimmunoassay systems have been successfully established. To this end, the general availability of intact human PTH and of its fragments has proved to be very helpful for the development of diagnostically useful radioimmunoassays.

1. Atkinson, M.J., Niepel, B., Jüppner, H., Butz, R., Casaretto, M., Zahn, H., Hehrmann, R., Hesch, R.D. (1981): J. Endocrinol. Invest. 4, 363.
2. Born, W., Dambacher, M.A., Meyrier, A., Ardaillou, R., Fischer, J.A. (1982): Clin. Endocrinol. (Oxf.) 17, 333.
3. Dambacher, M.A., Fischer, J.A., Hunziker, W.H., Moran, J., Roth, H.-R., Delvin, E.E., Glorieux, F.H. (1979): Clin. Sci. (Oxf.) 57, 435.
4. Fischer, J.A., Binswanger, U., Dietrich, F.M. (1974): J. Clin. Invest. 54, 1382.
5. Goldsmith, R.S., Furszyfer, J., Johnson, W.J., Fournier, A.E., Sizemore, G.W., Arnaud, C.D. (1973): J. Clin. Invest. 52, 173.
6. Marx, S.J., Sharp, M.E., Krudy, A., Rosenblatt, M., Mallette, L.E. (1981): J. Clin. Endocrinol. Metab. 53, 76.

Supported by Swiss National Science Foundation Grant 3.813-0.81

COMPARISON OF AMINO- AND CARBOXYL-TERMINAL ASSAY METHODS

Eduardo Slatopolsky

Renal Division, Department of Internal Medicine, School of Medicine, Washington University, St. Louis, Missouri

The main issue is not to compare an amino-terminal versus a carboxyl-terminal assay, but to characterize each individual assay. After we know the sensitivity and the affinity of a given antibody, then we can compare different assays. The total amount of radioimmunoassayable PTH in humans ranges between 300-400 pg/ml. Approximately 90% of this amount is C-terminal. Therefore, a C-terminal antibody should have sufficient sensitivity to detect 30-40 pg to be sensitive enough for clinical use. On the other hand, since the total amount of amino terminal PTH in serum is likely no greater than 30-40 pg/ml, an amino-terminal antibody should detect 3-4 pg to be sensitive enough for clinical use.

That is why, until recently, many of the amino-terminal immunoassays have been of little use in clinical medicine. Moreover, since it is known that the secretion of parathyroid hormone is pulsatile and the half-life of the amino-terminal portion of the PTH molecule is in the order of 3-5 minutes, one may obtain blood in a patient at at time when the levels may not be elevated.

In relation to patients with chronic renal insufficiency, the values obtained with a C-terminal radioimmunoassay gives to a physician an integrated value which assesses the chronic state of secondary hyperparathyroidism. Obviously, if a physician is interested in performing dynamic studies on a minute-to-minute basis in patients with chronic renal insufficiency, a C-terminal antibody will be of little use. However, from the practical point of view, patients could be followed on a monthly basis. There is good correlation between the levels obtained with a C-terminal antibody and bone histology. We have correlated bone histology and i-PTH utilizing our C-terminal antibody in normal volunteers and patients maintained on hemodialysis. There was a remarkable correlation in both groups between the levels of C-terminal radioimmunoassay for PTH and the number of osteoclasts, the degree of bone resorption and marrow fibrosis.

As I mentioned before, the C-terminal assay will not give us information on a minute-to-minute basis in uremic patients. However, it also will not take a month before we can see changes in PTH. When we have infused calcium intravenously and kept the levels between 11 and 12 mg/100 ml for a period of 72 hours, PTH decreased by approximately 70% of the original value.

I would like to emphasize a point that was previously made by Dr. Claude Arnaud. If one dialyzes a patient, there are rapid changes in ionized calcium, and we may greatly affect the levels of amino-terminal parathyroid hormone. Therefore, they may not correlate with the chronic state of secondary hyperparathyroidism and the degree of bone disease. This potential artifact does not occur with the use of a sensitive C-terminal antibody. As far as patients with primary hyperparathyroidism are concerned, we have now determined values in approximately 500 patients with surgically proven primary hyperparathyroidism. Our assay values have been elevated in 97% of these patients. Therefore, I feel, like Dr. Arnaud, that the use of a mid-region-C-terminal assay is very effective and practical in the management of patients with primary and secondary hyperparathyroidism.

DISCUSSION: CLINICAL APPLICATION OF PARATHYROID HORMONE

R. MARCUS: Some element of the rise in iPTH with age must have something to do with decreased clearance of intact hormone. Other elements of the rise may have something to do with secretion. I wonder whether the amino-terminal assay that Dr. Segre has described shows increased levels with age.

G. SEGRE: When we assayed immunoreactive PTH using this amino-terminal assay in a population from the Southwest, we found that the normal range of values in the older population were indistinguishable from those of young control subjects. In a similar study conducted in a small town near Boston, we found that the values in that population were approximately 20 pg/ml as opposed to approximately 12 pg/ml that we registered in the younger control population. The general subject is still under investigation. We think the most likely explanation is that elderly people living in New England do not receive as much sun exposure and do not ingest as much vitamin D. In fact, they seem to have an element of vitamin D deficiency and secondary hyperparathyroidism, but that remains to be documented.

A. TASHJIAN: Dr. Segre, I wonder whether your N-terminal PTH immunoassay measures the large molecular weight material that Dr. Goltzman described in patients with humoral hypercalcemia. Does your antiserum against that N-terminal sequence neutralize the biological activity of this material in the cytochemical bioassay?

G. SEGRE: We have not, as yet, chromatographed this material. To do this presents a problem because one would have to go through a concentration step prior to chromatography or following it. We would have concerns that apparent molecular size could change due to aggregation. The problem can be overcome but we haven't yet undertaken such studies of the material detected immunologically by the PTH assay in cancer patients. We do not know the molecular size of the material. Because it does not strip out with charcoal, we think it is probably a large molecule, but we cannot be certain.

In answer to your question about the cytochemical assay and whether we can neutralize the material, we have not explored this area. We have done collaborative studies with Dr. Broadus; in the *in vitro* studies that he described, the humoral agents that are released into the tissue culture media are not immunoprecipitated by our anti-PTH antiserum.

D. GOLTZMAN: We have not had the opportunity to use Dr. Segre's assay or antibody to do studies of the material which we detect with the cytochemical assay. When we initially reported our findings on the molecular size of this material, we attempted antibody neutralization with a commercial amino-terminal antibody, and did see a partial reduction in cytochemical bioactivity. We did not understand the meaning of this at the time, but I think that in view of Dr. Segre's current data, it is possible that there is some similarity of this material with PTH immunologically as well as in receptor binding capacity.

Consequently, a few, but not all, antisera to PTH may detect the malignancy factor.

J. O'RIORDAN: The cytochemical assay is an important advance, but it is difficult to perform. There are problems that have to be faced. For example, what is the normal range? It is variously reported by different groups to be from 8-30 pg/ml. While we are used to a much greater variation in immunoassays, we have to accept that even when using the same methods the results are often different. There will be a continuing problem in interpretation.

If we accept the fact that there are inhibitors in the cytochemical assay, then we are faced with the problem as to the correct results in physiological terms and whether these inhibitors are specific to the assay, or are physiologically important.

With regard to the immunoassays, if you divide 84 by 3, the result is 28. If you add 28 and 28, the result is 56. If you divide the molecule into three parts, the mid-region then ranges from 28 to 56. It means that we have a major semantic problem in that one investigator's mid-region assay becomes someone else's C-terminal assay, and maybe even an amino-terminal assay.

These semantic matters are minimized when one is talking about a research assay that is well-defined. When the same language is applied to commercial assays, it is difficult to know what one is measuring since these assays are less well-defined.

I agree with Dr. Segre that an amino-terminal assay can be extremely useful in the diagnosis of primary hyperparathyroidism, and also useful for physiological studies concerning the control of PTH secretion.

J. POTTS: By the way of summary, several important points have emerged this morning. First, although investigators have been working in the parathyroid immunoassay field for over 20 years, there is still a surprising degree of confusion regarding fundamental issues such as the central question of what is being measured by different assays. I think a number of our speakers, such as Dr. O'Riordan, have underscored the importance of referring to assays in terms of the specificity of what they measure. What is called an N- or a C-terminal assay has to be described carefully in terms of its antigenic recognition site, as well as its sensitivity. We have not had time to refer even to the important area of standards for the assays: these obviously influence the stated ranges of normal and abnormal values.

Assays that measure the mid- or carboxyl-region of the molecule are valuable for static measurements in differential diagnosis or in evaluating of long-term results of long-term therapy, as Drs. Arnaud and Slatopolsky emphasize. It is also clear, however, that for dynamic testing, an assay which recognizes only the short-lived, intact form of the hormone, such as amino-terminal assays with the requisite sensitivity can be used successfully. Assays of the type described by Dr. Segre may open new areas of study in pathophysiology.

There remains confusion about assay results in patients with tumor hypercalcemia (as discussed further in Session XV). Perhaps at the next of these symposia in a few years, most issues regarding clinical applications of parathyroid assays will be clear and simple, but I doubt it.

II ASSESSMENT OF TRABECULAR BONE STATUS

ASSESSMENT OF TRABECULAR BONE STATUS - INTRODUCTION

A. M. Parfitt

Bone and Mineral Metabolism Division, Henry Ford Hospital, Detroit, Michigan 48202, U.S.A.

At our last clinical symposium in 1972 (1) the assessment of cortical bone by radiogrammetry and by single energy photon absorptiometry was discussed in detail. The uses and limitations of these methods are now well established and they have provided an extensive body of data on age-related loss of cortical bone. We now need similar data for trabecular bone because of many differences between these two types (Table 1).

TABLE 1. Comparison of Cortical and Trabecular Bone.

	CORTICAL	TRABECULAR
Envelopes	Two	One
Proximity to bone marrow	Variable	Close
Surface/Volume	Low	High
Turnover	Low	High
Treatment Response	Slow	Rapid
Mineral Reservoir	Yes	No (!)
Relationship of Amount to Age	Curvilinear	Varies with method
Effect of Menopause	Acceleration	Varies with method
Fractures	Long bones	Vertebrae

1. In man, a temporary physiologic need for bone mineral during growth, pregnancy and lactation is met by increased cortical porosity (2), and the most important long-term response to increased parathyroid hormone secretion is cortical thinning (3).

The study of trabecular bone is attended by many more technical problems than the study of cortical bone, and some of the methods that have been used are given in Table 2.

TABLE 2. Methods for Measuring Trabecular Bone.

1. Histomorphometry (ilium, vertebra)
2. Photodensitometry (phalanges, vertebra)
3. Compton Scatter (calcaneum)
4. Single energy photon absorptiometry - single path (radius)
5. Single energy photon absorptiometry - multi path (radius)
6. Partial body neutron activation (trunk)
7. Dual energy photon absorptiometry (spine, femur, whole body)
8. Computed tomography (spine, distal radius, distal tibia)

Histomorphometry of trabecular bone is useful in population studies, but it is a cumbersome and inaccurate method for determining trabecular bone mass in individual subjects. Photodensitometry using an aluminum or potassium phosphate stepwedge is subject to several sources of error but needs no capital investment and could be used more widely (4). The description of the Compton Scatter technique at our last meeting aroused much excitement but almost a decade later a clinically useful procedure has still not been perfected (5). Single energy photon absorptiometry at the distal measurement site in the radius is frequently, but erroneously, believed to provide information on trabecular bone (6), but using single path instruments such as the Norland-Cameron, there is much less trabecular bone at this site than is commonly supposed, and what trabecular bone is there is metabolically inert and contributes little to the observed changes. The situation is slightly better with instruments capable of scanning at multiple levels, which can get closer to the active trabecular bone in the metaphysis (7). With partial body neutron activation, it is possible to measure the axial skeleton separately from the appendicular skeleton, and the measurement includes a higher proportion of trabecular bone than total body calcium (8). The last two methods are currently receiving most attention. In the proceedings of our last meeting dual energy photon absorptiometry (DPA) occupied less than half a page in a 700-page book, and quantitative computed tomography (QCT) had not been applied to bone at all.

Mazess further described the peculiarities of trabecular bone including its variable response to disease and treatment at different anatomic locations and consequent poorer site to site correlation than found in cortical bone. He once more drew attention to the problems caused by variable marrow composition, particularly for single energy QCT. Some of the surprisingly rapid loss reported after oophorectomy could in part be due to increase in marrow fat. Wahner reviewed the Mayo Clinic experience with DPA, described the relative immunity of this technique to changes in marrow fat and confirmed the apparent linear decline in spinal bone density with age and failure to observe a post-menopausal acceleration in bone loss with cross-sectional data. This may reflect in part the contribution of cortical bone in the vertebral appendages and probable increase in calcium deposition in paraspinal soft tissues and aorta with age. DPA of the spine discriminates between persons with and without vertebral compression fracture much better than single energy PA of the radius.

Genant reviewed the advantages of QCT for selective examination of trabecular bone and described how recent technical advances have reduced the error due to variable marrow fat. In contrast to DPA, a postmenopausal acceleration of trabecular bone loss is observed with QCT. Discrimination between persons with and without compression fracture appeared less satisfactory than with DPA, but this may have been the result of including some patients with wedging but without compression of a vertebra. However, as with DPA, discrimination is much better than with measurements of peripheral cortical bone. Ruegsegger described the application of QCT to trabecular bone of the extremities, particularly the distal radius and distal tibia. This technique has the highest precision of all the methods discussed, allowing the demonstration for the first time that bone loss in some patients occurs in abrupt steps rather than continuously. Because of its high precision, the technique is also ideally suited for monitoring the short-term response to a large number of potential therapeutic agents that could be used in accordance with the ADFR concept of Frost. Using a similar method Hangartner observed a significant correlation between trabecular bone density measured by QCT in the distal radius and in the spine, but with a prediction error of about 20%. As judged by the lack of discussion of these two papers, the implication of this new approach escaped many in the audience. Finally, Powell reported a rather low correlation between QCT and DPA measurements in the same subjects, although QCT correlated somewhat better than DPA with a semi-quantitative fracture index.

It was evidence from the presentations that a great deal of progress has been made in the non-invasive study of trabecular bone in the last ten years. There is still controversy about the size of the error due to variable marrow fat and how successful the different techniques are in coping with this error. Many more studies are needed directly comparing the two major techniques of

DPA and QCT in the same subjects, particularly serial measurements by both methods. Further improvement in both precision and accuracy is likely, but this must not be made an excuse for curtailing the duration of therapeutic studies, which is dictated by the biological characteristics of the remodeling system and not by technical factors in the methods of measurement (9). There is also much more to the study of trabecular bone than simply measuring its amount. The complex 3-dimensional structure of this tissue is clinically important for several reasons and is accessible to high resolution CT applied to iliac bone biopsy samples (10). Perhaps in another decade instrumental resolution will increase to the extent where similar information can be obtained from the intact patient, but this will probably require the application to bone of even newer methods such as NMR.

REFERENCES

1. Clinical Aspects of Metabolic Bone Disease, ed. B. Frame, A.M. Parfitt, H. Duncan. Excerpta Medica, Amsterdam, 1973.
2. Parfitt, A.M.: Integration of skeletal and mineral homeostasis. In: Osteoporosis: Recent Advances in Pathogenesis and Treatment. ed. H.F. DeLuca, H. Frost, W. Jee, C. Johnston, A.M. Parfitt, University Park Press, Baltimore, pp. 115-126, 1981.
3. Kleerekoper, M., A.R. Villanueva, C.H.E. Mathews, D.S. Rao, B. Pumo and A.M. Parfitt: PTH mediated bone loss in primary and secondary hyperparathyroidism. In: Clinical Disorders of Bone and Mineral Metabolism, this volume.
4. Colbert, C. and Bachtell, R.S. (1981): Radiographic absorptiometry (photodensitometry). In: Non-invasive Measurements of Bone Mass and Their Clinical Application, pp. 51-84, ed. S. Cohn, CRC Press, West Palm Beach, Florida.
5. Webber, C.E. (1981): Compton scattering methods. In: Non-invasive Measurements of Bone Mass and Their Clinical Application, pp. 101-120, ed. S.H. Cohn, CRC Press, West Palm Beach, Florida.
6. Hahn, T.J., V.C. Boisseau, and L.V. Avioli: Effect of chronic corticosteroid administration on diaphyseal and metaphyseal bone mass, J Clin Endocrinol Metab 39:274, 1974.
7. Christensen, M.S., C. Christiansen, J. Naestoft, P. McNair, I. Transbol: Normalization of bone mineral content to height, weight, and lean body mass: Implications for clinical use. Calc Tiss Int 33:5-8, 1981.
8. Harrison, J.E., K.G. McNeill, A.J. Hitchman, and B.A. Britt (1979): Invest Radiol 14:27-34.
9. Parfitt, A.M.: The morphologic basis of bone mineral measurements: Transient and steady state effects of treatment in osteoporosis. Editorial, Mineral & Electrolyte Metab 4:273-287, 1980.
10. Feldkamp, L.A., M. Kleerekoper, J.W. Kress, R. Freeling, C.H.E. Mathews, A.M. Parfitt (abstract): Calc Tiss Int (in press).

PROBLEMS IN MEASUREMENT OF TRABECULAR BONE

Richard B. Mazess

Department of Medical Physics, University of Wisconsin, Madison, WI, U.S.A.

The advent of new methods for measurement of trabecular bone over the past decade has raised several issues bearing on their clinical utilization. First, which skeletal locations indicate bone changes most sensitively? Conversely, are certain locations especially insensitive? Second, in what units (mass, density) are measurements best expressed? Third, what are the advantages and limitations of the available measurement methods? These topics are dealt with briefly in this summary.

ANATOMICAL LOCATION

Measurements on the compact bone of the limbs are correlated highly ($r>0.9$) with other limbs and with the total skeletal mass. In healthy controls total body bone mineral (TBBM by 153-Gd absorptiometry) or total body calcium (TBCa by neutron activation) was predicted with an error of about 8-10% from bone mineral content (BMC by 125-I absorptiometry) of the radius. In patients, however, the predictive error was 10-15%. The radius BMC also is predictive (15% error) of femoral neck BMC and spinal BMC in normals, but the predictive error is larger in patients (25%). Moreover, in osteoporotic men and women there was a different regression relationship between the radius and spine than in controls as a consequence of preferential spinal osteopenia in the patients. For this reason direct spinal measurements provide a very reliable diagnosis of early osteoporosis (patients under age 70 are 2 SD below controls) whereas radius BMC does not (5,7).

The spine, pelvis, and other areas of trabecular bone do not change more rapidly with normal aging than compact bone but there is evidence that (a) aging bone loss begins earlier in trabecular bone, and (b) trabecular bone is more responsive to a variety of stimuli (6). In osteoporosis the extent of bone loss in the spine and pelvis exceeds that occurring in the appendicular skeleton (Figure 1). Positive responses to therapy for osteoporosis have been noted almost exclusively in trabecular bone of the axial skeleton (PTH fragment, exercise, fluoride, calcitonin vitamin-D, metabolites) even where there has been slight or negative effects on compact bone.

All areas of trabecular bone are not as responsive as the bone of the axial skeleton. The average intercorrelation among various areas of trabecular bone is only about 0.7; this is comparable to the correlation between compact and trabecular bone. The correlation between the pelvis and spine is only 0.7 despite their physical proximity and similarity of marrow composition; the spine often shows greater osteopenia than is evident in iliac crest biopsies. Some areas, such as the distal radius, seem more highly correlated with the spine and pelvis while others such as the os calcis ($r = 0.3$ to 0.5) are not. In disease states this pattern of intercorrelation can be changed. For example, in immobilization the changes of the os calcis closely reflect those of the pelvis and spine (1%/week loss) but the distal radius does not. It is wishful thinking to assume that changes in any local area reflect changes of the spine.

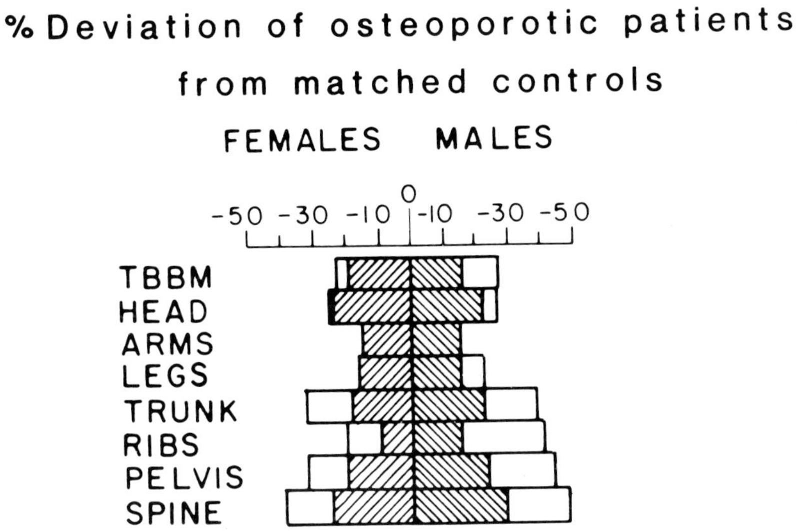

Figure 1. The deviation of total and regional bone mass (open) or density (hatched) in male (n=11) and female (n=18) osteoporotic patients based on dual-photon absorptiometry. The spine and pelvis are especially osteopenic.

UNITS OF MEASUREMENT

BMC measurements by 125-I absorptiometry are usually expressed in grams per centimeter axial length (even though the beam width is less than 1cm). When area measurements are done over an entire bone (vertebra, metacarpal) then the integrated result is given in grams. Such mass measurements do not compensate for variations in bone or body size, and cannot be compared to "density" measurements (which do compensate for size).

Volumetric density has been used in studies of skeletal specimens to eliminate chemical or biomechanical variations due to size. In samples of uniform size bone strength is proportional to density, however, density does not indicate the strength of an intact bone. There is a very large overlap in the spinal density of fracture and non-fracture cases. Rather integral mass of the spine or femoral neck is directly proportional to its strength (4,9). Use of density measures does reduce intra-individual variation but will provide a poorer indication of strength or fracture risk than mass. Mass measurements that are normalized for body size and bone size may have better diagnostic sensitivity in osteoporosis than density measures.

Both volumetric and area density are particularly useful for sequential monitoring on the same individual in order to minimize influences of sampling location which could readily influence a mass measurement.

MEASUREMENT METHODS

Various methods are available for measurement of trabecular bone (Table 1).

TABLE 1. Methods for measurement of trabecular bone; the errors of precision (Column A) and accuracy (Column B) are shown together with the apparent bone change induced by a 10% shift of marrow composition (Column C).

Method	Site	A	B	C
X-Ray CT	Distal radius, spine	3-5%	∿30%	3.5
Gamma-Ray CT	Distal radius, tibia	0.5%	1%	1.7
125-I Absorptiometry	Distal radius, os calcis	1%	2%	0.3
153-Gd Absorptiometry	Spine, femoral neck	3%	3%	0.3
Neutron Activation	Spine	5%	?	-
Compton Scattering	Distal radius, os calcis	20%	20%	2.5
Photodensitometry	Spine, femoral neck	5%	10-20%	0.8
Video Absorptiometry	Femoral neck, spine, distal radius	1%	2%	0.8

The X-ray CT methods using multiple slices are fairly precise (3 to 5%); those using only a few slices have a precision error of 20%. CT has a large accuracy error (25-75mg/cm^3 of mineral or from 20 to 80%) due in large part to variable marrow composition (1). Consequently single-energy X-ray CT cannot be used where bone composition (osteomalacia) or marrow composition varies. Gamma-ray CT (8) does not have this problem and is very precise (<0.5% error), but the equipment is costly and the peripheral sites measured probably do not reflect changes of the axial skeleton in disease and its treatment. Dual-energy X-ray CT of the spine seems an ideal clinical method if the large precision errors (15%) can be reduced.

125-I absorptiometry provides precise (1%) measures of the distal radius or os calcis (2) but again these locations do not change in the same way as the axial skeleton. The most distal part (5%) of the radius contains as much as 60% trabecular bone but slightly more proximal areas (10% from styloid tip) contain less (10-20%). 153-Gd absorptiometry is the only method giving precise and accurate (2-3% error) direct measurement of the axial skeleton. The radiation dose is quite low (<15mrem). The results are not influenced by composition of the marrow in the bone or of surrounding tissue. However, osteophytes could affect the results as could a calcified aorta. The same of course is true for local neutron activation of the spine. The high radiation dose (several rem) and cost of equipment will preclude use of that experimental method and also of Compton-scattering methods. Also Compton-scattering methods have very poor precision and accuracy on trabecular bone (0.04g/cm^3); the relative error for a typical determination is about 15-20%.

Radiographic photodensitometry was used about a decade ago for measuring the spine and femoral neck (10). The precision was comparable to that of X-ray CT (5%) but the accuracy was better (10-20%). Scattered radiation from thick body areas precluded accurate results on the axial skeleton. Video-absorptiometry minimizes that problem by using a series of scanning slits to reduce scattered radiation. A precision error of under 1% is readily obtained with a radiation dose of ∿125mrem (3). This method could be increasingly developed as an adjunct to digital radiography systems.

CONCLUSION

It is obvious that trabecular bone must be measured for diagnostic and monitoring purposes in bone disease but areas other than the axial skeleton may not reflect the processes occurring in that critical and active zone. The distal radius and the os calcis can be readily measured even with relatively simple methods, so it is imperative that changes at those locations be correlated with changes in the axial skeleton.

The units in which results are expressed will vary with the method used. Methodological comparisons must use common units; mass differs from density. Differences among methods, or laboratories, may reflect the units of measurement used. The area density frequently employed in dual-photon absorptiometry is different from the volumetric density used for CT and Compton-scattering methods. Mass and area density appear to be more useful for diagnosis than volumetric density, but area and volumetric densities appear more suited for serial monitoring than mass.

Several methods are available for measurement of trabecular bone. Single energy X-ray CT on the distal radius and/or the spine has been developed but though reasonably precise the method is subject to major accuracy errors associated with the varying composition of marrow and of bone. Single-energy X-ray CT will have to be carefully validated before it can be accepted for either clinical research or management. Dual-energy X-ray CT seems to overcome the most objectional shortcoming of the single-energy approach. Dual photon-absorptiometry is relatively errorfree and can be used for measuring the spine and femoral neck. However, the spine measurements are subject to errors due to osteophytes and to calcified aorta. Single-photon absorptiometry has been used on the distal radius and the os calcis but these locations may not correlate highly with the axial skeleton. Other methods, such as neutron activation of the spine, or Compton-scattering, involve high radiation dose and are relatively imprecise. Low-energy "gamma" CT of the radius and tibia is very precise and hence useful for research but the equipment is costly and presently available in only three research centers. As digital radiography systems become available in clinical practice we may expect new methods similar to videoabsorptiometry to be introduced for high-precision monitoring.

ACKNOWLEDGEMENT

Supported by NASA Contract GM-2-4506-416 and by NIH-AM-30202.

REFERENCES

1. Adams, J.E., Chen, S.Z., Adams, P.H. and Isherwood, I. (1982): J. Comput. Asst. Tomogr., 6, 601.
2. Christiansen, C. and Rodbro, P. (1975): Scand. J. Clin. Lab. Invest., 35, 323.
3. Dobbins J.T. III, Mazess, R.B. and Cameron, J.R. (1981): Med. Phys., 8, 563.
4. Hansson, T., Roos, B. and Nachemson, A. (1980): Spine, 5, 46.
5. Kruse, H.P., Kuhlencordt, F. and Ringe, J.D. (1976): In: Calcified Tissues 1975, p. 437. Editors: S. Pors Nielsen and E. Hjorting-Hansen. FADL Publishing, Copenhagen, Denmark.
6. Mazess, R.B. (1982): Clin. Orthop. and Rel. Res., 162, 239.
7. Riggs, B.L., Wahner, H.W., Dunn, W.L., Mazess, R.B., Offord, K.P. and Melton, L.J. III (1981): J. Clin. Invest., 67, 328.
8. Ruegsegger, P., Anliker, M. and Dambacher, M. (1981): J. Comput. Asst. Tomogr., 5, 384.
9. Vose, G.P. and Mack, P.B. (1963): Am. J. Roentgenol., 89, 1296.
10. Vose, G.P., Hoerster, S.A. and Mack, P.B. (1964): Am. J. Med. Elect., 3, 181.

DUAL-PHOTON ABSORPTIOMETRY: CLINICAL CONSIDERATIONS

Heinz W. Wahner, William L. Dunn, Kenneth P. Offord and B. Lawrence Riggs

Mayo Clinic and Mayo Foundation, Rochester, MN, U.S.A.

Measurement of bone mineral of the lumbar spine by dual-photon absorptiometry is a routine clinical test as well as a research tool. Technical developments in recent years, together with clinical experience from several laboratories, have produced a safe, nontraumatic laboratory test of high accuracy and precision, with modest demands on technician skill and with reliable instrumentation. This report discusses aspects of bone mineral measurements which are important for data interpretation and reviews clinical results.

INDICATIONS

The test can be performed without specific preparation on any patient able to remain in the supine position for about 45 minutes. There are a few contraindications: (1) patients with compression fractures in the scanning area should be excluded because compressed vertebrae do not reflect bone mineral in the lumbar spine (bone mineral may be higher, lower, or equal to the surrounding vertebra); (2) patients with metallic orthopedic devices or certain articles of clothing may alter bone mineral results (this is generally recognizable on inspection of the scan); (3) patients who have had a recent (3 to 5 days before) barium contrast radiograph of the gastrointestinal tract may have false results, regardless of whether barium overlies the spinal column or the background region; (4) patients with previous radioisotope tests such as bone scans will have false results for several days; and (5) patients with severe spinal deformity, severe degenerative disease, or previous surgery in the scanning region have measurements that are difficult to interpret; more experience is necessary in this area.

EFFECT OF INTRAOSSEOUS FAT ON RESULTS

Bone mineral measurements may be affected by changes in body fat. A nonuniform increase in fat surrounding the lumbar spine may show a decrease of bone mineral. The effect of changes in paraspinal fat has been reported by Krølner and Pors Nielsen (2).

We studied how changes in intraosseous and intramedullary fat affect bone mineral in the spinal column. To this end, pieces of freshly excised human bones were stepwise dried, dehydrated, defatted, and finally ashed. The treated pieces were then scanned repeatedly in 20 cm of water, with a layer of oil to recreate a soft-tissue absorption factor (RST) similar to that found in humans. Stepwise defatting resulted in a gradual increase in bone mineral values. The magnitudes of these changes are depicted in Table 1. A change in intraosseous fat of 10% of the total fat in the specimen had little effect on the measured bone mineral.

TABLE 1. The effect of fat on bone mineral (BM) measurements in lumbar vertebrae

Sample no.	Linear regression ($y = a + bx$)* a	b	Change in BM per 10% increase in total fat of specimen (gram)
V 858	43.4	-0.00072	-0.0072
V 943	56.9	-0.010	-0.10
V 003	24.5	-0.014	-0.14

*y = bone mineral in grams; x = percentage of total intraosseous fat in specimen. Total intraosseous fat is considered equal to ether-acetone extractable fat.

AGE-RELATED BONE LOSS

We studied patterns of bone loss in the axial and the appendicular skeleton in 187 normal volunteers (105 women and 82 men, ages 20 to 89 years) (3). In normal women, bone diminution from the vertebrae began in young adulthood and was linear throughout life. In the appendicular skeleton, however, bone diminution, as assessed by single-photon absorptiometry, did not occur until the age of 50 years, was accelerated from age 51 to 65, and then decelerated somewhat after the age of 65. Overall bone diminution throughout life was 47% for the vertebrae, 30% for the midradius, and 39% for the distal radius. For men, bone diminution was 15% for the lumbar spinal column and also was less for the midradius and distal radius. We believe that these different patterns may relate to differences in the proportional content of trabecular and cortical bone at the three scanning sites: the lumbar spinal column contains >66% trabecular bone, the midradius contains >95% cortical bone, and the distal radius contains 75% cortical and 25% trabecular bone.

We have initiated a longitudinal study to evaluate rates of bone loss in individual normal subjects. Preliminary data are consistent with our cross-sectional data in that bone loss was linear between the ages of 30 and 60 years, with no obvious postmenopausal acceleration. Prior to the age of 30 years, the trend was toward a gain of bone, and after the age of 60 years the trend was toward a flattening of the rate of bone loss. We are continuing to gather longitudinal data with the aim of defining rates of bone loss for each decade in women and in men. Until then, the questions of when bone loss begins in normal women and the extent to which it may be accelerated by menopause cannot be precisely defined.

Recently, Krølner (1) reported a seasonal influence on lumbar spinal bone mineral in a prospective study of 26 normal women, ages 19 to 66 years, using dual-photon absorptiometry of the lumbar spinal column. We evaluated differences in bone density in the winter-spring season and in the summer-fall season in 75 normal volunteers and found no evidence for a seasonal, cyclic pattern of bone loss. In the short-term study, 12.9% of subjects showed no change, 40% showed some increase, and 47.1% showed some decrease in area bone density relative to the baseline measurement. The differences between our data and those of Krølner could reflect differences in the latitude of Denmark and Minnesota or in the vitamin D intake of the respective populations.

TABLE 2. Separation of osteoporotic from normal subjects using different areas of the lumbar spine (L-1 to L-4)*

	Percentage below lower 5% cutoff	
	Normal (105 subjects)	Osteoporosis (76 pts)
Bone mineral area density (g/cm^2)		
L-1	3.8	17.8
L-2	4.8	39.5
L-3	4.8	47.5
L-4	4.8	32.0
L-1 to L-4	4.8	45.0
Mass (g)		
L-1 to L-4	4.8	37.5
L-2 to L-4	4.8	44.0
L-3	4.8	36.8

*The highest percentage of osteoporotic patients found below the 5% cutoff from the normal distribution gives the best separation, that is, the least overlap.

TABLE 3. Separation of osteoporotic from normal women, using different statistical approaches with respect to the normal data

Bone mineral area density (g/cm^2)*		Percentage below cutoff percentile			
		Normal (105 subjects)		Osteoporosis (76 pts)	
		Lower 5th	Lower 10th	Lower 5th	Lower 10th
Lumbar spine (L-1 to L-4)	A	4.8	9.5	44.7	51.3
	B			40.8	50.0
	C			30.3	48.7
Midradius	A			13.2	26.3
	B			13.2	26.3
	C			10.5	21.1
	D			17.1	31.6
Distal radius	A			3.9	23.7
	B			3.9	18.4
	C			3.9	17.1
	D			5.3	34.2

*A = based on a single linear regression for all ages; B = based on separate linear regressions for those 20-50 and over 51 years of age; C = based on separate linear regressions for 20-50, 51-65, and 66 years old or older; D = based on cubic regression on age. Note for lumbar spine, normal data are best expressed as a single linear regression; for the radius, a cubic regression on age was best.

OSTEOPOROSIS

The effectiveness of dual-photon absorptiometry to differentiate patients with idiopathic spinal osteoporosis (presence of nontraumatic compression fractures) from normal subjects was tested in a population of 105 normal women and 75 patients with osteoporosis. Both populations have previously been described (3).

Separation between the two populations was poor when measurements of bone mineral were based on one pass over the lumbar spine. Separation was best when the areas of L-1 to L-4 or L-3 alone were measured. We prefer to express the data in terms of area density (g/cm^2). Data expressed in mass units (g) were of about equal discriminating power in a limited number of subjects in whom this could be done appropriately. Frequently, a definite separation of individual vertebrae was not possible in patients with osteoporosis. In these, the confines within which the bone mass was to be determined were difficult to reproduce accurately. This does not constitute a problem in area measurements. A summary of these results is given in Table 2.

Using the L-1 to L-4 region and expressing the data as area density (g/cm^2), we obtained the best separation of the two populations when the normal data from the lumbar spine were expressed on the basis of a single linear regression for all ages. For midradius and distal radius, this was true when the data were expressed on the basis of a cubic regression on age. This is further shown in detail in Table 3.

Separation between the two groups could be improved further if a correction for loss of vertebral height in osteoporosis was introduced into the measurements of area density. Normalization of normal data for height, weight, and surface area did not result in better separation of the two populations. Osteoporotic women with compression fractures in the lumbar spine had a higher average bone mineral than did age-matched women with osteoporosis without lumbar compression fractures. Individual compression fractures were noted to have equal or higher area bone density than the neighboring nonaffected vertebrae.

METABOLIC BONE DISEASE

We studied patterns of bone loss in 100 patients with various types of endocrine dysfunction (4). The midradius and distal radius were studied by single-photon absorptiometry as sites containing predominantly cortical bone, and the lumbar spine was studied by dual-photon absorptiometry as a site representing predominantly trabecular bone. Mean bone density was expressed as positive or negative standard deviations from age- and sex-specific mean for normal persons (Table 4). For patients

TABLE 4. Mean bone mineral density for each scanning site, expressed as positive or negative standard deviations from the age- and sex-specific normal mean

Group	No.	Lumbar spine	Midradius	Distal radius
Normal subjects	187	0.00	0.00	0.00
Primary hyperparathyroidism	29	-1.15*	-0.45	-0.92†
Secondary hyperparathyroidism (chronic renal failure)	14	0.11	1.15‡	0.02
Hypercortisolism	17	-1.94*	0.29	-0.33
Hyperthyroidism	13	-0.82*	-0.70	-0.67
Acromegaly	7	0.68†	0.83	0.41
Postsurgical hypoparathyroidism	20	1.50*	0.70†	0.68‡

Significantly different from respective normal value: *$P<0.001$; †$P<0.01$; ‡$P<0.05$.

From Seeman, E., Wahner, H.W., Offord, K.P., Kumar, R., Johnson, W.J. and Riggs, B.L. (1982): J. Clin. Invest., 69, 1302. By permission of The American Society for Clinical Investigation.

with primary hyperparathyroidism, hypercortisolism, and hyperthyroidism, this deviation was negative, suggestive of a bone loss. For patients with secondary hyperparathyroidism due to chronic renal failure, acromegaly, and postsurgical hypoparathyroidism, the deviation was positive, suggestive of bone gain. There were significant ($\underline{P}$<0.001) differences in the response of bone among the different scanning sites (Table 4).

REFERENCES

1. Krølner, B. (1983): Calcif. Tissue Int., 35, 145.
2. Krølner, B. and Pors Nielsen, S. (1982): In: Non-Invasive Bone Measurements: Methodological Problems, p. 73. Editors: J.V. Dequeker and C.C. Johnston, Jr. IRL Press, Oxford.
3. Riggs, B.L., Wahner, H.W., Dunn, W.L., Mazess, R.B., Offord, K.P. and Melton, L.J., III. (1981): J. Clin. Invest., 67, 328.
4. Seeman, E., Wahner, H.W., Offord, K.P., Kumar, R., Johnson, W.J. and Riggs, B.L. (1982): J. Clin. Invest., 69, 1302.

Discussion of presentations by Parfitt, Mazess and Wahner:

DR. PARFITT: Dr. Mazess, your statement that measurements of cortical bone in the extremities are not useful in diagnosis rests on the assumption that only spinal osteoporosis is of interest. That seems to condemn other types of osteoporotic fractures, such as those of wrist or hip, to a secondary status.

DR. MAZESS: I agree that measurements on the peripheral skeleton can be used for screening, but I'm more concerned with how to evaluate the rapid changes that are occurring with therapy. The only way of doing that is by looking at trabecular bone, particularly in the axial skeleton.

DR. RAISZ: Dr. Wahner, have you looked at your data in relation to menopause?

DR. WAHNER: Our longitudinal study is only half completed. So far, we have seen no difference with respect to linearity in the pattern of bone loss.

DR. RAISZ: If you take out the patients who have a lot of osteophytosis or osteoarthritis, do you still fail to see perimenopausal acceleration of bone loss?

DR. WAHNER: We have not yet looked, but we agree that the presence of degenerative disease falsely increases the bone mineral content.

DR. NORDIN: First, I don't know where Dr. Mazess got the figure of a 23% error on single energy CT scanning from, but we have done repeated measurements by this method on the same vertebra in 30 normal people and the error is 9.1%.

Second, concerning the difficulty of distinguishing normal from osteoporotic patients, I would ask people to define what they mean by osteoporosis. 60% of normal women over 70 have got a wedged vertebra, but only 15% have got two crushed vertebrae. If you call the former group osteoporotic, you will not be able to identify them, because they are just variants of the normal population. But, as we showed at the Madison Osteoporosis meeting, if you confine your diagnosis of osteoporosis to patients with two or more crush fractures, they differ from normal people in virtually every measurement of bone mass.

Finally, concerning the menopause, 30% or more of American women are hysterectomized before the menopause, and a substantial proportion have both ovaries removed as well. Consequently, it is quite unacceptable to take a group of women aged 30 to 80, not ask them whether they've had their ovaries removed, call them normal, and plot spinal density against age. If the data were rearranged to allow for the menopause, then there is no loss of bone in premenopausal women as judged by CT scanning or forearm scanning. There is also no significant loss of bone in normal women after the age of 60 in the spine, and very little loss in the iliac crest. All the action takes place between the menopause and the age of 60.

DR. MAZESS: Dr. Nordin, your figure of 9% is for precision. I was referring to accuracy - the figure of 23% is one standard error of estimate of the regression of actual ash density on measured ash density, obtained recently by Laval Jeantet using a CGR. Incidentally, your definition of osteoporosis for clinical research is now widely accepted, and was used both in the Mayo Clinic studies and out own.

DR. DEQUEKER: How much of the bone in the spine is trabecular? I have seen several different figures in the literature. Laval Jeantet says 30% for the lumbar spine, I heard 70% today, and Dr. Wahner has reported 50%.

With dual energy photon absorptiometry, one includes the spinous processes and apophyseal joints, and I think there is much more cortical bone than many people assume.

DR. MAZESS: It depends on what you call trabecular. If you just scrape the surface of a vertebra, you'll see that most of it, even at the surface, is not really compact bone, although it may look so in a CT scan or radiograph. It's actually dense trabecular bone in organization. Even the spinous processes are trabecular, if one cuts them open. So it's a question of what you call trabecular and what you call compact.

DR. AVIOLI: Many investigators use measurements of metacarpal cortical thickness to monitor rates of bone loss and responses to treatment. If this index is getting better, can we assume that the spine is getting better?

DR. MAZESS: No.

QUANTITATIVE COMPUTED TOMOGRAPHY FOR VERTEBRAL MINERAL DETERMINATION

Harry K. Genant, Christopher E. Cann, Douglas P. Boyd, Felix O. Kolb, Bruce Ettinger, Gilbert S. Gordan

Departments of Radiology, Medicine, University of California, San Francisco, CA, U.S.A.

INTRODUCTION

Quantitative computed tomography (QCT) is now an established method (1,2-8,14-19,21,26) for the noninvasive assessment of bone mineral content in the vertebral spongiosum (and other anatomic locations) (20,23,27). Currently, QCT vertebral mineral determination has been implemented at 50 sites encompassing a wide geographic distribution and a wide array of commercial scanners (19).

The potential advantage of QCT over dual photon absorptiometry (DPA) (22,24,29) is its capability for precise 3-dimensional anatomic localization and for spatial separation of highly responsive cancellous bone from less responsive cortical bone. The lumbar vertebrae contains substantial amounts of compact bone, mostly in the laminae, pedicles and dense vertebral endplates (compact:trabecular ratio is approximately 1:2 in the young and 3:2 in the elderly) (9). Only part of the spinal mineral is high turnover trabecular bone, which has a turnover rate eight times that of compact bone (28). The sensitivity of a technique measuring an integral of compact and cancellous bone (such as area projection with DPA) may be low compared to QCT due to inclusion of low-turnover compact bone and extra-osseous mineral such as osteophytes or aortic calcification. The selective localization and the density measurement provided by QCT permit exclusion of these causes of low sensitivity or error and inclusion of purely trabecular bone.

TECHNICAL CONSIDERATIONS

QCT measurements (Fig. 1) are made on commercially available CT scanners using a mineral reference standard for simultaneous calibration, a computed radiograph (scout view) for localization, and either single- or dual-energy techniques (2,16,17,26). Representative volumes (approximately 4 cm^3) of purely trabecular bone at the midplane of 2 to 4 lumbar vertebral bodies are quantified and averaged, and the results are expressed in mineral equivalents of K_2HPO_4 in mg/cm^3. The examination takes 10-15 minutes and the radiation exposure is approximately 200 mrem (1/10 dose of routine CT study).

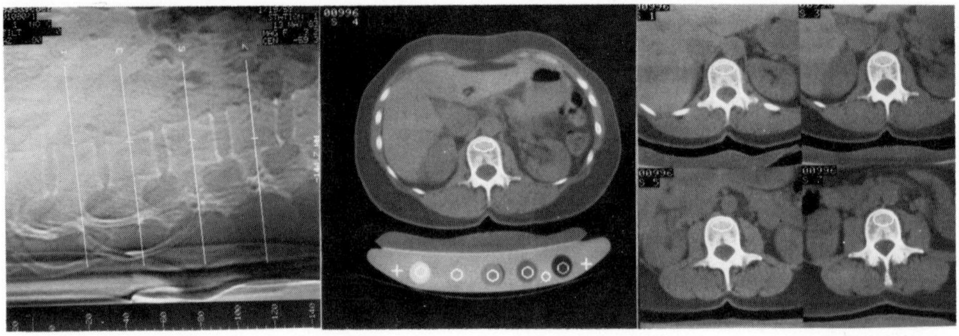

Figure 1. Advanced methodology for QCT vertebral mineral determination.

The precision (reproducibility) of vertebral QCT in humans is 1 to 3% for single-energy (80 kVp) and 3 to 5% for dual-energy (80 kVp/120 kVp) techniques (17). Recent improvements (8) in CT scanner technology (with the GE 9800 scanner) have further increased precision and reduced radiation exposure, i.e., a cadaver repositioned and scanned five times (at 100 mrem) resulted in a coefficient of variation of 0.32% for single-energy determination and 1.68% for dual-energy determination.

The accuracy of single-energy QCT is 1 to 2% for K2HPO4 solutions (14,15), 5% for monkey vertebral specimens (3), and 8% for human vertebral specimens spanning a wide age-range (Fig. 2) (26). These QCT accuracy figures compare favorably with the figures of approximately 10% currently reported (22) for spinal specimens using DPA.

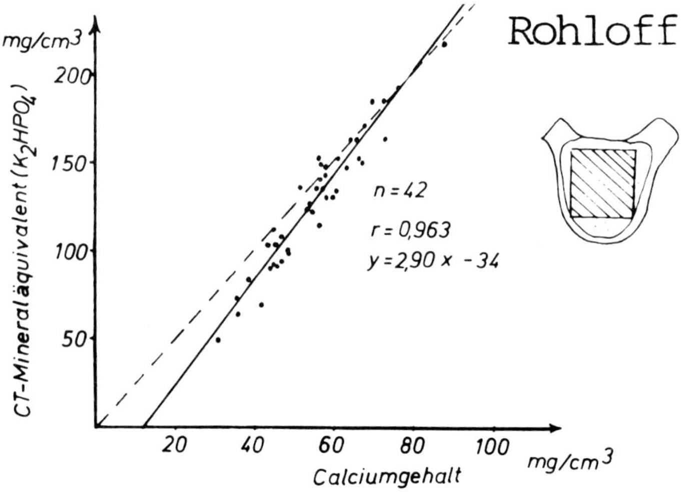

Figure 2.
Rohloff (26) showed high correlation and high accuracy (8% dispersion) for QCT measurement of human vertebrae versus ash weight.

The accuracy for QCT (and DPA), however, can be reduced to 20 to 25%, in the extreme, elderly osteoporotic population (14,15,21). In the case of DPA, vertebral compression with callous formation, angular and scoliotic deformity, hypertrophy of articular facets, discogenic sclerosis or marginal osteophytosis, and extra-osseous calcification, which are widespread in the elderly and are included in the integral measurement, may result in inaccurate as well as poorly reproducible vertebral measurements (9). In the case of QCT, the sources of error are different, but are correctable. The density of yellow marrow is less than that of red marrow because of the presence of fat, which reduces the measured spinal mineral equivalent by about 7 mg per 10% fat by volume (13,15). Extrapolating from available data (11) (Fig. 3) on vertebral body composition, the presence of marrow fat results in an under-estimation of 21 to 31 mg/cm^3 (from age 20 to 80 years) in the mineral value determined by QCT at 80 kVp (Fig. 4). This under-estimation can be eliminated by applying an age-related regression and including the fat variation in the estimated error of the mean. This leaves a residual uncertainty of 4-5 mg/cm^3 (1 S.D.), which is small compared with the normal biological variation of 30 mg/cm^3 (1 S.D.), i.e., the fat-induced inaccuracy is approximately one-sixth the biological variation (Fig. 4). Dual-energy QCT (1,13,14,21) using pre-processing or post-processing techniques can reduce the magnitude of this fat error in the elderly to 2 to 4%, but is considered unnecessary for most clinical applications, i.e., a high correlation (r = 0.98) and low dispersion (Sy/X = 7.37%) were found between single- and dual-energy measurements in 82 women aged 24 to 80 (Fig. 5).

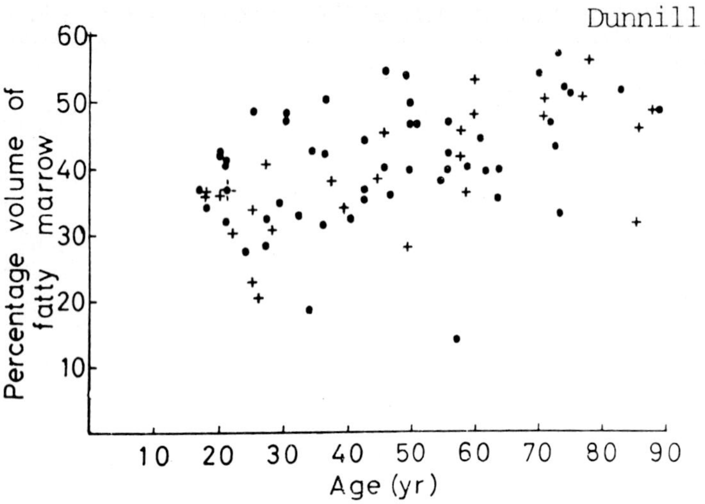

Figure 3. Dunnill (11) showed vertebral fat in humans increasing from an average 32% to an average 47% by volume from age 20-80, with a biological variation of approximately 15% (1 S.D.).

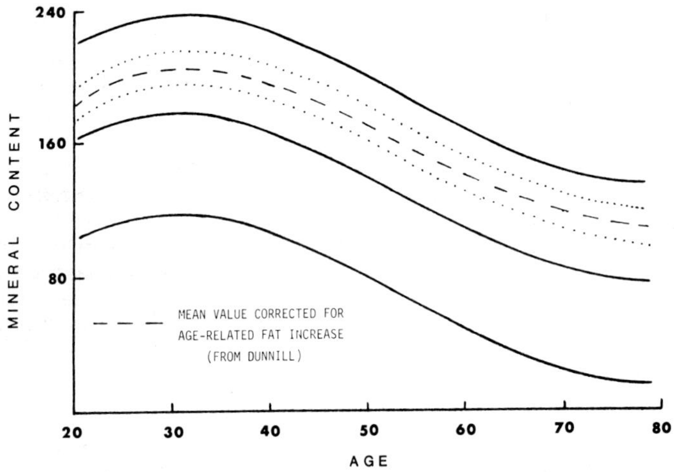

Figure 4. Normal female vertebral cancellous mineral content (in mg/cm³ K2HPO4 versus age. (——) mean and 95% confidence interval; and (– – –) corrected mean value and 95% confidence interval based upon age-related fat from Dunnill (11).

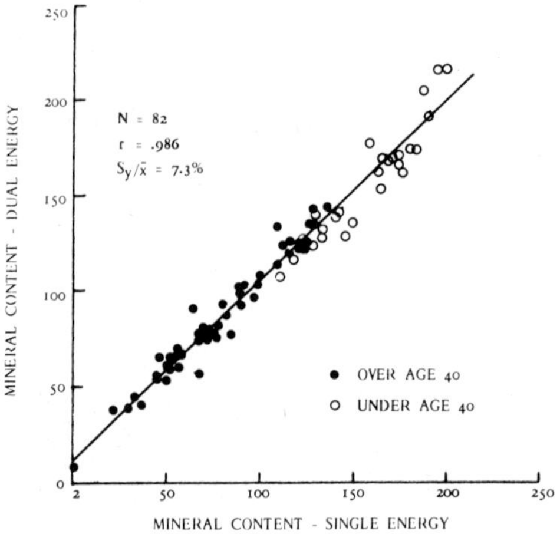

Figure 5. High correlation and low dispersion for dual-energy versus single-energy QCT measurement in women spanning a broad age range suggest that inaccuracy due to marrow compositional changes are not large and that single-energy determination may be adequate for most applications.

The interscanner coefficient of variation for two subjects using four different CT scanners was 3 to 4%, indicating that vertebral QCT results at one site may be extrapolated another. With a worldwide distribution of 2,000 advanced CT body scanners that are capable of performing QCT with minor modification and at relatively little cost, the potential now exists for widespread application of noninvasive vertebral mineral assessment (18,19).

CLINICAL APPLICATIONS

These QCT techniques have been used at UCSF to study vertebral mineral changes in osteoporosis and other metabolic bone diseases. Longitudinal and cross-sectional bone mass measurements have been obtained in over 1,500 patients seen during the past five years for clinical or research purposes (4-7,12-19).

The normal ranges of vertebral mineral and age-related bone losses were determined from cross-sectional studies (5) of 120 normal males and 203 normal females aged 20-80 years (Figs. 6 & 7). The normal mean value for young males and females was approximately 175 mg/cm³. Males, by linear regression, lost an average 0.84%/year, and females, by cubic regression, lost an average 1.2%/year, which was accelerated at menopause. Correcting for age-related marrow fat altered the observed rates of loss by only about 10%, e.g., in females, 1.08%/year versus 1.2%/year.

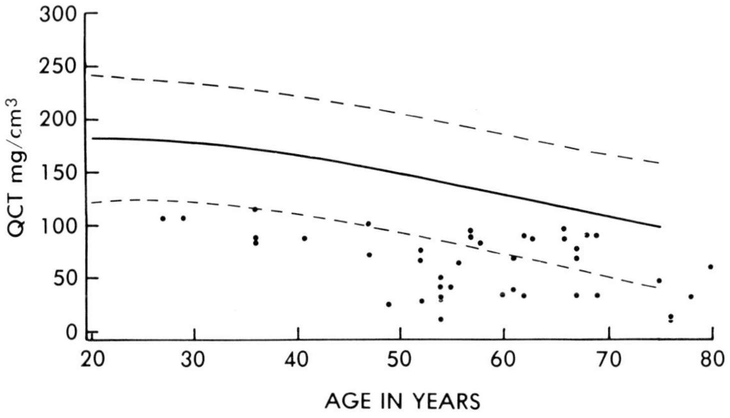

Figure 6. Normal male QCT vertebral mineral content versus age. Mean and 95% confidence interval are shown for cubic regression, which fits data only slightly better than linear regression ($p<.15$). Idiopathic osteoporotic males with vertebral fractures are plotted (•).

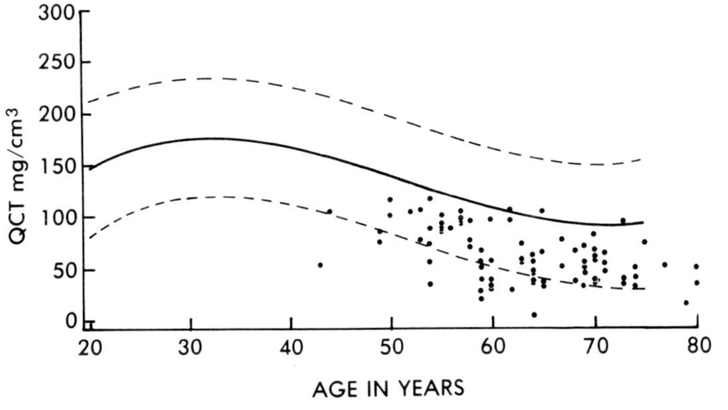

Figure 7. Normal female QCT vertebral mineral content versus age. Mean and 95% confidence interval are shown for cubic regression ($p<.05$). Osteoporotic females with wedged or crushed vertebrae are plotted (•).

Cross-sectional studies (6) in 25 young women with various forms of amenorrhea showed an average decrement from normal of 25% in vertebral mineral values and 10% in peripheral cortical values. Cross-sectional studies (12) in 80 perimenopausal women showed an average 5.6%/year vertebral cancellous mineral loss by QCT (Fig. 8) compared with 3%/year by photon absorptiometry and radiogrammetry of the peripheral cortex. Longitudinal studies (17) in 31 women following oophorectomy showed an average 9%/year vertebral cancellous loss, while integral vertebral loss (as in DPA) was only 4% (4) (Fig. 9), and peripheral cortical bone loss was 2 to 3%. The mininum protective dose of conjugated estrogen for preventing spinal bone loss following oophorectomy was 0.6 mg/day (17) (Fig. 10).

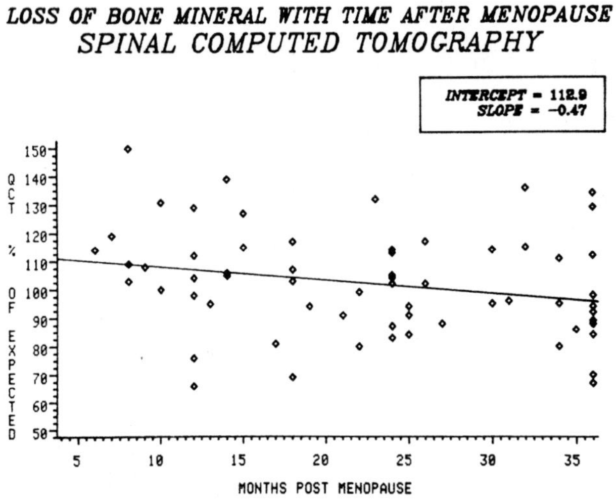

Figure 8. Cross-sectional studies (12) showing loss of QCT vertebral mineral with time after natural menopause.

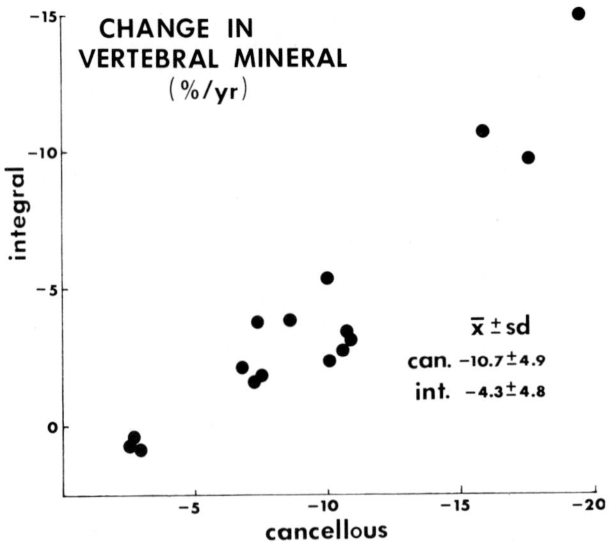

Figure 9. Comparison in 16 oophorectomized women of annual losses of vertebral mineral, integral versus cancellous measurement, both determined by QCT. Although losses by integral measurement (as with DPA) and by cancellous measurement (as with QCT) correlate, the latter demonstrates more than two-fold greater sensitivity.

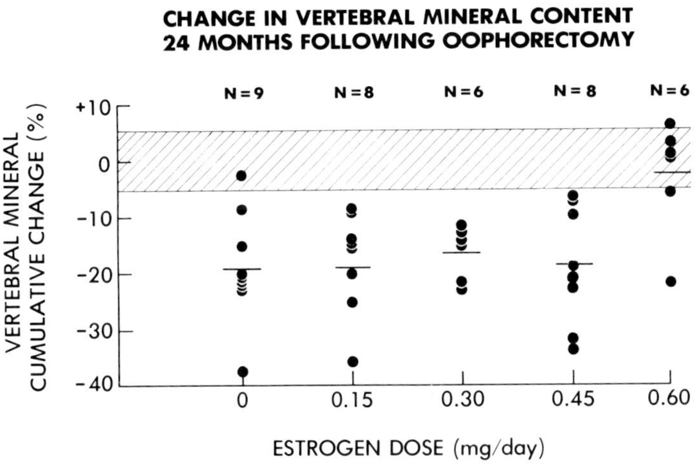

Figure 10. Dose response for vertebral QCT (17). Cross hatched area represents insignificant change.

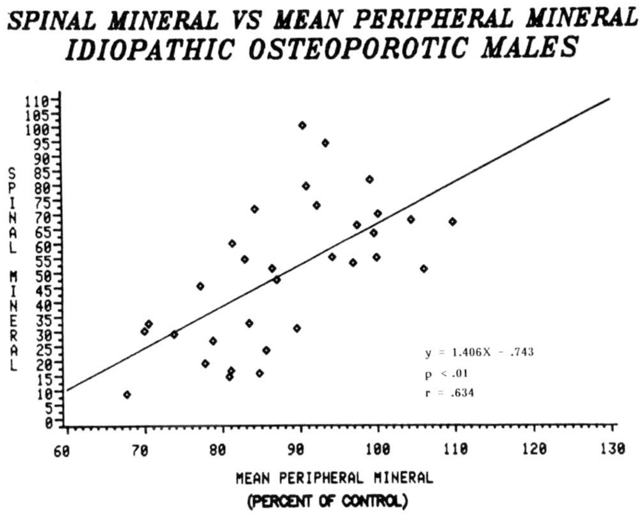

Figure 11. Idiopathic osteoporotic males showing larger decrement from normal for vertebral mineral QCT than for mean peripheral cortical mineral by radiogrammetry and photon absorptiometry.

Cross-sectional studies (7) in 48 males with idiopathic osteoporosis showed a mean decrement from normal of 48% in vertebral mineral and 15% in peripheral cortical mineral. When expressed as percent of normal, peripheral measurements in this group correlated (r = 0.63) with vertebral measurements, but did not provide a reliable individual estimate of vertebral mineral loss or of atraumatic spinal fractures (Fig. 11).

Vertebral QCT measurements in both males and females provided an index of fracture risk by revealing a threshold at approximately 110 mg/cm^3, above which fractures were rare and below which fractures were common (Figs. 6 & 7). In a related study (25), the correlation was high in 25 patients between an index of fracture severity and QCT vertebral mineral content (r = 0.66, $p < .01$), while the correlation between the fracture index and DPA was poor (r = 0.068, n.s.).

CONCLUSION

Quantitative computed tomography of the vertebral spongiosum is a rapid, sensitive, precise and acceptably accurate method for noninvasive measurement of bone mineral mass. The greatest advantages of spinal QCT (relative to DPA) lie in the high precision of the technique, the high sensitivity of the vertebral spongiosa measurement site, and the potential for widespread application.

ACKNOWLEDGEMENTS

Supported in part by NIH-AM27926, NASA-15899 and Ayerst Laboratories

REFERENCES

1. Adams, J.E., Pullan, B.R., Adams, P.H., et al (1982): J Comput Assist Tomogr. 6,204.
2. Cann, C.E. and Genant, H.K. (1980): J Comput Assist. 4,493.
3. Cann, C.E. and Genant, H.K., Young, D.R. (1980): Radiology, 134, 525.
4. Cann, C.E. and Genant, H.K. (1981): Calcif Tissue Int. 33, Suppl., 307.
5. Cann, C.E. and Genant, H.K. (1982): J Comput Assist Tomogr., 6,216.
6. Cann, C.E., Martin, M.C. and Genant, H.K. (1982): In: Proceedings, 64th Annual Endocrine Society Meeting.
7. Cann, C.E., Genant, H.K. and Kolb, F.O. (1982): Calcif. Tiss. Int. 34, 528.
8. Cann, C.E., Rutt, B.K. and Genant, H.K. (1982): In: Proceedings, 68th Scientific and Annual Meeting of the Radiological Society of North America.
9. Cann, C.E., Rutt, B.K. and Genant, H.K. (1983): In: Proceedings of the 5th Annual Meeting of the America Society for Bone Mineral Research.
10. Dunn, W.L., Wahner, H. and Riggs, B.L. (1980): Radiology, 136, 485.
11. Dunnill, M.S., Anderson, J.A., Whitehead, R (1967): J Pathol.,94, 275.
12. Ettinger, B., Genant, H.K. and Cann, C.E. (1983): J Comput Assist. Tomogr., In press.
13. Faul, D.D., Couch, J.L., Cann, C.E., Boyd, D.P. and Genant, H.K. (1982): J Comput Assist Tomogr., 6, 202.
14. Genant, H.K. and Boyd, D.P. (1977): Invest. Radiol., 12, 545.
15. Genant, H.K., Boyd, D.P., Rosenfeld, D., Abols, Y., and Cann, C.E. (1981): In: Noninvasive Measurements of Bone Mass and Their Clinical Applications, p. 121. Editor: S. H. Cohn. CRC Press, New York, N.Y.
16. Genant, H.K. and Cann, C.E. (1981): In, Osteoporosis: Recent Advances in Pathogenesis and Treatment, p. 37. Editors: H.F. DeLuca, H.M. Frost, W.S.S. Jee, C.C. Johnston and A.M. Parfitt. University Park Press, Baltimore, MD.
17. Genant, H.K., Cann, C.E., Ettinger, B. and Gordan, G.S. (1982): Ann. Inter Med. 97, 699.
18. Genant, H.K. (1983): Western J Med., July (In press).
19. Genant, H.K., Cann, C.E., Pozzi-Mucelli, R.S. and Kanter, A.S. (1983): J Comput Assist Tomogr., 6:548-567.
20. Hangartner, T.N. and Overton, T.R. (1982): J Comput Assist Tomogr. 6, 1156.
21. Laval-Jeantet, A.M., Roger, B. and Dallant, P. (1983): In: Proceedings, XVII European Symposium on Calcified Tissues, p. A2. Editors: U. Largiader and H. Fleisch. Springer International.
22. Marhard, L., Lindsay, R., Dempster, D.W., Pushparjn, N, King, D.W., Viliquett, G, Hawkins, W. (1983): Proceedings, Clinical Disorders of Bone and Mineral Metabolism, Detroit, Michigan.

23. Orphanoudakis, S.C., Jensen, P.S., Rauschkolb, E.N., Lang, R. and Rasmussen, H. (1979): Invest. Radiol. 14, 122.
24. Peppler, W.W. and Mazess, R.B. (1981): Calc. Tiss. Int. 33, 353.
25. Powell, M.R., Kolb, F.O., Genant, H.K., Cann, C.E. and Stebler, B.G. (1983): In, Proceedings, Clinical Disorders of Bone and Mineral Metabolism, Detroit, Michigan.
26. Rohloff, R., Hitzler, H., Arndt, W., and Frey, W. (1982): In, CT'82, p.126. Editors: J. Lissner and J. L. Doppman. Schnetztor-Verlag, Konstanz.
27. Ruegsegger, P., Elsasser, U., Anliker, M., et al (1976): Radiology, 121, 93.
28. Snyder, W. (1975): ICRP23, Oxford, Pergamon Press.
29. Wahner, H.W., Riggs, B.L., Beabout, J.W. (1977): J Nucl Med. 18, 432.

CLINICAL APPLICATION OF PERIPHERAL COMPUTED TOMOGRAPHY

Peter Rüegsegger and Maximilian Dambacher

Institute for Biomedical Engineering, University and Federal Institute of Technology Zurich, Switzerland
and
Research Laboratory for Calcium Metabolism, University of Zurich, Switzerland

Fractures in locations like the vertebrae, the proximal femur, and the distal forearm are clinical signs of a diminished bone mass either cortical or trabecular or both. Patients with crush fractures of the spine have low trabecular bone volume predominantly. Patients with fractures of the proximal femur may have normal trabecular bone volume, but a loss of cortical bone. Thus both bone compartments, cortical and trabecular are to be analyzed. However, because of the higher turnover of trabecular bone a rapid detection of bone loss is achieved in trabecular bone regions.

During the past ten years systematic efforts have been made (1) to develop special low dose CT-equipment for the precise quantitation of small changes in peripheral bones. The principal motivation of these efforts is to provide the means and the methodology to analyze quantitatively the gradual development of osteoporosis and also the success of therapeutic countermeasures in individual patients.

MATERIALS AND METHODS

Our special purpose low dose CT-system for bone densitometry is based on a miniaturized translational/rotational type scanner. The first clinical prototype of such a scanner was equiped with an Iodine isotope source (2) (effective energy 29 keV), a newer system utilizes a highly filtered X-ray tube (3) (effective energy 41 keV). Single photon detection, low energy of the photons and the restriction to peripheral measuring sites allow low dose measurements, the radiation dose per CT-examination being less than 5 mrem.

Standard measuring sites for bone evaluations are the distal tibia and the distal radius. Due to the non-homogeneous distribution of bone, precise longitudinal evaluations require the reproducible selection of the same sample volumes in the trabecular bone regions. This problem is solved by making use of digital radiograms and measurement of stacks of CT-scans. In evaluating the bone parameters from the CT-scans (4), the computer isolates the tibia - or the radius - from the surrounding tissue, peels off 50% of the picture element so that a core of 50% of the bone cross section remains and calculates the mean linear attenuation coefficient of this region (trabecular bone parameter). The average linear attenuation coefficient taken over 100% of the bone cross section contains compact and trabecular bone (total bone parameter). The precision of the trabecular bone parameter in actual examinations has been determined to be 0.3% for the old isotope CT-system. For the new X-ray system it is 0.1%. The volumetric ratio of bone marrow to bone trabeculae is such that their contributions to the trabecular bone parameter are approximately equal. Provided that there are no considerable changes in the bone marrow composition during a longitudinal examination, a precision of 0.1% in the determination of the trabecular bone parameter thus allows the detection of a 0.3% change in trabecular bone density from two successive CT-examinations. Drastic bone marrow changes would induce inaccuracies in the bone density determination (a 10% increase in fat content causes a shift in normal bone density of 1%). At peripheral measuring sites such changes are not likely to occur - however, in future applications, this source of inaccuracy has to be eliminated by dual energy CT-examinations.

RESULTS

Peripheral trabecular bone appears to be a good indicator for trabecular bone of the skeleton. Measurements of the third lumbar vertebra and the distal radius from cadavers aged 22 to 73 years yielded an excellent correlation (1) ($r = 0.92$; $N = 16$). A surprisingly good correlation was also found (5) between the volume density of bone samples from the iliac crest and the trabecular bone parameter of the distal tibia ($r = 0.72$; $N = 14$). Furthermore the trabecular bone densities of the distal radius and the distal tibia of a large population of normal and osteoporotic females (6) correlate well ($r = 0.88$; $N = 159$).

Cross-sectional data of a population of normal females show no significant age dependency between age 20 and menopause. After menopause healthy women loose 0.81% trabecular bone per year. The trabecular bone density of an average osteoporotic female at age 70 is 42% lower than that of an average healthy female at age 50. Calculated from cross-sectional data the average osteoporotic female looses 2.5% trabecular bone per year after menopause (assuming that osteoporosis is the result of an excessive bone loss after menopause). Following trabecular bone changes of individual females for a period of three years we found that postmenopausal normal women as a group loose 0.95% trabecular bone per year, whereas postmenopausal women with clinically proven but untreated osteoporosis as a group loose bone at a rate of 2.7% per year. Thus the average bone loss evaluated from longitudinal examinations coincides with the average bone loss predicted from the cross sectional data.

Trabecular bone density provides a better separation of the osteoporotics from the normals than total bone (trabecular and cortical bone) or the Garn-Index (cortical bone). For a group of 44 normal females and 25 osteoporotics in the age range 50 to 70 years all three bone parameters had been examined. The discrimination power of the three parameters is as follows: For the trabecular bone density 2 of 25 osteoporotics are in the normal range, for the total bone density 14 of 25, and for the Garn-Index 15 of 25 respectively.

Following individual cases of postmenopausal osteoporosis we observed an enormous variety of temporal pattern of trabecular bone loss (Fig. 1). Three of twelve osteoporotic females did not show any bone loss for two years or longer. Nine lost bone from 2% to 20%. In general, bone was lost in a steplike pattern. Phases of stability were followed by phases of acute bone loss. The duration of bone loss ranged from three to nine months. The duration of relative stability is less well documented. We anticipate a duration of one year or longer.

Sodium fluoride (80 mg/day) was given for up to three years to a group of patients with clinically proven postmenopausal osteoporosis (7). As in the untreated cases peripheral trabecular bone had been measured in intervals of three months. Under treatment we observed phases of trabecular bone gain in seven of 16 patients (four of these patients had a significantly higher trabecular bone density after two years than initially). Five of the patients remained completely unchanged during the whole period of observation. Five patients lost bone - again in a steplike pattern like the untreated patients. An evaluation of the total bone parameter (trabecular and cortical bone) indicates that cortical bone is not increased by the NaF treatment. So far the loss of cortical bone is not significantly different in the treated and

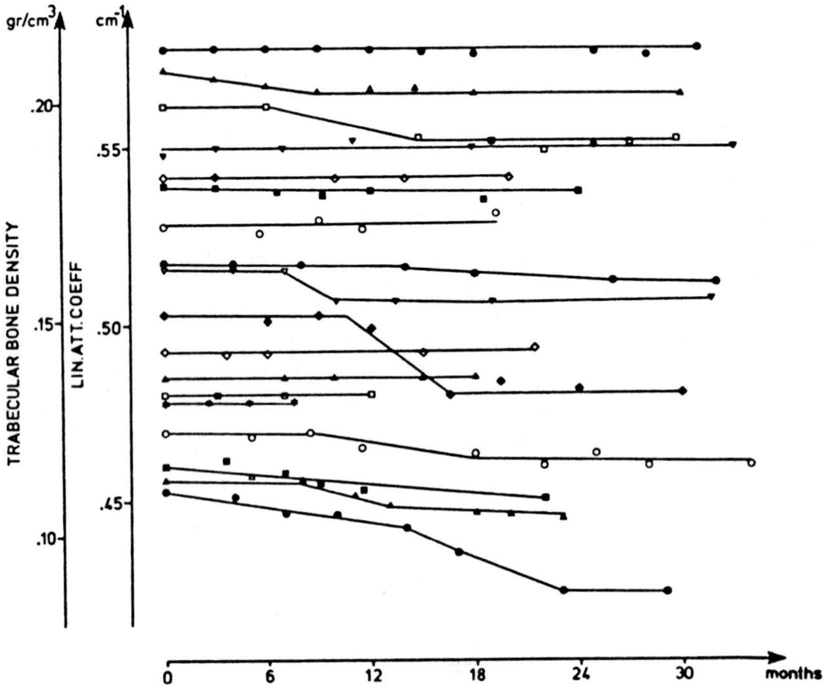

Figure 1. Individual loss of trabecular bone (distal tibia) of patients with untreated postmenopausal osteoporosis.

the untreated group. NaF therefore probably stimulates the formation of trabecular bone but not that of cortical bone.

Corticosteroid induced bone loss was also successfully quantitated with peripheral CT (8). We followed twenty patients with bronchial asthma during the first year of chronic alternate day treatment. The documented trabecular bone loss is considerable: 25 mg PREDNISONE given every other day causes an average trabecular bone loss of 3.5% within one year. Bone loss is dose and age dependent. Young patients at 50 mg/2d loose up to 17% trabecular bone within one year. An evaluation of the total bone parameter (trabecular and cortical bone) shows, within one year, a decrease of 1.1%, the maximum individual loss was 4.5%. This reduction of total bone might be attributed to the loss in the trabecular bone compartment. Thus, in general cortical bone loss seems to be insignificant after one year of treatment. Trabecular bone loss had been monitored at the distal tibia and the distal radius. Albeit not identical for each individual we found that bone loss correlates well (r = 96; N = 20) at these two measuring sites.

Quantitative computed tomography of the peripheral skeleton has proven to be valuable in quantitating gradual bone changes. Conceivably the documentation of individual temporal patterns of trabecular and cortical bone loss may provide insight into the dynamics of osteoporosis and the pathology involved. Furthermore QCT will help in working out efficient treatment regimes in metabolic bone diseases.

REFERENCES

1. Rüegsegger, P., Anliker, M. and Dambacher, M. (1981): J Comput Assist Tomogr, 5, 384-390.
2. Rüegsegger, P., Elsasser, U. and Anliker, M. (1976): Radiology 121, 93-97.
3. Stebler, B., Steiger, P. and Rüegsegger, P. (1982): J Comput Assist Tomogr, 6, 201-202.
4. Rüegsegger, P., Stebler, B., Dambacher, M. (1982): Mayo Clinic Proceedings 57 (Suppl), 96-103.
5. Olah, A.J., Rüegsegger, P., Dambacher, M.A. (1983): Comparison of Histomorphometry and Computed Tomography in Quantitating Trabecular Bone (this conference).
6. Rüegsegger, P., Dambacher, M.A., Rüegsegger, E., Fischer, J.A. and Anliker, M. (1983): Bone Loss in Pre- and Postmenopausal Women - a Cross Sectional and Longitudinal Study Using QCT (submitted for publication).
7. Dambacher, M.A., Rüegsegger, P., Fischer, J.A. and Anliker, M. (1983): Bone Loss in Osteoporosis as Quantified by Computed Tomography (this conference).
8. Rüegsegger, P., Medici, T.C. and Anliker, M. (1983): Corticosteroid-induced Bone Loss - a Longitudinal Study of the Alternate Day Therapy in Patients with Bronchial Asthma Using QCT (submitted for publication).

Discussion of presentations by Genant and Ruegsegger:

DR. MAZESS: With regard to the accuracy of quantitative computed tomography, at least six studies (three in the past year) have shown very large inaccuracies (50-75%) on bones that are not macerated, so that the marrow is still present. In all studies where the marrow was removed, the accuracy was very good as Dr. Genant showed. But the presence of marrow of variable composition is a significant source of inaccuracy. In normal people marrow fat changes little and the difference between the single and dual energy CT is perhaps 7-8%, but marrow fat may go up to 70% in osteoporosis and to 80 or 90% in immobilized individuals or those receiving corticosteroids. Variable amounts of osteoid could introduce similar errors.

DR. GENANT: Three of these studies that you have widely quoted represent work that was done in the late 1970's without using adequate calibration, without precise localization, and without beam hardening corrections. All of these technical problems have been reduced in recent years. Several of the other studies represent worse case examples. In the femur the amount of fat is roughly two to three times that in the vertebral body, and the amount of mineral in the elderly population is reduced by about one-half. The inaccuracy of about 30% for the distal femur of elderly subjects shown by Adams would extrapolate to about 6% in the spine over a broad age range.

It is true that with very severe demineralization a small absolute inaccuracy corresponds to a large relative inaccuracy, which on occasion can approach 20 or even 30%. But we do not feel that this invalidates the procedure as a diagnostic tool - the difference between measurements 3.0 and 3.2 standard deviations below normal is unlikely to be of clinical importance. Nevertheless, we recognize the potential for inaccuracy, and have developed the dual energy technique that is now becoming more widely available.

DR. RAISZ: If the entire vertebral trabecular bone mass was decreasing at 10% per year, the negative balance would be between 100 and 200 mg. daily, but in normal postmenopausal women the negative balance is increased by only about 20-25 mg. per day, so presumably the changes you observe are localized or transient.

DR. GENANT: The very rapid loss followed oophorectomy in women who previously were normally menstruating. Abrupt estrogen withdrawal probably leads to more rapid loss than the gradual withdrawal of normal menopause. We do not have any calcium balance studies, but peripheral cortical bone responds much less dramatically.

DR. REEVE: Dr. Charles, using a new method, found that calcium loss from the spine is much higher than generally supposed, and could account for the difference between the two estimates of the rate of loss.

DR. WILLIE: What is the cost of these techniques? Will the cost fall with wider use, and will CT really be a clinical tool in the future?

DR. GENANT: It costs approximately a million dollars for a new CT scanner, but there are already two thousand in the world capable of doing spinal measurements. Scheduling 3-4 patients per hour, the cost would be $100-$150 per study. To get started, you need a phantom costing about $500.

DR. SHAPIRO: Many pediatric studies use single energy photon absorptiometry of the radius; for example, looking at developmental abnormalities in small for date children or the effect of feeding various formulas on bone mineral accumulation. I'm concerned about the anatomical features that were presented earlier and problems in positioning.

DR. GENANT: We are becoming increasingly aware of bone mineralization problems in the pediatric population, and you are correct that there are many unsolved difficulties with all measurement techniques in terms of adequate immobilization and the effects of growth and increasing size on serial measurements.

DR. JOHNSTON: With quantitative CT measurement, the radiation dose may be high. For example, on our machine it is about 750 milliroentgen. This is acceptable for diagnosis but too high for serial measurements in normal individuals.

DR. GENANT: The dose is somewhat scanner and manufacturer dependent. Averaging in a small volume as we do, the dose is lower than with conventional CT imaging by a factor of at least 10, but this is not possible with all scanners. With the GE scanner, which has the widest distribution, the dose of 100-200 millirem is substantially less than for a conventional abdominal x-ray. In contrast, to carry out dual-photon absorptiometry (DPA) in the elderly without obtaining a radiograph can be misleading because of uncertain localization, unrecognized osteophytosis, minor compressions and Schmorl's nodes, so the total radiation dose may be less for CT than for DPA.

COMPARISON OF TRABECULAR BONE DENSITY AT AXIAL AND PERIPHERAL SITES USING COMPUTED TOMOGRAPHY

Thomas N. Hangartner, Thomas R. Overton, Wynne M. Rigal

Departments of Applied Sciences in Medicine and Surgery, University of Alberta, Edmonton, Alberta, Canada.

INTRODUCTION

Investigations based on conventional X-ray techniques suggest that bone loss in osteoporosis is first visible in the spine. Radio-lucent areas and crush fractures have been quantitised in order to introduce some objective measure of bone loss. Recently, computed tomography (CT) was adapted to produce quantitative values for spinal bone density by expressing the linear attenuation coefficients as equivalents to simultaneously measured K_2HPO_4 test solutions (1). The precision of these measurements is given as ±3%, which means that a difference of 6% between two measurements is needed to be significant. In its present development dual energy CT provides a poorer precision than single energy CT (2) but has the advantage of producing results with an approximately 5 times better accuracy.

Dual photon absorptiometry (3) has been used to measure certain regions of the spine. The results, however, express total mineral content rather than mineral density and are therefore dependent upon the measured, unknown bone volume. It is not possible with this method to separately obtain data for trabecular bone. A problem common to single energy CT and dual photon absorptiometry is the unknown composition of bone marrow which influences the values of bone density or mineral content in a similar way.

Special purpose CT with low energy isotope sources (4,5) has been applied to the measurement of peripheral bones, particularly the distal part of the radius. The reproducibility of trabecular bone measurements is better than 1%. Due to the low energy spectrum used and the small expected variations in marrow-fat composition at these peripheral sites the accuracy of the measurements is also in the order of 1%. The lower precision and accuracy of spinal compared to peripheral CT measurements is based on inherent limitations of the whole body CT instrumentation.

Given the variety of technological approaches to bone evaluation and the several different skeletal sites used for these measurements, it is important to determine if peripheral and axial bone measurements reflect a similar skeletal status. Since no one technique can measure both axial and peripheral bone density in vivo with acceptable precision, this present study concerns the measurement of trabecular bone density in excised bones obtained at post mortem, which are evaluated using the gamma-ray CT system (5).

MATERIALS AND METHODS

24 pairs of radii/vertebrae (L3) were obtained at postmortem from subjects without any disease known to affect bone. The specimens were immediately frozen and subsequently measured in our γ-CT system.

For the vertebral bodies CT measurements were made in a coronal plane at 3mm intervals with a 2mm slice thickness. Each section was analysed by excluding the outer area containing compact bone and then averaging the bone density values over the remaining trabecular bone area. Fig. 1 shows the density variation of three vertebral bodies from ventral to dorsal. For the purpose of comparing axial bone density with peripheral bone density it is important to obtain a bone density parameter averaged over all sections of a particular sample in order to avoid errors

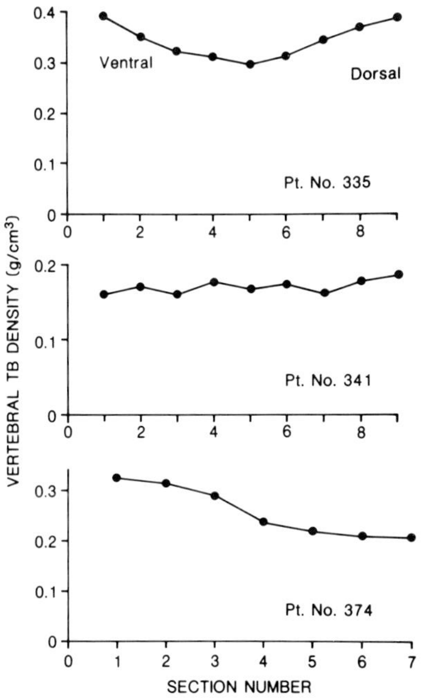

Fig. 1: Variation of trabecular bone density in three typical vertebral bodies measured in a coronal plane with 2 mm thick slices at 3 mm intervals.

due to the significant inhomogeneities which are present.

The radii were measured transaxially with 2mm slice thickness. The scans covered the bone volume in the distal 10% length and were spaced at 2mm intervals. The bone cross-sections were analysed with our standard procedure (5) and the average trabecular bone density for every slice was obtained. Since the trabecular bone density at the distal end of the radius is varying similarly to that in vertebral bodies averaging over all sections is necessary in order to obtain representative density values.

RESULTS AND DISCUSSION

The correlation between vertebral and radial trabecular bone density is shown in Fig. 2. The fitted line indicates that the trabecular bone at the axial site is generally half as dense as at the radial site. The correlation coefficient r=0.706 indicates a good correspondence between trabecular bone at the axial and peripheral sites. Considering the distribution of the single data points it seems unlikely that the correlation coefficient would change drastically with a larger sample since there are no extreme data points at either end of the fitted line that dominate the correlation.

The bone density is expressed as physical density in g/cm^3 rather than in linear attenuation coefficients (1/cm). This makes the data independent of the energy of the gamma-ray photons employed to produce the CT projection data; however, assumptions are needed for the composition of bone marrow. Without specific composition values available for each measured bone, standard values have been assumed. This is reflected by the fact that the regression line crosses the y-axis at a positive value rather than at zero. The vertebrae used in this study (subject ages 19 to 93) likely contain more hematopoietic marrow than the radii thus slightly increasing the calculated value for vertebral bone density. The effect on the correlation, however, should be small since the error involves only a systematic shift of the vertebral data.

Although the correlation coefficient is fairly high (r=.706, $p < 0.001$) the trabecular bone density value measured at either the axial or the peripheral site is not useful for predicting the value at the other site with a precision comparable to that of the measurement procedure; this is seen in the magnitude of the prediction error which is ± 20%. It may, however, not be

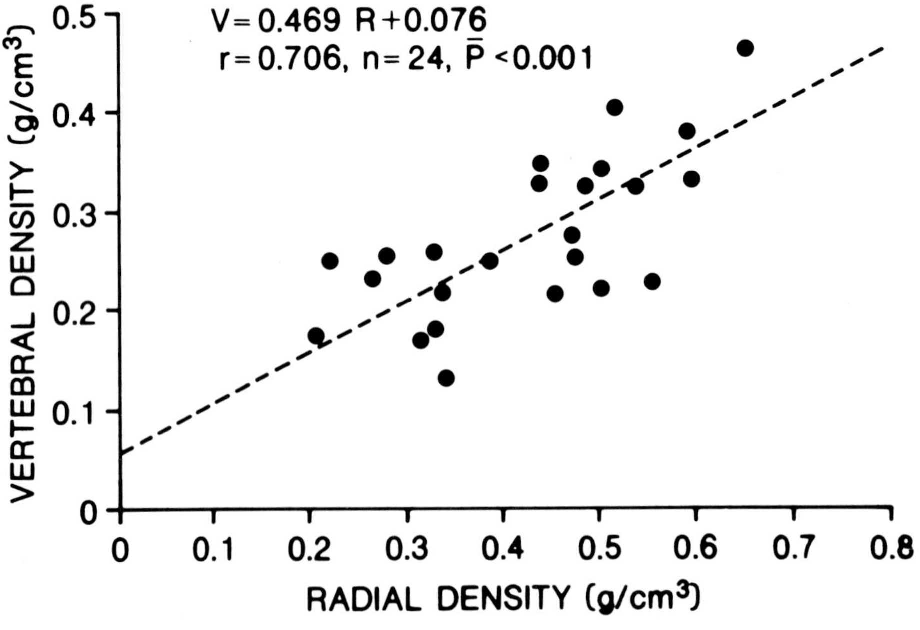

Fig. 2: Correlation of trabecular bone density between vertebral body (L3) and distal end of the radius.

very important to observe a high correlation (and hence good predictive capability) between axial and peripheral bone density. Due to the high inter individual variations in bone density, even in normals in the same age group, a separation between normals and osteoporotics, for example, is unlikely to be successful if based only on one measurement, particularly in early stages of the disease. It is probably more important to establish the rate of bone loss in longitudinal measurements. The critical question is now: does bone density in the axial skeleton change in a similar way to bone density in the peripheral skeleton? We have designed a study involving chronic renal failure patients who receive a pulse dose of 1,25 $(OH)_2D_3$. The patients are measured periodically on a whole body CT scanner in order to obtain trabecular bone density values for the spine and on a γ-CT scanner for evaluating the distal end of the radius. First results indicate that axial and peripheral bones change in a similar way.

REFERENCES

1. Cann, C.E. and Genant, H.K. (1980): J. Comput. Assist. Tomogr., 4, 4, 493-500.
2. Genant, H.K. and Boyd, D. (1977): Invest. Radiol. 12, 6, 545-551.
3. Peppler, W.W. and Mazess, R.B. (1981): Calcif. Tissue Int. 33, 353-359.
4. Rüegsegger, P., Elsasser, U., Anliker, M., et al. (1976): Radiology, 121, 93-97.
5. Hangartner, T.N. and Overton, T.R. (1982) J. Comput. Assist. Tomogr. 6, 6, 1156-1162.

COMPARISON OF DUAL PHOTON ABSORPTIOMETRY AND QUANTITATIVE COMPUTED TOMOGRAPHY OF THE LUMBAR SPINE IN THE SAME SUBJECTS

Malcolm R. Powell, Felix O. Kolb, Harry K. Genant, Christopher E. Cann, and Benno G. Stebler

Departments of Medicine and Radiology, University of California, San Francisco, CA, U.S.A.

Vertebral mineral may be measured by two non-invasive methods that appear likely to become generally available. Quantitative computed tomography (QCT) measures the average volume density of 3.5 cm^3 samplings of 2 vertebral bodies selected to avoid compressive changes.(1) Usually, L1 and 2 are measured. Dual photon absorptiometry (DPA) measures area density of entire lumbar vertebral segments, excluding the transverse processes.(2),(3) Only segments not superimposed over other bones are measured, conventionally L1 through 4. Compressed segments may be excluded. These methods measure different bone regions, QCT data limited to trabecular bone of the vertebral body and DPA data including the cortical and trabecular components of the whole vertebral segment plus extra-vertebral mineral in the area projection of the vertebral segment. We compared data obtained by each method on the same vertebral segments and also with single photon absorptiometry (SPA) measurements of the non-dominant radius.

MATERIALS AND METHODS

Retrospective comparison was made in 26 patients measured first by QCT and second by DPA at intervals of 7 to 28 months (mean 15.9±5). All but 5 patients had their measurements compared in L1 and L2. DPA was performed using a new commercial instrument manufactured by Lunar Radiation Corporation of Madison, Wisconsin. This instrument provides mineral analyses using edge detection adjusted to correspond to the edge finder used at the Mayo Clinic.(4) QCT estimations are expressed in mg/cm^3, DPA estimations as g/cm^2 and as mg/cm^3 after approximation of volume from vertebral segment area (referred to by the instrument manufacturer as the "corpus" measurement), and SPA as bone mineral content (BMC) in g/cm or g/cm^2 (BMC/W).

Comparisons were also made using a fracture index wherein each vertebra from T3 through L5 was graded 0 = no compression, 0.5 = equivocal, 1 = mild, 2 = moderate, and 3 = severe compression. Scores were totaled for all segments and an overall grade was added to indicate trabecular loss and other factors. The total scores ranged from 1 to 25 with a mean of 7.3.

Analysis was by Pearson product moment correlation coefficient calculation, assuming linear relationships of variables.

RESULTS

As might be expected with a wide variety of demineralizing disease processes, there were wide ranges of observed bone mineral values (Table 1). One patient was excluded from further review because only L3 and L4 DPA data were obtained. Correlation coefficients were first calculated on data obtained in the various spine and non-dominant radius measurements (Table 2). Subsequently, correlations with the fracture indices were made for bone mineral data obtained by each method (Table 3, n = 25).

TABLE 1.	Data Ranges	Means
QCT volume density, 2 segments averaged	3-164 mg/cm^3	77.2
DPA area density, same 2 segments averaged	.416-1.059 g/cm^2	.831
"corpus" volume density,2 segments averaged	86-202 mg/cm^3	146
bone mineral, 2 segments	10.1-29.6 g	22.0
lowest area density of 4 segments	.343-1.058 g/cm^2	.781
Fracture Index, summed T3 through L5	1-25	7.4

TABLE 2. Correlations Among QCT, DPA and SPA

	r	p
QCT vs. DPA area density	0.40	<.05
QCT vs. DPA volume density	0.43	<.05
QCT vs. DPA bone mineral	0.25	
QCT vs. lowest DPA area density	0.50	<.02
Radius BMC/W vs. QCT	0.48	<.02
Radius BMC/W vs. DPA area density	0.56	<.01

Scattergrams reveal considerable disparity with a somewhat bimodal distribution of fracture indices (Figure 1). There are 5 data sets with fracture indices averaging 20 and 20 data sets with fracture indices averaging 4.2. The 5 high fracture index data sets average 6.3 standard deviations from the mean of the low fracture index group. Re-analysis of correlations among the lower fracture index data sets showed stronger correlations (Table 3, n = 20).

TABLE 3. Fracture Index Correlations with QCT, DPA and SPA

n=25	r	p
Fracture Index vs. QCT	-.66	<.01
Fracture Index vs. DPA area density	-.068	
Fracture Index vs. DPA corpus	-.16	
Fracture Index vs. DPA bone mineral	0.033	
Fracture Index vs. lowest DPA area density	-.12	
Fracture Index vs. radius BMC/W	0.072	
n = 20		
Fracture Index vs. QCT	-.83	<.01
Fracture Index vs. DPA	-.50	<.02

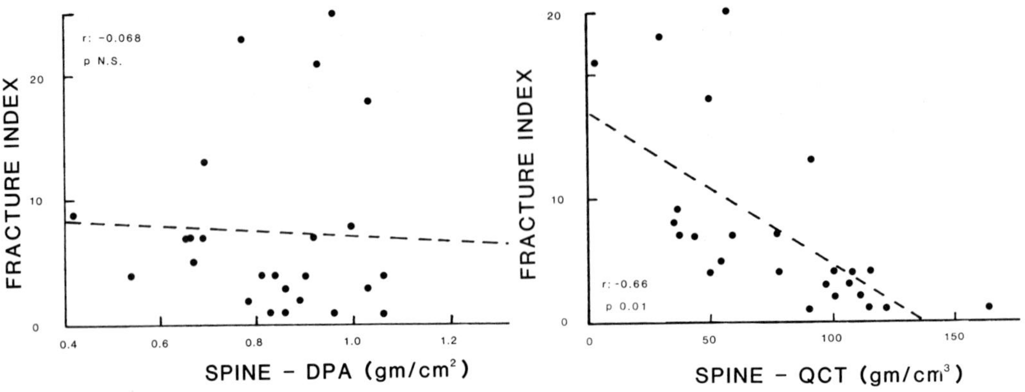

Figure 1. Scattergrams of Fracture Index vs. QCT and DPA

These patients with an apparent subset of very high fracture indices were idiopathic osteoporosis (3 patients with fracture indices 13, 23 and 25) and long term steroid therapy for collagen disease and regional enteritis with malabsorption (fracture indices 18 and 23). They tended to have well preserved posterior vertebral elements and shell-like vertebral bodies. Their QCT measurements were relatively much lower as a group (3,30,50,57 and 91 mg/cm^3) than the corresponding DPA measurements (.796, .768, 1.028, .837, and .687 g/cm^2 for respective fracture indices of 21,23, 18, 25 and 13).

DISCUSSION

It is apparent that QCT and DPA show general correlation in estimation of spine mineral in most patients. However, they do measure different bone regions, QCT vertebral body trabecular bone, and DPA the entire vertebral segment except the transverse processes. Some patients show regional demineralization of the trabecular bone of the vertebral bodies, causing more striking abnormality in QCT measurements than in DPA measurements on the whole vertebra. The most appropriate applications of each method will probably be determined in terms of utility of regional versus total vertebral assessment and in terms of precision and accuracy of measurement that are obtained in general use of each method.

REFERENCES

1. Cann, C.E., and Genant, H.K. (1980): J Computer Assist Tomography, 4,493.
2. Mazess, R.B., Ort, M., Judy, P., and Mather, W. (1970): in Proceedings, Bone Measurement Conference, J.R. Cameron editor, U.S. Atomic Energy Commission, Conf 700515, 300.
3. Wilson, C.R., and Madsen, M. (1977): Invest Radiol., 12,180.
4. Riggs, B.L., Wahner, H.W., Dunn, W.L., Offord, K.P., and Melton, L.J.III. (1981): J Clin Invest., 67,328.

Discussion of presentations by Hangartner and Powell:

DR. CHESNUT: We found no significant correlation between total body calcium by neutron activation and spinal CT in patients with osteoporosis, but a significant correlation with dual photon absorptiometry.

DR. GENANT: In the elderly osteoporotic population the relative amount of cancellous to cortical bone, particularly in the spine, has diminished considerably and the extent of extraosseous mineral has increased, so your observation is not surprising and is consistent with the data presented by Dr. Powell.

DR. WAHNER: One has to sample the skeleton at the site of interest; if you are interested in spinal fractures, sample the spine. The prediction of total body calcium from radius measurement is good because the percentage of trabecular and cortical bone is the same in the radius and in the total skeleton. There is a difference between the femoral neck and the lumbar spine in the pattern and rate of bone loss. Finally, in dual-photon absorptiometry we are moving towards a smaller sampling size and a shorter test. The 40 minutes we are presently using for measurements of L1 to L4 is probably an overkill.

DR. REVAK: I'd like to raise the question of equilibrium between cortical and trabecular bone. Trabecular bone responds faster because it has more surface area, but is only 20% of the total skeletal mass. When trabecular bone is lost, is cortical bone resorbed and mineral redeposited in trabecular bone?

DR. PARFITT: I am not sure what you mean by equilibrium, but with increasing age the inner third of the cortex in some bones is converted to a structure that topologically resembles trabecular bone, with a higher surface-to-volume ratio, and less than 50% of the tissue volume occupied by bone, but this occurs by subendosteal resorption, not by redeposition of mineral.

DR. NORDIN: In young osteoporotics cortical bone measurements are mostly in the normal range, but in elderly osteoporotics who are no longer losing trabecular bone rapidly, cortical bone mass is falling more rapidly than in normal subjects. The older the patient, the greater the difference in cortical bone from normal controls.

III VITAMIN D IN CLINICAL MEDICINE

VITAMIN D IN CLINICAL MEDICINE - OVERVIEW

John G. Haddad

Department of Medicine, University of Pennsylvania School of Medicine, Philadelphia, PA, U.S.A.

With the availability of stereospecific assays for vitamin D and its metabolites, many clinicians now appraise the role of these sterols in the pathogenesis and treatment of diseases affecting mineral and skeletal homeostasis. Some of these assays have been commercially available for quite sometime, and it seems very appropriate to reflect on what they measure and how to interpret the results. Much new information has been published over the past 10-12 years, and attempts to sort out the clinically relevant features of vitamin D metabolism can be confusing. Other sections of this Symposium deal specifically with certain diseases affecting vitamin D metabolism, but Professors Haussler, Stanbury, DeLuca and Rasmussen deal more directly with the biological relevance of sterol production, quantitation and the interpretation of the sterol assay data in light of the presumed activities of the vitamin's metabolites.

As indicated by Haussler and colleagues, the competitive protein binding assays (CPBA) have had greatest usage, but we must be aware of the improved technology suggested by the novel cytoreceptor assay (1), polyclonal RIA (2), monoclonal RIA (3) and innovative, facile preparative approaches to CPBA (4). Continuing progress in the development of selective, sensitive, precise and convenient assays seems likely in the current climate. Although available, quantitation of the vitamin D carrier protein (DBP) has not gained wide usage in the interpretation of "bound" or "free" sterol (5). If the role of DBP in blood sterol transport is indeed passive, and not one of carrier-mediation into tissues, it seems likely that estimates of "free" sterol could be useful in situations wherein sterol transport is compromised or augmented.

Two of the more controversial areas in the establishment of a consensus regarding the interpretation of sterol values have been the role(s) of sterols other than 1,25-$(OH)_2D$, and the relevance of the extra-renal production of 1,25-$(OH)_2D$. These areas are directly addressed herein, and Stanbury and Mawer's emphasis on 1,25-$(OH)_2D$ tacitly underscores their alignment with the view that this sterol is the cardinal metabolite in the expression of the vitamin's "traditional" biological activity. The clear-cut alliances of several relevant diseases with 1,25$(OH)_2D$ underproduction, overproduction and resistance appear to ramify this position. Extra-renal 1,25-$(OH)_2D$ synthesis currently appears to be clinically significant in sarcoidosis and certainly of interest in pregnancy, but, as Professor DeLuca indicates, of uncertain <u>in vivo</u> significance in other tissues.

The uniqueness of 1,25-$(OH)_2D$ biosynthesis in kidney appears to have withstood challenges far better than those directed toward searching for new "target tissues" for this potent sterol.

A large number of reports have convincingly demonstrated the presence of high affinity, selective 1,25-$(OH)_2D$ receptors in tissues not usually associated with major translocations of mineral ions (6). This latter review also states the case for 24,25$(OH)_2D$'s role in various activities, but Haussler and co-workers presently reveal their inability to confirm some of these findings. An exciting development by Pike (7) has been the production of monoclonal antibodies to the 1,25-$(OH)_2D$ receptor, providing a new probe to reveal the topography and relevance of the sterol-receptor association. The exciting influence of 1,25$(OH)_2D$ on cellular differentiation, calcium-mediated or not, shall clearly attract future investigators.

Very interesting clinical observations by Stanbury and Mawer suggest the importance of several factors in carefully interpreting sterol assay values. Clearly, nutritional or photobiological, hormonal and, possibly, ionic and autoregulatory influences can condition blood sterol concentration. In recent years, others have begun to appraise the clearance of sterol(s) from blood, and alterations in sterol degradation might characterize certain conditions, such as the augmented loss of water-soluble sterol conjugates into the urines of patients with cholestatic liver disease (8).

Perhaps a major clinical focus for the controversy surrounding 1,25-$(OH)_2D$'s importance has been the observations that osteomalacia can develop in the presence of slightly high, normal or low blood concentrations of this sterol, and this comes up in the discussion. Several factors would appear to be relevant here, including substrate (25-OHD) availability, dietary mineral content, age of the patient or rate of growth, degree of secondary hyperparathyroidism, renal function, etc. In other words, absolutely normal 1,25-$(OH)_2D$ blood levels may be inappropriately low in a situation demanding very high levels in order to provide sufficient intestinal mineral transport for mineralization of the skeleton. The exciting observations of 5-6 fold higher 1,25$(OH)_2D$ blood levels during the healing of vitamin D deficiency further suggest the possibility of a non-PTH, 1α-hydroxylase-stimulator of skeletal origin.

Session III provided a lively, albeit too brief, formal and informal review of central considerations in the clinical interpretation of vitamin D assays, metabolism and action. The real message of the Symposium was, I think, exemplified by this session. Clinical studies and laboratory observations are both valuable in formulating and testing hypotheses, and the precious dialogue between these disciplines should be maintained.

REFERENCES

1. Manolagas, S., Culler, F., Howard, J., Brickman, A., and Deftos, L. (1983): J. Clin. Endo. & Metab., 56, 751.
2. Clemens, T., Hendy, G., Papapoulos, S., Fraher, L., Care, A., and O'Riordan, J. (1979): Clin. Endocrinol. (Oxford), 11, 225.
3. Perry, H., Chappel, J., Clevinger, B., Haddad, J., and Teitelbaum, S. (1983): Program of 5th ASBMR Meeting, San Antonio, Texas, p. A65.
4. Reinhardt, T., Horst, R., Orf, J., and Hollis, B. (1983): Program of 5th ASBMR meeting, San Antonio, Texas, p. A66.
5. Bouillon, R., Van Assche, F., Van Baelen, H., Heyns, W., and DeMoor, P. (1981): J. Clin. Invest., 67, 589.
6. Norman, A., Roth, J., and Orci, L. (1982): Endocrine Reviews,

3, 331.
7. Pike, J., Donaldson, C., Marion, S., and Haussler, M. (1982): Proc. Nat. Acad. Sci., 79, 7719.
8. Jung, R., Davie, M., Siklos, P., Chalmers, T., Hunter, J., and Lawson, D. (1979): Gut, 20, 840.

VITAMIN D METABOLITES: NEW PHYSIOLOGIC AND CLINICAL INSIGHTS

Mark R. Haussler, Shigeharu Dokoh, David J. Mangelsdorf, Carol A. Donaldson and J. Wesley Pike

Department of Biochemistry, University of Arizona Health Sciences Center, Tucson, AZ, U.S.A.

Vitamin D's paramount role in the control of blood calcium is well recognized. The vitamin's primary function appears to be the stimulation of intestinal calcium absorption, with an additional action in bone mineral resorption. The final bioactivation of vitamin D to 1,25-dihydroxyvitamin D (1,25$(OH)_2$D), the accepted hormonal form of the sterol, occurs in the kidney. The vitamin D metabolic pathway is becoming increasingly complex with the identification of a number of side-chain modifications of both the intermediate 25-hydroxyvitamin D (25(OH)D) and the 1,25$(OH)_2$D hormone. These side-chain metabolites include 24,25-dihydroxyvitamin D (24,25$(OH)_2$D), a putative "bone mineralizing" sterol. The biological activities of these side-chain derivatives are diminished compared to the parent forms, indicating that they probably constitute a pathway for degradation of 25(OH)D and 1,25$(OH)_2$D. Interestingly, these enzymatic modifications are stimulated by 1,25$(OH)_2$D, suggesting that this dynamic hormone regulates its own metabolic elimination. Finally 1,25$(OH)_2$D is now known to bind to receptors in the nucleus of a wide array of target tissues beyond intestine, bone and kidney. These findings raise the exciting possibility that 1,25$(OH)_2$D may have uncharacterized roles in cellular regulation which may or may not involve calcium economy as a common denominator.

ASSAYS FOR VITAMIN D METABOLITES IN HUMANS

Sensitive and rigorous assays for serum vitamin D and its major metabolites have been devised in the past decade. The most widely used methodology is that of competitive protein binding, usually coupled with selective extraction and HPLC isolation of the metabolite of interest (1). Serum 25(OH)D (normal = 15-60 ng/ml) appears to be an excellent index of vitamin D status--reflecting the sum of dietary and sunlight derived vitamin D pools. Serum 1,25$(OH)_2$D (normal = 20-60 pg/ml) is indicative of the rate of renal biosynthesis of the hormone, which is estimated to be about 2 μg/day. Circulating 1,25$(OH)_2$D is affected by physiological states of mineral stress, with enhanced levels of the calcemic hormone occurring in active growth, pregnancy and lactation. 1,25$(OH)_2$D levels are compromised in chronic renal failure, tumor-induced osteomalacia and vitamin D-dependent rickets Type I. Striking healing of rickets occurs when patients with D-dependency rickets Type I are treated with small doses ($\leq$ 1 μg/day) of 1,25$(OH)_2D_3$, supporting the conclusion that these patients possess a defect in the renal 1α-OHase enzyme.

SIGNIFICANCE OF 24,25$(OH)_2$D

24,25$(OH)_2$D (normal = 2-4 ng/ml) represents a controversial vitamin D metabolite. Clinically, 24,25$(OH)_2D_3$ elicits beneficial effects in certain osteomalacic syndromes that are refractory to normal doses of 1,25$(OH)_2D_3$, but only when administered in combination with the 1,25$(OH)_2D_3$ hormone. Although tenuous, this has led to the notion that 24,25$(OH)_2$D has unique bone mineralizing qualities and there have been preliminary reports of putative "receptors" for 24,25$(OH)_2$D in cells pertinent to bone formation like chondrocytes (2). We have examined this question at the molecular level to determine the mode of action of 24,25$(OH)_2$D. 24,25$(OH)_2$D circulates in blood bound to D-binding protein (DBP) in a total concentration of 10^{-8}M--100 times that of the 1,25$(OH)_2$D-DBP complex. However, because of its very high affinity for DBP, the free 24,25$(OH)_2$D available for entry into target cells is limited. Combining this with the relatively low affinity of 24,25$(OH)_2$D for the intracellular vitamin D receptor, it is evident that normal blood levels of 24,25$(OH)_2$D do not readily associate with the 1,25$(OH)_2$D receptor.

With respect to putative receptors uniquely specific for binding 24,25$(OH)_2$D, we have employed methodology similar to that of Binderman and associates (2), who reported that chick limb bud cells (differentiating chondrocytes) contain such a receptor. Basically, cytosols are incubated for a short period (90 min) at 0°C with 24,25$(OH)_2[^3H]D_3$ (87 Ci/mmol) at a concentration of 2 nM in the absence or presence of a 100-fold excess of radioinert vitamin D metabolite competitors; receptor-like binding is then quantitated via charcoal separation (1). Table 1 shows that our results with limb bud cytosol are similar, but not identical to those of Binderman and associates: 24,25$(OH)_2D_3$ indeed is seemingly the most effective competitor, followed by 25(OH)D_3 and then 1,25$(OH)_2D_3$. Although these data suggest a specific 24,25$(OH)_2$D receptor exists in chondrocytes, we can obtain a dramatically similar pattern of competition using either serum DBP or a 1,25$(OH)_2D_3$-receptor preparation from chick gut cytosol (Table 1). Independent experiments (Dokoh *et al.*, submitted for publication) show that limb buds contain a small amount of the 1,25$(OH)_2$D receptor and respond to 1,25$(OH)_2D_3$, but not 24,25$(OH)_2D_3$, to increase proteoglycan biosynthesis. Therefore, in our hands, chondrocytes derived from chick limb bud cells neither contain a distinct receptor for 24,25$(OH)_2$D nor respond to this sterol in culture. We conclude that the apparent receptor-like binding observed in limb buds by others (2) results from the combined association of 24,25$(OH)_2[^3H]D_3$ with serum DBP (contamination) and the 1,25$(OH)_2$D receptor under non-equilibrium conditions occurring in a 90 min incubation. Moreover, the concept that 24,25$(OH)_2$D "receptors" are artifactual leads us to conclude that, *in vivo*, 24,25$(OH)_2$D is either functioning by being metabolized to a 1,25$(OH)_2$D analog like 1,24,25$(OH)_3$D, or that 24,25$(OH)_2$D administration to patients potentiates the action of 1,25$(OH)_2$D by altering its disposition in the body. 24,25$(OH)_2$D could prolong the half-life of 1,25$(OH)_2$D by influencing the side-chain metabolizing enzymes which normally degrade the hormone.

TABLE 1. Apparent receptor-like binding of $24,25(OH)_2D_3$

Preparation	$24,25(OH)_2[^3H]D_3$ Binding			
	No Competitor	$25(OH)D_3$	$1,25(OH)_2D_3$	$24,25(OH)_2D_3$
Chick limb bud cytosol*	100%	93%	100%	16%
Chick limb bud cytosol	100%	46%	61%	40%
Serum DBP (fetal calf)	100%	63%	95%	30%
Embryonic chick gut cytosol	100%	18%	55%	13%

*Binderman and associates, Biochem. Biophys. Res. Communs. 106, 644 (1982).

RECEPTOR FOR $1,25(OH)_2D$

In contrast to the situation with $24,25(OH)_2D$, receptors for $1,25(OH)_2D$ are well documented in all known vitamin D target tissues and their detection in cultured fibroblasts from humans (3) means that their clinical relevance can be probed. We have recently generated monoclonal antibodies against the chick intestinal $1,25(OH)_2D_3$ receptor and several of these cross-react with the human $1,25(OH)_2D_3$ receptor (4). Using these monoclonal antibodies, we have devised a radioligand-immunoassay for the human $1,25(OH)_2D$ receptor (Dokoh *et al.* and Pike *et al.*, submitted for publication) and are currently investigating fibroblasts from patients resistant to $1,25(OH)_2D$ at the target tissue level (vitamin D-dependent rickets Type II) for the presence of binding defective species of the receptor protein. The combined use of radioreceptor assay for circulating $1,25(OH)_2D$ and radioligand-immunoassay for the $1,25(OH)_2D$ receptor represents an essential tool in differentiating Types I and II of vitamin D-dependency rickets as well as defining subgroups of kindreds with vitamin D-dependent rickets Type II.

$1,25(OH)_2D$ AND CELL DIFFERENTIATION

Recent work by Abe *et al.* (5) indicates that mouse myeloid leukemia cells differentiate into macrophages when challenged with $1,25(OH)_2D_3$ in culture. We have similarly studied the human promyelocytic leukemia cell line, HL-60, and observed that it also undergoes maturation along the monocyte-macrophage pathway in the presence of physiologic levels of $1,25(OH)_2D_3$ (Mangelsdorf *et al.*, submitted for publication). This differentiation process is mediated by the specific $1,25(OH)_2D_3$ receptor, but other aspects of the process await further biochemical characterization. The clinical significance of these observations will require trials in humans, but there exists the extraordinary possibility that $1,25(OH)_2D_3$ may act as a natural antileukemogenic agent in acute myelogenous leukemia. Of equal importance to basic physiology is the probability that $1,25(OH)_2D_3$'s action to cause differentiation in HL-60 cells is a manifestation of the normal action of this hormone to elicit maturation of myeloid stem cells into macrophages. Because macrophages are thought to be the precursor of the bone resorbing osteoclasts, this is a logical mechanism whereby $1,25-(OH)_2D$ brings about calcium resorption via recruitment of cells competent in bone remodeling. Moreover, PTH is thought to act both directly to stimulate osteoclast production from myeloid precursors (6), and on T-lymphocytes to cause the elaboration of putative osteoclast enhancing factors (7). Thus, as is summarized in Fig. 1, we propose that $1,25(OH)_2D$ and PTH probably operate in concert to create and enlist the cells that resorb and remodel bone. Clearly, these calcemic hormones not only regulate mineral homeostasis, but they also participate directly in bone turnover by orchestrating the population of cells within bone.

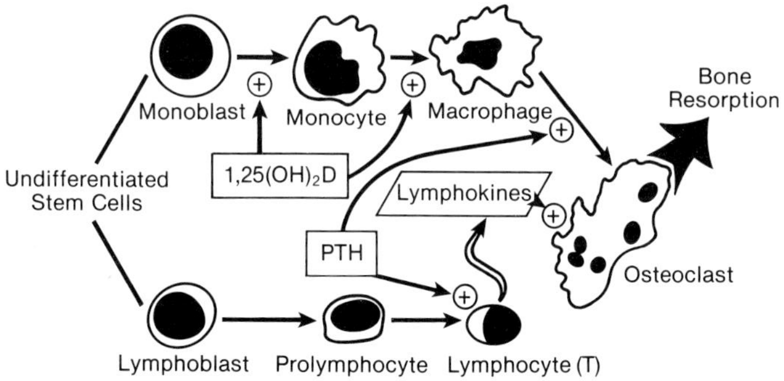

Figure 1. Proposed new pathway for the mediation of bone remodeling by the calcitropic hormones.

REFERENCES

1. Dokoh, S., Llach, F. and Haussler, M.R. (1982): In: Vitamin D-Chemical, Biochemical and Clinical Endocrinology of Calcium Metabolism, p. 743. Editors: A.W. Norman, K. Schaefer, D.v. Herrath and H.-G. Grigoleit. de Gruyter, Berlin.
2. Somjen, D., Somjen, G.J., Harell, A., Mechanic, G.L. and Binderman, I. (1982): Biochem. Biophys. Res. Commun., 106, 644.
3. Eil, C. and Marx, S.J. (1981): Proc. Natl. Acad. Sci. USA, 78, 2562.
4. Pike, J.W., Marion, S.L., Donaldson, C.A. and Haussler, M.R. (1983): J. Biol. Chem. 258, 1289.
5. Abe, E., Miyaura, C., Sakagami, H., Takeda, M., Kunno, K., Yamazaki, T., Yoshiki, S. and Suda, T. (1981): Proc. Natl. Acad. Sci. USA, 78, 4990.
6. Roodman, G.D., Ibbotson, K.J., McManus, L.M. and Mundy, G.R. (1983): Clin. Res. 31, 395A.
7. Yamamoto, I., Potts, J.T. and Segre, G.V. (1983): J. Clin. Invest. 71, 404.

VITAMIN D METABOLISM IN MAN: CONTRIBUTIONS FROM CLINICAL STUDIES

S. W. Stanbury and E. Barbara Mawer

Department of Medicine, University of Manchester, The Royal Infirmary, Manchester, U.K.

Our studies of the metabolism of an i.v. pulse dose of cholecalciferol (D_3) - in vitamin D (D) deficient, replete and deliberately D-treated subjects - indicated that the quantitative formation of both 25-(OH)D_3 and 1,25-$(OH)_2D_3$ was apparently determined by the prevailing D-status of the individual; more of each metabolite was produced the greater the degree of D-deficiency. Based largely on animal experiment, it is now the orthodox belief that formation of 25-(OH)D_3 is determined by the availability of its precursor and not subject to regulation; whereas production of 1,25-$(OH)_2D_3$ is 'tightly regulated' essentially independently of the concentration of its precursor plasma 25-(OH)D_3.

REGULATION OF PLASMA [25-(OH)D]IN MAN

In patients taking daily oral doses of D, Stamp & Haddad demonstrated a direct power-function relationship between intake and plasma [25-(OH)D] but there are no available data relating plasma [D] to plasma [25-(OH)D] in similar circumstances. To permit measurement of both plasma [D_3] and plasma [25-(OH)D_3], radioactive D_3 was injected i.v. into D-deficient subjects together with increasing doses (0.06 - 40 ug/kg in different subjects) of stable D_3 (1,2). There was a direct power-function relation between plasma [25-(OH)D_3] and plasma [D_3], over a several hundred-fold variation of the latter, but the fractional 25-hydroxylation of the dose was related inversely to the plasma [D_3]. Liver perfusion studies (Mawer & Reeve) and other observations in D-deficient patients (Davies & Mawer) suggested that elevation of the concentration of D_3 in the plasma (or,more probably, in the liver) exerted a quantitative constraint on 25-hydroxylation. It was also demonstrated (Davies) that a 2.5 mg s.c. or i.m. depot of D_3 could produce a significant sustained increase of plasma [25-(OH)D_3]with barely detectable associated increase of plasma [D_3]. These various observations, and especially the demonstrated efficiency of 25-hydroxylation at low levels of plasma [D_3], led us to postulate that the physiological production of 25-(OH)D_3 may be through a slow release of D_3 from skin and its quantitative clearance from the blood by 25-hydroxylation (2). Moreover, since prolonged whole-body exposure to effective sunlight appears not to elevate plasma [25-(OH)D_3] above 50-80 µg/l - as compared with values an order of magnitude higher resulting from massive oral dosage with D - it seemed necessary to invoke also some mechanism that limited the quantitative release of D_3 from the skin.

Supported by a Grant from the British Medical Research Council.

Holick (3) demolished this hypothesis by showing that 'sun-burning' doses of UVI to the whole body rapidly increased plasma [D_3], in proportion to the dose of irradiation, to produce levels as high as 140 µg/litre: and we have found (unpublished) that sunbathing without burning can elevate plasma [D_3] to ~40 µg/l. Thus photobiogenically produced D_3 appears to have free access to the blood. The immunity from D-intoxication after solar exposure would seem to require that some factor - limited available precursor, photodegradation or pigmentation - ensured that the D_3 entering the blood was always quantitatively less than may be absorbed from massive therapeutic oral dosage. However, the decay of plasma D_3, after stopping either artificial UV- or solar exposure is at about the same rate ($t_{\frac{1}{2}}$ 2-4 days) as is seen with an i.v. pulse dose of D_3 (1). This implies that most of the D_3 from skin will be sequestrated rapidly in indifferent tissues, outside the metabolic pool and thus unavailable for immediate 25-hydroxylation. Orally administered D is absorbed in chylomicron form and, although this can and does transfer to the plasma D-binding globulin, some fraction of those chylomicrons are likely to be taken up by the liver. It is conceivable that the slow hepatic cellular processing of such chylomicrons results in sustained, unphysiologically high concentrations of D at the site of 25-hydroxylation.

Irrespective of such speculation, measurements in a random group of 30 individuals showed values of plasma [D] between 0 and 1.5 µg/l in 21, with levels up to ~50 µg/l in the others (unpublished). There was no correlation between plasma [D] and plasma [25-(OH)D]. Sunbathing increased both plasma [D] and [25-(OH)D] but, in the 3-6 weeks after stopping exposure, there was an 8-fold change in plasma [D] without significant accompanying change of plasma [25-(OH)D]. Thus plasma [D] and plasma [25-(OH)D] were not correlated, either in cross-sectional measurements in a population in an apparently steady state, or in longitudinal dynamic observations in a single individual. There seems to be much still to be learned about the relationships between 25-(OH)D and its precursor.

REGULATION OF PLASMA 1,25-$(OH)_2$D IN MAN

It has been shown in man that the plasma [1,25-$(OH)_2$D] varies reciprocally with the calcium (Ca) intake in the diet (Lemann) and in response to acutely induced changes of serum [Ca] (Bilezekian). These results are compatible with parathyroid hormone (PTH) being the principal trophic stimulus to 1,25-$(OH)_2$D production in humans as in animals. Our own finding, of an inverse relation between the vitamin D status and the amount of 1,25-$(OH)_2D_3$ produced from a pulse dose of D_3, might also be explained by corresponding differences of PTH secretion. However, the mean plasma [1,25-$(OH)_2$D] in D-replete patients with primary hyperparathyroidism (ly HPT) is about twice the normal mean level, and individual values are unrelated to the prevailing plasma [iPTH] (Broadus). Infusions of PTH adequate to elevate plasma [Ca^{2+}] also approximately double plasma [1,25-$(OH)_2$D] (Slovik).

In contrast, treatment of hypocalcaemic D-deficiency osteomalacia with small (200-500 IU) daily oral doses of D rapidly corrects the low plasma [1,25-$(OH)_2$D], which then increases with the plasma [25-(OH)D] to reach values 4-6 times the normal mean level; supranormal concentrations of plasma

1,25-$(OH)_2D$ are sustained for weeks as the osteomalacia heals. During the first 50 days of such therapy when, with the dosage used, plasma [25-(OH)D] may not exceed 10 μg/l, plasma concentrations of the two sterols are closely positively correlated(4). In the hypercalcaemic osteomalacia that can develop when 1y HPT is complicated by D-deficiency, similar D-treatment produces identical effects and plasma [1,25-$(OH)_2D$] increases to levels much higher than are encountered in D-replete 1y HPT (5). In chronic renal failure, a large increase of plasma [25-(OH)D] may restore the low plasma [1,25-$(OH)_2D$] to normal; but, in the exceptional case complicated by D-deficiency osteomalacia, moderate increases of plasma [25-(OH)D] may produce supranormal levels of plasma [1,25-$(OH)_2D$] (unpublished). Fig. 1 summarizes

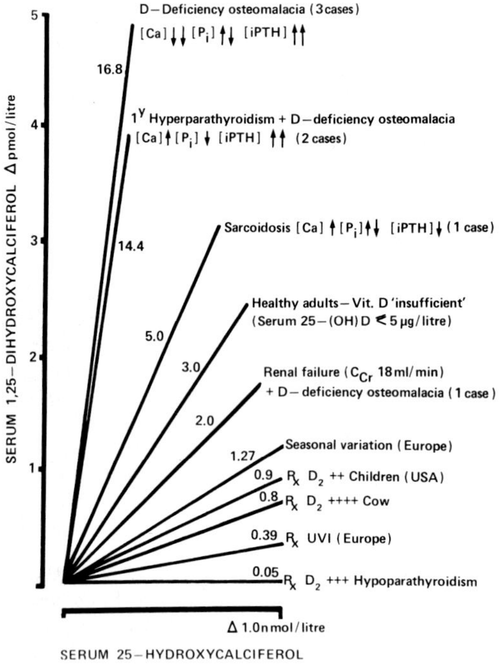

Figure 1

these and other human studies in which plasma [1,25-$(OH)_2D$] has been observed to increase as an apparently direct consequence of a primary increase of plasma [25-(OH)D]. Degrees of precursor-dependence can occur irrespective of plasma [Ca], [P_i] or [iPTH]: but, whereas in hypoparathyroidism a 1 nmol/l increase of plasma [25-(OH)D] may be associated with an increment in plasma [1,25-$(OH)_2D$] of 0.05 pmol/l, the corresponding increment in D-deficiency osteomalacia may be 15 pmol/l. Thus, in D-deficiency osteomalacia there is some factor operating that greatly facilitates the formation of 1,25-$(OH)_2D$ from low concentrations of plasma 25-(OH)D.

Despite this factor, it appears not possible to increase plasma [1,25-$(OH)_2D$] in healing osteomalacia to more than 5-6 times the mean normal by increasing further the plasma [25-(OH)D]; there appears to be a constraint on the excessive production of

$1,25\text{-}(OH)_2D$ and a finite limit to the tolerated elevation of its plasma concentration. In contrast, in type 2 vitamin D-dependency, therapeutically induced greatly elevated levels of plasma [25-(OH)D] can be associated with concentrations of plasma $1,25\text{-}(OH)_2D$ some 50-100 times the normal mean level (5). In this syndrome, the quantitative restraint on the production of $1,25\text{-}(OH)_2D$ from its precursor is not evident, and the difference from simple D-deficiency cannot be explained by differences of plasma [Ca], [P_i] or [iPTH]. It is,however, established (Liberman) that cellular receptors for $1,25\text{-}(OH)_2D$ are defective in this syndrome - and we suggest that defective receptors in the renal tubule impair the process of 'self-inhibition' or 'autoregulation' of $1,25\text{-}(OH)_2D$ production.

This aberrant behaviour of type 2 vitamin D-dependency, with its defective receptors, strongly suggests that 'autoregulation' may contribute to the physiological control of plasma [$1,25\text{-}(OH)_2D$] in man. Fig. 2 compares 2 groups of healthy and clinically normal individuals; 24 with plasma [25-(OH)D] $\leq$ 5 µg/l and 30 with mean plasma [25-(OH)D] 7.5 times as high. In the

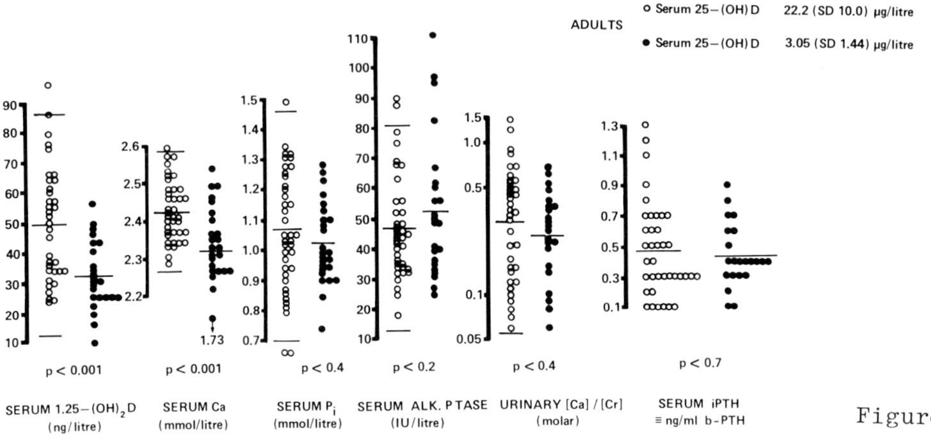

Figure 2

25-(OH)D deficient individuals, the plasma [$1,25\text{-}(OH)_2D$] is significantly lower; but most individual values are within the control range, implying a more efficient production of $1,25\text{-}(OH)_2D$ from reduced available precursor. The mean plasma [Ca] is also lower suggesting that these individuals could have 2y HPT - but no evidence of this was apparent in the measurements of plasma [iPTH] or in indirect indices of parathyroid function. Could this indicate that the initial response to a reduction of plasma [$1,25\text{-}(OH)_2D$] is an autoregulatory increase of 1α-hydroxylase activity - and that 2y HPT comes into operation when this local mechanism fails?

In 13 psoriatic and control subjects, Mawer & Sommer (in press) observed the effects of a 3 week course of UVI (Fig. 3). The mean increment of plasma [$1,25\text{-}(OH)_2D$] was related - 1) inversely with initial (pre-treatment) plasma [25-(OH)D]; 2) positively (NS) with the mean increment of plasma 25-(OH)D and 3) significantly inversely with the initial plasma [$1,25\text{-}(OH)_2D$]. The data are compatible with 'D' playing a direct role in regulating its own metabolism.

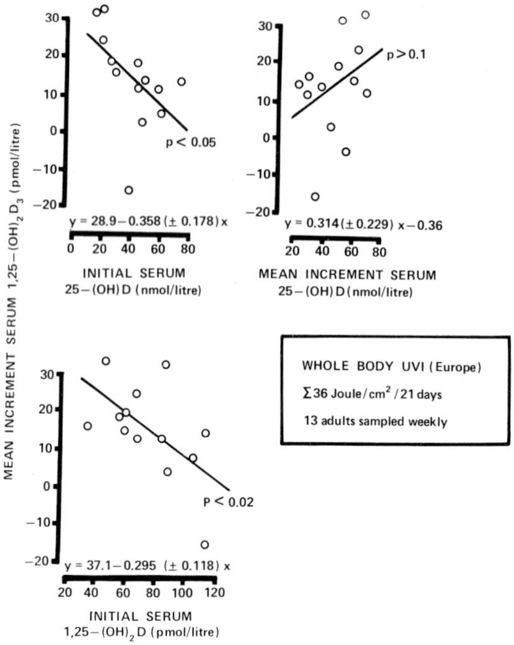

Figure 3

REFERENCES

1. Mawer, E.B. (1980): In: Vitamin D; molecular biology and clinical nutrition, p.149. Editor: A.W. Norman, Marcel Decker, New York.
2. Stanbury, S.W., Mawer, E.B., Taylor,C.M. and Silva, P. de. (1980): Mineral Electrolyte Metab., 3, 51.
3. Adams, J.S., Clemens, T.L., Parrish, J.A. and Holick, M.F. (1982): New Eng. J. Med., 305, 722.
4. Stanbury, S.W., Taylor, C.M., Lumb, G.A., Mawer, E.B., Berry, J., Hann, J. and Wallace, J. (1981): Mineral Electrolyte Metab., 5, 212.
5. Stanbury, S.W. (1981) J.Roy.Coll.Phys. London, 15, 205.

Discussion following papers by M. Haussler and W. Stanbury:

D. SHERRARD: Just a comment in defense of 24,25(OH)$_2$D. We now have treated at least seven patients, some of whom were reported at the Vitamin D meetings last year, with 24,25(OH)$_2$D alone, who had the refractory osteomalacia of renal failure. They did respond. Of course, some patients don't respond, but seven clearly responded to that drug without any other D metabolite. Some were anephric, too.

M. HAUSSLER: Were those patients given 1,25(OH)$_2$D also?

D. SHERRARD: No, they were not given 1,25(OH)$_2$D. This is a group of seven who did not receive 1,25(OH)$_2$D while they were getting 24,25(OH)$_2$D. They failed to respond to 1,25(OH)$_2$D before receiving 24,25(OH)$_2$D.

M. HAUSSLER: Of course, one of the possible ways in which 24,25(OH)$_2$D could act is to alter the disposition of 1,25(OH)$_2$D in the body when there is combination therapy. Your point about successful therapy with $24,25(OH)_2D$ alone is new information to me.

L. DEFTOS: The findings you reviewed about malignant leukocytes can also be observed in normal leukocytes. My laboratory has observed that $1,25(OH)_2D$ promotes the development of normal human monocytes to macrophage-like cells. Also, this effect is characterized by the appearance of the $1,25(OH)_2D$ receptors in these cells, suggesting that this receptor may be one of the nutritive receptors, which subserve a more general nutritive need of cells as they are developing immunologic functions. My question is, whether you have noticed any quantitative or qualitative changes in the $1,25(OH)_2D$ receptors during the histologic progression of the cells that you studied?

M. HAUSSLER: Not in the HL-60 cells that we studied. They start out with about 4,000 copies of the $1,25(OH)_2D$ receptor per cell which doesn't seem to change with $1,25(OH)_2D$ treatment. We have measured $1,25(OH)_2D$ receptors on HL-60, a malignant cell type, by the radioligand immunoassay. I think your findings are important because they are with normal cells.

H. MALLUCHE: I have a question for Dr. Haussler who concluded that $1,25(OH)_2D$ stimulates or differentiates osteoclasts. If that theory is correct, should we not see after long-term therapy with $1,25(OH)_2D$ an increased bone turnover? In our own experience, we see a different histologic picture on long-term treatment with this metabolite, i.e., a decrease of osteoblastic and osteoclastic activity. How can we reconcile this with your theory?

M. HAUSSLER: Let me turn the issue around. There are instances, i.e., uremia, where cell-mediated immunity is suppressed and increased infections occur in patients with D deficiency. There is also evidence that a deficiency of $1,25(OH)_2D$ may be associated with malfunctioning macrophages. So, there may be a basal effect of $1,25(OH)_2D$ on a certain proportion of myeloid stem cells being recruited for osteoclasts. Now, you ask about increasing $1,25(OH)_2D$ above normal. Although, it's my understanding that $1,25(OH)_2D$ therapy does cause increased bone remodelling in patients, it may be that $1,25(OH)_2D$ is involved in the basal physiological response and there are other controls to prevent too much osteoclast recruitment by excess $1,25(OH)_2D$.

L. AVIOLI: I'm intrigued by your observation, Dr. Haussler. I wonder if you have done another experiment relative to the effects of $1,25(OH)_2D$ on cells? It has been shown that in vitro treatment of macrophages with $1,25(OH)_2D$ increase their ability to engulf foreign particles. And, in vitro treatment of leukocytes with $1,25(OH)_2D$ increase their ability to phagocytize E. coli, suggesting an effect of $1,25(OH)_2D$ on some cyto-skeletal structure. Have you measured any of these phenomena in your system?

M. HAUSSLER: We have not. We presented our data as a basic cell differentiation phenomenon, but we're not precluding the fact that macrophages could respond further. They do have $1,25(OH)_2D$ receptors. For instance, as you suggest, some actin or cyto-skeletal effect of $1,25(OH)_2D$ is a possibility with regards to the macrophages. It's amazing how we keep discovering new effects of $1,25(OH)_2D$. I suspect that if $1,25(OH)_2D$ recruits and creates macrophages, it might stimulate them as well.

M. PARFITT: Dr. Stanbury, have you considered the possibility that the rise in vitamin D produced in the skin and the rise produced by oral administration may be accompanied by different binding proteins that might alter their ability to be converted to 25-hydroxy-D?

W. STANBURY: You have speculated on the probable role of binding proteins in subserving some regulatory functions. The snag is, I know of no native data to suggest that the property of the common place D binding protein changes in any circumstance. Do you?

M. PARFITT: No, but there might be other binding proteins that we don't know about.

W. STANBURY: Indeed. And, it could well be that there is something particular about D binding proteins within the liver that makes the liver capable of recognizing the fact that the D-3 level has risen too high and the 25-hydroxylation should be inhibited. But, that's only guesswork.

THE CARDINAL ROLE OF 1,25-DIHYDROXYVITAMIN D_3 IN MINERAL HOMEOSTASIS

Hector F. DeLuca

Department of Biochemistry, College of Agricultural and Life Sciences, University of Wisconsin-Madison, Madison, WI, U.S.A.

Although there is little doubt that vitamin D must be metabolically activated before it can function, some disagreement still exists regarding the functional forms of the vitamin. There is almost uniform agreement that 25-hydroxylation of the vitamin must occur predominantly in the liver before the vitamin can serve in a functional capacity. Most, but not all, scientists in the calcium field agree that 1α-hydroxylation must also occur before the functions of vitamin D can be satisfied. Until recently, it was believed that the kidney is the sole site of 1α-hydroxylation, giving substance to the idea that the kidney is an endocrine organ that secretes the steroid hormone, 1,25-dihydroxyvitamin D_3 (calcitriol), that then functions to elevate plasma calcium and phosphorus by facilitating intestinal calcium and phosphorus absorption, bone calcium mobilization, and perhaps renal reabsorption of calcium.

Recently, there has been a question raised regarding the exclusivity of the renal production of calcitriol. Certainly, there is no doubt that in the pregnant animal, nephrectomy does not eliminate production of calcitriol, and in fact, it is now quite clear that the placenta is a site of 1α-hydroxylation. More recently, there has been the report that cells explanted from bone and other sites can carry out 1α-hydroxylation *in vitro*. These studies were used to imply that bone and other tissues might be the site of significant 1-hydroxylation *in vivo*. If this were true, the endocrine nature of the kidney in regard to the vitamin D system would be severely compromised. A re-examination of the intestinal and bone calcium mobilization responses of anephric animals most clearly reveals that animals without kidneys do not elicit a response to physiologic doses of 25-hydroxyvitamin D_3 (25-OH-D_3, calcidiol). On the other hand, animals that have uremia brought about by ureteric ligation but nevertheless retain their kidneys in circulation retain their response to physiologic doses of calcidiol. To examine the question of extrarenal synthesis of calcitriol more closely, we have repeated experiments carried out previously in our laboratory and that of Professor Kodicek's using anephric, vitamin D-deficient animals as compared to sham-operated controls and animals that have their ureters ligated to produce the same degree of uremia as is present in the anephrics (1). We injected these animals with radiolabeled calcidiol of 160 curries/mmole and 20 hours later the animals were sacrificed, their tissues extracted and chromatographed first on Sephadex LH-20 followed by straight-phase HPLC and finally by reverse-phase HPLC. The radioactivity found in the calcitriol region was measured and the amount of calcitriol that might be present in each of the tissues was computed. The results show no measureable production of calcitriol in anephric animals (<1 pg/animal), while massive amounts are produced in sham-operated animals and in ureteric ligated animals (1). Thus, using the most sensitive method of detection available, *no* calcitriol could be detected. Therefore, in agreement with the target organ response experiment, we must conclude that in the non-pregnant mammal the kidney is for all practical purposes the exclusive site of calcitriol synthesis, restoring confidence in the kidney as the endocrine organ for the vitamin D system. Although the experiments with tissue cultures are interesting, they should not be interpreted as implying significant in vivo production of calcitriol at extrarenal sites.

Besides calcitriol, it has also been suggested that other metabolites of vitamin D might be involved in the target organ responses. It has been especially claimed that 24-hydroxycalcidiol ($24R,25\text{-}(OH)_2D_3$), another metabolite discovered by us in 1972, might be a functional form in the mineralization of bone, in the suppression of parathyroid hormone secretion, or in embryonic development. Because the function might be of a subtle nature, we have used 24,24-difluorocalcidiol to test whether the functions of vitamin D require 24-hydroxylation. We have carried out extensive experiments to show that no $24R,25\text{-}(OH)_2D_3$ can arise from the difluoro compound (Tanaka, Ikekawa, Kobayashi & DeLuca, submitted). Furthermore, from an electronic point of view, the fluoro grouping is less like an hydroxyl than even hydrogen, and hence the idea that the fluoro groups could act as a hydroxyl has no chemical basis. Experiments with binding proteins, especially the chick intestinal cytosol receptor for calcitriol, show that the fluoro groups act as an analog of hydrogen and not hydroxyl. We have taken rat pups from vitamin D-deficient mothers and grown them to maturity exclusively on one of the following forms of vitamin D: A. calcidiol by mouth; B. calcidiol delivered subcutaneously by osmotic minipump; C. calcitriol delivered by osmotic minipump; D. $24,24\text{-}F_2$-calcidiol given by mouth. These animals were grown to maturity and the females were then mated with normal males and the pups from these animals were grown to maturity. These pups were then examined in several ways. The animals given the forms of vitamin D described were all equal in their growth and in all aspects of their appearance (2). In no case was any pathology seen in either the difluorocalcidiol group or the calcitriol group. Bones were removed and subjected to biochemical analysis, revealing that they had mineralized normally (3). In addition, double tetracycline labeling was carried out, and the bones from these animals submitted to Dr. Michael Parfitt in a coded manner. These were studied by histomorphometric methods, resulting in the conclusion that the bones from the animals given the vitamin D compounds were indistinguishable and well mineralized (Parfitt, Mathews, Brommage, Jarnagin & DeLuca, submitted). Thus, no evidence through two generations of growth and reproduction for a role for $24R,25\text{-}(OH)_2D_3$ could be found in the rat. In the view of the authors, therefore, we believe that $24R,25\text{-}(OH)_2D_3$ is not a functional form of vitamin D. We have also carried out experiments using the $24,24\text{-}F_2$-calcidiol in birds to illustrate that 24-hydroxylation is certainly not required for embryonic growth and development as has been suggested before (4). $26,26,26,27,27,27\text{-}F_6$-Calcidiol is also equally active with calcidiol in all of the known functions of vitamin D (5). This hexafluoro compound does not undergo conversion to the calcidiol 26,23-lactone or to the 26-hydroxylated vitamin D compounds. Therefore, all known side chain modified forms of vitamin D that have been discovered appear not to be important in the functional aspects of vitamin D.

In contrast to the 24 and 26 positions, introduction of fluoro groups in the 1 position or in the 25 position of vitamin D_3 on the other hand markedly diminishes biological activity of the vitamin D compounds (6,7). These experiments, together with the difluoro and hexafluoro experiments shown above, act in a sense as controls to illustrate that 1 and 25 hydroxylation of vitamin D_3 is essential for function, whereas 26 and 24 modifications are not required.

An important aspect of calcium homeostasis is the drain on plasma calcium by the mineralization process. There has been considerable question whether vitamin D might function in the transfer of mineral from plasma to the calcification sites. Evidence has been mixed, although experiments recently from Holtrup and Baylink's groups have argued against a role for vitamin D in this area. We have recently developed methods whereby mobile animals can be infused with calcium and phosphorus in quantities that can maintain normal plasma calcium and phosphorus levels in truly vitamin D-deficient animals for a period of at least 10 days. With the system devised in our laboratory by Ms. Johnnie Underwood, the catheters are placed through a plastic skull cap subcutaneously and inserted into the carotid artery. These animals are then connected through a swivel and can eat, drink and move about their cages in a normal fashion. Table 1 shows bone growth and mineralization of these animals. It is clear that these animals are able to mineralize their bones in a normal fashion at least as measured biochemically, and in fact bone growth is normal in the absence of vitamin D during this 10 day period. No evidence could be found for a failure of

Table 1. Mineralization and bone growth does not require vitamin D if bone is supplied with calcium and phosphorus

	Not Infused		Infused	
	-D	+D	-D	+D
Serum Ca (mg/dl)	5.1*	10.2	10.4	10.4
Serum P (mg/dl)	6.2*	8.5*	9.8	9.7
Femur Length (nm)	22.2*	24.5	25.1	25.8
Femur Ash (%)	36.7	46.2	52.1**	47.5
Femur Ash (mg)	52.3*	89.6	117.5**	95.1

* Lower than other groups; $P < 0.001$
** Higher than corresponding +D; $P < 0.001$

mineralization by the absence of vitamin D, provided plasma calcium and phosphorus are maintained in the normal range. These bones have been labeled with tetracycline and submitted for bone histomorphometry to Dr. Weinstein at the Medical College of Georgia. Preliminary results reveal that the mineralization process is normal in these animals. Thus, we can remove doubt from the idea that mineralization will proceed normally without vitamin D, provided plasma calcium and phosphorus levels are normal. This eliminates the idea that vitamin D plays a direct role in this process. On the other hand, there seems little doubt that vitamin D plays an essential role in bone, both for mobilization of calcium in calcium homeostasis and in the bone modeling and remodeling sequences. These, however, have not been fully defined, although it now seems that the vitamin must function primarily in the resorption aspect of these sequences.

There is no doubt, therefore, that vitamin D through calcitriol plays an important role in the regulation of plasma calcium and phosphorus. In 1971, Boyle, Gray & DeLuca provided strong evidence that plasma calcium level in some fashion regulates production of calcitriol by the kidney. Subsequent work by Garabedian, Tanaka, Holick & DeLuca and Fraser & Kodicek provided evidence that the calcium regulation of calcitriol production is mediated by the parathyroid hormone. There has been the suggestion without adequate proof that calcium may directly regulate the calcitriol production in the kidney. Recently, we have been able to develop a series of methods involving direct measurement of the renal 1α-hydroxylation and renal 24-hydroxylation in the mammalian kidney (8). Endocrine manipulations are much easier in the case of mammals, and hence direct examination of the role of parathyroid hormone could be made. Parathyroidectomy results in a fall in calcitriol production as has previously been demonstrated *in vivo* (8). However, it is clear that plasma calcium levels change very rapidly in the parathyroidectomized animal long before a change results in the renal 1α-hydroxylase and plasma 1,25-$(OH)_2D_3$ levels. When parathyroid hormone is administered to the parathyroidectomized animal, again plasma calcium responds very quickly to the parathyroid hormone, but the alteration in renal 1α-hydroxylation is very much slower.

These results demonstrate two important facts: (1) Plasma calcium is not likely to be a regulator of the renal 1α-hydroxylation *in vivo*, and (2) The vitamin D endocrine system does not play a significant role in the minute-to-minute regulation of plasma calcium concentration. This must be relegated primarily to the parathyroid hormone and to calcitonin. The vitamin D endocrine system is more involved in the calcium economy of the body, stimulating intestine to absorb calcium when it is needed. It also plays an important role in increasing the calcium transport machinery in bone and kidney making it more sensitive to parathyroid hormone. Calcitriol must also play an important role in stimulating osteoclastic-mediated bone resorption when dictated by modeling and remodeling sequences.

In conclusion, calcitriol is the only form of vitamin D that has a proven physiologic function. Calcitriol plays an important role in intestinal calcium absorption, intestinal phosphorus absorption, the mobilization of calcium from bone, and perhaps renal reabsorption of calcium. It does not appear to play an important role in the mineralization process of bone, but probably plays an important role in the modeling and remodeling sequences of bone. Parathyroid hormone is the primary calcium homeostatic hormone with calcitriol, functioning to permit parathyroid hormone regulation of plasma calcium by its function in kidney and bone. Most important, calcitriol plays an essential role in the calcium economy of the body by playing an essential role in regulating intestinal calcium absorption.

REFERENCES

1. Reeve, L., Tanaka, Y. and DeLuca, H. F. (1983): J. Biol. Chem., in press.
2. Jarnagin, K., Brommage, R., DeLuca, H. F., Yamada, S. and Takayama, H. (1983): Am. J. Physiol., 244, E290.
3. Brommage, R., Jarnagin, K., DeLuca, H. F., Yamada, S. and Takayama, H. (1983): Am. J. Physiol., 244, E298.
4. Ameenuddin, S., Sunde, M., DeLuca, H. F., Ikekawa, N. and Kobayashi, Y. (1982): Science, 217, 451.
5. Tanaka, Y., Pahuja, D. N., Wichmann, J. K., DeLuca, H. F., Kobayashi, Y., Taguchi, T. and Ikekawa, N. (1982): Arch. Biochem. Biophys., 218, 134.
6. Onisko, B. L., Schnoes, H. K., DeLuca, H. F. and Glover, R. S. (1979): Biochem. J., 182, 1.
7. Paaren, H. E., Fivizzani, M. A., Schnoes, H. K. and DeLuca, H. F. (1981): Arch. Biochem. Biophys., 209, 579.
8. Tanaka, Y. and DeLuca, H. F. (1981): Proc. Natl. Acad. Sci. USA, 78, 196.

THE ROLE OF 1,25$(OH)_2D_3$ IN THE PATHOGENESIS OF OSTEOMALACIA

Howard Rasmussen

Departments of Internal Medicine and Cell Biology, Yale University School of Medicine, New Haven, CT, U.S.A.

With the discoveries that 1,25$(OH)_2D_3$ acted to increase bone resorption and the intestinal absorption of calcium and phosphate, it is widely assumed that the active metabolite of vitamin D had been discovered (1). With this assumption went the prediction that osteomalacia developed as a result of a deficiency of 1,25-$(OH)_2D_3$. This prediction appeared to be verified when it was shown that patients affected with vitamin D dependency rickets had an impaired ability to synthesize this renal hormone, 1,25$(OH)_2D_3$. However, the results of studies conducted in the past decade lead to the conclusion that in man and experimental animals there is no simple relationship between the appearance of rickets and/or osteomalacia and a deficiency of 1,25$(OH)_2D_3$.

To discuss these results, it is useful to begin by reviewing briefly what this decade of study has revealed concerning the physiological role of 1,25$(OH)_2D_3$. Then a consideration of the role of 1,25$(OH)_2D_3$ in the pathogenesis of osteomalacia will be considered in three parts: a) factors other than 1,25$(OH)_2D_3$ that regulate intestinal calcium absorption; b) plasma 1,25$(OH)_2D_3$ concentrations in osteomalacia; and c) 1,25$(OH)_2D_3$ in the treatment of osteomalacia. After this, the role of other metabolites in the pathogenesis of osteomalacia will be discussed.

ROLE OF 1,25$(OH)_2D_3$

From work in the past decade, it is clear that 1,25$(OH)_2D_3$ is a major component of the parathyroid gland-kidney-gut system responsible for the maintenance of plasma calcium homeostasis. When plasma calcium falls, PTH rises. This increase in PTH acts both by a

This research was supported by a grant from the National Institutes of Health (AM-28437).

short and long feedback loop to restore plasma calcium concentration (3). The short loop is between parathyroid gland and distal renal tubule. When PTH rises, distal tubular calcium reabsorption increases as a means of restoring the plasma calcium concentration to normal. The long loop is between parathyroid gland, kidney and intestine. When PTH rises, the proximal tubular synthesis of $1,25(OH)_2D_3$ concentration leads to an increase in intestinal calcium absorption as a means of restoring the plasma calcium concentration to normal and thereby signalling the parathyroid gland to reduce its rate of PTH secretion. It is also clear that dietary phosphate deficiency or that occurring as a result of a renal phosphate leak lead to an increase in plasma $1,25(OH)_2D_3$ (3). Hence, this hormone is involved in both calcium and phosphate homeostasis.

ROLE OF $1,25(OH)_2D_3$ IN SKELETAL HOMEOSTASIS

One of the problems in coming to an understanding of the role of $1,25(OH)_2D_3$ in mammalian physiology is a failure to distinguish between plasma calcium homeostasis and skeletal mineral homeostasis. For example, it is clear that the process of bone mineralization can take place normally when the plasma calcium concentration is as low as 5 mg/dl or as high as 15 mg/dl. Hence, simply regulating the plasma calcium concentration near a value of 10 mg/dl is not essential to the process of bone mineralization. Conversely, it is clear that osteomalacia can develop in patients with a normal plasma calcium concentration. Thus, the fact that $1,25(OH)_2D_3$ plays a vital role in plasma calcium homeostasis does not mean necessarily that it plays a significant role in skeletal homeostasis.

A way to put this problem into even sharper focus is to consider the changes in mineral metabolism induced by the administration of growth hormone to a growth hormone deficient human adolescent (4). Administration of growth hormone to such an individual leads to an increase in positive calcium balance of approximately 150 mg/d. Only 30 mg of this can be accounted for by enhanced renal conservation. The remainder must reflect an increase in intestinal calcium absorption. Based upon our knowledge of the PTH-$1,25(OH)_2D_3$ calcium control system, one would predict that if the primary event in this growth hormone-treated child is a net movement of 120 mg/d of calcium into the skeleton, this should lead to an increase in plasma PTH and secondarily $1,25(OH)_2D_3$. However, neither change occurs. Instead, intestinal calcium absorption increases without a change in either plasma PTH or $1,25(OH)_2D_3$ concentration. These results, and others, lead to the conclusion that skeletal mineral homeostasis is governed by a different messenger system than plasma mineral homeostasis. The most likely messenger is some signal directly from bone to intestine which tells the intestine how much calcium the growing skeleton needs, and allows skeletal growth and mineralization to proceed without disrupting plasma mineral homeostasis. Clearly, these results suggest that factors other than $1,25(OH)_2D_3$ regulate intestinal calcium absorption, and skeletal mineral homeostasis.

A second way to approach the same question is to determine whether there is any correlation between plasma $1,25(OH)_2D_3$ concentration and the rate of bone mineralization. There are two parts to this question: Do mineralization defects appear in the face of normal or high concentrations of plasma $1,25(OH)_2D_3$, and does normal mineralization occur under situations where $1,25(OH)_2D_3$ concentrations are low? The answer to both parts is yes.

Patients with hypo- or pseudohypoparathyroidism have normal rates of bone mineralization even when plasma $1,25(OH)_2D_3$ concentrations are low. Most striking are some patients with pseudohypoparathyroidism in whom secondary hyperparathyroidism with high rates of bone turnover are seen (5). If there is any circumstance under which $1,25(OH)_2D_3$ deficiency should lead to osteomalacia, this is it, but osteomalacia does not occur. A similar situation is seen in many patients with renal failure, low plasma $1,25(OH)_2D_3$, severe hyperparathyroidism and osteitis fibrosa cystica with little or no osteomalacia. Clearly, there are states in which high rates of bone turnover are seen in which no mineralization defect develops even though plasma $1,25(OH)_2D_3$ concentration is abnormally low.

Likewise, it is now clear that patients with simple vitamin D deficiency (6) anticonvulsant-induced osteomalacia (7), or with D-deficiency secondary to intestinal disease (5) are observed in which osteomalacia develops in spite of normal or high plasma concentrations of $1,25(OH)_2D_3$. One suggested explanation for the lack of apparent correlation between plasma $1,25(OH)_2D_3$ and intestinal calcium absorption is that the $25(OH)D_3$ level is low in D-deficiency so that there are more binding sites for $1,25(OH)_2D_3$ on plasma D binding protein. However, this explanation seems unlikely (4). Furthermore, another situation has been reported where there is a similar lack of correlation between plasma $1,25(OH)_2D_3$ and intestinal calcium absorption in which normal plasma $25(OH)$-D_3 concentrations are found. This is dietary-induced phosphate depletion in the rat (8,9,10). The plasma $1,25$-$(OH)_2D_3$ increases, but there is no increase, or only a transient increase, in intestinal calcium absorption, measured by either balance or transport techniques. These data are also suggestive that a signal from skeleton to gut may play a role in skeletal mineral homeostasis, and that this signal is related to the availability of bone mineral ions.

The most controversial aspect of the relationship between $1,25(OH)_2D_3$ and osteomalacia concerns the effectiveness of $1,25(OH)_2D_3$ as a therapeutic agent in the treatment of osteomalacia. Some investigators report incomplete or little effect (11), others complete healing (12). It is not possible to discuss these various reports in detail, but it is telling that careful studies in man (11), chicks (13,14), and rats (15) have led to the conclusion that $1,25(OH)_2D_3$ alone will not correct the bone lesions of vitamin D deficiency.

ROLE OF OTHER METABOLITES

In approaching the question of the role of other metabolites of vitamin D in skeletal homeostasis, it is essential to clarify one very important point. Traditional views of the action of vitamin D are that this agent has two major physiological effects: it increases mineral ion absorption in the intestine, and it increases the resorption of mineral ions from bone (1). Both effects are seen within a few hours, both are produced by $1,25(OH)_2D_3$. Ergo, $1,25(OH)_2D_3$ is <u>the</u> active metabolite of vitamin D. This central dogma has and continues to obscure the fact that vitamin D increases bone growth, bone mass, and mineralization by some direct effect on the formation-mineralization side of bone modeling and remodeling (16). Unfortunately, bone growth is a slow and complex process, difficult to study. The bone that is removed in a few days is replaced in months. A totally different time scale is involved. The same rules of evidence cannot apply to the events in formation that apply to those involved in resorption. A hormone that regulates this process would be expected to change slowly in concentration, not rapidly as does $1,25(OH)_2D_3$.

Whether $24,25(OH)_2D_3$ is such a hormone continues to be a matter of debate. What is no longer debatable are the following facts: 1) $24,25(OH)_2D_3$ has biological effects *in vivo* and *in vitro* that are qualitatively different from those of $1,25(OH)_2D_3$; 2) the plasma concentration of $24,25(OH)_2D_3$ falls during vitamin D restriction long before $1,25(OH)_2D_3$ concentration does; 3) the factors that control $24,25(OH)_2D_3$ synthesis differ, in part, from those that regulate $1,25(OH)_2D_3$ synthesis (5,17,18).

One of the major pieces of evidence against a specific physiological role of $24,25(OH)_2D_3$ is that D-deficient animals fed the 24-difluro analog of $25(OH)D_3$ show no signs of D-deficiency (19), from which it has been concluded that hydroxylation of the 24 position is not essential for any of the biological effects of vitamin. This argument is considerably weakened by the observation, made by the same group of investigators, that difluro 25,24-hydroxyvitamin D also serves as a substitute for vitamin D. By their logic, one is led to the conclusion that the 25-position is also not essential for the biological actions of vitamin D, a position with which few would agree.

Although many different studies have attempted to define the role of $24,25(OH)_2D_3$, only three will be discussed because they lead to the same general conclusion but are done in different species, and even different levels of organization. The first is that of Bordier *et al.* in man (11); the second that of Endo *et al.* in chick bone in culture (14) and the third that of Hanson *et al.* in the rat (7).

Bordier *et al.* (11) showed that a combination of $1,25(OH)_2D_3$ and $24,25(OH)_2D_3$ was more effective than either metabolite alone in increasing the rate of bone mineralization in humans with vitamin D-deficiency osteomalacia.

Endo *et al.* (14) reported that a combination of parathyroid hormone, $1,25(OH)_2D_3$ and $24,25(OH)_2D_3$ was necessary in order to stimulate the rate of mineralization of embryonic chick bone *in vitro*. Any combination of D metabolites without PTH was ineffective, as was any single metabolite with PTH.

Parenthetically, it is of more than passing interest that patients with renal osteodystrophy of the osteomalacia type (as opposed to the hyperparathyroid type) of bone disease have low plasma PTH (20), $1,25(OH)_2D_3$ and usually low $24,25(OH)_2D_3$ plasma concentrations and do not respond to treatment with $1,25(OH)_2D_3$ alone as do most patients with the hyperparathyroid type of bone disease, but do respond to a combination of $1,25(OH)_2D_3$ and 24,25-

$(OH)_2D_3$ (21).

In the growing but D-deficient chick, Ornoy et al. (13). have shown that a combination of $24,25(OH)_2D_3$ with 1,25-$(OH)_2D_3$ is more effective than either metabolite alone in correcting the abnormalities of bone growth and structure seen in these animals.

Tam, Hanson and associates (15,22,23) studied the correlation between $1,25(OH)_2D_3$ and $24,25(OH)_2D_3$ and the appearance of osteomalacia in adult rats placed on a D-restricted diet. They showed that bone apposition rate declined after several weeks on such a diet, and the decline correlated with a fall in the plasma concentrations of $24,25(OH)_2D_3$ and $25(OH)D_3$ but a sustained normal level of $1,25(OH)_2D_3$. If animals were fed a phosphate restricted diet as well, the plasma $1,25(OH)_2D_3$ was several times normal and intestinal calcium absorption was increased in spite of which the histological signs of rickets developed.

In adult animals made D-deficient, the fall in bone apposition rate could be corrected by the administration of $25(OH)D_3$ but not by that of $1,25(OH)_2D_3$. If animals were made D-deficient and were parathyroidectomized, then neither PTH nor $24,25(OH)_2D_3$ alone were effective in restoring apposition rate to normal, but the combination was effective.

These data from man, chick, and rat lead to the same conclusions: a) $24,25(OH)_2D_3$ is a bone-active vitamin D metabolite; b) the mineralization of bone is regulated by the interplay of at least three humoral factors, PTH, 1,25-$(OH)_2D_3$ and $24,25(OH)_2D_3$ and c) bone mineralization is controlled not simply by the plasma mineral ion product but directly by a complex hormonal system which means that the factors responsible for skeletal mineral ion homeostasis are different from those responsible for plasma mineral homeostasis but there is a significant overlap--PTH and $1,25(OH)_2D_3$ are components of both homeostatic systems.

The other conclusion is that multiple factors may play a role in the pathogenesis of osteomalacia in man. In simple vitamin D deficiency, these appear to be largely a deficiency of $24,25(OH)D_2$ [and $25(OH)D_3$] and a reduced mineral ion product; in vitamin D dependency rickets a reduced mineral ion product and a reduced plasma $1,25(OH)_2D_3$ concentration, in the osteomalacia form of ROD low plasma concentrations of PTH, $1,25(OH)_2D_3$ and $24,25(OH)_2D_3$ may all contribute.

CONCLUSION AND PERSPECTIVE

At the very least, it is now clear that there is no

simple correlation between the circulating concentration of 1,25$(OH)_2D_3$ and the rate of bone mineralization. This means that we do not yet understand why osteomalacia develops as a consequence of vitamin D deficiency. If we agree that changes in skeletal mineral deposition, and in plasma concentrations of calcium and phosphate may occur shortly after the onset of a restricted intake of vitamin D, at a time when 1,25$(OH)_2D_3$ is either normal or high, then the question arises as to why these changes have occurred. If the only action of 24,25$(OH)_2D_3$ is to stimulate bone mineral apposition, then a decrease in 24,25$(OH)_2D_3$ should lead to a decrease in the net uptake of calcium by bone. This change would not lead to a fall in mineral ion product. Alternative explanations which must be exploited are: a) 25$(OH)D_3$ and/or 24,25$(OH)_2D_3$ have a direct effect upon the efficiency of proximal tubular reabsorption of calcium and phosphate; b) 24,25-$(OH)_2D_3$ [and/or 25$(OH)D_3$] influence the responsiveness of the intestine to the action of 1,25$(OH)_2D_3$; or c) 24,25-$(OH)_2D_3$ [and/or 25$(OH)D_3$] regulate the synthesis of a bone-derived factor (hormone) which regulates intestinal calcium absorption at sites other than those influenced by 1,25$(OH)_2D_3$. Exploration of these possibilities should provide new insights into the role of the vitamin D endocrine system in skeletal homeostasis. This knowledge should, in turn, provide us with a clearer undersaanding of the factors involved in the pathogenesis of osteomalacia.

REFERENCES

1. DeLuca, H.F. (1976): Ann. Inter. Med., 85, 367.
2. Rasmussen, H. and Anast, C. (1983): In: The Metabolic Basis 1 of Inherited Disease, p. 1743. Editors: J.B. Stanbury, J.B. Wyngaarden, D.S. Fredrickson, J.L. Goldstein and M.S. Brown. McGraw-Hill Book Co., New York.
3. Broadus, A., Horst, R.L., Lang, R., Littledike, E.T. and Rasmussen, H. (1980): New Engl. J. Med. 302, 421.
4. Gertner, J.M., Horst, R.L., Broadus, A.E., Rasmussen, H. and Genel, M. (1979): J. Clin. Endocrinol. Metab. 49, 185.
5. Rasmussen, H., Baron, R., Broadus, A.E., DeFronzo, R., Lang, R. and Horst, R.L. (1980): Am. J. Med. 69, 360.
6. Eastwood, J.R., de Wardener, H.E., Gray, R.W. and Lemann, J.L., Jr. (1979): Lancet 1, 1377.
7. Jubuz, W., Haussler, M.R., McCain, T.A. and Tolman,

K.G. (1977): J. Clin. Endocrinol. Metab. 44, 617.
8. Rader, J.I., Baylink, D.J., Hughes, M.R., Safilian, E.F., and Haussler, M.R. (1979): Am. J. Physiol. 236, E118.
9. Leu, D.B.N., Brautbar, N., Walling, M.W., Silis, V., Coburn, J.N. and Kleeman, C.R. (1979): Am. J. Physiol. 236, E451.
10. Brautbar, N., Levine, B.S., Walling, M.W. and Coburn, J.W. (1981): Am. J. Physiol. 241, G49.
11. Bordier, P., Rasmussen, H., Marie, P., Miravet, L., Gueris, J. and Ryckewaert, A. (1978): J. Clin. Endocrinol. Metab. 46: 284.
12. Nagant de Deuxchaisnes, C., Ronbout-Lindermanns, C., Huaux, J.P., Wilhops, H. and Meersenaan, F. (1979): In: Molecular Endocrinology, p. 375. Editors: I. MacIntyre and J. Szelke. North-Holland Biomedical Press, Amsterdam.
13. Ornoy, A.D., Goodwin, D., Noff, D. and Edelstein, S. (1978): Nature 276, 5.
14. Endo, H., Kyoki, M., Kawashima, K., Nayuchi, T. and Hashimoto, Y. (1980): Nature 286, 262.
15. Tam, C.S., Heersche, J.N.M., Jones, G. and Murray, T.M. (1983): Endocrinology. In press.
16. Rasmussen, H. and Bordier, P. (1974): The Physiological and Cellular Basis of Metabolic Bone Disease. Williams and Wilkins, Baltimore.
17. Garabedian, M., Lieberherr, M., N'Guyen, T.M., Corovol, M.T., Bailly de Bois, M. and Balsan, S. (1978): Clin. Orthop. and Rel. Res. 135, 241.
18. Massry, S.G., Tuma, S., Dira, S. and Goldstein, D.A. (1979): J. Lab. Clin. Med. 94, 152.
19. Halloran, B.P., DeLuca, H.F., Barthell, E., Yamada, S., Ohmori, M. and Takayama, H. (1981): Endocrinology 108, 2067.
20. Hodsman, A.B., Sherrard, D.J., Wong, E.G.C., Brickman, A.S., Lee, D.B.N., Alfrey, A., Singer, F.R., Norman, A.W. and Coburn, J.W. (1981): Ann. Int. Med. 94, 629.
21. Hodsman, A.B., Wong, L.G.C., Sherrard, D.J., Brick man, A.S., Lee, D.B.N., Singer, F., Norman, A.W. and Coburn, J.W. (1983): Am. J. Med. 74, 407.
22. Harrison, J.E., Hitchman, A.J.W., Jones, G., Tam, C.S. and Heersche, J.N.M. (1982): Metabolism 32, 1121.
23. Tam, C.S., Jones, G. and Heersche, J.N.M. (1981): Endocrinology 101, 1448.

Discussion following papers of Rasmussen and De Luca

A. NORMAN: With all the attention on the question of whether 24R, 25 $(OH)_2D_3$ does or does not have biological activity, I feel compelled to reiterate some of our data in support of that possibility and then to ask Dr. DeLuca a question.

In a second generation experiment, studying the phenomenon of egg hatchability, we compared the contribution of $24R,25(OH)_2D_3$ with the naturally occurring isomer of the dihydroxymetabolite with $24S,25(OH)_2D_3$ both given in conjunction with $1,25(OH)_2D$. It was only when the naturally occurring 24R, $25(OH)_2D_3$ was given in conjunction with $1,25(OH)_2D$ that normal egg hatchability in the quail was sustained.

These results when taken with the demonstration from our laboratory of a receptor for $24,25(OH)_2D$ in the parathyroid glands and that of Somjen, et al, in the chondrocytes, still supports the possibility there may be biological activity unique to $24,25(OH)_2D$. Dr. Rasmussen's comments lends support to this possibility.

My question is, with the knowledge that there is a $23,25(OH)_2D$, it seems possible that all your efforts at blocking the 24 position by preparing a difluoro derivative may have forced the metabolite to become 23-hyroxylated; thus you may have generated an analogue of $24,25(OH)_2D_3$ namely, 23,25 dihydroxyvitamin D. I don't see how, looking at the difluoro and hexafluoro data, you can exclude the contribution of a possible 23-hydroxylated compound to replace the role of $24,25(OH)_2D_3$.

H. DE LUCA: We have 23,23 difluoro 25 hydroxy-D that is under test right now. Dr. Norman, we will give you that answer soon. Now, with regards to the question about the natural isomer, versus the unnatural one, one of the important findings thatDr. Tanaka did with the two isomers is that the unnatural isomer is only very poorly one-hydroxylated in the bird. So I don't think that really constitutes evidence against that possibility.

Secondly, the difluoro compound, I think is a pretty potent argument. How about the injection experiments where you can inject $1,25(OH)_2D_3$ back into those eggs and return them to normal hatchability. I don't know that we can ever exclude some function for $24,25(OH)_2D$ that we are missing because of its subtlety. We obviously can only go to the limit of our experiments and detection methods. So, to absolutely say that there is no role for any other metabolite of vitamin D, other than $1,25(OH)_2D_3$, is premature.

I must say also that I have not seen convincing evidence that anyone has shown a role for another metabolite of vitamin D, other than $1,25(OH)_2D$.

C. NORDIN: I don't think Dr. Rasmussen need have been so surprised at seeing osteomalacia in the presence of normal $1,25(OH)_2D$ levels. We reported at Berlin, four or five years ago, that calcium absorption in normal women of various ages correlates weakly with the 25-hydroxy level and weakly with the 1,25 level but much more strongly if both levels were taken into account. When you consider that you can get osteomalacia with low 1,25 levels and normal 25 hydroxys or with normal 1,25 levels and low 25 hydroxys, the simplest and most rational explanation is that these two hormones both act on the receptor. The $1,25(OH)_2D$ is a thousand times as potent as 25 hydroxy D. Normally it is the sum of the two that is doing the job and one picomole of $1,25(OH)_2D$ is approximately equivalent to 1 nanomole of 25 hydroxy D_3,

H. RASMUSSEN: I agree with Dr. DeLuca in one sense. No one has proved that $24,25(OH)_2D$ has an unique role. But there are certain problems with the hypothesis which demands that there is a simple correlation between $1,25(OH)_2D$ and osteomalacia; or between the plasma calcium and phosphate concentration and osteomalacia. There are patients with severe osteomalacia who have a normal calcium and phosphate concentration, and there are patients with osteomalacia and high levels of plasma $1,25(OH)_2D$.

I think Dr. Nordin's comments are appropriate. One possibility, in fact, is the importance of the sum of the vitamin D metabolites. There are a number of situations clinically where changes in bone mineralization, whatever way you want to measure it, do not correlate with changes in $1,25(OH)_2D$. Maybe it is 25(OH)D and not $24,25(OH)_2D$ that acts as a hormone in its own right, but it's just more effective when it's $1,25(OH)_2D$.

H. DE LUCA: I will agree with the possibility that somewhere in the phylogenetic scale, we will find a function for 25 hydroxy D, and it may well have some vestigial role in man. I don't know, but I haven't seen the evidence that convinces me yet.

If the rat is a reasonable mammalian model, we can grow these animals for two generations on $1,25(OH)_2D$. Unless we're going to say that $1,25(OH)_2D$, at that very low concentration, serves as an analogue of 25-hydroxy D, I don't see how we can escape the conclusion that it looks like $1,25(OH)_2D$ is the most critical metabolite.

H. RASMUSSEN: We accept your data, Dr. DeLuca. However, a possibility to be considered is that under unusual conditions $1,25(OH)_2D$ is being converted into another analog like 1,24,25D which is doing something important. I don't think you've checked that possibility to my knowledge.

H. DE LUCA: Oh, I'm sure that there's some 1,24,25D in these animals that are given $1,25(OH)_2D$ only, but not in the ones given the difluoro compound.

H. RASMUSSEN: Now, the second point is that your data doesn't address the issue that I've been talking about which Dr. Nordin also addressed. How do you account for the fact that you have a patient with severe osteomalacia, a normal serum calcium and phosphate level and a $1,25(OH)_2D$ of 100 picograms/ml or more?

H. DE LUCA: I think Dr. Stanbury's data is probably instructive in this regard. Whenever you have a surfeit of uncalcified bone, the normal level of $1,25(OH)_2D$ is not 100 picograms/ml, but is much higher. One of the major errors I think we make in discussing 1,25 dihydroxy D_3 levels is we speak of a normal value without defining the circumstances. There is a normal value only when you specify all of the parameters that are known to control $1,25(OH)_2D$ levels. Now, if you have a large amount of uncalcified osteoid, as in the case of osteomalacic patients, the normal adaption is to make lots of 1,25 $(OH)_2D$ until the bone is healed. That's a normal level for that circumstance.

H. RASMUSSEN: I don't follow that argument at all.

H. DE LUCA: It's very simple. In order to heal rickets or osteomalacia, the normal event is to raise blood $1,25(OH)_2D$ levels to super values which stay high until the bone is mineralized. That's all I'm saying.

H. RASMUSSEN: No, but let's take the patient whose $1,25(OH)_2D$ stayed normal or actually increased while he is developing osteomalacia; how did he develop osteomalacia in the face of having a normal or elevated 1,25 level?

H. DE LUCA: If that person is developing osteomalacia, the plasma 1,25 is not responding appropriately to a given circumstance.

H. RASMUSSEN: But why is he developing osteomalacia in the first place?

H. DE LUCA: All I'm saying is that the $1,25(OH)_2D$ level has to respond appropriately when an uncalcified matrix is being synthesized. You have given me one point about the blood level at a time when there is osteomalacia and you say that it hasn't changed. Well, I don't know if it has changed or not. You've given me only one point in time.

M. HAUSSLER: Two questions for Dr. DeLuca. First of all, what do you recommend as your second-generation $1,25(OH)_2D$, the 24,24-difluoro analog or the 26,27-hexafluoro compound? That is to say, which one is going to be the best long-acting $1,25(OH)_2D$ for patients?

H. DE LUCA: Or the 23,23-difluoro? I can't tell, they all have about equal biological activity. The hexofluoro compound seem to produce a more lasting effect.

M. HAUSSLER: The other question is, have you looked for $24,25(OH)_2D$ receptors, since Dr. Norman brought this controversial point up again?

H. DE LUCA: Yes we have, and we cannot see any evidence for them.

J. HADDAD: Professor Stanbury, could I lean on you a bit and ask you about the whole concept of osteomalacia with an inappropriately low $1,25(OH)_2D$ level? Is dietary calcium important perhaps? Would you like to comment on that? Specifically, could $1,25(OH)_2D$ levels that appear normal or even slightly high, be inappropriately low, given a set of clinical conditions?

W. STANBURY: When we encounter osteomalacia due to simple vitamin D deficiency, plasma levels of 25-hydroxyvitamin D are low; plasma 1,25-dihydroxy-vitamin D may be immeasurably low, within a lower part of the normal range, or actually normal. If you take the obvious prototype, the patient with plasma $1,25(OH)_2D$ too low to be measurable, giving a single dose of 400 units of vitamin D may restore normal levels of this metabolite without necessarily altering the low plasma 25-hydroxyvitamin D. We suspect that a similar phenomenon occurs 'spontaneously' in the vitamin D deficient patients we see among our immigrant Asian population. If the women pull the veil aside for half an hour on a sunny day, they may derive sufficient 25-hydroxyvitamin D to increase their originally very low $1,25\text{-}(OH)_2D$ level to normal - and it seems probable that these individuals oscillate between a state of total $1,25\text{-}(OH)_2D$ deficiency and its repletion. Such acquisition of a normal plasma $1,25\text{-}(OH)_2D$ by a patient with osteomalacia does not, of course, immediately alter the clinical or radiological features of that disease (nor eliminate the wide osteoid seams). Consequently, a patient with all the clinical features of vitamin D-deficiency osteomalacia can have either a low or normal plasma $1,25\text{-}(OH)_2D$. Giving a little extra vitamin D, sufficient perhaps to increase plasma 25-hydorxyvitamin D from 2 to 4 ng/ml, will then induce supranormal levels of plasma $1,25\text{-}(OH)_2D$ which may be sustained for weeks until the bone disease has healed. What the mechanism is that tells the kidney to produce $1,25\text{-}(OH)_2D$ at that level is uncertain.

J. REEVE: Perhaps Dr. DeLuca provided his own answer when he presented data that vitamin D may have little or nothing to do with actual mineralization. For mineralization of the excess osteoid that has previously been accumulated, you have to supply mineral and there are two facets to that. One is how much mineral is in the diet, and the other is how much mineral is being absorbed. Until it is shown that Dr. Rasmussen's problem patients had adequate supplies of mineral in the diet, I think for the moment Dr. DeLuca is off the hook.

IV ASSESSMENT OF MINERAL AND MATRIX TURNOVER

ASSESSMENT OF MINERAL AND MATRIX TURNOVER

Moderator: Stephen M. Krane

Department of Medicine, Harvard Medical School and Massachusetts General Hospital, Boston, Massachusetts, U.S.A.

In order to understand the pathophysiology of skeletal diseases and evaluate the results of therapy, it is essential to have markers for bone cell function and means to accurately measure the synthesis and degradation of the extracellular matrix of bone. As our knowledge has advanced concerning the structure and composition of bone, and pathways of biosynthesis of the skeletal components, new markers have become available for this purpose. In addition, it is of value to place in perspective the utility of techniques which have been used for years to quantitate bone formation and resorption.

Bone is a two-phase material comprised of an inorganic mineral phase (∿ 65% of weight) and an organic matrix (∿35% of weight). The calcium-phosphorus mineral phase, at least part of which is organized with respect to the collagenous portion of the organic matrix, consists of poorly crystalline hydroxyapatite (1). The composition of the organic matrix of bone is shown in Table 1.

TABLE 1. Composition of the organic matrix of bone

I. Type I collagen - 90-95% of total

II. Non-collagenous proteins
- A. "True" matrix constituents (osteoblast-derived)
  1. Osteonectin
  2. Bone sialoprotein
  3. Bone proteoglycan
  4. Other glycoproteins
  5. Phosphoproteins
- B. Bound to mineral phase (osteoblast-derived)
  1. Bone GLA protein (osteocalcin)
- C. Serum-derived
  1. α_2-HS glycoprotein
  2. Other serum proteins

The collagen of bone is almost exclusively type I, identical in primary structure to the type I collagen in other organs (2). There are differences, however, in certain posttranslational modifications between the type I collagens in skin and bone particularly with respect to content of hydroxylysine, hydroxylysine glycosides and the hydroxylysine-derived hydroxypyridinium crosslinks (3). The distinctive collagenous product of the osteoblast can thus be ascribed to the expression of genes coding for proteins other than the component $\alpha1(I)$ and $\alpha2(I)$ chains.

Over the past several years, several non-collagenous proteins, unique to bone, have been identified and characterized. The isolation of several of these, such as the γ-carboxyglutamic acid (GLA) protein (osteocalcin), osteonectin and bone proteoglycan has been made possible by avoiding artefacts introduced by mechanical shearing forces and release of proteases during demineralization and extraction. Osteonectin is a good example (4,5). It represents ∿25% of the noncollagenous proteins of bovine bone. It is made by osteoblasts, and can bind to apatite, as well as denatured collagen. In addition, osteonectin may have a functional as well as structural role in regulation of collagen and protein synthesis. When radioimmunoassays are developed for this protein it should serve as another marker for matrix protein metabolism in humans.

In the process of bone formation, mineral ions enter the inorganic phase; these ions are then removed in the process of bone resorption. The kinetics of radiocalcium and radiostrontrium uptake by the skeleton thus provide a means for quantitation of bone formation and resorption. Validation of the derived rates is best accomplished by employing an independent method. In this Symposium, J. Reeve and associates have successfully used histomorphometric methods with double tetracycline labeling to calculate local bone formation rates and correlate these with whole body radiotracer data properly corrected for long term exchange processes.

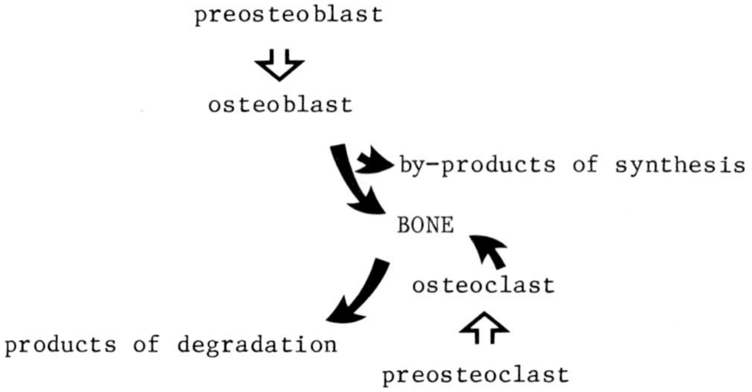

Figure 1. Schematic representation of bone formation and resorption.

As suggested in Fig. 1, the synthetic activities of osteoblasts might be monitored without direct bone sampling, were byproducts of the matrix components that become part of bone quantitatively released and easily measured. Moreover, the release of degradation products of bone resorption could provide an accurate index of these processes. Considerable effort has been devoted to measurements of collagen-related markers, particularly total urinary hydroxyproline excretion. Many investigators have relied on this measurement in the evaluation of metabolic bone diseases. Unfortunately, total urinary hydroxyproline represents only 10-20% of that released from collagen degradation since free hydroxyproline released from collagen-derived oligopeptides is oxidized to a number of other products. In individuals excreting relatively low amounts of urinary hydroxyproline, e.g. osteoporotics, a minor change in catabolism, resulting from therapy, could account for major changes in hydroxyproline excretion. Furthermore, significant amounts of urinary hydroxyproline are derived from collagen sequences other than bone, particularly in those individuals excreting <40 mg/day. For these reasons, other measurements have been used such as hydroxylysine and its glycosides which more accurately reflect the amount as well as the source of collagen degradation. These methods are tedious but are constantly being modified. K. Kivirikko reviews this subject and in addition discusses measurements of serum levels of posttranslational collagen-modifying enzymes in disease states.

Collagens are synthesized as procollagens, molecules with extra sequences at either end which must be cleaved when the mature fibril is formed extracellularly. L.S. Simon discusses preliminary observations on the use of radioimmunoassays for two of the procollagen extensions to evaluate changes in Paget's disease and other conditions. The procollagen extensions are examples of byproducts of synthesis shown in Fig. 1, but it should be noted that the aminoterminal peptides may also have a regulatory role in feedback control of collagen formation.

One of the recently developed markers for the noncollagenous proteins of bone involves radioimmunoassay for bone GLA protein. This 49-amino acid polypeptide is produced by osteoblasts and the rate of its synthesis is subject to endocrine control. It is probably synthesized at some stage in bone formation later than that of such noncollagenous proteins as osteonectin, and its role in bone remains to be defined. Nevertheless, this GLA protein is unique to bone and circulates in normal human plasma. Moreover, as discussed by L. Deftos and associates, circulating levels change in bone diseases and in response to alterations in parathyroid hormone secretion. Whether levels of bone GLA protein primarily reflect bone formation or resorption remains to be determined.

Several of the noncollagenous proteins of bone are not produced by bone cells but become part of the extracellular matrix in the course of bone formation. Albumin and α_2-HS glycoprotein are two examples. The α_2-HS glycoprotein is synthesized in the liver, released into the circulation and selectively taken up by bone. Thus, levels of this protein in plasma might reflect, inversely, rates of bone formation. R. Smith and associates discuss the results they have obtained using a radioimmunoassay for α_2-HS glycoprotein in patients with metabolic bone diseases. This direction of changes in the levels of the protein are as predicted, although their magnitude is not great enough for this measurement to be widely utilized.

In order to adequately quantitate bone formation a measurement that reflects osteoblastic activity directly would be highly desirable. Measurements of circulating alkaline phosphatase activity have been available for over 50 years, since it had been shown that bone is rich in this enzyme and that it is localized predominantly in osteoblasts. Despite this evidence, the role of alkaline phosphatase in bone formation has yet to be defined. The enzyme in bone can be distinguished from that in other tissues using immunological and kinetic methods, as discussed by M.P. Whyte.

It is apparent that considerable progress has been made in development of markers for bone formation and resorption that are not dependent on bone biopsy. Many of the methods for measurement of these markers are currently being developed and should in the future provide accurate and quantitative information for diagnosis and understanding of the pathophysiology of metabolic bone diseases and evaluation of therapy.

REFERENCES

1. Glimcher, M.J., Bonar, L.C., Grynpas, M.D., Landis, W.J. and Roufosse, A.H. (1981): J. Crystal growth, 53, 100.

2. Krane, S.M. and Simon, L.S. (1981): In: The Chemistry and Biology of Mineralized Connective Tissues, p. 185. Editor: A. Veis. Elsevier/North Holland, Amsterdam.

3. Eyre, D.R. (1981): In: The Chemistry and Biology of Mineralized Connective Tissues, p. 51. Editor: A Veis. Elsevier/North Holland, Amsterdam.

4. Termine, J.D., Belcourt, A.B., Conn, K.M. and Kleinman, H.K. (1981): J. Biol. Chem., 256, 10403.

5. Termine, J.D., Kleinman, H.K., Whitson, S.W., Conn, K.M., McGarvey, M.L. and Martin, G.R. (1981): Cell, 26, 99.

TRACER MEASUREMENTS OF BONE REMODELLING AND THEIR SIGNIFICANCE IN INVOLUTIONAL OSTEOPOROSIS

Jonathan Reeve, *Monique Arlot, Richard Hesp, Marisol Tellez and *Pierre J. Meunier

M.R.C. Clinical Research Centre, Harrow, U.K.
and *Unité INSERM 234, "Pathologie des tissus calcifiés", Lyon, France.

The evolutionary significance of bone remodelling in adult man is not completely clear. Recent concepts of plasma calcium homeostasis have emphasised the predominant role of the 'bone fluid compartment' (BFC) in contributing to the short-term stability of the extra-cellular fluid calcium concentration (1). The remodelling process may, however, contribute to plasma calcium homeostasis during prolonged unavailability of dietary calcium in the face of obligatory faecal losses. Remodelling probably also contributes to survival by optimizing the ratio of required skeletal strength to skeletal weight.

Remodelling has received considerable attention because it becomes abnormal in most metabolic bone disorders. Efforts have been directed towards measuring rates of new bone formation and resorption, both locally and in the skeleton as a whole. All in vivo techniques have involved the use of tracers, either of bone mineralization, osteoid formation (2) or cell kinetics (3). In the clinical setting, only measurements of mineral uptake have proved practicable. Kinetic information on related processes such as rates of osteoid formation, osteoblast proliferation and osteoclastic resorption has had to be inferred indirectly using collateral information.

The first studies with bone seeking tracers were performed by Hevesy and his collaborators using ^{32}P. In his 1944 Nobel lecture (4), Hevesy pointed out that ^{32}Phosphate could exchange at bone surfaces accessible to the bloodstream as well as being incorporated into new bone. In order to measure local rates of new bone formation, he administered tracer so as to keep the plasma specific activity constant and determined local bone specific activities of tracer at varying times after commencement of tracer administration. Unfortunately, ^{32}P is an energetic β-emitter and is therefore only poorly localised by autoradiography. It is also extensively taken up by soft tissues, so that no assumptions could be made regarding its partition between hard and soft tissues without their direct examination. Calcium-45 can be better localised autoradiographically than ^{32}P, so it has been used in animal studies to discriminate between exchange and bone forming processes.

The chief use of calcium tracers (^{45}Ca, ^{47}Ca, ^{85}Sr) in man, in whom radiation doses must be restricted, has been to estimate bone turnover non-invasively. Taking advantage of the fact that 99% of calcium is in the skeleton, mathematical models were devised to separate tracer uptake in the exchangeable pools of bone and soft tissues from that taken up by bone formation ('accretion') (5). The experimental data required were serial measurements of plasma specific activity of tracer following an intravenous injection of tracer and the cumulative excretion of tracer with time. These models differed in mathematical detail, being based on largely heuristic considerations rather than independently identified physiological systems of pools and compartments with pre-determined volumes and interconnections. Although this approach generated widespread initial enthusiasm, scepticism arose as evidence accumulated which pointed to the physiological inadequacy of the mathematical models employed.

Criticism of these techniques has been based on one or more of the following criteria. Firstly, long-term calcium exchange processes were documented autoradiographically by Rowlands (6) in quiescent bone which were too slow to be included in the 'exchangeable pools' of any then current kinetic model. This Marshall attributed to solid state diffusion (7), a physico-chemical process also first studied radioisotopically in lead by Hevesy (4). Secondly, the mathematically simpler compartmental models only fitted the data over a limited timespan, a problem which led to the development of increasingly complex compartmental models and new non-compartmental models. The former often proved incapable of adequate measurement precision given the imprecision of real biological data (8). Finally, all the models reviewed and critically compared by Jung (8) overestimated bone turnover as measured independently by studies of radioactive contamination of normal skeletal tissue or by histomorphometry (7). This prompted the development of a new technique for measuring whole body bone formation and resorption rates which gave more realistic estimates of turnover (9). It depended on the use of ^{85}Sr and the acquisition of data for much longer periods than hitherto employed so as to estimate long-term exchange.

Meanwhile, Frost had studied the tetracyclines as in vivo markers of calcification in bone biopsy specimens (10). Tetracyclines complex calcium and are laid down at sites of new bone formation as well as exchanging at blood-accessible bone surfaces. If time is allowed for the tetracycline at non-bone forming sites to exchange back into the circulation, only sites of osteoid mineralization remain labelled. Following two short courses of tetracycline, the distance between labels gives a measure of the thickness of osteoid mineralized in the interval between courses. It has also been suggested that osteoid of normal thickness not taking a double label is mineralizing at a slow or imperceptible rate. However, various doubts remained concerning such interpretations. The gastrointestinal absorption of the drug may be variable, and the bone exposure to a tetracycline depends on its renal excretion and local bone blood flow. The brightness of the labels can depend on tissue fixation and processing, and finally tetracycline is not an 'ideal' tracer in that its metabolic behaviour does not exactly mimic its tracee molecules of calcium and phosphate.

A need remained to validate the discrimination of tetracycline labelled osteoid surfaces from unlabelled osteoid in diseases such as osteoporosis. We had recently shown that in osteoporosis, calculated rates of whole body bone formation correlated significantly with calcium balance data when corrected for 'long-term' exchange but not when calculated without this correction (11). The former result was consistent with recent histomorphometric studies suggesting that bone formation could be reduced substantially in idiopathic osteoporosis (12,13); and for the first time it linked depressed bone formation to a simultaneous loss of bone mineral. It was therefore also essential to determine which of the two kinetic models was correct.

We have now studied 26 patients suffering from idiopathic osteoporosis, who had previously given informed consent, with 8 mm trans-iliac biopsies (preceded by double tetracycline labelling) and near-simultaneous 18-day calcium balance studies. The balances were designed to simulate the patients' normal dietary intake of calcium and phosphate. Measured faecal excretion of calcium was corrected by using the continuously administered marker Cr_2O_3. Undecalcified sections of the biopsies were quantitated for osteoclast numbers ($OCmm^{-2}$), trabecular resorption surfaces (RS%), trabecular osteoid surfaces (OS%), trabecular osteoid surfaces taking a double label (DLS%), the linear apposition rate (CR, µm/day) and osteoid thickness index. The activity of the osteoblasts in forming new bone, relative to the osteoid surfaces they nourished, was calculated as (DLSxCR)/OS; (AOB). AOB, RS and OC all correlated weakly with calcium balance. Much better results were obtained using bivariate regression analysis to allow for the effects of coupling between formation and resorption, so correlating calcium balance independently with one formation and one resorption index. These correlations were significant at the 2% level for the formation activity index (AOB) and at the 1% level for both resorption indices (OC and RS). A separate index of the duration of the reversal phase, during which osteoclasts are replaced by osteoblasts on the resorption surfaces, was devised (RS/OC). This did not correlate significantly with calcium balances.

These results suggest that reduced osteoblast activity can be revealed by a reduced proportion of osteoid taking a tetracycline label as well as by a reduced calcification rate (CR) (14); and that either or both may contribute significantly to bone loss in osteoporosis. Bone loss is also more rapid in patients with a higher activation frequency of new trabecular basic multicellular units as revealed by higher resorption indices.

Most of these patients had simultaneous 6-month studies of ^{85}Sr kinetics from which rates of whole body bone 'formation' were calculated, both corrected and uncorrected for long-term exchange (9). To investigate whether the observed (Fig. 1) early loss of 'accreted' calcium tracer is due to exchange processes rather than rapid resorption of new bone (as some investigators originally postulated (5)), we compared the relative extent of trabecular resorption surfaces (RS%) in the biopsies with the fraction of 'accreted' tracer lost in the first six months after bone uptake.

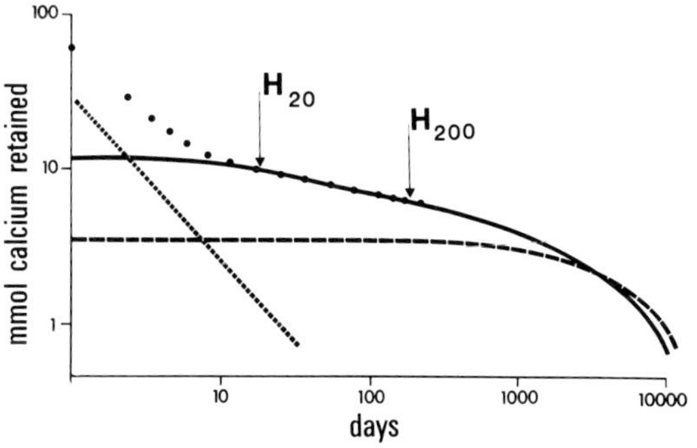

Figure 1. Solid line - single passage retention of one day's uptake of calcium in fixed bone in a normal subject (as traced by ^{85}Sr, for method see ref. 9). The retention in the conventionally accepted (rapidly) exchangeable pools is shown thus .... In the absence of diffuse uptake (6) and long-term exchange (7), a different shaped fixed bone curve would be expected------, unless new bone is preferentially resorbed which seems unlikely (see below). In the absence of preferential resorption, fractional loss of 'accreted' calcium by long-term exchange in the first six months is closely approximated by $(H_{20} - H_{200}) / H_{20}$ (11).

There was no significant correlation ($r=0.21$), suggesting that preferential resorption of new bone does not occur. However, when doubly labelled osteoid surfaces were compared with the fraction of 'accreted' tracer retained at six months, a good correlation was obtained, which did not apply to the unlabelled osteoid (Fig. 2). We also found a better correlation between doubly-labelled osteoid surfaces and exchange-corrected whole body bone formation rates ($n=18$, $r=0.69$, $P<0.002$) than between doubly-labelled surfaces and uncorrected rates ($r=0.49$, $P<0.05$).

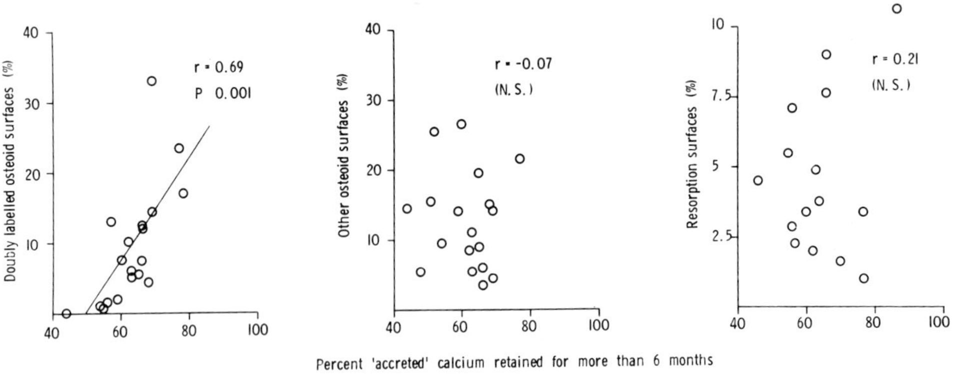

Figure 2. Relationships between three histomorphometric indices in iliac trabecular bone and the percentage of calcium taken into the fixed bone pools which is retained there for at least six months (calculated as 100 H_{200}/H_{20}). The results suggest that retention is better when 'accreted' calcium is subsequently overlaid by new bone as indicated by more extended doubly labelled osteroid seams. Note also the absence of an inverse relationship between resorption surfaces and percentage retention.

These results have two implications. Firstly, the simultaneous use of two independent tracers of local and whole body bone formation has allowed us to validate further the use of double tetracycline labelling for measuring actively mineralizing osteoid surfaces and to demonstrate the importance of making corrections for long-term exchange processes in deriving true rates of bone formation from whole body studies with calcium tracers. Secondly, they support the concept that premature maturation of osteoblasts from the 'cuboidal' to the 'terminal' form, or else their premature death and replacement by flat osteocytes, is an important mechanism contributing to further bone loss in involutional osteoporosis.

It also appears from these and our earlier results (11) that the long-term exchange component of the accretion rate is not only substantial but very variable and depends on osteoblastic activity. It therefore seems justified to advocate the use of our procedure for correcting for this long-term exchange (9) in future studies of bone formation and resorption when a non-invasive approach is required.

REFERENCES

1. Parfitt, A.M. and Kleerekoper, M. (1980): In: Clinical Disorders of Fluid and Electrolyte Medtabolism, p. 269. Editors: Maxwell and Kleeman. McGraw Hill, New York.
2. McLean, F.C. and Budy, A. (1964): Radiation, Isotopes and Bone. Academic Press, New York.
3. Jaworski, Z.F.G., Kimmel, D.B. and Jee, W.S.S. (1983): In: Bone Histomorphometry, p. 225. Editor: R.R. Recker. CRC Press, Boca Raton, Florida.
4. von Hevesy, G. (1944, reprinted 1962): In: Adventures in Radioisotope Research, p. 928. Pergamon Press, New York.
5. Pearson, O.H. and Joplin, G.F. (1964) (Eds.): Dynamic Studies in Metabolic Bone Disease. Blackwell, Oxford.
6. Rowland, R.E. (1964): In: Bone Biodynamics, p. 335. Editor: H.M. Frost. Little Brown, Boston.
7. Marshall, J.H. et al (1973): Health Phys., 24, 125.
8. Jung, A., Bartholdi, P., Mermillod, B., Reeve, J. and Neer, R. (1978): J. Theoret. Biol., 73, 131.
9. Reeve, J., Hesp, R. and Wootton, R. (1976): Calcif. Tiss. Res., 22, 191.
10. Frost, H.M. (1970): Calcif. Tiss. Res., 3, 211.
11. Reeve, J., Green, J.R., Hesp, R. and Hulme, P. (1982): Clin. Sci., 63, 153.
12. Darby, A.J. and Meunier, P.J. (1982): Calcif. Tiss. Int., 33, 199.
13. Parfitt, A.M. et al (1981): In: Osteoporosis, p. 321. Editors: H.F. DeLuca et al. University Park Press, Baltimore.
14. Meunier, P.J., Briancon, D., Vignon, E., Arlot, M. and Charhon, S. (1981): In: Osteoporosis, p. 293. Editors: H.F. DeLuca et al. University Park Press, Baltimore.

Discussion following paper of J. Reeve.

S. KRANE: This has been a discussion in the use of isotope tracers to measure rates of bone formation and resorption, which in the absence of bone biopsies may be useful in evaluating the effects of the movement of mineral into and out of the skeleton.

C. NORDIN: I don't understand why you reached the conclusion that both your Mark One model (Calcif. Tiss. Res., 20, 121, 1976) and the Leed's model, which gave the same answer, overestimated bone turnover. The average value we get with our method is about 250mg a day and that works out to about 2g a week c 100g a year. In a 1000g skeleton that gives a life span of about 10 years.

The evidence from radium and the radiostrontium work suggests that the mean life span of the bone is very close to something like ten years. I think the values that you used and we still find are compatible with all the other observed data.

J. REEVE: The summarized data published by John Marshall et al (Health Physics, 24, 125, 1973) suggested that the radiation exposure work gave a figure of up to double that for the whole skeleton.

Now I appreciate that there is considerable room for discussion as to the fractional turnover rate for trabecular bone, which probably turns over twice as fast in the iliac crest as in the vertebral bodies. Nevertheless, cortical bone probably turns over at a considerably lower rate than 10% a year, probably a third of that. We have not found any evidence of preferential resorption which could explain our kinetic data in terms of the turnover rate that you are suggesting. Do you suggest that there is preferential resorption of newly-formed bone?

C. NORDIN: Whatever your other analyses may show, I'm just going back to your original statement. You said that the long-term radiation data showed that the isotopic methods overestimate the rate of bone turnover; I don't think they do. They may slightly underestimate it, but they don't overestimate it.

J. REEVE: I was merely giving the reason for doing the work in the first place. We now have data which shows that these methods do overestimate bone turnover, unless there is preferential resorption of new bone.

S. KRANE: There may be a preferential resorption of old matrix versus new matrix. There is evidence in animals of a preferential resorption of new matrix. It would be nice if we could have independent methods to validate a method for mineral which would also measure matrix turnover.

EXCRETION OF URINARY HYDROXYPROLINE PEPTIDES IN THE ASSESSMENT OF BONE COLLAGEN DEPOSITION AND RESORPTION

Kari I. Kivirikko

Department of Medical Biochemistry, University of Oulu, Oulu, Finland

Hydroxyproline is found in vertebrate proteins almost exclusively in collagens and a few other proteins with collagen-like amino acid sequences. This amino acid is derived from proline that is hydroxylated only in a peptide-bound form, and essentially all the endogenous free hydroxyproline and peptides containing this amino acid present in biological fluids are derived from the degradation of various forms of collagens. The biosynthesis of these proteins is a complex process and involves a number of intracellular and extracellular post-translational modifications of the newly synthesized polypeptide chains. Isotopic studies have demonstrated that a considerable portion of newly synthesized collagen is rapidly degraded in part inside the cell and in part in the extracellular space. A portion of slightly older collagen is also degraded before being incorporated into the mature collagen fibers, and even the collagen fibers are subject to continuous turnover: they are synthesized and degraded in the body continuously.

The relationship of the urinary hydroxyproline to the metabolism of collagen is thus complex, as changes in the excretion of this amino acid reflect changes in both the rate of collagen synthesis and the rate of collagen degradation. Only about 10% of the hydroxyproline released by the breakdown of collagen in the tissues is found in the peptide-bound form, about 90% being degraded to the free amino acid. The peptides containing hydroxyproline are rapidly excreted into the urine, whereas practically all the free amino acid is reabsorbed in the kidneys and degraded further, eventually to carbon dioxide and urea. The urinary hydroxyproline thus represents only about 10% of the hydroxyproline released by collagen breakdown, over 95% of this amino acid excreted being in the peptide-bound form. Most of these peptides are of small size, but some urinary hydroxyproline is present in nondialyzable polypeptides. The nondialyzable polypeptides containing hydroxyproline appear to be derived mainly from the breakdown of newly synthesized collagens, and therefore fractionation of urinary hydroxyproline into dialyzable and nondialyzable forms may give useful information in some cases (for reviews on urinary hydroxyproline, see refs. 2,4,5).

Measurements of hydroxyproline excretion in patients with certain diseases are now performed in many clinical laboratories on a routine basis. The normal values for hydroxyproline excretion are dependent on age, sex, body size, and dietary intake of hydroxyproline. When the values are determined on gelatin-free diets or in spot urine samples obtained after an overnight fast and are corrected for body surface area or creatinine excretion, the effect of the variables can be minimized. Normal values reported by a number of laboratories using adequate methods for assays of urinary hydroxyproline are in good agreement (2,4). These values can be converted to the amount of collagen degraded in the body by knowing the average content of hydroxyproline in various collagens and by assuming that only about 10% of the hydroxyproline released by collagen breakdown is found in the urinary peptides. Such calculations indicate that the amount of collagen degraded per year in a body of a healthy adult is about 0.4-1.2 kg, and may be as high as 5 kg during normal puberty. These values indicate that the rate of collagen turnover is quite significant even in adults. In diseased states these values can be markedly higher.

Since about half of the body collagen is located in the bones, altered urinary hydroxyproline values are found especially in diseases with bone collagen involvement or in conditions affecting collagen metabolism systemically, such as endocrine disorders. An altered hydroxyproline excretion is thus found in Paget's disease of bone, in neoplastic bone disease, in rickets and osteomalacia, in hyper- and hypothyroidism, in acromegaly, in hyperparathyroidism, in the Marfan syndrome and in some patients with connective tissue disorders. Assays of urinary hydroxyproline may be useful in research on all these disorders. Earlier these assays were also used on a routine basis in the diagnosis and/or follow-up of the bone and endocrine disorders mentioned above and to confirm the diagnosis of the Marfan syndrome. Due to the direct assays currently available for the hormone concentrations, measurements of the hydroxyproline excretion are now only rarely carried out in the endocrine disorders. Therefore the main reasons for hydroxyproline assays for practical purposes are nowadays the bone disorders in which these measurements may be useful in both the diagnosis and the follow-up. It should be especially noted that the hydroxyproline excretion is not usually increased in ordinary physiological osteoporosis, and thus a high urinary hydroxyproline excretion in this condition is highly suggestive of a pathological process.

Hydroxylysine is another amino acid unique to collagens and proteins with collagen-like amino acid sequences. This amino acid is present in part as galactosylhydroxylysine and in part as glucosylgalactosylhydroxylysine, the relative proportion and total content of the two glycosylated hydroxylysines being different for different collagens. These two hydroxylysine glycosides are also found in urine. They are probably not metabolized to the same extent as hydroxyproline, and therefore they may be more quantitative markers of collagen turnover than hydroxyproline. The excretion of hydroxylysine glycosides is altered in the same diseases as the excretion of hydroxyproline, but as the ratio of glucosylgalactosylhydroxylysine to galactosylhydroxylysine is different in different collagens, the ratio in the urine may give information of the origin. For example, the ratio in bone collagen is distinctly lower than that in normal urine. Therefore, in conditions accompanied by an increased hydroxyproline excretion due to bone collagen involvement there is a distinct decrease in the ratio of glucosylgalactosylhydroxylysine to galactosylhydroxylysine, the ratio approaching that found in bone collagen (see 3,5). On the other hand, when patients with Paget's disease of bone and a low urinary ratio of glucosylgalactosylhydroxylysine to galactosylhydroxylysine are given calcitonin, the ratio increases at the same time as the excretion of urinary hydroxyproline decreases (3).

During recent years attempts have been made to develop methods for the estimation of changes in ongoing collagen synthesis in tissues using serum samples. These methods include measurement of three of the post-translational enzymes involved in collagen synthesis: the concentration of the immunoreactive prolyl 4-hydroxylase protein, and the activities of galactosylhydroxylysyl glucosyltransferase and lysyl oxidase. In addition serum assays are available for certain propeptides of procollagens. All these new serum assays may give useful information in some disorders on changes in collagen synthesis (see 1).

REFERENCES

1. Bolarin, D.M., Savolainen, E.-R. and Kivirikko, K.I. (1982): Int. J. Cancer, 29, 401.
2. Kivirikko, K.I. (1970): Int. Rev. Connect. Tiss. Res., 5, 93.
3. Krane, S.M., Kantrowitz, F.G., Byrne, M., Pinnell, S.R. and Singer, F.R. (1977): J. Clin. Invest., 59, 819.
4. Laitinen, O. (1974): Acta Med. Scand., Suppl. 577, 1.
5. Smith, R. (1980): Clin. Sci. 59, 215.

Discussion following the paper of K. Kivirikko

L. RIGGS: It is known that half of collagen resides in bone and half in soft tissue. Of course, these two compartments have different rates of turnover. Could you estimate for us how much of the urinary hydroxyproline is derived from bone and how much from soft tissue?

K. KIVIRIKKO: It is relatively difficult to give such an estimate in normal conditions. However, because half of the body collagen is located in bones, while the other half is located in a number of tissues, diseases with changes in bone collagen turnover are usually accompanied by large changes in hydroxyproline excretion. On the other hand, diseases that are limited to a single tissue other than bone usually show only minor changes in urinary hydroxyproline.

PROCOLLAGEN EXTENSION PEPTIDES AS MARKERS OF COLLAGEN SYNTHESIS

Lee S. Simon and Stephen M. Krane

Department of Medicine, Massachusetts General Hospital and New England Deaconess Hospital, Boston, MA.

Bone is a dynamic organ continually remodelled during life through complex processes of organized cellular activity. Remodelling is initiated by osteoclasts which resorb old bone and is followed by deposition of new bone by osteoblasts. Resorption and formation are tightly coupled in the normal state so that the mass of bone does not change (1). Bone formation involves the synthesis of new organic matrix, in which type I collagen is the most abundant component.

Collagens are synthesized intracellularly as precursor molecules, procollagens, which contain both aminoterminal and carboxyterminal globular extensions. Probably prior to fibril formation these extension peptides are cleaved from the molecule by specific endopeptidases yielding the helical trimers (2). Of the different types of procollagens identified so far, two abundant species are the interstitial types I and III procollagens. The former is the precursor for the predominant collagen type found in bone. Type III procollagen is particularly abundant in vascular and intestinal smooth muscle, skin and uterine tissue, as well as fetal and newborn tissues, but it is not a component of mineralized tissues (3).

Type I procollagen consists of two identical $\alpha1$ (I) chains and one $\alpha2$(I) chain (4). The carboxyterminus (pColl-I-C), one of the extensions of these chains, once cleaved is stabilized by interchain disulfide bonds as a molecule with M_r ∿100,000 (Fig. 1). pColl-I-C circulates in human serum and its levels can be determined by radioimmunoassay (5,6,7).

Type III procollagen consists of three identical $\alpha1$(III) chains, with aminoterminal and carboxyterminal extensions. The aminoterminus (pColl-III-N) once cleaved is stabilized by interchain disulfide bonds proximal to the cleavage site (Fig. 1). pColl-III-N also circulates in human serum as a molecule with M_r ∿45,000. A radioimmunoassay has also been developed to measure levels of this peptide in human serum (5,8,9).

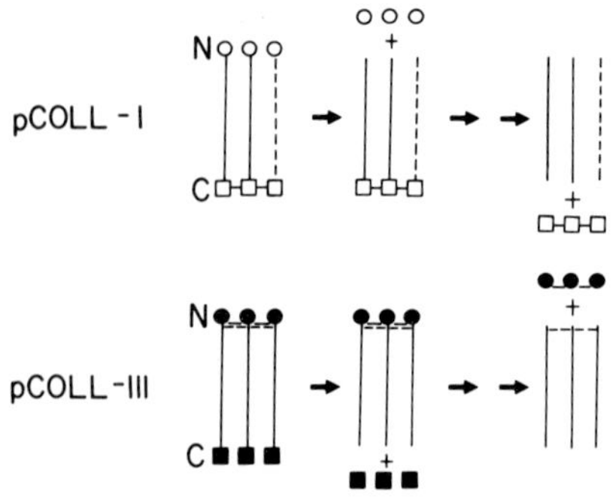

Figure 1. Processing of types I and III procollagens. This schematic diagram

describes the postulated processing of type I (pColl-I) and type III (pColl-III) procollagens. pColl-I is probably processed at the aminoterminus (N) and then at the carboxyterminus (C). Conversely, pColl-III is probably processed first at the carboxyterminus (C) and then at the aminoterminus (N) (8).

We have been studying mechanisms of control of collagen turnover we have used the radioimmunoassays to measure levels of these peptides in serum in different conditions, examples of which will be described. Antigen and antibody for the pColl-I-C assay were obtained from B. Goldberg, and kits for the pColl-III-N assay were obtained from Hoechst.

EFFECTS OF PARATHYROID HORMONE

It has been demonstrated in organ or cell cultures and cell-free translation systems that parathyroid hormone (PTH) inhibits collagen synthesis. Evidence indicates that control is at the level of transcription since levels of translatable type I procollagen mRNA are decreased in bone pretreated with PTH (10). PTH also increases the activity of the 25(OH)vitamin D-1α hydroxylase enzyme resulting in increased levels of $1,25(OH)_2D$; $1,25(OH)_2D$ also decreases collagen synthesis in vitro (11). We therefore asked whether measurement of serum levels of procollagen extension peptides would provide information about effects of PTH in vivo.

Our approach was to infuse synthetic human PTH 1-34 intravenously for 24 hours in two normal and six osteoporotic individuals and measure at intervals serum levels of pColl-I-C, pColl-III-N, ionized calcium and $1,25(OH)_2D_3$. In all instances, serum levels of pColl-I-C fell (nadir between 16-20 hours of infusion; mean nadir 56% [range 39-82%] of initial values) and returned toward initial values 14 h after discontinuing PTH (to mean 92% [range 76-108%] of initial values) (12). In contrast, pColl-III-N levels did not fall, but tended to rise to mean 153% [range 120-189%] of initial values, 14 h after discontinuing PTH. The changes were observed whether or not levels of $1,25(OH)_2D$ rose with the PTH, while levels of pColl-I-C were negatively correlated with ionized calcium in each subject (mean r= -0.77 [range -0.63 to -0.99]). The levels of pColl-III-N reached their peak at the time when ionized calcium returned towards preinfusion levels.

These results are consistent with PTH suppression of bone collagen synthesis, since the decreases in serum levels of the procollagen peptides were observed only for the type I peptides. We do not yet know the significance of the rise in the type III peptides. Perhaps it could be related to the replacement of marrow with the reticular stroma (probably type III collagen) that characterizes the bone disease of hyperparathyroidism.

PAGET'S DISEASE OF BONE

Paget's disease of bone is a useful model for studying bone resorption and formation in humans, since the changes are often of great magnitude and the pagetic process is responsive to pharmacological manipulation. We have corroborated previous data of elevated levels of pColl-I-C in sera of pagetic patients compared to normal subjects (13). We found that in 11 normal subjects, ages 21-55, the mean levels of pColl-I-C were 89 ng/ml with a maximum value of 190 ng/ml, while 22/26 pagetic subjects had levels in excess of 190 ng/ml and mean levels of 314 ng/ml. Unexpectedly, we also found high levels of pColl-III-N in pagetic sera. The mean in these same subjects was 27.4 ng/ml with levels in 20/21 patients greater than 12 ng/ml, contrasted with a mean level of pColl-III-N in 11 normal subjects of 9.7 ng/ml with a maximum of 12.0 ng/ml (13). The elevation of levels of pColl-I-C correlated with the extent of increased bone turnover as estimated by measurements of urinary hydroxyproline excretion or serum alkaline phosphatase activity.

Since the turnover of pagetic bone can be modified by drugs, we also assessed the acute effects of salmon calcitonin and the chronic effects of dichloromethylene diphosphonate. Administration of salmon calcitonin, resulted in decreases in serum levels of pColl-I-C which paralleled the fall in urinary hydroxyproline excretion. The levels of pColl-III-N also decreased but to a lesser degree (14). In other subjects, treatment with dichloromethylene diphosphonate produced a fall in the levels of pColl-I-C which were correlated with a fall in serum levels of alkaline phosphatase (13). Serum levels of pColl-III-N also fell, but did not reach the normal range. Our assumption is that the levels of pColl-I-C in Paget's disease reflect the synthesis of bone collagen proper whereas those of pColl-III-N reflect the synthesis of the reticular stroma found interspersed among the bone spicules. If our results accurately describe these processes, then this therapy does not completely suppress the abnormality of increased synthesis of reticular stroma.

We cannot be certain whether these changes observed in levels of pColl-I-C or pColl-III-N are indices of decreases in collagen resorption, new collagen synthesis, or both. Salmon calcitonin decreases osteoclast functions and presumably secondarily decreases osteoblast functions through putative local coupling factors (15,16). Glucocorticoids have previously been found to suppress activity of Paget's disease (17). We have found that single doses of 30 mg of prednisone suppress serum levels of pColl-I-C and pColl-III-N without a decrease in urinary hydroxyproline excretion (18). This presumptive dissociation of osteoclastic function (no change in urinary hydroxyproline excretion) from suppressed osteoblastic function (decreasing serum levels of pColl-I-C and pColl-III-N) is some evidence that the serum procollagen peptides are derived from collagen synthesis rather than resorption.

CORRELATION OF CIRCULATING PROCOLLAGEN PEPTIDES WITH HISTOMORPHOMETRY

We have initiated a pilot project in collaboration with M. Parfitt, Henry Ford Hospital, to measure serum levels of pcoll-I-C and pColl-III-N in patients in whom bone histomorphometric data are available. Six osteoporotic subjects had "low turnover" osteoporosis by biopsy criteria. All of these had low serum levels of pColl-I-C (mean 44 ng/ml ± 17.9 ng/ml SD; range 29-77 ng/ml). The levels of pColl-III-N were normal (mean 7.1 ng/ml ± 1.0 ng/ml SD; range 6.3 - 9.1 ng/ml). In other individuals with increased bone turnover, high levels of pColl-I-C were found.

SUMMARY

Serum levels of pColl-I-C as well as pColl-III-N are increased in states of increased bone turnover, such as Paget's disease, and decrease with therapy. The changes in the circulating procollagen extension peptides probably reflect changes in collagen synthesis. The alterations in levels of pColl-I-C probably reflect changes in new bone type I collagen synthesis while the alterations in levels of pColl-III-N probably reflect changes in tissues other than bone per se. In Paget's disease and hyperparathyroidism serum levels of pColl-III-N may be derived from increased marrow fibrosis interspersed among pagetic bone spicules. Measurements of these procollagen fragments should continue to provide markers for bone matrix useful for understanding pathophysiology and results of therapy of metabolic bone diseases.

REFERENCES

1. Krane, S.M. (1981): In: Pathophysiology, the Biological Principles of Disease, p. 755. Editors: L.H. Smith and S. Thier. W.B. Saunders, Philadelphia, PA.

2. Prockop, D.J., Kivirikko, K.I., Tuderman, L., and Guzman, N.A. (1979): New Engl. J. Med. 301, 13, 77.
3. Gay, S. and Miller, E.J. (1978): Collagen in the Physiology and Pathology and Pathology of Connective Tissue. Gustav Fischer, Stuttgard and New York.
4. Hofman, H., Fietzek, P.P., and Kühn K. (1980): J. Mol. Biol. 141, 293.
5. Nowack, H., Olsen, B.R., and Timpl, R. (1976): Eur. J. Biochem. 70, 205.
6. Goldberg, B., and Scherr, C.J. (1973): Proc. Natl. Acad. Sci. (U.S.A.) 70, 361.
7. Taubman, M.B., Goldberg, B., and Scherr, C.J. (1974): Science 186, 1115.
8. Fessler, L.I., Timpl, R., and Fessler, J.H. (1981): J. Biol. Chem. 256, 2531.
9. Rohde, H., Vargas, L., Hahn, E., Kalbfleisch, H., Briguera, M., and Timple, R. (1979): Eur. J. Clin. Invest. 9, 451.
10. Kream, B.E., Rowe, D.W., Gworek, S.C., and Raisz, L.G. (1980): Proc. Natl. Acad. Sci. (U.S.A.) 77, 5654.
11. Rowe, D.W., and Kream, B.E. (1982): J. Biol. Chem. 257, 8009.
12. Simon, L.S., Slovick, D.M., Wortman, P.D., Neer, R.M., and Krane, S.M. (1982): Clin. Res. 30, 476A.
13. Taubman, M.B., Kammerman, S., and Goldberg B. (1976): Proc. Soc. Exp. Biol. Med. 152, 284.
14. Simon, L.S., Kovitz, K.L., Krane, I.M., Krane, S.M. (1981): Arthritis Rheum. 24 (suppl), S58.
15. Canalis, E., Peck, W.A., and Raisz, L.G. (1980): Science 210, 1021.
16. Farley, J.R., Masuda, T., Wergedal, J.E., and Baylink, D.J. (1982): Biochemistry 21, 3508.
17. Albright, F. and Henneman, P.H. (1955): Trans. Assoc. Am. Physc. 68, 238.
18. Simon, L.S., Kovitz, K.L., Krane, I.M., Wortman, P. and Krane, S.M. (1982): Calcif. Tiss. Int. 34(suppl), S35.

Discussion following paper by L. Simon

L. RAISZ: The changes in the blood level could, of course, reflect a change in clearance. Is there any way you can assess how this material is cleared from the body? Does any of it appear in the urine or is it degraded by the liver or kidney?

L. SIMON: We have done studies to look for levels of the carboxy-terminal portion of Type I procollagen in urine and have not found any. We presume that the molecule must be degraded in the kidney or bladder.

G. PALMIERI: Do patients with Paget's disease who have elevated procollagen Type III have normal parathyroid function? What is the explanation for elevation of Type III procollagen when Paget's disease involves bone?

L. SIMON: Tests for parathyroid function have been normal. We presume, although we do not have any data to prove it, that the Type III amino terminal peptide is derived from the increased marrow fibrosis juxtaposed to areas of increased bone turnover.

K. KIVIRIKKO: Studies of O. Niemela and others in our laboratory have indicated that antigens related to the amino-terminal propeptide of Type III procollagen are found in at least three different peaks in gel filtration and that these forms do not give identical displacement curves in radioimmunoassay. Accordingly, one of the next steps in studies of these antigens should be attempts to improve the radioimmunoassay so that one is measuring only one of the three serum forms.

S. KRANE: The idea is that these peptides, too, are metabolized in measuring the heterogeneous pool of metabolizable peptides.

BGP AND BONE METABOLISM

Leonard J. Deftos and Bayard D. Catherwood

The Endocrine Section of the University of California and the San Diego Veterans Administration Medical Center, La Jolla, California, U.S.A.

The skeletal system is involved by many disease processes. Although the pathogenesis of these diseases is complex and multifactorial, two basic abnormalities of bone metabolism seem to be present - abnormalities of bone resorption and abnormalities of bone formation (1, 2). However, identifying and quantitating the skeletal abnormalities for diagnosis and treatment have been difficult because of the lack of sensitive, specific, and convenient methods to evaluate bone metabolism.

Many procedures have been used to assess bone metabolism. These include radiological, radionuclear, radiogrammetric, and densitometric evaluation of the skeleton; histological examination of biopsy specimens; scanning and radionuclide procedures; measurements of collagen and related substances; and the measurement of alkaline phosphatase. Although these procedures have been very useful and have provided important information about skeletal metabolism, each of these methods has its limitations in regard to specificity, sensitivity, and/or practicality. Newer procedures for evaluating skeletal status are continually being introduced and some seem quite promising (3-9). However, despite their improvement in sensitivity, even these methods do not have the specificity and convenience that a serum or urine biochemical marker for bone metabolism would.

Alkaline phosphatase and hydroxyproline and other collagen-related substances have been widely used as biochemical markers for bone metabolism. Although they have been useful and can be quantitated better than the previously mentioned procedures, they too have significant limitations (1,2).

A radioimmunoassay for bone Gla protein (BGP) has been recently developed and applied to measurements of this protein in the serum of a series of normal subjects and patients with a wide variety of bone diseases (10,11). BGP is our name for the 49-amino acid protein which contains up to three γ-carboxyglutamic acid (Gla) residues and which comprises a significant percent of total bone protein (12-16). This protein has been also referred to in the literature as Gla-protein and osteocalcin (17-21). The biological function of this protein has not been established and is the subject of active research. BGP seems to be produced by the osteoblast and Gla residues are produced at specific sites by post-translational carboxylation, conferring on the peptide an affinity for binding divalent cations and hydroxyapatite (22-25). BGP synthesis is regulated by the calcitropic hormones (11, 25-26). Thus, BGP may be involved in the mineralization process although its exact role is not clear (18,26). The carboxylation of the glutamic acid residues of BGP seems to play an important role in the biological properties of this protein (12). Carboxylation confers upon BGP its property of binding to calcium, other divalent cations, and hydroxyapatite; thus, carboxylation may be important in determining the function of BGP in the formation and/or maturation of bone (12-13, 26). Human BGP is unique among all species of the peptide thus far characterized in demonstrating heterogeneity of γ-carboxylation (14). Since Gla residues are absolutely required for binding to hydroxyapatite, it is possible that this heterogeneity plays an important role in the predisposition of humans to metabolic bone disease compared with lower mammals and other vertebrates. Although the exact details of this process have not been worked out, it is of obvious importance to be able to recognize the carboxylated versus the non-carboxylated forms of BGP.

In general, those bone diseases that are characterized by increased bone turnover are accompanied by an increased blood level of BGP (10, 25). The serum concentrations of BGP correlate in a general way with plasma alkaline phosphatase determinations (25). However, there are important examples of the dissociation between these two measurements and there are several examples in which the measurement of BGP seems to be a better index of bone disease than alkaline phosphatase. For example, significant changes could be detected in the plasma BGP concentrations during treatment of several bone diseases whereas significant changes in serum alkaline phosphatase do not occur (10). In addition, BGP has the important advantage over alkaline phosphatase in that it is a specific marker for bone disease. Thus, unlike alkaline phosphatase, its plasma levels are not contributed to by any other organs. We have also demonstrated that BGP is a more sensitive index of bone metabolism than is calcitonin, and glucocorticoids under conditions where alkaline phosphatase does not change (10,11,27). As a radioimmunoassay procedure, the detection of BGP can be readily adapted to measurements in a large number of plasma samples. Therefore, there is every reason to anticipate that the radioimmunoassay of BGP will become an important procedure in assessing skeletal metabolism (10, 25).

Most of the evidence indicates that BGP is produced by the osteoblast and thus reflects bone formation (24,26,28). However, the response of BGP to $1,25(OH)_2D$, estrogens and glucocorticoids, and especially the rapid response to calcitonin, all suggest that BGP reflects bone resorption. The administration of calcitonin and the steroids, both inhibitors of bone resorption, decreased serum BGP (27,29,10,30). Whereas, the effect of steroids on BGP may be explained by coupling of resorption and formation, the effect of calcitonin on BGP is so rapid (11) that a direct (rather than coupled effect) is more likely. A slight increase in BGP formation seems to occur in some patients with osteoporosis and is also consistent with this view (11). One laboratory has also recently reported an increase with age of BGP in females and this is more consistent with a correlation of BGP and bone resorption (30). This can be contrasted with reports supporting the formation hypothesis from two laboratories that BGP decreases with age (10,17). Therefore, the issue of whether BGP reflects bone formation or bone resorption remains unresolved. The development of techniques which could separately identify changes in bone formation and bone resorption could provide a powerful tool for the independent and separate study of these two processes and their perturbations in disease and therapy.

In order to improve the clinical value of radioimmunoassays for hBGP we are developing a series of assay systems based on peptide fragments of the molecule. We have already demonstrated the feasibility of such an approach by developing a radioimmunoassay based on a 13-amino-acid carboxy-terminal peptide of bovine BGP (27,29). This peptide was coupled with carbodiimide to keyhole limpet hemocyanin and used to raise antibodies in rabbits. The peptide was radiolabelled by the glucose oxidase method and subsequently purified by high pressure liquid chromatography. The purified tracer was then used to screen antibodies and one of the antibodies was found to result in a sensitive radioimmunoassay. This assay has preferential sensitivity and specificity for detecting changes in human plasma BGP which reflect alterations in bone metabolism.

Supported by the National Institutes of Health, The American Cancer Society, and the Veterans Administration.

REFERENCES

1. Avioli, L.V. (1977): Am J Physiol 242:E82.
2. DeLuca, H.F., Frost, H.M., Jee, W.S.S., Johnston, C.C., Jr., and Parfitt, A.M. (1981): Clin Chim Acta 27:2002.
3. Chesnut, C.H., III, Nelp, W.B., Baylink, D.J., and Denny, J.D. (1977): Metabolism 26:267.
4. Cohn, S.H., Zanzi, I., Waswani, A., Wallach, S., Aloia, J., and Ellis, K.J. (1975): In: Nielsen S.P. and Hjorting-hansen, E. (eds). Calcified Tissues 1975, pg. 375. FADL Publishing Co., Copenhagen.
5. Greenfield, M.A., Carven, J.D., Huddleston, A., Kehrer, M.K., Wishko, D., and Stern, R. (1981): Radiology 138:701.
6. Huddleston, A.L. (1978): Phys Med Biol 23:523.
7. Lurye, D.R., Castronovo, F.P., Jr., and Potsaid, M.S. (1977): J Nucl Med 18:1069.
8. Pullan, B.R. and Roberts, T.E. (1978): Br J Radiol 51:24.
9. Wallace, J.D. (1974): J Am Med Assoc 230:447.
10. Price, P.A., Parthemore, J.G., and Deftos, L.J. (1980): J Clin Invest 66:878.
11. Deftos, L.J., Parthemore, J.G., and Price, P.A. (1982): Calcif Tis Intl 34:121.
12. Gallop, P.M., Lian, J.D., and Hauschka (1980): New Engl J Med 302:1460.
13. Lian, J.B., Carnes, D., and Holtrop, M.E. (1982): Proceedings of the Fourth Annual Mtg of the American Society for Bone and Mineral Research Abstract #S51.
14. Poser, J.W., Esch, F.S., Ling, N.C., and Price, P.A. (1980): J Biol Chem 255:8685.
15. Price, P.A. and Nishimoto, S.K. (1980): Proc Natl Acad Sci 77:2234.
16. Price, P.A., Poser, J.W. and Raman, N. (1976): Proc Natl Acad Sci 73:3374.
17. Gundberg, C.M., Lian, J.B. and Gallop, P.M. (1982): Proceedings of the Fourth Annual Mtg of the American Society for Bone and Mineral Research, Abstract #S31.
18. Lian, J.B., Reit, B., Roufosse, A.H., Glimcher, M.J., and Gallop, P.M. (1979): IN: Suttie, J.W. (ed.) Vitamin K Metabolism and Vitamin K-Dependent Proteins, pg 237. University Park Press, Baltimore.
19. Patterson-Allen, P., Brautigam, C.E., Grindeland, R.E., Asling, C.W., and Callahan, P.X. (1982a): Analyt Biochem 120:1.
20. Patterson-Allen, P.E., Callahan, P.X., and Young, D.R. (1982b): Proceedings of the Fourth Annual Mtg of the American Society for Bone and Mineral Research, Abstract #S12.
21. Slovik, D.M., Gundberg, C.M., Lian, J.B., and Neer, R.M. (1982): Proceedings of the Fourth Annual Mtg of the American Society for Bone and Mineral Research, Abstract #S15.
22. Hauschka, P.V. and Carr, S.A. (1982): Biochemistry 21:2538.
23. Hauschka, P.V., Lian, J.B. and Gallop, P.M. (1975):Proc Natl Acad Sci 72:3925.
24. Nishimoto, S.K. and Price, P.A. (1979): J Biol Chem 254:437.
25. Price, P.A. and Baukol, S.A. (1980):J Biol Chem 255:8685.
26. Price, P.A. and Baukol, S.A. (1981): Biochem Biophys Res Commun 99:928.
27. Catherwood, B.D. (1982): Proceedings of the Fourth Annual Mtg of the American Soceity for Bone and Mineral Research, Abstract #S29.
28. Price, P.A., Lothringer, J.W., Baukol, S.A. and Reddi, A.H. (1981a); J Biol Chem 256:3781.
29. Catherwood, B.D.: J Clin Elect Met, submitted.
30. Delmas, P.D., Stenner, D., Wahner, H.W. Mann, K.Gl, Riggs, B.L.: Proceedings of the Fourth Annual Mtg of the American Society for Bone and Mineral Research, pg. S-4.

Discussion following the paper of L. Deftos

A. TASHJIAN: Could you tell us how the concentrations of bone GLA protein in plasma change with the patient's vitamin K status? What happens to patients being anticoagulated with coumarin-type drugs?

L. DEFTOS: In the normal clinically applicable coumarin doses, there are no changes in concentration. If you give experimental animals large doses of coumarin, you can lower the BGP levels.

PLASMA ALPHA 2HS GLYCOPROTEIN AND BONE FORMATION

R.Smith, S.Vipond and B.A.Ashton

MRC Bone Research Laboratory and Nuffield Orthopaedic Centre, Headington, Oxford, U.K.

Alpha 2HS glycoprotein is a circulating polypeptide (MW 49 000 daltons) which is synthesised in the liver and concentrated selectively into mineralising bone about 100 times with respect to other plasma proteins, probably by preferential adsorption from tissue fluid into forming hydroxyapatite surfaces (1). After injury or inflammation its plasma concentration falls, probably due to a fall in hepatic synthesis. Additionally, alpha 2HS glycoprotein has the properties of a non-specific opsonin; it promotes phagocytosis by neutrophils and macrophages, enhances the endocytosis of DNA by macrophages and binds via a specific receptor to EBV-transformed lymphocytes (4). In a previous study (2) we could detect no significant difference with age or sex in the alpha 2HS concentration in 58 normal adults (104% ± 2.4 of a standard plasma containing 63 mg per 100 ml); Dickson, Bagga and Paterson (3) have recently recorded similar values but note that they are higher in men (mean 64.8 mg per 100 ml, age 20-60) than in women of comparable age, in whom there was a progressive decline in mean values from 63.2 mg per 100 ml at 21-30 years to 57.3 mg per 100 ml at 51-60 years).

In 24 adults with Paget's disease of bone the mean alpha 2HS concentration was significantly lower than normal(2). There was also a significant inverse correlation between the plasma alkaline phosphatase and alpha 2HS glycoprotein concentrations; and on treatment with calcitonin or the phosphonate EHDP the alpha 2HS glycoprotein increased as that of alkaline phosphatase fell. It was concluded that the abnormally low pretreatment values of alpha 2HS glycoprotein could be quantitatively accounted for by the known increase in bone formation (mineralisation) rate in Paget's disease; but the rapidity and extent of the change in concentration of this glycoprotein during effective treatment was not explained by the reduced formation rate which such treatment eventually produced. It was considered possible the alpha 2HS degradation was reduced at the site of bone resorption, or that hepatic synthesis was increased.

Subsequently we have measured the circulating alpha 2HS concentrations in a variety of bone disorders and examined the changes in individual patients during treatment. The results suggest further ways in which changes in bone physiology may affect the concentration of alpha 2HS glycoprotein.

PATIENTS AND METHODS

Patients studied included those with acquired and inherited disorders of bone matrix (osteoporosis and osteogenesis imperfecta), with excessive skeletal bone formation (osteopetrosis, melorheostosis and Engleman's disease), with ectopic ossification (fibrodysplasia ossificans progressiva), with defective mineralisation (osteomalacia and fibrogenesis imperfecta ossium) and with excessive bone resorption (hyperparathyroidism). Patients with Paget's disease (Fig 1) were treated with dichloromethylene diphosphonate (Cl_2 MDP), and those with disorders of mineralisation with vitamin D or its metabolites.

RESULTS

Apart from patients with Paget's disease no consistent abnormalities were found in other bone disorders, but the numbers studied were small. Treatment of 10 patients with Paget's disease with Cl_2 MDP produced a significant increase in plasma alpha 2HS glycoprotein.

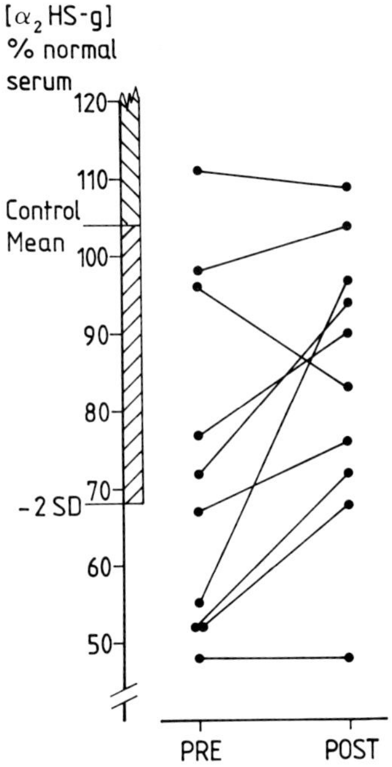

Figure 1. Plasma alpha 2HS glycoprotein concentration (expressed as percent of normal) in 10 patients with Paget's disease, before and after 3 months treatment with Cl_2 MDP. Significance of difference between the two groups, P less than 0.05 (Wilcoxon matched pairs signed-ranks test).

Two adults with the clinical and histological features of fibrogenesis imperfecta ossium were given 1 alpha hydroxycholecalciferol. This produced a temporary decrease in alpha 2HS glycoprotein concentration which closely mirrored the increase in total urinary hydroxyproline excretion, an indicator of bone resorption (Fig 2), and less so that of plasma alkaline phosphatase. Similar changes occurred in a patient with post-gastrectomy osteomalacia given parenteral 24,25 dihydroxycholecalciferol.

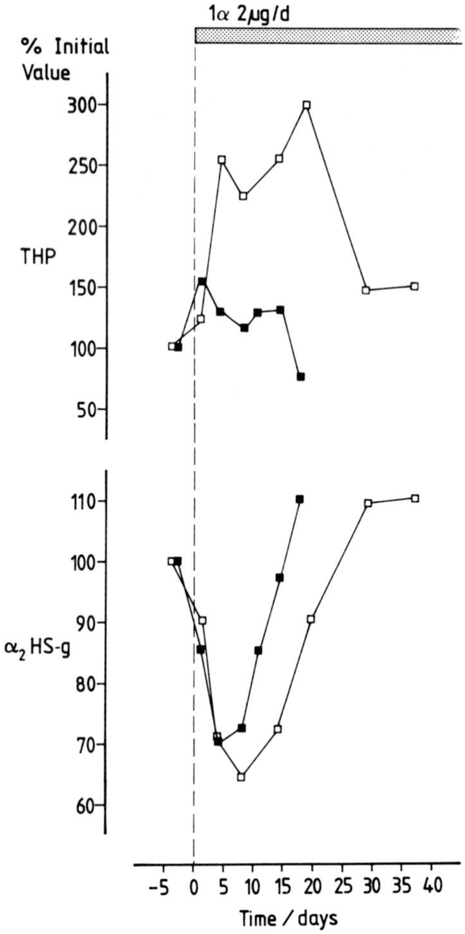

Figure 2. Changes in the concentration of plasma alpha 2HS glycoprotein and the urinary total hydroxyproline excretion in two patients with defective mineralisation treated with 1 alpha hydroxycholecalciferol. Values expressed as percent of pretreatment measurements.

DISCUSSION

Since alpha 2HS glycoprotein is known to be incorporated into mineralising bone (1), low plasma concentrations are not unexpected when there is a prolonged increase in bone formation rate, as in Paget's disease. Our current results on patients with Paget's disease confirm previous findings (2), but the preliminary sequential data obtained during the treatment of patients with disorders of mineralisation suggest that changes in bone resorption rate may affect the plasma alpha 2HS glycoprotein concentration.

The acute effect of calcitonin therapy on patients with Paget's disease is to decrease bone resorption rate, and coincidentally to increase plasma alpha 2HS glycoprotein levels (2). Conversely this study has shown that in the early stages of healing osteomalacia, when bone resorption is known to be elevated, there is a concomitant reduction in the alpha 2HS glycoprotein concentration in plasma. It is not known whether this association between the resorption rate and plasma alpha 2HS glycoprotein levels is due to actual utilisation of the glycoprotein by the resorbing cells (in the same way as alpha 2HS glycoprotein is consumed during phagocytosis), or to the removal of alpha 2HS glycoprotein from tissue fluid by adsorption on to the mineral surfaces recently exposed by resorption. A cyclic action of osteoclasts stripping alpha 2HS glycoprotein from mineral surfaces, resorbing mineral, and then resting during which time alpha 2HS glycoprotein would be adsorbed on to the exposed hydroxyapatite surfaces, could be a major pathway of alpha 2HS glycoprotein turnover. Measurement of changes in alpha 2HS glycoprotein concentration in other bone disorders where bone formation and resorption are temporarily dissociated, as after parathyroidectomy, could be of use in testing these hypotheses. While measurement of the basal plasma concentration of alpha 2HS glycoprotein in most bone diseases has, so far, been clinically unrewarding, it has opened new avenues for the consideration of the interaction between bone mineral, interstitial fluid proteins and bone cells.

REFERENCES

1. Ashton, B.A., Hohling, H.J. and Triffitt, J.T. (1976): Calcif. Tiss. Res, 22, 27
2. Ashton, B.A. and Smith, R. (1980): Clin. Sci, 58, 435
3. Dickson, I.R., Bagga, M. and Paterson, C.R. (1983): Calcif. Tissue. Int. 35, 16
4. Lewis, J.G., Crosier, P.S. and Andre, C.M. (1982): FEBS Lett, 138, 37

Discussion following paper by Roger Smith

S. KRANE: I guess since a_2S glycoprotein makes up about 25% of the non-collagenous proteins in bone, it must be taken up from plasma in some regular percentage because the numbers are fairly tight. Do you think it could be taken up in the process of bone formation?

R. SMITH: Yes. I think that was the original idea. Certainly in growing animals it is taken up in bone formation. However, I do not think there is a good estimate of how much is taken up in man.

S. KRANE: From the serum levels that you were measuring?

R. SMITH: Yes.

S. KRANE: These measurements are going to be around for some time and workers are going to be sorting out the data to determine what they mean in relationship to bone disease.

ALKALINE PHOSPHATASE AND THE MEASUREMENT OF BONE FORMATION

Michael P. Whyte

Division of Bone and Mineral Metabolism, Departments of Medicine and Pediatrics, Washington University School of Medicine and Metabolic Research Unit, Shriners Hospital for Crippled Children; St. Louis, Missouri, U.S.A.

ROLE FOR ALKALINE PHOSPHATASE IN BONE FORMATION?:

Since the discovery of alkaline phosphatase (AP) by Robison in 1923, considerable evidence has linked this enzyme with formation of the skeleton (1). Robison's pioneering work revealed that growing bone is especially rich in phosphatase activity and that the pH optimum of the enzyme is alkaline. He suggested that AP promoted skeletal mineralization by liberating inorganic phosphate (Pi) from phosphate esters, and that the local increase in Pi concentration led to the deposition of calcium-phosphate salts in bone matrix. Additional circumstantial evidence for a role for AP in bone mineralization began to accumulate rapidly with Kay's report in 1930 that assay of AP activity in blood revealed increased values in a variety of bone disorders, and that the magnitude of the increased activity generally reflected the severity of the skeletal disease. However, it was in 1948 that Rathbun provided what has, in my opinion, come to be the strongest evidence for a direct role of AP in bone formation. Rathbun suggested that the severe rickets which affected an unusual infant patient could be attributed to the paucity of AP activity noted in the child's blood and bone - a disorder he called "hypophosphatasia" (2). Subsequently, AP activity in bone, liver, and kidney (but not intestine or placenta) has been found to be reduced in the severe recessive infantile form of this disorder. Recent biochemical studies - which reveal that three separate genes code for a placental, intestinal, and "bone/liver/kidney" AP isoenzyme - complement Rathbun's findings and indicate that hypophosphatasia is an "inborn-error-of-metabolism" characterized by some defect(s) in the production of the bone/liver/kidney family of "secondary" AP isoenzymes. Severe rickets as the clinical expression of an inherited autosomal recessive defect characterized by profound deficiency of the bone/liver/kidney AP isoenzyme, therefore, provides firm evidence that AP plays a critical role in bone formation.

MECHANISM OF ALKALINE PHOSPHATASE ACTION IN SKELETAL MINERALIZATION:

The prevalent hypothesis concerning how AP promotes bone mineralization centers on three discoveries of the 1960's (2): i) Anderson and coworkers found that the initial site of bone mineral deposition occurs in extracellular "matrix vesicles" produced by osteoblasts and chondrocytes; ii) Fleisch and colleagues demonstrated that inorganic pyrophosphate (PPi) was an inhibitor of hydroxyapatite crystal formation and dissolution, and iii) Russell and coworkers documented that blood and urine PPi levels were increased in patients with hypophosphatasia. As a result, AP is currently believed to promote mineralization in matrix vesicles when its PPiase action releases Pi for bone salt deposition while hydrolyzing the inhibitor (PPi) of hydroxyapatite crystal formation (2). However, controversy concerning the precise role of AP in bone mineralization persists. It stems, in part, from studies where steriospecific inhibitors of AP have been used in vitro to assess mineralization. Toxic effects of these substances are difficult to distinguish from direct effects due to AP inhibition.

Although there is controversy concerning the precise role of AP in bone mineralization - and evidence that the physiological role of AP may be more complex than to act simply as a PPiase (1) - assay of circulating total AP (TAP) activity remains an inexpensive, reproducible, and readily available parameter which clinicians have found helpful to investigate and follow patients with a variety of skeletal diseases. The question I have been asked to address briefly in this review is whether or not assay of circulating AP activity is a useful way to assess underlying rates of bone formation.

CIRCULATING ALKALINE PHOSPHATASE ISOENZYMES:

Before one interprets the clinical significance of a level of circulating TAP activity or considers TAP in an attempt to predict the bone formation rate in a given individual or in a group of patients, it should be recalled that circulating AP activity is generally the sum of the activity of two or more AP isoenzymes (1). TAP activity measured in the blood of normal adult subjects represents approximately equal contributions by two AP isoenzymes - one presumeably derived from bone (BAP), the other from liver (LAP). Infants and children normally have high circulating TAP activity because of increased BAP. However, a considerable number of pertubations other than bone disease can increase the circulating TAP activity by introducing or increasing the activity of AP isoenzymes other than BAP. These factors include fatty meals (which increase blood levels of the normally small amount of circulating intestine AP isoenzyme), pregnancy (where a placental AP isoenzyme appears in the blood during the last trimester), a large number of medications and a variety of hepatic diseases (which increase circulating LAP activity), and finally a variety of malignancies which produce "ectopic" forms of AP, e.g. (Regan isoenzyme). Also, it is of considerable importance to remember that circulating BAP (TAP) activity can increase in diseases which characterize both extremes of skeletal formation rates, i.e. disorders associated with accelerated bone remodeling - whether local (Paget's bone disease) or generalized (hyperthyroidism or hyperparathyroidism) - and those characterized by a mineralization defect (e.g. most types of rickets and osteomalacia). Fortunately, assay of blood TAP activity largely reflects BAP in individuals with uncomplicated bone disease, and disorders characterized by extremes in skeletal remodeling activity are generally easily distinguished. Therefore, assay of TAP remains a useful biochemical parameter to follow during therapy for many metabolic bone diseases. Even here, however, there are pitfalls i.e., circulating TAP activity (BAP) may increase transiently with initiation of effective therapy as skeletal mineralization is normalized (e.g. treatment of vitamin D deficient rickets or osteomalacia) or following fracture. Despite all of these potential difficulties in the interpretation of circulating AP activity, several studies have suggested that blood AP activity does indeed reflect the underlying rate of bone formation.

CIRCULATING *TOTAL* ALKALINE PHOSPHATASE ACTIVITY AND BONE FORMATION RATES:

Net bone formation rates can be assessed indirectly by a variety of techniques including serial radiologic procedures (radiographs, neutron-activation-analysis, dual-photon-absorptiometry, and computerized-axial-tomography), metabolic balance studies, and radioisotope accretion rates, or directly by histomorphometric analysis of undecalcified bone biopsy specimens following sequential tetracycline "labels". Assay of urine hydroxyproline (HP) remains a standard technique to indirectly measure bone resorption, but is also used to assess bone formation rates since skeletal mineralization and resorption are generally "coupled".

Paget's bone disease - characterized by focal acceleration of bone remodeling - has been associated with the highest recorded levels of circulating TAP activity. Several studies suggest that the blood TAP activity reflects the rate of bone formation in this disorder. Circulating TAP generally parallels the extent and activity of Paget's disease, i.e. patients with polyostotic disease usually have higher serum TAP activity than those with monostotic disease, and patients with sclerotic or "healed" lesions often have relatively low levels. Furthermore, when bone formation is assessed indirectly (assuming coupled rates of bone remodeling) by assay of urine HP, a close correlation has been found between circulating TAP activity and urine HP excretion. Also, studies of Ca^{47} accretion have revealed that circulating TAP activity correlates well with calculated rates of skeletal mineralization in Paget's bone disease.

Not all studies, however, have concluded that the activity of circulating TAP activity reflects the underlying rate of bone formation. In 1970, Shifrin reported failure of serum TAP activity to predict the results of direct measurement of bone formation in rib biopsy specimens from patients with a variety of metabolic diseases (3). He concluded that "no useful correlation was found between serum alkaline phosphatase values and lamellar bone formation in 67 patients with metabolic and other bone diseases". However, his study contained numerous problems in design including: i) use of hand-ground sections of bone which were frequently labeled once instead of twice with tetracycline, ii) study of subjects who had recently undergone fracture, iii) a patient population which included 11 individuals with osteomalacia, and iv) "there were so many associated medical conditions, and such a variety of past and present medications, that the influence of these findings or the results cannot be statistically determined".

In an excellent study reported in 1977, Lauffenburger and colleagues investigated 15 patients with "low" skeletal turnover (postmenopausal osteoporosis) and six with "high" turnover (Paget's bone disease) (4). A variety of static histomorphometric parameters of bone formation (determined with iliac crest specimens) as well as Ca^{47} accretion were found to be highly correlated with blood TAP activity for each disease group (e.g., $r=0.94$, $p<0.01$ and $r=0.69$, $p<0.01$ for the relationship between TAP and Ca^{47} accretion in untreated Pagetic and osteoporotic patients, respectively) and especially when data from both groups were combined. My colleagues and I, however, found a poor correlation ($r=0.15$) between circulating TAP activity and a direct measurement of bone formation (cellular rate of mineralization) in 26 women with untreated postmenopausal osteoporosis who had received two tetracycline labels prior to biopsy (5).

CIRCULATING *BONE* ALKALINE PHOSPHATASE ACTIVITY AND BONE FORMATION RATES:

The utility of assaying circulating TAP levels to predict bone formation rates in the less extreme abberations of skeletal remodeling is compromised because of the problem of multiple circulating AP isoenzymes. A quick and accurate quantitative method to assay BAP activity is not available (1). The two principle circulating forms of AP (LAP and BAP) are "secondary" isoenzymes which differ from one another only by post-translational modification and are, therefore, difficult to quantitate separately. Consequently, fewer studies have been published where circulating BAP activity has been painstakenly assessed by heat inactivation, electrophoretic, and/or chemical inhibition studies and then compared with bone formation rates.

Stepan and coworkers, however, reported in 1978 that when circulating BAP activity is quantitated using inactivation/inhibition procedures, it has a strong positive correlation with urine HP excretion not only in a variety of bone diseases - including osteoporosis ($r=0.80$), primary hyperparathyroidism ($r=0.84$), Paget's disease ($r=0.95$), metastatic bone disease ($r=0.86$), and osteomalacia ($r=0.94$) - but in control subjects as well ($r=0.82$) (6).

CONCLUSIONS:

AP plays a critical role in bone mineralization. The few studies which have examined the relationship between circulating TAP (or BAP) activity and bone turnover suggest that the activity of this enzyme is positively correlated with bone formation. However, the presence of several circulating AP isoenzymes and the potential for a variety of pertubations to mask basal circulating BAP activity minimizes the utility of a single TAP assay in the individual patient. Furthermore, assay of BAP activity is currently an expensive and time consuming research procedure. Recently, generation of monoclonal antibodies to placental and intestinal AP, and recently to the bone/liver/kidney isoenzyme, hold promise that circulating BAP may soon be quickly and accurately quantitated by immunological methods. When better assays for BAP become available, studies to determine their precision in reflecting bone remodeling kinetics, especially in patients with osteoporosis, will be an important area for research.

REFERENCES:

1. McComb RB, Bowers GN Jr., Posen S: Alkaline Phosphatase, Plenum Press, New York, 1979.

2. Rasmussen H: Hypophosphatasia, in The Metabolic Basis of Inherited Disease 5th Ed., edited by J.B. Stanbury, J.B. Wyngaarden, D.S. Fredrickson, J.L. Goldstein, M.S. Brown. 1983, McGraw-Hill Book Company, New York, pp. 1497-1507.

3. Shifrin LZ: Correlation of serum alkaline phosphatase with bone formation rates. Clin. Orthop. 70: 212-215, 1970.

4. Lauffenburger T, Olah AJ, Dambacher et al: Bone remodeling and calcium metabolism: a correlated histomprhometric, calcium kinetic, and biochemical study in patients with osteoporosis and Paget's disease. Metabolism 26: 589-606, 1977.

5. Whyte MP, Bergfeld MA, Murphy WA, Avioli LV, Teitelbaum SL: Postmenopausal osteoporosis: a heterogeneous disorder as assessed by histomorphometric analysis of iliac crest bone from untreated patients. Am. J. Med. 72: 193-202, 1982.

6. Stepan J, Pacovsky V, Horn V, et al: Relationship of the activity of the bone isoenzyme of serum alkaline phosphatase to urinary hydroxyproline excretion in metabolic and neoplastic diseases. Eur. J. Clin. Invest. 8: 373-377, 1978.

Discussion following paper by M. Whyte

S. KRANE: Alkaline phosphatase, which has been around for a long time, may be one of the better markers for osteoblast activity.

L. RAISZ: How certain are we that the enzymes from liver and bone are really different?

M. WHYTE: I think the evidence is quite good that there is a single alkaline phosphatase gene in man for the bone, liver and kidney isoenzyme. Nevertheless, electrophoretic, heat denaturation and inhibition studies have shown that the bone and liver isoenzyme in man are quite different. These differences are due to post-translational modifications. I do not think anyone knows whether or not there may be additional differences in disease states; for example, if circulating alkaline phosphatase in Paget's disease is precisely the same bone alkaline phosphatase that we assay in growing children.

S. KRANE: What is the nature of the post-translational modification that distinguishes the isoenzymes?

M. WHYTE: It has not been well characterized but the alkaline phosphatases contain a considerable amount of carbohydrate.

M. PARFITT: If you examine the evolution of vitamin D deficiency at the stage when patients have secondary hyperparathyroidism and not osteomalacia, the alkaline phosphatase is high and the bone formation rate measured by the tetracycline method is high. However, when the disease progresses to a more advanced stage with osteomalacia, the bone formation rate measured by tetracycline decreases and the alkaline phosphatase increases even further. How do you explain this clear-cut discrepancy between the formation of mineralized bone and the alkaline phosphatase level?

M. WHYTE: I do not have a good explanation but the clinical observation is that circulating alkaline phosphatase activity increases when there seems to be an attempt, successful or unsuccessful, to enhance bone mineralization.

R. WEINSTEIN: Perhaps one of the best illustrations of the alkaline phosphatase relation to mineralization and turnover of bone is in renal osteodystrophy. There is data to suggest that the level of the alkaline phosphatase activity in the serum relates directly to the mineralization rate as measured by double tetracycline labeling and when osteomalacia occurs in renal osteodystrophy the alkaline phosphatase levels are inappropriately low. This may be a worrisome biochemical sign in a patient with subperiosteal resorption and renal failure. I think this observation supports the role of alkaline phosphatase in mineralization more than almost any other evidence.

M. WHYTE: I agree. Your data show that in renal osteodystrophy the blood alkaline phosphatase activity does reflect bone formation rates assessed by iliac crest biopsy after double tetracycline labeling. In the study from St. Louis by Hruska and coworkers, it was especially predictive of peritrabecular fibrosis and bone resorption, rather than formation.

L. DEFTOS: It may be that the increase in alkaline phosphatase is due to its underutilization, if it does in fact play a role in the mineralization process. I would like to ask Dr. Whyte if he thinks that monoclonal antibodies offer any advantages over polyclonal antibodies in the development of simple radioimmunoassay procedures for alkaline phosphatase?

M. WHYTE: I think they will. For example, polyclonal antibodies have not been successful in distinguishing bone and liver isoenzymes.

L. DEFTOS: No, they have not, but I think that there are successful radioimmunoassays for alkaline phosphatase based on polyclonal antibodies and that the problems will be the same for both methods.

V PATHOGENESIS OF HYPERPARATHYROIDISM

PATHOGENESIS OF HYPERPARATHYROIDISM

Louis M. Sherwood

Departments of Medicine and Biochemistry, Albert Einstein College of Medicine, Bronx, New York 10461, U.S.A.

Primary hyperparathyroidism, with the advent of routine screening procedures for calcium, has been recognized as an extraordinarily common disorder, often increasing in frequency in the elderly. Secondary hyperparathyroidism is associated with chronic renal failure and may also occur in patients with malabsorption, vitamin D deficiency and other causes of a low serum calcium. The papers in this session deal with various aspects of normal parathyroid cell biology and biochemistry and abnormalities that have been identified in hyperplastic or adenomatous glands. Although recognition of the clinical disorders is relatively straightforward and diagnosis by radioimmunoassay relatively simple (despite the caveats of PTH radioimmunoassay), there is much that needs to be learned about normal and abnormal control mechanisms, and we have limited specific information on pathogenetic factors, particularly in primary hyperparathyroidism.

During the past two decades, PTH from man, the cow, and a number of other species has been purified, sequenced and the critical features of peptide structure necessary for biologic activity determined. The biosynthesis of hormone and its precursor forms has been elaborated, the precursor has been synthesized in cell-free systems, and the complete sequence of DNA coding for hormonal mRNA and most of the genomic DNA identified. These issues are reviewed in the discussion by Sherwood and colleagues. There is extraordinarily little information at present on control mechanisms operating at the biosynthetic level, but the first evidence has been provided by our laboratory for a direct effect of calcium on levels of mRNA in the parathyroid cell. Certainly, a great deal of new information needs to be obtained, but the sophisticated tools of molecular biology are now readily available, and these issues should be approachable within the near future. With the paucity of data on regulation of biosynthetic mechanisms in normal glands, there is no data at all on these issues in adenomatous or hyperplastic glands. That should also be forthcoming.

Much more has been learned about regulation of hormone secretion, and these issues have been explored extensively in vitro and in in vivo by a number of workers including Sherwood, Brown, Cohn, Fischer, Mayer, Aurbach, Potts, Williams and others. The use of isolated parathyroid cells to study aspects of normal and abnormal secretion will be reviewed by Brown, and a definition of parameters of secretion such as maximal secretory rate, set point, slope of the curve at its midpoint and minimal secretory rate defined. It has been well-documented that minimal secretion occurs both in vivo and in vitro despite calcium concentrations higher than normal, and this factor contributes to overall secretory rate in hyperparathyroidism. Increases in set point (calcium level at which 50% suppression of PTH secretion occurs) in some patients with primary hyperparathyroidism is considered a significant factor in the oversecretion of hormone. The relative contributions of "set point" and "minimal secretory rate" (related to cell number) are discussed. A variety of agents other than low calcium have now been defined as secretogogues for PTH, including beta agonists, dopamine, histamine, secretin and prostaglandins, and these appear to

Supported in part by USPHS Grant Number AM 28556

work through adenylate cyclase and cyclic AMP, but their physiologic importance has not been defined. Likewise, it has not been demonstrated convincingly that beta blockers or histamine receptor antagonists are useful in controlling secretion of hormone from patients on any chronic basis, lessening the potential significance of these agents as agonists of secretion. The mechanisms by which low calcium, other divalent cations such as magnesium and the other agonists that work through cyclic AMP stimulate secretion are being defined. There is some data on the interaction of calcium and other regulators in abnormal parathyroid glands, but it is incomplete.

Finally, almost no information is present in the area of regulation of cell growth and number, both benign (hyperplasia, adenoma) and malignant (carcinoma). Jackson describes an interesting approach to assessing pathogenesis in terms of the measurement of glucose 6-phosphate hydrogenase in parathyroid adenomas. Although these fascinating studies suggest that adenomas are polyclonal in origin and imply that there may be stimulatory factors that result in primary hyperplasia, the nature of such factors at present is very obscure. The only factor known to cause parathyroid hyperplasia is a low serum calcium, which readily produces such changes in animals maintained on a low calcium diet and in patients with renal failure and other disorders such as malabsorption or vitamin D deficiency in which the serum calcium is low. Such individuals usually have a low or normal serum calcium, unless they have such marked hyperplasia of the glands that a hypercalcemic state results. The latter has been described with chronic renal failure and malabsorption, but it is unusual. Much more common, however, is the hypercalcemia that occurs in the post renal transplant state. These individuals, who have developed marked secondary hypertrophy and hyperplasia of their glands as a result of hypocalcemia and vitamin D deficiency and also have resistance to PTH action, then have correction of renal function by transplantation. The hyperplastic parathyroid tissue is still present, and with the loss of resistance to PTH action, and the restoration of normal vitamin D metabolism, hypercalcemia commonly results. The parathyroid tissue, when tested, is usually not autonomous, but behaves like hyperplastic glands. It is impressive that many of these patients have persistent hyperplasia for years post transplant, and it is not at all clear that hyperplastic glands, once developed, regress adequately. A similar model has been produced by the transplantation of multiple normal parathyroid glands into a single rodent.

We know so little about the factors that generate parathyroid hyperplasia, particularly at the subcellular or membrane level, or the factors that might lead to regression. This session is intended to provide an introduction to this area and to open up a number of provocative issues which will be dealt with more adequately at subsequent conferences as new data unfolds.

CELL BIOLOGY OF THE PARATHYROID GLAND AND ITS RELATIONSHIP TO HYPERPLASIA

Louis M. Sherwood, John Russell and Girija Bhargava

Departments of Medicine and Biochemistry, Albert Einstein College of Medicine, Bronx, New York 10461, U.S.A.

In recent years, there has been considerable progress in understanding the biochemistry of parathyroid hormone and its biosynthesis, storage and secretion. The focus of this discussion will be on aspects of normal parathyroid cell anatomy, biochemistry and physiology that are potentially relevant to cell regulation in the hyperplastic or adenomatous gland.

ANATOMY OF THE CELL

The normal parathyroid contains several cell types, although the most active is the chief cell. This cell consists of both active and inactive variants, with inactive cells predominating (14). In the resting phase, parathyroid cells are large, have relatively straight membranes and abundant glycogen, lipid and lipofuscin bodies. Granular endoplasmic reticulum and free ribonucleoprotein particles are dispersed. There is limited Golgi and relatively few peripheral secretory granules. During hormone synthesis, the cells become smaller in size, increased membrane tortuosity develops, and there is enlargement of the Golgi as well as aggregation of the endoplasmic reticulum. As secretion begins, mature granules fuse with the cell membranes and release hormone. The cells then increase their size and reaccumulate glycogen and lipid, followed by a decrease in Golgi and return to the involuted state. In hyperplastic glands, on the other hand, a much larger portion of the cells are in the active, rather than the inactive phase (14).

REGULATION OF HORMONE SYNTHESIS, STORAGE AND SECRETION

The subcellular events in the parathyroid gland have been well characterized. The first event in hormone synthesis involves transcription of DNA to heterogeneous nuclear RNA, which is processed further to mRNA which codes for the sequence of pre-proPTH (5). Pre-proPTH consists of 115 amino acids, including the sequences of pre-proPTH, proPTH and PTH. The "leader or signal" sequence is cleaved as the newly-synthesized hormone is transported through the endoplasmic reticular membrane into the subcellular transport system. It then moves to the Golgi apparatus where it is packaged into pro-secretory granules, and conversion of proPTH to PTH occurs (5). Although there are theoretically several sites of potential calcium regulation during translation and processing to PTH, there has been no evidence as yet to document any effect of calcium. Moran et al (12) showed increased amino acid incorporation into proPTH with low calcium, but other studies (9) show that low calcium increases nonspecifically the synthesis of all proteins in the parathyroid cell. Heinrich et al (9) were not able to detect any effect at 7 hours of high or low calcium on hybridizable mRNA. Recent studies by our group (15), using similar techniques, showed a direct effect of high calcium on decreasing mRNA

Supported in part by USPHS grant number AM28556.

over a 12-72 hour period. Further studies, using the sophisticated and sensitive tools of molecular biology, both _in vitro_ (isolated cells and tissue culture) as well as in glands manipulated _in vivo_, should be helpful in elucidating the regulatory control of biosynthesis.

REGULATION OF PTH BIOSYNTHESIS AND SECRETION

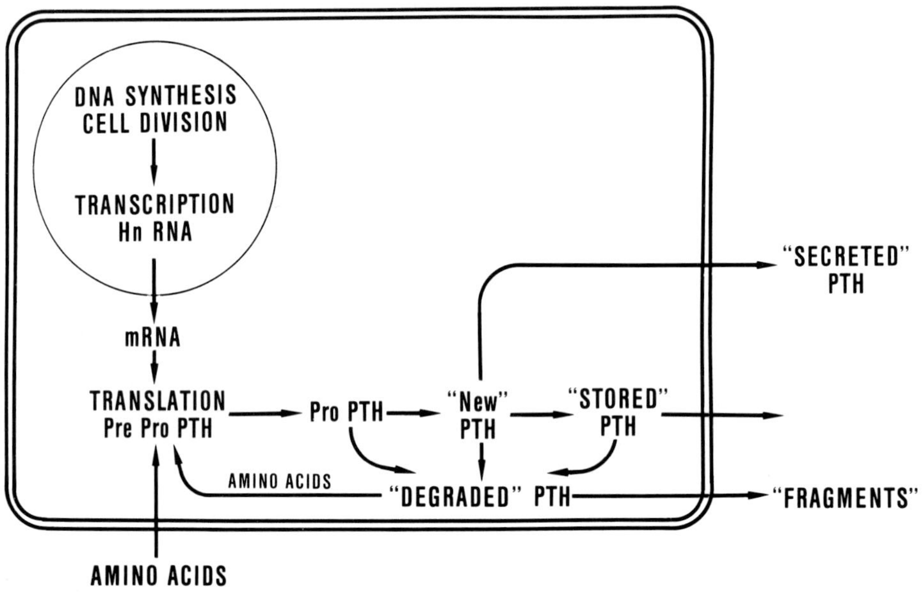

Figure 1. Potential control points in the biosynthesis, storage, degradation and secretion of PTH.

Studies by Cohn et al (4) and our own group (8) suggest that there are two pools of PTH in the gland. Agents that stimulate beta receptors and increase adenylate cyclase activity seem to discharge stored hormone, whereas low calcium enhances the release of both newly-synthesized as well as stored hormone. The relationship between extracellular calcium and secretion of hormone has been well studied, both _in vivo_ and _in vitro_ (3,4,6-8,16).

There is considerable evidence that calcium enhances the degradation of hormone intracellularly (6,7). This process leads not only to generation of small peptides and amino acids, but also to the direct release of fragments into the circulation, particularly at high calcium (7). Whether these fragments are the same as those generated in the periphery from the metabolism of PTH remains to be determined, but heterogeneity in peripheral blood may result both from extracellular and intracellular degradation. Whether the effects of calcium regulation are through cytosolic calcium or membrane effects has not yet been determined. Despite extensive data on regulation of secretion in normal and abnormal glands, there is a paucity of data on biosynthesis, which now depends on the new techniques of molecular biology.

PARATHYROID SECRETORY PROTEIN

During in vitro PTH synthesis, incorporation of amino acids into secreted peptides larger than PTH was identified. Kemper et al (10) first showed that there was a predominant polypeptide of 70,000 daltons, and that there was an inverse correlation between release of this protein (parathyroid secretory protein or PSP) and calcium. Majzoub et al (11) demonstrated a "leader sequence" of 18 amino acids in the protein precursor, and it was suggested that PSP was in the secretory granules (4). We have recently purified bovine PSP (18), shown by radioimmunoassay that it is released in parallel with PTH during a variety of in vitro manipulations (17) and have identified it as a phosphorylated protein, phosphorylation being inversely related to calcium (1). A similar protein, chromogranin A, appears to be in the adrenal medulla (2) as well as other endocrine tissues. Although the exact function and biologic importance of the peptide is not known, it appears to be a protein present in secretory cells. Its active phosphorylation suggests that it may be an important protein in relation to control of hormone secretion.

HYPERPLASIA OF THE PARATHYROID AND ABNORMAL SECRETION

The normal human parathyroid gland is approximately 30mg in weight (14). Even a modest parathyroid adenoma may double the amount of tissue. In children the parathyroid is composed of rather uniform sheets and cords of chief cells, with relatively few fat cells. At birth, the total weight is less than 10mg, and there is continuous growth in both total and parenchymal weight up to age 25-30, where these plateau (parenchymal weight being approximately three-quarters of total weight). Throughout life there is an increasing number of stromal fat cells, which in older persons may occupy 60-70% of the gland.

The pathogenesis of parathyroid hyperplasia is at present obscure. Except for the well-known effects of a low calcium diet in stimulating hyperplasia, and the hyperplasia that occurs in patients with chronic renal failure and malabsorption, pathogenetic factors responsible for cell division are poorly understood. There are genetic disorders in which hyperparathyroidism is present, and these consist primarily of the multiple endocrine neoplasia syndromes I and II. The histologic abnormality of the parathyroids is always hyperplasia; presumably this abnormality is on a genetic basis, but there may be other environmental or local factors. A second factor identified in some patients with hyperparathyroidism is childhood irradiation to the head and neck (13). Not only thyroid carcinoma, but also carcinoma of the salivary glands and parathyroid adenomas may occur. While this is a risk factor in those who received irradiation, it is not a factor in the majority of patients. One can only speculate concerning humoral, metabolic or growth factors responsible for hyperplasia. In addition to low calcium, agents such as beta agonists, dopamine, histamine, secretin and prostaglandins stimulate secretion (3,4,8,16). These effects are generally short-term and from a limited pool of hormone, and there is no evidence that these agents cause hyperplasia. At the same time, one must be open to the possibility that certain humoral or metabolic factors will be identified which could account for the hyperplastic response.

CRITICAL QUESTIONS

Finally, in pursuing issues of parathyroid hyperplasia related to cell biology, one would raise several important questions:

1. What subcellular signals regulate the biosynthesis of PTH, and what links between hormone secretion and biosynthesis exist?
2. What subcellular signals cause hyperplasia to occur during chronic stimulation of the gland, and over what time frame does this occur?

3. What factors other than low calcium cause parathyroid hyperplasia?
4. What abnormalities in the control of hormone synthesis and secretion are present in abnormal glands?
5. Why is hyperplastic tissue once developed so slow to regress? This is particularly a problem in patients with chronic renal failure who have secondary hyperparathyroidism and who have renal allografts.
6. What factors, genetic or metabolic, are responsible for hyperplasia in the familial syndromes?

REFERENCES

1. Bhargava, G., Russell, J. and Sherwood, L.M. (1983): Proc. Natl. Acad. Sci., 80, 878.
2. Bhargava, G. and Sherwood, L.M. (1983): Clin. Res., 31, 469A.
3. Brown, E.M., Hurwitz, S. and Aurbach, G.D. (1977): Endocrinology, 100, 1696.
4. Cohn, D.V. and MacGregor, R.R. (1981): Endocr. Rev., 2, 1.
5. Habener, J.F. (1981): Ann. Rev. Physiol., 43, 211.
6. Habener, J.F., Kemper, B. and Potts, J.T., Jr. (1975): Endocrinology, 97, 431.
7. Hanley, D.A., Takatsuki, K., Sultan, J.M., Schneider, A.B. and Sherwood, L.M. (1978): J. Clin. Invest., 62, 1247.
8. Hanley, D.A., Takatsuki, K., Birnbaumer, M., Schneider, A.B. and Sherwood, L.M. (1980): Calcif. Tissue Int., 32, 19.
9. Heinrich, G., Kronenberg, H.M., Potts, J.T., Jr. and Habener, J.F. (1983): Endocrinology, 112, 449.
10. Kemper, B., Habener, J.F., Rich, A. and Potts, J.T., Jr. (1974): Science, 184, 167.
11. Majzoub, J.A., Kronenberg, H.M., Potts, J.T., Jr., Rich, A. and Habener, J.F. (1979): J. Biol. Chem., 254, 7449.
12. Moran, J.R., Barn, W., Tiechschmid, C.R. and Fischer, J.A. (1981): Endocrinology, 108, 2264.
13. Rao, S.D., Frame, B., Miller, M.J., Kleerekoper, M., Black, M.A. and Parfitt, A.M. (1980): Arch. Intern. Med., 140, 205
14. Roth, S.I. (1979): In: Endocrinology, pp. 587-592. Editor: L. DeGroot Grune and Stratton, New York.
15. Russell, J., Lettieri, D. and Sherwood, L.M. (1983): Clin. Res., 31, 546A.
16. Sherwood, L.M., Hanley, D.A., Takatsuki, K., Birnbaumer, M.E., Schneider, A.B. and Wells, S.A. (1977): In: Proceedings of the Sixth Parathyroid Conference, p. 301. Excerpta Medica, Amsterdam.
17. Sherwood, L.M., Takatsuki, K., Porat, A., Shin, K.Y. and Jackimek, A. (1981): Clin. Res., 29, 579A.
18. Takatsuki, K., Schneider, A.B., Shin, K.Y. and Sherwood, L.M. (1981): J. Biol. Chem., 256, 2342.

THE TWO-HIT THEORY OF NEOPLASIA: IMPLICATIONS FOR THE PATHOGENESIS OF HYPERPARATHYROIDISM

Charles E. Jackson

Division of Clinical Genetics, Department of Medicine, Henry Ford Hospital, Detroit, Michigan, U.S.A.

The advent of routine serum calcium screening (2) has demonstrated that hyperparathyroidism is a surprisingly common condition and yet its pathogenesis remains largely an enigma. The cause of most cases of hyperparathyroidism is unknown although cellular environmental factors as with chronic renal failure and malabsorptive states are obvious factors in some cases. Mutation in a neoplastic process must also be implicated in those cases of hyperparathyroidism associated with radiation (10) and in those patients with hereditary hyperparathyroidism (6) and the multiple endocrine neoplasia syndromes.

Albert Einstein is quoted (3) as stating in 1926, "on principle, it is quite wrong to try founding a theory on observable magnitudes alone. In reality the very opposite happens. It is the theory which decides what we can observe." Knudson (8) in 1971 proposed a two-mutational-event theory for the initiation of neoplasia and postulated that a comparison of ages of onset of hereditary and sporadic retinoblastoma was compatible with such a model. In his theory both events occur in somatic cells in sporadic or non-hereditary patients and the tumors are generally solitary. In hereditary neoplasms, the first event is a germinal or genetic mutation that makes many cells susceptible to tumorigenesis, presumably by way of a second event which is probably a somatic mutation that transforms a mutant cell into a tumor cell. The purpose of this presentation is to discuss the contributions this theory can make towards a better understanding of the pathogenesis of the parathyroid cell proliferation associated with hyperparathyroidism.

Although hereditary hyperparathyroidism is known to have a generally earlier age of onset than the sporadic conditions (6), it has not been possible to compare age of onset curves as did Knudson (8) with retinoblastoma. However, data regarding this theory have been obtained by studying parathyroid tumors utilizing the X chromosome-linked enzyme glucose-6-phosphate dehydrogenase (G-6-PD) to determine the number of cells from which the tumors arose. Studies of three G-6-PD heterozygous females (5), showed both G-6-PD enzymes in all parathyroid tumors as evidence of their multicellular development. Multicellular origin of parathyroid tumors was reported later in 7 additional patients with hyperparathyroidism (7). As a consequence of inactivation of one X chromosome in XX somatic cells, women heterozygous at

Supported in part by PHS grant number CA22595 awarded by the National Cancer Institute, DHHS.

the X-linked enzyme G-6-PD locus for the usual gene (Gd^B) and a variant (Gd^A) have two cell populations, one synthesizing B-type G-6-PD and the other, A-type enzyme. Normal tissues or non-neoplastic hyperplasia of normal tissues show both enzyme types, but neoplasms that develop clonally show a single-enzyme phenotype (B or A). The majority of neoplasms studied with G-6-PD have had single-enzyme phenotypes (4) suggesting that they developed clonally.

Knudson & Meadows (9) suggested that benign hereditary tumors that might result from a single inherited mutation would also be expected to be multicellular in origin since that event could have affected all of the precursor cells before X chromosome inactivation took place (Fig. 1). For a malignancy to develop in a cell of this type of hereditary tumor, a second mutational event would be expected to be initiated in only one cell of multiple hyperplastic cells so that it should develop clonally and therefore manifest only one G-6-PD type. The parathyroid tumors of only one G-6-PD heterozygous woman with hereditary hyperparathyroidism have been studied (7). In this patient each of the three glands removed showed both A and B G-6-PD enzymes in ratios similar to those found in normal tissues. This is compatible with the parathyroid tumors being manifestations of only the first or the genetic mutational event in Knudson's two-mutational-event theory on the initiation of cancer (8).

If hereditary hyperparathyroidism is the result of a first (genetic or germinal) mutational event in Knudson's theory, one would expect that, as a result of a second somatic mutational event, parathyroid cancer would be observed more frequently in families with hereditary hyperparathyroidism and that parathyroid cancer would be expected to occur at an earlier age in those familial cases than with sporadic parathyroid cancers. Support for Knudson's theory is provided by the observations on the age of onset of the eight cases of parathyroid cancer occurring within five families with hereditary hyperparathyroidism in the literature - an earlier average age of onset (35.2 years) was seen compared with 45.3 years in the sporadic cases of parathyroid cancer (7). The reporting of eight cases of such a rarely occurring cancer in five families with hereditary hyperparathyroidism does suggest that individuals with hereditary parathyroid tumors may be at increased risk of developing this type of malignancy. No studies of G-6-PD heterozygous patients with parathyroid cancer in hereditary hyperparathyroidism have been reported.

The finding of multicellular origin is not unexpected in hereditary hyperparathyroidism (7). However, the multicellular origin of sporadic cases is unexpected if they were a result of a mutagenic event. Multicellular origin would be compatible with most hyperparathyroidism being a result of a non-neoplastic process in which unknown factors have stimulated many cells in the parathyroid glands. These findings suggest that parathyroid hyperplasia and adenomas that are difficult to distinguish from each other pathologically may also be similar biologically (5). G-6-PD studies of the parathyroid glands in an appropriate woman with familial hypocalciuric hypercalcemia, in patients with secondary hyperparathyroidism, or in patients with radiation-induced parathyroid tumors would be of interest. Clonal development would be surprising in the first two instances but would be expected in the radiation-induced tumors (7) (Fig. 1).

The G-6-PD data reported by Baylin and coworkers (1) in four

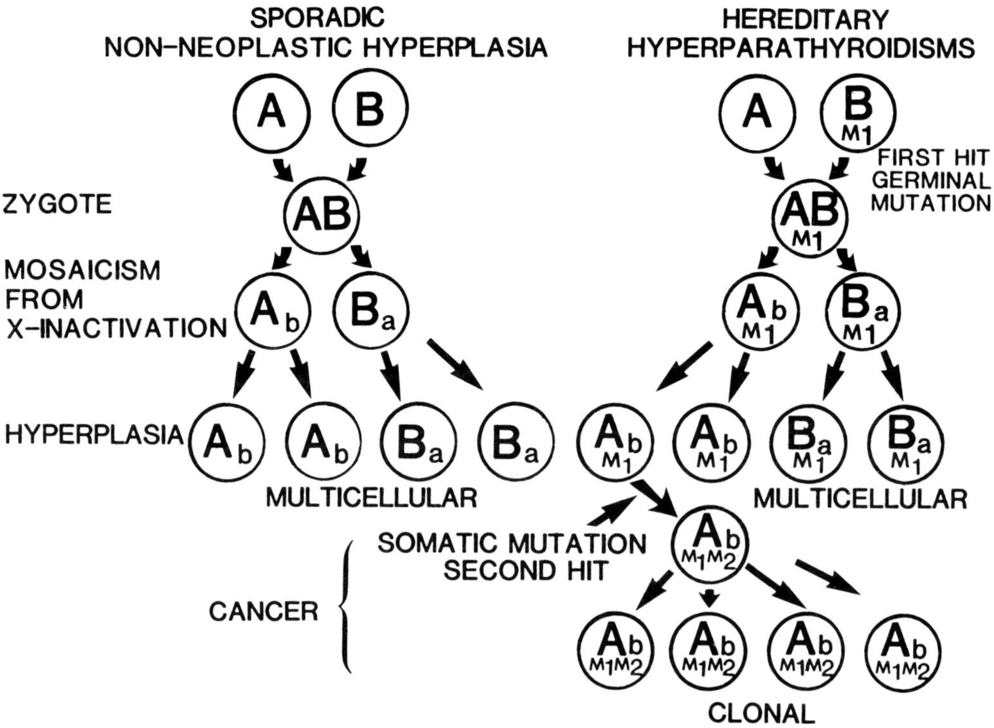

Fig. 1 Schematic representation of proposed events causing an increased parathyroid cell mass in hyperparathyroidism (HPT) - modified from Knudson & Meadows' illustration (9) of the postulated steps on the initiation of neoplasia in general.
Small case a and b = G-6-PD type of an inactivated X.
M_1 = the first mutation (genetic in hereditary HPT and somatic in sporadic mutationally-induced HPT).
M_2 = the second mutation (somatic in both). This results in one cell of a group of hyperplastic cells being converted into a malignant cell.
This model predicts multicellular development of hyperplasia in non-neoplastic HPT and hereditary HPT and is supported by G-6-PD studies(5,7) Clonal development would be expected in hyperplasia of radiation-induced HPT and in parathyroid cancer.

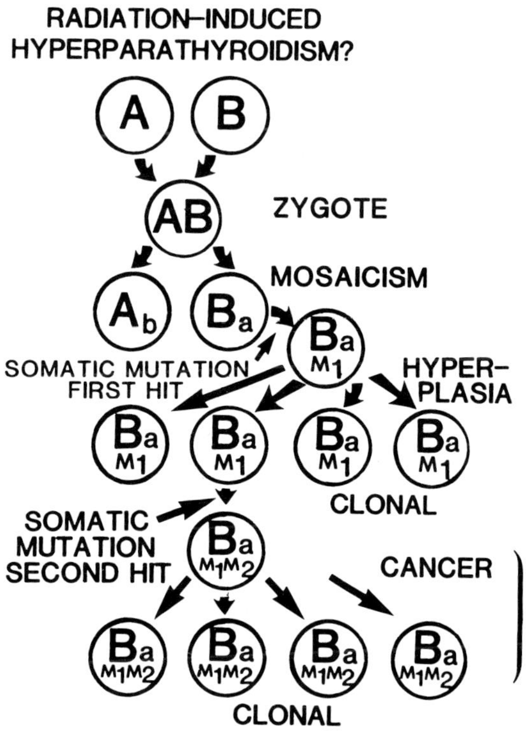

patients with multiple endocrine neoplasia syndrome type 2 (MEN-2) suggest that the medullary thyroid cancers and the one pheochromocytoma studied developed clonally. In one MEN-2 patient they found a tumor with type A in one thyroid lobe and a tumor with type B in the opposite lobe suggesting that the mutations arose in single cells of multiple clones of susceptible cells (C-cell hyperplasia) as would be predicted by Knudson's theory. G-6-PD studies of parathyroid tumors in MEN-2 have not been reported.

The postulated expectations regarding G-6-PD data in non-neoplastic hyperplasia, in hereditary hyperplasia, in sporadic or non-hereditary mutagen-induced hyperplasia, and in parathyroid cancer are illustrated in figure 1. This figure was modified from a similar scheme for neoplasia in general presented by Knudson & Meadows (9). It can be seen that sporadic hyperplastic lesions resulting from mutation as with radiation or possibly chemical mutagens would be expected to be of clonal origin whereas non-neoplastic hyperplasia and hereditary hyperparathyroidism would be expected to be of multicellular origin as has been observed in the G-6-PD studies (7). Since mutation is involved in both the hereditary and the radiation-induced hyperparathyroidism, this model would predict that parathyroid cancer would be more likely in those types than in the common sporadic non-neoplastic hyperparathyroidism (7). It would predict that these cancers should be of earlier age of onset in hereditary hyperparathyroidism since the mutation is present at birth rather than occurring at the time of radiation (or other mutagen exposure) as has been found in comparing the age of onset of sporadic parathyroid cancer with that occurring in the 5 families of hereditary hyperparathyroidism reported (7). Although radiation and possibly chemical mutagens are etiological factors in some cases of hyperparathyroidism, the G-6-PD evidence of multicellular development suggests that generalized non-neoplastic effects of cell growth factors are more commonly important.

REFERENCES

1. Baylin, S.B., Hsu, S.H., Gann, D.S., Smallridge, R.C. and Wells, S.A. Jr. (1978): Surgery, 199, 429.
2. Boonstra, C.E. and Jackson, C.E. (1962): Ann. Intern. Med., 57, 963.
3. Einstein, A. Quoted by Brush, S.G. (1974): Science, 183, 1164
4. Fialkow, P.J. (1976): Biochim. Biophys. Acta, 45, 283.
5. Fialkow, P.J., Jackson, C.E., Block, M.A. and Greenawald, K.A. (1977): N. Engl. J. Med., 297, 696.
6. Jackson, C.E. and Boonstra, C.E. (1967): Am. J. Med., 43, 727.
7. Jackson, C.E., Cerny, J.C., Block, M.A. and Fialkow, P.J. (1982): Surgery, 92, 875.
8. Knudson, A.G., Jr. (1971): Proc. Nat. Acad. Sci, USA, 68, 820.
9. Knudson, A.G., Jr. and Meadows, A.T. (1980): N. Engl. J. Med., 302, 1254.
10. Rao, S.D., Frame, B., Miller, M.J., Kleerekoper, M., Block, M.A. and Parfitt, A.M. (1980): Arch. Intern. Med., 140, 205.

THE INTERACTION BETWEEN ABNORMAL CELLULAR PROLIFERATION AND SECRETION IN PRIMARY HYPERPARATHYROIDISM

Edward M. Brown, Meryl S. LeBoff, Dolores Shoback and Richard E. Wilson
Departments of Medicine and Surgery, Brigham and Women's Hospital, and Harvard Medical School, Boston, MA, U.S.A.

Primary hyperparathyroidism is thought to result from inappropriate hypersecretion of PTH despite hypercalcemia, unlike secondary hyperparathyroidism where the increase in PTH secretion is a compensatory response to a physiological stimulus (presumably hypocalcemia). There is no recognized extraparathyroid abnormality which is the proximate cause of primary hyperparathyroidism (analogous to Vitamin D deficiency or renal insufficiency in secondary hyperparathyroidism). Studies of the pathophysiology and pathogenesis of this disorder, therefore, have focused on the parathyroid glands *per se*. This does not imply, however, that there may not be environmental (i.e. radiation) or other factors (as in multiple endocrine neoplasia) which lead to abnormal proliferation and/or function of pathologic parathyroid tissue in primary hyperparathyroidism.

Evidence for hypersecretion of PTH in this disorder is primarily indirect. Most patients with primary hyperparathyroidism show elevated circulating levels of immunoreactive PTH. These radioimmunoassays generally recognize fragments of PTH as well as the intact hormone, leading to considerable uncertainty about the true circulating levels of intact PTH in both hyperparathyroid and normal subjects. Recently, ultrasensitive cytochemical bioassays (1) and sensitive aminoterminal radioimmunoassays (2), which probably measure predominantly intact PTH, have confirmed elevated circulating levels of PTH in most patients with primary hyperparathyroidism. Although these techniques quantify circulating concentrations of PTH rather than secretion rates *per se*, it is likely that primary hyperparathyroidism is associated with increases in secretion rate at least equivalent to the elevations in circulating levels of PTH in this disorder.

The maintenance of an inappropriately increased rate of PTH release, despite the development of hypercalcemia, appears to be central to the pathophysiology of primary hyperparathyroidism. Two factors which have been emphasized as potentially contributing to the development of hypersecretion of PTH in primary hyperparathyroidism are an increase in the total mass of parathyroid tissue and/or qualitative change in the functional characteristics of the individual parathyroid cell (i.e. resistance to the suppressive effects of extracellular calcium on hormonal secretion).

In most cases of primary hyperparathyroidism, there is an increase in the total mass of parenchymal parathyroid tissue. In occasional cases, however, hypercalcemia may be cured by removal of an abnormal parathyroid gland whose mass is comparable to that of the combined mass of four normal parathyroid glands. Thus, an increased total mass of parathyroid tissue may not be an absolute prerequisite for the development of hypercalcemic hyperparathyroidism. Both hypertrophy and hyperplasia contribute to the increase in mass of parathyroid tissue in patients with primary hyperparathyroidism. The diameter of normal chief cells is 6-8 microns, while the diameter of chief cells in parathyroid adenomas, on the other hand, varies from 8-14 microns (3). Cellular hypertrophy alone, therefore, could account for a several fold increase in tissue mass. The remaining increase in the mass of hyperplastic parathyroid glands is presumably accounted for by an increase in cell number.

Data from studies in vivo as well as in vitro suggest that the release of intact PTH from the parathyroid cell is not completely suppressible by calcium even with high extracellular calcium (4). A persistent, non-suppressible component of PTH release might lead to hypercalcemia, therefore, if there were a sufficiently great increase in the mass of even normal parathyroid tissue. The development of hypercalcemia in rats autotransplanted with 20-80 normal rat parathyroid glands may represent, in fact, an animal model of hypercalcemic hyperparathyroidism due to this phenomenon (5).

Early studies demonstrated that parathyroid tissue from most, but not all, patients with primary hyperparathyroidism was responsive to changes in the extracellular calcium concentration in vivo (6) as well as in vitro (7). Hypercalcemia in this disorder, therefore, could not be explained simply by autonomy of PTH secretion but was perhaps related to a more subtle secretory abnormality, such as a change in sensitivity to extracellular calcium (6). Subsequent studies, in fact, have demonstrated that tissue from most patients with primary hyperparathyroidism does, in general, show a decreased sensitivity to calcium (8,9). Thus, abnormal parathyroid tissue senses an elevated calcium concentration as normal, contributing to inappropriate hypersecretion of PTH.

In contrast to the changes in set-point (the calcium concentration half-maximally inhibiting secretion) in pathological parathyroid cells, maximal PTH release at low calcium concentrations on a per cell basis is slightly reduced, on the average, in cells from pathological glands (10). In most cases, therefore, an increase in the maximal secretory capacity for PTH in primary hyperparathyroidism results from changes in the number of cells rather than in the maximal output per cell. In some cell preparations, however, there are several-fold increases in maximal secretory rate per cell which might contribute to hormonal hypersecretion (10).

To evaluate the relative importance of cellular hypertrophy and hyperplasia vs qualitative changes in secretory function in promoting hormonal

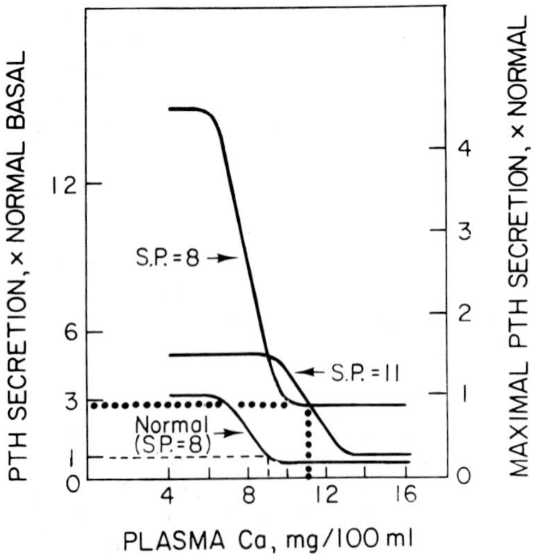

Figure 1. Effect of set-point on PTH hypersecretion. Note that at a calcium of 11 mg/dl only a 1.5-fold increase in maximal secretory rate is necessary to produce a 3-fold rise in the normal basal secretory rate with a gland having an elevated set-point (S.P. = 11 mg/dl ≅ 1.3 mM), while a 4.5-fold increase in

maximal secretory rate is necessary with a normal set-point (S.P. = 8 mg/dl ≅ 1.0 mM).

hypersecretion, we have developed a model of the relationship between PTH secretion and the extracellular calcium concentration in normal and abnormal parathyroid tissue (11). This model fits data from studies in vitro or in vivo according to sigmoidal curves described by four parameters-maximal secretory rate, slope of the curve at its midpoint, set-point, and minimal secretory rate. It should be pointed out that this is not a kinetic model, but one which predicts the effects of calcium on PTH release under conditions of apparent steady state in vitro. Additional models are required to describe the complex kinetics of the acute secretory response to hypocalcemia which is observed in vivo.

This sigmoidal model provides excellent fits to experimental data from studies in vitro (11). Moreover, it fits the data according to parameters which are useful for examining the importance of changes in maximal hormonal secretion (i.e. tissue mass) and set-point for calcium. By systematically varying these parameters, it is possible to examine the changes in secretory rate which occur when they are varied individually and also to study the way in which they interact to affect hormonal secretion.

At any given calcium concentration, secretory rate is directly proportional to the maximal secretory rate of the tissue. Because of the steepness of the curves relating PTH release to the extracellular calcium concentration, on the other hand, even a fairly subtle (10-20%) increase in set-point can produce a large increase in secretory rate at extracellular calcium concentrations in the hypercalcemic range without any change in maximal secretory rate (11). If both set-point and maximal secretory rate change, the effect of an alteration in the former is that a smaller increase in tissue mass is necessary to achieve a given degree of hormonal hypersecretion. The nature of this interaction is illustrated schematically in Figure 1. From a practical point of view since most cases of primary hyperparathyroidism show increases in both set-point and tissue mass, it is likely that both parameters contribute to the pathophysiology of the increased secretion of PTH in this disorder.

In normal parathyroid tissue, the enhanced secretory response to chronic hypocalcemia is presumably related both to an increase in the mass of parathyroid tissue and to a rise in hormonal output per cell. While the inverse relationship between PTH release and the extracellular calcium concentration at the level of the individual cell is widely recognized, experimental support for a similar regulation of cellular proliferation by calcium is more fragmentary. The latter includes data that indices of cellular proliferation such as gland weight, number of mitoses, or thymidine incorporation are increased by low calcium concentrations. The increased mass of parathyroid tissue in primary hyperparathyroidism suggests that the proliferative response of the parathyroid cell to calcium is abnormal in this disorder. It is possible, therefore, that primary hyperparathyroidism represents a linked disorder in the regulation of PTH release and cellular proliferation with both processes insensitive to the suppressive effects of extracellular calcium. There are as yet, however, no data directly examining the relationship of parathyroid cellular proliferation to the extracellular calcium concentration in primary hyperparathyroidism.

A major hindrance to studying further the control of parathyroid cellular proliferation by calcium has been the lack of a suitable experimental system. We have recently devised techniques for culturing dispersed bovine parathyroid cells in an attempt to develop such a system (12). While they are morphologically intact and secrete more immunoreactive PTH per cell than acutely dispersed parathyroid cells, these cultured cells show a progressive loss of suppressibility of secretion by calcium with time. After four days in culture, immunoreactive PTH release is inhibited only 20% by 3.0 mM calcium compared with 70-80% in acutely dispersed cells. Cultured cells also show a loss of the high-calcium-induced suppression of agonist-stimulated cAMP accumulation and their proliferation is unaffected by high calcium concentrations (doubling time of about four days at both 1.0 and 3.0 mM calcium). Thus, cultured bovine parathyroid cells develop a generalized resistance to extracellular calcium which is more severe than that seen with most pathologic parathyroid glands in primary hyperparathyroidism. Further understanding of the abnormal cellular function in cultured bovine parathyroid cells might provide clues to the types of abnormalities underlying the development of primary hyperparathyroidism.

The cellular mechanisms by which extracellular calcium regulates parathyroid function are not known. If there is a similar inverse relationship between the effects of calcium on PTH secretion and cellular proliferation, it is possible that both processes are regulated by some common intracellular mediator. cAMP and cytosolic calcium have both been suggested as potential second messengers for the effects of extracellular calcium on PTH secretion (4). The regulation of both of these functions, therefore, represent possible loci for the abnormal control of cell function in primary hyperparathyroidism. The development of better techniques for studying parathyroid cellular proliferation and further studies of the cellular mechanisms underlying secretion and cell division on this cell type may provide clues to basis for the disordered cellular function in primary hyperparathyroidism.

REFERENCES

1. Goltzman, D., Henderson, B. and Loveridge, N. (1980): J. Clin. Invest., 65, 1309.
2. Segre, G.V., Harris, S.T., Neer, R. and Potts, Jr., J.T. (1981): Calcif. Tis. Int'l., 33, Suppl., 317.
3. Castleman, B. and Roth, S.I. (1978): Tumors of the parathyroid glands. Armed Forces Institute of Pathology, Washington, D.C.
4. Brown, E.M. (1982): Min. and Elect. Metab., 8, 130.
5. Gittes, R.F. and Radde, I.C. (1966): J. Urol., 95, 595.
6. Murray, T.M., Peacock, M., Powell, D. and Potts, Jr., J.T. (1972): Clin. Endocrinol. Metab., 1, 235.
7. Birnbaumer, M.E., Schneider, A.B., Palmer, D., Hanley, D.A. and Sherwood, L.M. (1977): J. Clin. Endocrinol. Metab., 45, 105.
8. Brown, E.M., Brennan, M.F., Hurwitz, S., Windeck, R., Marx, S.J., Spiegel, A.M., Koehler, J.A., Gardner, D.G. and Aurbach, G.D. (1978): J. Clin. Endocrinol. Metab., 46, 267.
9. Habener, J.F. (1978): J. Clin. Invest., 62, 436.
10. Brown, E.M., Gardner, D.G., Brennan, M.F., Marx, S.J., Spiegel, A.M., Attie, M.F., Downs, Jr., R.W., Doppman, J.L. and Aurbach, G.D. (1979): Am. J. Med., 66, 923.
11. Brown, E.M. (1983): J. Clin. Endocrinol. Metab., 56, 572.
12. Le Boff, M.S., Rennke, H. and Brown, E.M. (in press), Endocrinology.

DISCUSSION OF PATHOGENESIS OF HYPERPARATHYROIDISM

Drs. Sherwood, Jackson, Brown
(Moderator: Dr. Sherwood)

J. POTTS: Dr. Sherwood, I won't comment about the molecular biology reviewed, because in a sense the details of that are a little beyond the scope of the meeting. The significance of the molecular biology studies ultimately is to understand the response of the parathyroid cell. It is our feeling that we will want to look at the changes in messenger RNA levels and what they are telling us about the response of the gland to chronic low calcium stress, studying the glands removed from animals manipulated in vivo. What's interesting is that your data and that of others suggest that the parathyroid biosynthetic rate does not change very rapidly, neither up nor down, in response to suppression or stimulation, unlike many other endocrine tissues in which there is a sudden activation of gene activity such as estrogen induction of certain target organs (e.g., proteins in the oviduct).

What is interesting to this audience, is what determines the hyperplastic response of the cells. This issue is pertinent to both the polyclonal etiology of primary hyperparathyroidism that Dr. Jackson suggested, and in secondary hyperparathyroidism, whether and why the gland stays hyperplastic. In other words, it is the pathogenesis of abnormal cell proliferation that we are really interested in. If you were to study animal models of vitamin D deficiency, for example, one might find that the cells become hyperplastic as their way of increasing hormone output, because their basic biosynthetic rate per cell was near maximum at all times. As you pointed out, what regulates gland hormone content is both secretion and degradation of intracellular stores; a three to four change in hormone content is the maximum variation. The parathyroid cell may be designed to undergo very rapid hyperplastic change, as the principal adaptation to chronic hypocalcemic stress. Could that underlie certain of the cellular responses that we see, particularly in renal failure and secondary hyperparathyroidism? I would like to hear what Dr. Sherwood has to say about cell biology and also ask Dr. Jackson what he thinks the implications of his findings are for the surgical treatment of primary hyperparathyroidism.

L. SHERWOOD: I think that Dr. Pott's point is well taken and that we need to look in vivo at what happens to animals with chronic renal failure, a low-calcium diet or with vitamin D deficiency, using all the tools of molecular biology. This is now feasible in the rat and perhaps other species, but hard to do in cows. There is old animal data which suggests that the hyperplastic response of the parathyroid glands to renal failure occurs early. I would like very much to know what subcellular signal(s) causes the parathyroid cells to divide. I agree that the parathyroid cells are operating close to or at maximal capacity, and somehow a low ambient calcium or other factors produce a subcellular or membrane signal which causes them to divide and increase their biosynthetic capacity. We are still some distance from knowing what that signal is.

C.E. JACKSON: I agree that there are cellular growth factors, some of which we are unaware of at present. To answer Dr. Potts' other question about the implications regarding surgery and the possibility of parathyroid carcinoma being present in mutation-induced hyperparathyroidism, perhaps we should consider surgery on patients with hereditary hyperparathyroidism and radiation-induced hyperparathyroidism because of some concern about parathyroid carcinoma. This is probably premature, but I think the G6PD findings do imply that we should give some thought to this approach.

L. SHERWOOD: I believe that Dr. Potts was interested in knowing whether your findings of polyclonal hyperplasia in primary hyperparathyroidism might suggest that there is generalized hyperplasia for which we should be more aggressive in our surgical management. This would be difficult to do when the vast majority of the data from the literature supports the concept that removal of a single adenoma cures the disease in most patients.

A.M. PARFITT: Just a comment to sharpen the dilemma posed by Dr. Potts. It seems that the same cells in the parathyroid gland have both the capacity to secrete hormone and the capacity to undergo cell division. There is no evidence for an anatomically separate cell compartment responsible for cell renewal. The limited histologic data suggests that when mitoses occur, they are randomly distributed throughout the gland. This means that some cells are clever enough to ignore the stimulus to increase hormone secretion, to stop making hormone and to reprogram themselves for mitosis. This is the crucial issue in the development of parathyroid hyperplasia, and the techniques that are now being developed should be applied to this problem.

L. SHERWOOD: We need an established line of human parathyroid cells in culture where one can look at cell cycles to study the problem of hormone production versus cell division. Unfortunately, such cell lines have not yet been developed.

L. DEFTOS: I would like to make a comment about your discussion of PSP. PSP or chromogranin A containing cells are found in the calcitonin-secreting cells of the thyroid gland. Dr. O'Connor of our institution, has shown such cells to be present in the insulin-secreting cells of the pancreas, in the pituitary gland, and in the argentaffin cells of the gastrointestinal tract. This is a ubiquitously-occurring protein whose role in the secretory process is uncertain. I think that name PSP or even chromogranin A is misleading and perhaps ESP, endocrine secretory protein, might be a better term.

M. KLEEREKOPER: Dr. Jackson, if radiation is indeed mitogenic to the parathyroid tissue, why don't we see a higher incidence of parathyroid hyperplasia in radiation-induced hyperparathyroidism than we do in the naturally-occurring disease.

C.E. JACKSON: This would mean that radiation is affecting more than one cell, because we do often have hyperplasia of more than one gland in radiation-induced hyperparathyroidism.

M. KLEEREKOPER: But no more often with radiation-induced hyperparathyroidism than with naturally-occurring or sporadic hyperparathyroidism.

C.E. JACKSON: It would mean that many cells were radiated, and that the hyperparathyroidism was clonally derived from several different cells. I think we can get this question if we find a G6PD heterozygote female who has radiation-induced hyperparathyroidism with more than one gland involved. I would suspect that we would see one gland of A origin and another gland of B origin as has been seen in medullary thyroid carcinoma in the reports of Baylin and Associates (in which there is a tumor on one side that is of A origin and on the other side of B origin). Studies on such a patient would give us information as to whether or not the adenoma or hyperplasia was clonal in nature, each tumor originating in different cells in the parathyroids.

S. MARX: The definition of primary hyperparathyroidism can be expanded somewhat beyond what Dr. Brown suggested. Dr. Parfitt suggested that one could classify hypercalcemia as an equilibrium or a nonequilibrium form of hypercalcemia with the equilibrium form being a chronic steady rate in which there were no acute changes occurring in any of the major calcium compartments. If we accept this definition, it would then be possible to have a form of hypercalcemia that is supported by normal levels of PTH in plasma, but where the inappropriate function of the parathyroid gland is not hypersecretion of parathyroid hormone but failure to suppress PTH secretion below the normal level in response to chronic hypercalcemia. I think this might be important because it allows the possibility that one could have primary hyperparathyroidism with normal biologically-active levels of PTH in plasma. This would account for some of the overlaps which continues to be seen with all radioimmunoassays. I think it also is an appropriate way of thinking about what is going on in familial hypocalciuric hypercalcemia (where there is proliferation of parathyroid cells with normal circulating levels of PTH).

VI MANAGEMENT OF HYPERCALCEMIC HYPERPARATHYROIDISM

THE MANAGEMENT OF PRIMARY HYPERPARATHYROIDISM: OVERVIEW

M. Kleerekoper, M.D.

Bone and Mineral Division, Department of Medicine
Henry Ford Hospital, Detroit, MI, U.S.A.

In the hands of a skilled parathyroid surgeon, parathyroidectomy (PTX) is a curative procedure for primary hyperparathyroidism (PHPT) more than 95% of the time. Why then is there a need to discuss further the management of PHPT? Why are not all patients in whom the diagnosis is firmly established on clinical and biochemical grounds sent to a skilled parathyroid surgeon for elective PTX? The question is really a philosophical one that tries to address the questions of what is meant by "cure" of PHPT and which patients with PHPT have a disease that needs a "cure"?

The past two decades have been a period when many patients with PHPT have had the diagnosis considered because of a chance finding of hypercalcemia on a biochemical screen, done either as a routine measure in a well patient or in an ill patient when the screening test was ordered for other reasons. It is likely that the majority of patients with PHPT present in this way, rather than as the more classic patient with "stones, bones and abdominal groans." Most consultants who are referred patients with PHPT develop arbitrary criteria that mandate PTX at the time of diagnosis. These include signs or symptoms directly referable to hypercalcemia, nephrolithiasis, skeletal disease, peptic ulcer disease, pancreatitis, impaired renal function etc. Most physicians have a cut-off point for hypercalcemia, above which all patients are referred for PTX. This arbitrary criterion varies among physicians with most accepting a limit of 11.5 to 12.0 ng/dl.

In the now classic study conducted at the Mayo Clinic, a large number of patients with mild asymptomatic PHPT was followed prospectively up to 10 years following the initial diagnosis. The salient features of that study were that 20% of patients were lost to follow-up during the period of observation and 20% of the patients had progression of the disease so that PTX was felt to be indicated. In retrospect it was apparent that a substantial number of patients in whom the disease was considered to have progressed were initially misclassified and that the rate of progressive disease may be less than was observed in that study. A major defect in the design of the study was its failure to assess the effect of successful PTX on the natural history of the disease. Additionally, this study was undertaken before sophisticated techniques for measuring bone mass and the effect of PTH excess on bone mass were available. These problems were addressed by two papers presented at the symposium.

The first of these was a retrospective analysis of 128 patients reviewed an average of 7.8 years following "successful" PTX. This study, performed by Posen and his colleagues in Sydney, Australia, provided some surprising and challenging observations. Fifteen per cent of the patients had died during the follow-up period, but in only one case could the death be attributed to surgery. Whether this simply reflects the fact that the prevalence of PHPT increases with age or whether PHPT contributed to irreversible deterioration in function prior to surgery, could not be ascertained from this study. PTX did not appear to have an entirely protective effect against the development of nephrolithiasis in contrast to other studies. No patient who was free of stones prior to PTX developed stones during the postoperative follow-up. However, in the 70% of patients who had nephrolithiasis prior to surgery, a significant reduction in the number of patients who developed recurrent stones during follow-up was not apparent. Successful PTX did not have an appreciably favorable effect on hypertension that was present in 40-50% of the patients preoperatively, nor did it result in restoration of impaired renal function. Using crude radiographic assessment, PTX was also without any improvement in the prevalence or degree of osteoporosis.

Neer and his colleagues from the Massachusetts General Hospital in Boston presented quite similar observations on 45 patients followed prospectively for 3 years following successful PTX. These patients were all considered to have mild, asymptomatic PHPT prior to surgery. The decision to operate was based on the presence of impaired renal function or, more frequently, on the presence of osteopenia (bone mineral content >2 standard deviations below expected for age, sex and race). Two patients developed kidney stones during the follow-up period. As a group, there was no improvement in blood pressure or in renal function, nor was there any restoration of the deficit in bone mineral content. Perhaps of greater importance was the failure of PTX to slow the rate of bone loss when the group was considered as a whole, although this was observed in some patients.

The Australian group also reported findings on 32 patients observed on average of 6.6 years following unsuccessful PTX. There were 4 deaths in this group (12.5%), one of which resulted from progressive vertebral fractures and respiratory failure - presumably a manifestation of progressive osteitis fibrosa. As was the case with the successfully treated patients, kidney stones did not occur in those patients who were stone free preoperatively. There was no other evidence for progression of PHPT.

A noteworthy and challenging observation was the seemingly high prevalence of non-parathyroid malignancy in those patients who remained hypercalcemic following surgery. In the successfully treated group, 8 out of 128 (6%) developed a variety of malignancies. However, 7 of the unsuccessfully treated group (22%) did develop malignancy, a statistically higher prevalence in this group ($p < 0.01$). There have been several reports of an increased prevalence of non-parathyroid malignancy in PHPT when compared to the general population, but it has never been clearly established whether this is more than the chance occurrence of two relatively common conditions in an aging population. This observation by Posen et al must focus attention on this potential "complication" of PHPT. If hypercalcemia, elevated PTH, or perhaps PHPT is in some way "mitogenic" it is somewhat surprising that this was not found in the 10 year prospective study carried out at the Mayo Clinic. The prevalence of malignancy in the group of 74 patients Posen and colleagues followed, in whom surgery was not performed, is apparently not known, but would be of interest.

If successful PTX is without obvious benefit in patients with mild PHPT so treated, has anything new been learned since the Mayo Clinic study of patients who were not operated upon? Neer and his colleagues reported their 3 year experience in this regard in a small number of patients. Like the Mayo Clinic experience, the drop-out rate was relatively high (12%) which must be carefully considered whenever a decision to "follow" a patient with PHPT is undertaken. The Boston group did not detect any significant progression of the disease over a 3 year period, with regards to serum calcium and inorganic phosphate, urine calcium excretion, renal function and bone mineral content. There are several anecdotal reports of patients with established mild PHPT developing sudden and marked rises in serum calcium while under observation. Since there is currently no known means of predicting this albeit rare, life-threatening complication, every attempt must be made to ensure continuous observation of all patients with PHPT in whom a decision not to recommend elective PTX is made at the time of initial diagnosis.

The type of surgery required for patients with primary HPT was presented by Wells and Leight, highlighting their experiences at Duke University in North Carolina and Washington University in St. Louis. Most surgeons prefer to identify all four parathyroid glands at the time of initial neck exploration.

The surgeon should rely on his own skills at identifying parathyroid tissue and resect those glands that appear macroscopically enlarged (> 50 mg). The role of the pathologist at the time of surgery is to confirm that the resected tissue is indeed parathyroid and the surgeon should place little reliance on the descriptive terms "parathyroid adenoma" and "parathyroid hyperplasia" at the time of surgery.

Of 350 patients accrued over a 5 year period, 68% had single gland enlargement, 22% had two or three gland enlargement and 10% had four gland enlargement. No patient with single gland enlargement, and only one patient with two or three gland enlargement, had recurrence of primary HPT during a 4 year follow-up. Patients with four gland enlargement have been managed by total parathyroidectomy and autotransplantation of tissue in the forearm muscle. The incidence of graft failure was less than 5%. Thirty-six percent of patients with four gland enlargement had familial hyperparathyroidism. The incidence of recurrent hypercalcemia in this group was 65% and included 4 patients who had familial hypocalciuric hypercalcemia. The incidence of recurrent hypercalcemia in patients with four gland enlargement without familial hyperparathyroidism was 15%.

There remains a small group of patients with primary HPT in whom elective surgery would normally be recommended but who are considered too great a risk for elective surgery because of other medical considerations. There is also a growing group of patients in whom surgery is recommended but who choose to decline surgical intervention. Dr. John Bilezikian from Columbia University, New York outlined medical alternatives for these patients. General principles of management include maintaining adequate hydration and avoidance of immobilization and thiazide diuretics. There is only limited evidence that restriction of dietary calcium is of benefit. However, if one can demonstrate an increased intestinal absorption of calcium or elevated 1-25 dihydroxy cholecalciferol levels, dietary restriction of calcium theoretically should be of benefit.

Drug therapy to inhibit parathyroid secretion (e.g. beta-blockers and H_2 receptor antagonists) or to inhibit the action of PTH on bone (e.g. estrogens, calcitonin, diphosphonates) have not been especially helpful in most centers. However, there are scattered case reports of a short-term reduction in serum calcium with some of these drugs. Estrogens appear to have the most potential benefit, particularly in postmenopausal women with primary HPT. While the serum calcium may not be "normalized" the rate of bone loss may be decreased by administration of estrogen to this group.

SUMMARY AND CONCLUSIONS

It is clear that in the hands of a skilled parathyroid surgeon elective parathyroidectomy is a simple, safe and effective means of curing PHPT in more than 95% of cases. It is equally clear that there is as yet no equally effective medical therapy for this disease, although the administration of estrogens to postmenopausal women with PHPT holds promise of decreasing the rate of bone loss. There are many patients, perhaps the majority, who derive no clinical benefit from having their disease "cured" by PTX. What is not currently available from the data, either in the published literature or in the material presented at this symposium, is the means of accurately predicting, at the time of diagnosis, which patient is likely to develop complications if not "cured." To the classic list of "stones, bones and abdominal groans" that has been known to complicate PHPT must be added a possible increased occurrence of non-parathyroid malignancy in untreated patients. If close observation during follow-up after diagnosis can be asssured, only a small number of patients will develop major complications such as life-threatening hypercalcemia if left untreated. Careful observation must remain an important caveat because two prospective studies have documented a 12 and 20% drop-out rate during 3 and 10 year follow-up periods respectively.

THE SURGICAL MANAGEMENT OF PATIENTS WITH PRIMARY HYPERPARATHYROIDISM

Samuel A. Wells, Jr. and George S. Leight
Departments of Surgery, Duke University Medical Center, Durham, NC
and the Washington University Medical Center, St. Louis, MO, USA

Currently, it is the policy of most clinicians to advise neck exploration for patients who are diagnosed as having primary hyperparathyroidism (PHP). Primarily due to the studies of Purnell and associates (1) this almost routine practice is being questioned, especially in asymptomatic patients with a serum calcium concentration below 11 mg/dl. The natural history of "mild primary hyperparathyroidism" and its associated risks are unknown since few patients with this entity have been studied for long periods. In our clinic, neck exploration is advised for virtually all patients with primary hyperparathyroidism unless there is a medical contraindication.

Almost always, neck exploration is an elective procedure and should be performed when convenient once the diagnosis has been made. The operation is always performed under general anesthesia and the method of exposing the operative field is standardized. Most surgeons prefer to identify all four parathyroid glands before removing those which are enlarged. Wang and associates (2) have preferred a more conservative technique. If at the initial unilateral exploration, an enlarged parathyroid gland and a normal parathyroid gland are found, both are resected. If the enlarged gland has pathologic findings characteristic of a parathyroid adenoma and the normal size gland appears normal histologically, the opposite side of the neck is not explored. Conversely, if at the initial unilateral exploration, macroscopically normal parathyroid glands are identified, the opposite side of the neck is explored. If a large and a small gland are identified, they are removed and the operation is terminated. In Wang's series, there was a very low incidence of "double adenomas" (on separate sides of the neck) if, at the initial exploration, a large and a normal parathyroid gland were found unilaterally.

The previously descriptive terms "parathyroid adenoma" and "parathyroid hyperplasia" used by pathologists have not been helpful in guiding the surgeon at the time of neck exploration. Whether or not a given parathyroid gland should be removed depends on its size. We recently studied 100 consecutive patients with PHP in whom all 4 parathyroid glands were identified at neck exploration. Those glands which appeared large macroscopically (>50 mg) were resected. Sixty-five of the 100 patients with PHP had a single enlarged parathyroid gland. Fifteen patients had 2 enlarged glands, 10 patients had 3 enlarged glands, and 10 patients had 4 enlarged glands. Therefore, the incidence of multiglandular enlargement in patients with PHP is higher than previously reported.

In a larger study of 350 patients with PHP accrued over a 5 year period, 237 (68%) had single gland enlargement, 77 patients (22%) had 2 or 3 gland enlargement, and 36 (10%) had 4 gland enlargement. None of the patients with PHP due to single gland disease has developed persistent or recurrent hyperparathyroidism (mean period of followup 4 ± 3.4 years). Only one of the patients with PHP due to 2 or 3 gland enlargement has developed recurrent hypercalcemia. In an evaluation of 143 parathyroid glands removed from the 77 patients with PHP due to 2 or 3 gland enlargement, the histologic interpretation was correlated with the gland weight.

Twenty-nine glands appeared normal histologically even though the mean weight was 128.4 mg. Eighty-four of the enlarged glands were interpreted histologically as "parathyroid hyperplasia"; the mean weight of these parathyroids was 301 mg. Thirty glands were interpreted as being "parathyroid adenomas"; the mean weight of these glands was 1,334.3 mg.

Unlike the patients with PHP due to 1, 2, or 3 gland enlargement, patients with PHP due to 4 enlarged parathyroid glands are much more difficult to manage surgically. We have chosen to manage patients with PHP due to generalized parathyroid enlargement by total parathyroidectomy and autotransplantation of tissue to the forearm muscle. The incidence of graft failure is less than 5%. Should these patients develop recurrent hypercalcemia following total parathyroidectomy and autotransplantation, a portion of the graft can be removed under local anesthesia obviating the necessity for the patient to undergo a repeat neck exploration.

Of the 36 patients in this category, 13 (36%) had familial hyperparathyroidism (either multiple endocrine neoplasia type I, multiple endocrine neoplasia type II, or familial hypocalciuric hypercalcemic hyperparathyroidism). The incidence of recurrent hypercalcemia in this group was 65%. Four of these patients had familial hypocalciuric hypercalcemic hyperparathyroidism and each of the 4 developed recurrent hypercalcemia after surgery. The incidence of recurrent hypercalcemia in patients with nonfamilial hyperparathyridism due to 4 gland enlargement has been 15% (3).

In patients who are being reexplored for recurrent or persistent PHP after an initial failed operation, noninvasive or invasive localization studies may be indicated. Most often we do not utilize selected venous sampling or selective arteriography prior to reoperative surgery. If an enlarged parathyroid gland is found at reoperation, and one is unsure whether a normal parathyroid gland remains, the resected parathyroid can be sliced into small pieces and viably frozen in dimethylsulfoxide, autologous serum and tissue culture media (4). The tissue can be cryopreserved in liquid nitrogen for several months. If in the postoperative period it becomes obvious that the patient has been rendered aparathyroid, the autologous parathyroid tissue can be thawed and grafted into the forearm under local anesthesia. This methodology offers the surgeon substantial versatility in managing patients with persistent or recurrent disease.

REFERENCES

1. Purnell, D.C., Scholz, D.A., Smith, L.H., et al.: Treatment of primary hyperparathyroidism, Am. J. Med, 56:800, 1974.

2. Wang, C.A.: Surgery of the parathyroid glands, Adv. Surg., 5:109, 1971.

3. Wells, S.A., Farndon, J.R., Dale, J.K., Leight, G.S., and Dilley, W.G.: Long-term evaluation of patients with primary parathyroid hyperplasia managed by total parathyroidectomy and hetertopic autotransplantation. Annals of Surgery, 192:451, 1980.

4. Wells, S.A., and Christiansen, C.: The transplanted parathyroid gland: Evaluation of cryopreservation and other environmental factors which affect its function, Surgery, 75:49, 1974.

IS PARATHYROIDECTOMY OF BENEFIT IN PRIMARY HYPER-PARATHYROIDISM?

Solomon Posen, Phillip Clifton-Bligh, Thomas S. Reeve. Clare Wagstaffe, Margaret Wilkinson

Endocrine Unit, Royal North Shore Hospital, St. Leonards, New South Wales, 2065, Australia

It is generally believed that patients with primary hyperparathyroidism benefit from parathyroidectomy. In order to verify this belief we studied 265 patients with primary hyperparathyroidism who had been referred over a 22 year period and who had received 3 different types of treatment on a non-randomized basis: (1) "Successful" operation. There were 142 hypercalcemic individuals who became and remained normocalcemic after the surgical removal of histologically verified parathyroid tissue. (2) "Unsuccessful" operation. There were 33 hypercalcemic individuals with elevated serum immunoreactive parathyroid hormone (iPTH) values who remained hypercalcemic and whose serum iPTH remained elevated after neck exploration. Included in this group were 9 patients whose original operation had been performed in other units and 10 individuals who became normocalcemic for varying periods after surgery but who subsequently became hypercalcemic again. (3) No operation. In 90 hypercalcemic individuals with elevated serum iPTH values neck exploration was either not recommended or refused.

In each group, females outnumbered males approximately 2:1 and in each group males were significantly younger than females. Patients with serum creatinine values of 0.3 mmol/l or greater at presentation were excluded. Patients with malignancies were excluded unless either removal of parathyroid tissue led to normocalcemia or a parathyroid adenoma was found at autopsy or the time sequence of the malignant lesion made its relationship with hypercalcemia extremely unlikely.

All patients were sent a circular letter inviting them to attend. A total of 154 patients were examined by one of us while 45 patients were examined by their own physicians who supplied relevant information, X-ray films and sera. Twenty-two patients were contactable and allegedly well but unwilling to see either one of us or their own physicians. Thirty-seven patients had died and 7 could not be traced. The proportions of patients who attended were similar in the 3 groups.

In 13 cases the original decision not to operate was changed. In 3 patients (all males) there were spectacular rises in serum calcium with symptoms attributed to hypercalcaemia. Three patients showed minor rises in serum calcium during the period of observation while in 1 patient, surgery was recommended on account of recurrent calculi. In 6 patients the decision to operate was based on pressure from the patients or from colleagues. Each of these 13 patients was classified only with the group in which he/she spent most of the period of observation.

During the interview the patients were asked specific questions relating to symptoms of urinary calculi (8), cerebrovascular disease and major abdominal episodes dating from the time when the decision had been taken to operate or not to operate. A blood pressure reading was taken after the patient had been seated for 10 minutes and details of anti-hypertensive and other drug therapy were recorded.

Blood was taken for the measurement of serum calcium, serum creatinine, and serum immunoreactive parathyroid hormone (iPTH). The patient was given a container for the measurement of 24 hour urine calcium and 5 radiographs were taken (lateral lumbar spine, lateral thoracic spine, hands, chest and pelvis). These were subsequently assessed for the presence or absence of osteoporosis on a semiquantitative basis and the results recorded on a 0-2 scale for each film, with 0 indicating no osteoporosis and 2 indicating "definite" osteoporosis.

RESULTS

Table 1 shows that patients not submitted to surgery were significantly older than patients in the other 2 groups, that their hypercalcemia was less severe, that they had a lower prevalence of renal calculi and that they were followed-up for a significantly shorter period.

Serum iPTH values (not shown) were also significantly lower in the unoperated group than in the other 2 groups. Serum creatinine and 24 hour urine calcium values were similar in the 3 groups.

TABLE 1. Differences between operated and unoperated patients.

	Mean age (yr)*	Mean serum calcium (mmol/l)*	Prevalence of renal stones(%)*	Mean duration of follow-up (yr)
Successful operation	50.8	3.15	69.7	7.8
Unsuccessful operation	50.2	3.16	48.5	6.6
No operation	56.3**	2.89**	27.8**	5.3**

* At time of decision
** p value for difference from operated groups <0.001

The prevalence of malignant disorders was higher in the "unsuccessful" (7/32) than in the "successful" (8/138) patients ($p<0.01$) even though these 2 groups were matched for age and sex.

Table 2 shows the status of the patients on the "follow-up day" (March 31st 1983). The percentages of patients who had died did not differ significantly between the groups. Except for one patient in the "successful" group who died from intractable cardiac failure 72 hours after parathyroidectomy and 1 patient in the "unsuccessful" group who died of respiratory failure due to progressive osteoporosis with multiple spontaneous fractures, there were no deaths directly attributable to hyperparathyroidism.

TABLE 2. Current status of 3 groups of hyperparathyroid patients

	Alive	Dead	Unknown
Successful operation	118	21 (15.1%)	3
Unsuccessful operation	28	4 (12.5%)	1
No operation	75	12 (15.6%)	3

In all 3 groups of patients the prevalence of renal stones at the time of follow up was greater amongst patients who had shown evidence of stones (8) at the time of the decision than amongst those who had not. While "improvement" in renal stone status during the time of observation was more common amongst patients who had been rendered normocalcemic and "worsening" of stone status was more prevalent amongst those with persistent hypercalcemia, these differences were not statistically significant. Hypertension, defined as a diastolic blood pressure of 100 or more and/or the regular consumption of antihypertensive medication, was found at follow-up in 40-50% of members of each group.

TABLE 3. Mean biochemical values at the time of follow-up in 3 groups of hyperparathyroid patients

	Serum calcium (mmol/l)	Serum iPTH (ng/ml)	Serum creatinine (mmol/l)	Urine calcium (mmol/24hr)
Successful operation	2.38	0.32	0.13	3.41
Unsuccessful operation	2.88*	1.45*	0.14	6.41*
No operation	2.74*	1.02*	0.11	5.70*

* Significantly ($p<0.001$) different from successful group but not from each other

Table 3 shows the biochemical status of the 3 groups of patients at the time of follow-up. Mean serum calcium, serum iPTH and urine calcium had become normal in the "successful" group whereas these values remained abnormal in the other 2 groups. There were no significant differences between the groups relating to serum creatinine values or relating to the osteoporosis "scores". While each group contained several individuals who were obviously osteoporotic with crush fractures of vertebrae, the majority showed no abnormalities.

DISCUSSION

As the patients in the unoperated group were not matched with the other two groups it is not possible, from this study, to give a statistical assessment of the benefits of parathyroidectomy in primary hyperparathyroidism. However, it is clear from our experience and from several other published and unpublished series (Table 4) that untreated hyperparathyroidism is compatible with long survival and a lack of demonstrable deleterious effects on kidney or bone. If chronic hypercalcemia and/or chronic parathyroid hormone excess aggravate the atheromatous process such aggravation is not apparent from our studies.

We recognise that parathyroid surgery is relatively free of morbidity (4), that chronic hypercalcemia is associated with characteristic cardiac lesions (10), that severe hypercalcemia may lead to renal damage and death and that parathyroid carcinomas can not be diagnosed with certainty in unoperated patients (12). For these reasons we generally recommend surgery in young patients, in patients with symptoms attributable to the hyperparathyroid state and in patients with serum calcium values in excess of 3.0 mmol/l (12 mg/dl).

TABLE 4. Other series describing patients with "untreated" hyperparathyroidism

	N	Mean follow-up period (yr)	Deaths (N)
Scholz & Purnell (11)	86	10 (approx)	35
Adams (1)	31	4.0	4
Van't Hoff et al. (13)	32	4.2	3
Harrop et al. (7)	39	2.5	2
This paper	118	5.7	16

Total: 306 patients observed for 1883 patient-years

However, there is very little evidence that parathyroidectomy cures anything other than hypercalcemia, the symptoms of hypercalcemia, parathyroid osteopathy and, rarely, muscular weakness. Renal calculi persist in 50% of patients, even after successful parathyroidectomy (Posen unpublished). Pancreatitis (2) and hypertension (3) occur with equal frequency in operated and unoperated patients. Renal impairment, evidence of arterial disease and radiological signs of osteoporosis were no more prevalent in the unoperated and "unsuccessful" groups than in patients who had undergone a successful parathyroidectomy (5). The reputed toxicity of parathyroid hormone to peripheral nerves (6) and bone marrow (9) did not give rise to clinical problems in this group of patients with unoperated primary hyperparathyroidism.

We have therefore become increasingly conservative in older, asymptomatic patients and in patients who have previously had unsuccessful neck explorations. Morover, we have also adopted a more tolerant approach towards patients who do not want a neck exploration even if these patients are young and even if serum calcium values are in excess of 3 mmol/l. To-date we have not had cause to regret this tolerance.

REFERENCES

1. Adams, P.H. (1982) J. Roy. Coll. Phys. Lond., 16, 184.
2. Bess, M.A., Edis, A. J., Van Heerden, J.A. (1980) J.A.M.A., 243, 246.
3. Britton, D.C., Thompson, M.H., Johnston, I.D.A., Fleming, L.B. (1971) Lancet, 2, 74.
4. Cowie, A.G.A. (1982) J. Roy. Soc. Med., 75, 942.
5. Dixon, J., Smith, J.F. (1981) J. Clin. Path., 34, 730.
6. Goldstein, D.A., Chui, L.A., Massry, S.G. (1978) J. Clin. Invest., 62, 88.
7. Harrop, J.S., Bailey, J.E., Ingle, A.R., Matthews, H.L. (Personal communication)
8. Lavan, J.N., Neale, F.C., Posen, S. (1971) Med. J. Aust. 2, 1049.
9. Meytes, D., Bogin, E., Ma, A., Dukes, P.P., Massry, S.G. (1981) J. Clin. Invest., 67, 1263.
10. Roberts, W.C., Waller, B.F. (1981) Am. J. Med., 71, 371.
11. Scholz, D.A., Purnell, D.S. (1981) Mayo Clin. Proc., 56, 473.
12. Shane, E., Bilezikian, J.P. (1982) Endocrine Reviews, 3, 218.
13. Van't Hoff, W., Ballardie, F.W., Bicknell, E.J. (Personal communication)

MEDICAL APPROACHES TO THE MANAGEMENT OF PRIMARY HYPERPARATHYROIDISM

John P. Bilezikian

Departments of Medicine and Pharmacology, College of Physicians and Surgeons, Columbia University, New York, NY, U.S.A.

More widespread recognition of primary hyperparathyroidism over the past fifteen years has been accompanied by earlier detection and the frequent presence of asymptomatic mild hypercalcemia (1-2). For the growing population of patients with primary hyperparathyroidism, clear-cut indications for surgical removal of the abnormal gland(s) are frequently not present. If the serum calcium is greater than 1 mg/dl above the upper limits of normal, or if there are symptoms or signs of hyperparathyroidism, regardless of the degree of hypercalcemia, surgical removal of the adenomatous or hyperplastic tissue constitutes proper management. When attempting to establish the presence of signs or symptoms, the multisystem potential and the variable natural history of primary hyperparathyroidism compound the difficulty of ascertaining who is truly asymptomatic and, moreover, who may eventually suffer from one or more of the potential adverse consequences of the disease (3). Uncertainty about whether surgery should be performed in this increasingly large number of patients with primary hyperparathyroidism, who are discovered most commonly in the course of a routine multichannel screening test, has led to non-surgical considerations of care (4). Other subgroups of patients with primary hyperparathyroidism for whom medical management might conceivably be beneficial are those who should undergo surgery but refuse it; patients with major, coexisting medical problems; and patients with persistent or recurrent disease despite previous neck surgery.

GENERAL PRINCIPLES OF MANAGEMENT

An important general principle of management is adequate hydration. Without sufficient fluid intake, dehydration could lead to a greater increase in the serum calcium. Diuretics, therefore, are used with great caution in these patients. Thiazide diuretics, in particular, should be avoided because they reduce urinary calcium excretion and thus, may contribute to worsening hypercalcemia (5). Along with maintaining adequate hydration, ambulation should be encouraged in order to prevent negative calcium balance associated with immobilization.

It is not clear whether dietary calcium restriction is a useful general recommendation. In those patients who demonstrate increased absorption of calcium from the gastrointestinal tract and elevated levels of 1,25-dihydroxyvitamin D (6), a restricted calcium diet has a potential role, especially if one can demonstrate concomitant reductions in serum and urinary calcium and no further increase in the parathyroid hormone level.

SPECIFIC APPROACHES: INHIBITION OF PARATHYROID HORMONE SECRETION

A specific, non-surgical approach to the management of primary hyperparathyroidism is to inhibit the secretion of parathyroid hormone. In view of recent information implicating the beta-adrenergic catecholamines and histamine in the regulation of parathyroid hormone secretion (7), it was reasonable to consider the possibility that their inhibitors, beta-adrenergic blocking drugs and H_2 receptor antagonists, respectively, might be efficacious. The majority of reports, however, have failed to substantiate a significant effect of the prototype beta-adrenergic inhibitor, propranolol, or the H_2 receptor antagonist, cimetidine, on serum calcium or parathyroid hormone levels in patients with primary hyperparathyroidism (4).

SPECIFIC APPROACHES: INHIBITION OF PARATHYROID HORMONE ACTION ON BONE

Several agents with the potential to inhibit the actions of parathyroid hormone on bone have been investigated as therapeutic options in this disorder. It has been reported in numerous papers over the past fifty years that oral phosphate administration may help to lower the serum calcium in primary hyperparathyroidism. Very recently, Broadus et al. observed in a small number of hyperparathyroid subjects with increased 1,25-dihydroxyvitamin D levels, that oral phosphate lowers serum and urine calcium, 1,25-dihydroxyvitamin D levels, and indices of calcium absorption (8). However, these patients also demonstrated significant increases in parathyroid hormone and nephrogenous cyclic AMP levels, an undesirable consequence of therapy. In addition to this potential concern of phosphate therapy is another possible disadvantage, namely ectopic calcification in soft tissues. This latter concern has limited the use of oral phosphate in primary hyperparathyroidism.

The effect of estrogens to inhibit the actions of parathyroid hormone on bone has still not been studied systematically in primary hyperparathyroidism. Reports so far have been uncontrolled and not considered from the viewpoint of potential risks of estrogen use. Similarly unimpressive is the evidence that calcitonin, an inhibitor of osteoclast activity, might be a useful adjunct in the medical management of primary hyperparathyroidism. No systematic investigation has yet shown calcitonin to be efficacious as a chronic form of therapy in primary hyperparathyroidism. It is unlikely that calcitonin will be shown to be useful and practical because of its expense, the need for parenteral administration, and the transitory nature of its effects in other hypercalcemic conditions.

Finally, the diphosphonates have been investigated in primary hyperparathyroidism. These compounds inhibit osteoclast-mediated bone resorption and have been shown to be efficacious in many disorders characterized by excessive osteoclast-mediated bone resorption (9-11). A particulary promising agent is dichloromethylene diphosphonate. Two recent reports have shown significant reductions in serum and urine calcium in hyperparathyroid patients following the administration of dichloromethylene diphosphonate without concomitant elevations in parathyroid hormone or urinary cyclic AMP levels (12-13). These observations were made over approximately three months; it remains to be seen whether dichloromethylene diphosphonate will be effective as a chronic suppressant of the hypercalcemia and hypercalciuria of primary hyperparathyroidism.

SUMMARY

In summary, there are currently no established medical or pharmacological alternatives to surgery for primary hyperparathyroidism. Patients who are surgical candidates should undergo parathyroidectomy, if at all possible. Regular and careful medical observation is essential for the early detection of complications, should they develop, in patients with mild asymptomatic primary hyperparathyroidism who do not undergo surgery. Continued observation and medical follow are reserved for patients who remain asymptomatic.

ACKNOWLEDGMENT

A few of the results cited were obtained through support from grant RR 00645 from the National Institutes of Health.

REFERENCES

1. Heath, H.III, Hodgson, S.F. and Kennedy, M.A. (1980): N. Eng. J. Med., 302, 189.
2. Mundy, G.R., Cove, D.H. and Fisken, R. (1980): Lancet, 1, 1317.
3. Mallette, L.E., Bilezikian, J.P., Heath, D.A. and Aurbach, G.D. (1974): Medicine (Baltimore), 53, 127.
4. Bilezikian, J.P. (1982): Ann. Intern. Med., 96, 198.
5. Middler, S.A., Pak, C.Y.C. and Bartter, F.C. (1972): N. Eng. J. Med., 287, 199.
6. Broadus, A.E., Horst, R.L., Lang, R., Littledike, E.T. and Rasmussen, H. (1980): N. Eng. J. Med., 302, 421.
7. Heath, H.III (1980): Endocr. Rev., 1, 319.
8. Broadus, A.E., Magee, J.S., Mallette, L.E., Horst, R.L., Lang, R., Jensen, P.S., Gertner, J.M. and Baron, R. (1983): J. Clin. Endocrinol. Metab., 56, 953.
9. Jacobs, T.P., Siris, E.S., Bilezikian, J.P., Baquiran, D.C., Shane, E., and Canfield, R.E. (1981): Ann. Intern. Med., 94, 312.
10. Jung, A., Van Ouwenaller, C., Chantraine, A. and Courvoisier, B. (1981): Cancer., 48, 1922.
11. Douglas, D.L., Duckworth, T., Kanis, J.A., et al. (1980): Arthritis Theum., 23, 1185.
12. Shane, E., Baquiran, D.C. and Bilezikian, J.P. (1981): Ann. Intern. Med., 95, 23.
13. Douglas, D.L., Kanis, J.A., Paterson, A.D., Beard, D.J., Cameron, E.C., Watson, M.E., Woodhead, S., Williams, J. and Russell, R.G.G. (1983): Brit. Med. J., 286, 587.

ESTROGEN THERAPY FOR POSTMENOPAUSAL WOMEN WITH PRIMARY HYPERPARATHYROIDISM

Robert Marcus, Phillip Madvig, Marilyn Crim, John Kosek and Alan Pont

Aging Study Unit, VA Medical Center, Stanford University, Palo Alto, California, U.S.A.

We are conducting a prospective clinical trial of conjugated estrogens in the management of primary hyperparathyroidism in postmenopausal women. To date we have enrolled 14 patients, in whom the diagnosis was established on the basis of sustained hypercalcemia without other apparent cause, elevated circulating concentrations of parathyroid hormone, and a bone biopsy showing changes characteristic of hyperparathyroidism, that is, increased prevalence of osteoid seams. Patients are subjected to a comprehensive metabolic evaluation on entry into the study, and following 2 months of each of the three doses of estrogen used (see Table 1). If normalization of hypercalcemia is achieved, that dose of conjugated estrogens is maintained for a full year, at which time the metabolic assessment and iliac crest bone biopsy are repeated. The effect of estrogen therapy on serum calcium is shown in the table. Serum calcium dropped to 10.2 ± 0.07 mg/dl in the 10 "responders," who have remained eucalcemic for periods of 6 to 20 months. In two patients temporary interruption of therapy led to rapid emergence of hypercalcemia.

24-hour urine calcium excretion fell significantly from 360 ± 40 mg pretreatment to 240 ± 45 mg on therapy ($p<0.05$). There was a similar reduction in basal urinary calcium excretion from 0.25 ± 0.07 mg/dl GFR to 0.15 ± 0.005 mg/dl GFR ($p<0.05$). There was no consistent change in serum PTH on therapy with the mean value on therapy not significantly different from the pre-treatment value. However, urine cyclic AMP rose significantly during therapy from 5.00 ± 0.31 nM/dl GFR to 6.5 ± 0.5 nM/dl GFR ($p<0.05$). We interpret this result to suggest that sensitivity of the renal adenylate cyclase system to PTH may have been increased by estrogen.

Estrogen therapy reduced the serum alkaline phosphatase from 90 ± 4 iu/l to 64 ± 2 iu/l ($p<0.01$). Serum 1-25 dihydroxycholecalciferol levels were elevated initially and remained stable and unchanged on treatment. Once again this suggests that the impact of the estrogen was not primarily on the nephron, but appeared to be on bone.

Pre- and post-treatment iliac crest biopsies are available in 4 patients. Trabecular bone volume remained stable in all patients but in no patient was there any dissipation of the hyperosteoidosis that was characteristic of the pre-treatment biopsy. This is in contrast to the complete resolution of this hyperosteoidosis 6 months following successful surgery for primary hyperparathyroidism in one of the "non-responders."

We conclude that estrogen therapy can provide long-term control of serum and urine calcium in postmenopausal women with hyperparathyroidism. Therapy does not alter the fundamental lesion of this disorder, the excessive production of parathyroid hormone, but does appear to achieve a partial resolution of the increased bone turnover, as shown by a reduction in alkaline phosphatase. Estrogen therapy may constitute an effective form of long-term management for patients who are unwilling or unable to undergo surgical therapy.

TABLE

THE EFFECT OF ESTROGEN THERAPY ON SERUM CALCIUM

	Initial	Treated	Dose, Mg
RESPONDERS	11.2±0.21	10.2±0.11	2.5
	10.7±0.16	10.2±0.07	1.25
	10.8±0.29	10.3±0.13	0.625
	10.8±0.21	10.4±0.15	1.25
	10.8±0.11	10.3±0.08	1.25
	11.2±0.14	10.4±0.12	1.25
	10.7±0.22	10.0±0.07	1.25
	11.1±0.30	9.8±0.09	1.25
	11.0±0.23	10.4±0.11	1.25
	10.7±0.16	9.8±0.18	0.625
	10.9±0.07	10.2±0.07	
NON-RESPONDERS	10.8±0.20	10.6±0.11	SURGERY
	10.8±0.24	10.8±0.20	SURGERY
	11.5±0.24	12.0±0.50	SURGERY
	11.4±0.30	11.6±0.30	SURGERY
	11.1±0.19	11.3±0.33	
TOTAL	11.0±0.07	10.5±0.16	

MANAGEMENT OF HYPERCALCEMIC HYPERPARATHYROIDISM

Discussion following papers by S. Posen, S. Wells, J. Bilezikian, R. Marcus

L. RIGGS: I don't think there is any question that parathyroid hormone is bad for bone. Other than the traditional reasons for operation, probably the most important reason for surgery in most patients with primary hyperparathyroidism in postmenopausal women who represent a large group of patients with primary hyperparathyroidism, is the presence of osteoporosis. You won't see osteoporosis by measuring only appendicular bone density, but it will be seen if you measure bone density of the spine. In our studies using dual-photon absorptiometry, patients with primary hyperparathyroidism as a group had mean bone mineral density values of the lumbar spine of almost two standard deviations below the normal mean. Also, we have shown by a case control study that patients with primary hyperparathyroidism as a group have an increased number of vertebral compression fractures, which is even more evident in postmenopausal women. I also think the decision to operate is going to depend largely on whether or not one is fortunate enough to have access to an expert parathyroid surgeon. I think everyone agrees, including Dr. Posen, that there are some patients that will develop serious complications, including accelerated hypercalcemia; and it's not possible to predict in advance who those patients might be. If you are not going to operate, you have to follow each patient every year for the rest of their life; and parathyroid surgery, if done by an expert, as Dr. Wells pointed out, is effective in curing the disease in better than 95% of cases and is not associated with significant mortality or morbidity.

S. POSEN: Thank you, Dr. Riggs. First, I ought to reply to your remark that there is more vertebral bone disease in patients with hyperparathyroidism than in controls. This statement is based on a widely quoted paper from the Mayo Clinic by Dauphine et al that was published in the Annals of Internal Medicine about 1975. That paper describes a number of patients who arrived at the Mayo Clinic, referred for parathyroid surgery, and whose spinal x-rays were compared with a number of patients referred to the orthopedic section at the Clinic for laminectomy. It is my strong belief that the controls were in fact selected because they did not have bone disease.

L. RIGGS: I would like to say that the control groups were selected so that they had the same referral pattern in order to get around the bias of referral.

C. NORDIN: I have a word of warning about this business of leaving patients unoperated, particularly leaving postmenopausal women unoperated, There were certain facts that didn't emerge from Dr. Neer's presentation which I would like to mention as we have followed a number of these patients for many years. The first is that postmenopausal women with hyperparathyroidism always have a higher urinary hydroxyproline than postmenopausal women without hyperparathyroidism. The second is that if you follow their cortical bone measurements sequentially they are losing bone at a substantially faster rate than the normal postmenopausal population. The third is that when they are parathyroidectomized, the urine hydroxyproline decreases, and they stop losing cortical bone. The fourth is that of the 10 patients we reported about ten years ago whose plasma calcium decreased on estrogen, many of those have now been followed for a long time, with a number added, and it is perfectly clear that postmenopausal hyperparathyroid women on estrogen do not lose cortical bone; in fact, they may gain bone. The final point is that among our series of 130 femoral neck fracture patients in Leeds, I think there were five patients with primary hyperparathyroidism, which is much higher than you would expect by chance alone. So my word of warning is that everything in the garden looks lovely as far as short-term follow up is concerned, but in 20 or 30 years' time, a significant proportion of these unoperated and untreated patients will suffer femoral neck fractures. It is perfectly acceptable to leave many of these women unoperated, but if they are postmenopausal women, they are entitled to a small dose of estrogen. The fact is that about half the hypercalcemia is from bone resorption and half of it is from increased tubular reabsorption of calcium. You can reduce the bone resorption component with estrogen. You lower the plasma calcium by about 0.5 mg. per 100 ml., the bone loss stops, and I think you are protecting the patient against fractures in the future.

R. NEER: It seems to me clear that hyperparathyroidism is indeed bad for the skeleton. Many hyperparathyroid patients evaluated by us and by others have been found to have premature osteopenia. If one uses sensitive techniques for detection of osteopenia, nearly 50% of operated patients will have this complication. We presume they have lost bone more rapidly than normal because they have premature osteoporosis but they are not, as a group, losing bone so rapidly that one can demonstrate it in a period of three years. Within that overall group are individuals with hyperparathyroidism who are losing bone detectably faster than normal, and we have operated on all such patients. Looking at all the patients with mild hyperparathyroidism, however, it becomes more difficult to demonstrate a rapid rate of bone loss. It is only selected individuals within that population who are losing bone rapidly.

C. NORDIN: No, forgive me, I'm talking about sequential multiple metacarpal measurements on postmenopausal mild hyperparathyroid patients. As a group they are losing cortical bone significantly faster than age-matched controls.

L. AVIOLI: I'd like to share with the panel what I consider to be an intriguing set of observations made by others at this meeting today: a) I am sure the panel will agree that this disease, primary hyperparathyroidism, is a disease with greater frequency in women over the age of 50 to 55, b) we are being confronted with data that in normal women there seems to be a tendency for PTH to rise with age, specifically over the age of 50, c) we heard some data at this meeting last evening reflecting the difference between vertebral crush fractures and femoral neck fractures; namely, that in the latter population there seemed to be a degree of osteoclastosis and elevations in PTH, d) we have been reading for some time that if you treat postmenopausal women with estrogens, their blood calcitonin increases following estrogen administration, and now we've heard today and as previously reported by Dr. Nordin, that if you give estrogen to patients with primary hyperparathyroidism, a number of them respond with a fall in serum calcium. One of the questions I have for the panel is how are we going to separate a normal woman, who seems to have a predisposition to femoral neck fractures because her serum PTH is higher, from a woman who has primary hyperparathyroidism?

R. NEER: I think your question really is how do define normocalcemic primary or secondary hyperparathyroidism. It seems to me the best approach will be calcium suppression tests of the sort discussed yesterday by Dr. Segre, using an amino-terminal-specific PTH assay. Parathyroid hormone levels that cannot be suppressed by induced hypercalcemia presumably indicate parathyroid glandular abnormalities. There have been recent reports of osteoporotic patients whose bone mass increased following parathyroidectomy for secondary hyperparathyroidism with a normal serum calcium concentration. How frequently such patients exist is an important question.

M. KLEEREKOPER: Wouldn't a bone biopsy tell you whether the parathyroid hormone is contributing to the osteopenia in such a patient?

R. NEER: No, I don't think so. Administration of exogenous parathyroid hormone in low doses will increase bone turnover 2-3 fold without causing any changes in calcium balance. More severe hyperparathyroidism causes increased bone turnover with a negative calcium balance. So I would be very reluctant to conclude on the basis of a bone biopsy that a patient's hyperparathyroidism is causing or isn't causing negative calcium balance and osteopenia.

M. PARFITT: Our own serial data in treated hyperparathyroidism shows a definite increase in the bone mineral content in the first 6-12 months after operation, but I agree with Dr. Neer that the magnitude of increase is small and represents only about 10% of the deficit; however, if you follow the patients long enough I agree with Dr. Nordin that the rate of bone loss in these people does seem to be greater than you would expect for their age. I would like to ask a question of the panel members whether they believe in the existence of what Dr. G. Gordan reported several years ago as menopausal hypercalcemia. It has been shown by many workers that there is an increase in the mean serum calcium after menopause and one would expect that in a large group this would produce in a few individuals values that conform to the definition of hypercalcemia. I have seen two patients who I believe fit this picture. They had hypercalcemia in the early postmenopausal period, which subsided spontaneously with the passage of time. Now my question is, if there is such an entity as menopausal hypercalcemia, how does one differentiate this from hyperparathyroidism both in terms of how to treat that patient and whether the patient should be included in the kind of clinical study that Dr. Marcus presented.

M. GARCIA: With regards the action of Cimetidine in primary hyperparathyroidism, I have to clarify several points. Number one, the protocol that we follow is different than shown here. The infusion lasts for 50 minutes and we give a bolus injection of 600 mg. We found that the peak action of the drug occurs at 15 minutes and thereafter disappears gradually. Also, one has to take into consideration the fact that the activity of the drug is very short. It does not last more than two hours. We have now studied about 83 primary hyperparathyroid patients in five years, and we have seen these changes in all cases.

A. KORKOR: What is the role of CT before surgical treatment of primary hyperparathyroidism? The second question concerns the role of parathyroid cryopreservation? It's not only that we have a problem convincing our surgeons, but it is very expensive. Based on available data there is not really much difference between the results of a 3 1/2 gland parathyroidectomy and total parathyroidectomy with the cryopreservation, in terms of long-term effects.

S. WELLS: Regarding your first question, we do not do any initial localization studies in patients with primary hyperparathyroidism, once the biochemical diagnosis is made. I think CT has been most helpful in patients with a recurrent or persistent postoperative hyperparathyroidism as well as to evaluate the mediastinum. It is noninvasive and has distinct advantages over arteriography and venography. Regarding cryopreservation, we only do that in patients before reoperation. We do not routinely cryopreserve parathyroid tissue in patients with four gland disease. We used to, but not now, because of the extremely low incidence of graft failure. Cryopreservation of tissue, is the technique to use if you are going to do a large volume of reoperative surgery. It is an expensive technique if you are going to do it correctly. Cryopreservation costs between $5,000 and $10,000; but, at the moment, there is no other way. Rapid freezing and DMSO, another preservative, have really not been as effective as slow freezing techniques.

E. SLATOPOLSKY: With regard to the effects of Cimetidine, studies were done in St. Louis by Dr. Cunningham in normal volunteers and patients with renal failure. Dr. Cunningham obtained blood before and after treatment with H_2 blockers. PTH was measured by Dr. Segre with his amino-terminal assay and by ourselves with a mid region/C-terminal assay. Neither Dr. Segre nor we were able to detect any effect on PTH secretion.

J. COBURN: I'd like to ask Dr. Posen about his patients who are having recurrent stones. I wonder are these patients passing stones that already existed or are they forming new stones?

S. POSEN: We didn't attempt to differentiate between old stones and new stones and anyone who has had contact with stone-forming patients must be aware of the difficulties in making such distinctions.

R. NEER: I would like to comment on that too. One of the startling differences between Dr. Posen's study and our study is the difference in the incidence of stones. He has a very large number of people who have stones; we had only two. The Mayo Clinic's ten-year follow-up study also had a large number of patients with stones. The Mayo Clinic study and Dr. Posen's study included from the outset individuals who had a past history of stone or had a stone in the abdomen at the time of presentation. Our study did not include any such individuals. The guarded inference is that the best predictor of whether you're going to have stones in the future is whether you have had them in the past.

D. SLOVIK: A question to Dr. Wells. I realize that in the hands of a skilled surgeon the postoperative complications from a four-gland exploration is very low, but do you advocate four-gland exploration for a patient who has clearly a very large adenoma on one side and a very small gland on the same side?

S. WELLS: No, I don't see anything basically wrong with that. There was a study reported from Sweden within the last few months, comparing these two techniques. It was not a randomized control study, but patients were evaluated who had unilateral exploration with those who had bilateral exploration and biopsy. In the latter group there was a day or two longer hospitalization and the calcium stayed low somewhat longer. I just don't feel safe leaving one side unexplored. We find patients, less than 5%, who have bilateral disease, that is, a large gland on each side of the neck. We are only talking about ten minutes or so of additional operating time.

D. SLOVIK: I am concerned about surgeons who operate only occasionally on parathyroid glands. They may perform extensive neck surgery in trying to identify small glands in aberrant locations when the incidence of postoperative complications such as hypoparathyroidism and recurrent laryngeal nerve palsies would be increased.

S. WELLS: Well I guess you could argue that way, but that may be the surgeon that really ought to explore the other side. I mean the occasional parathyroid surgeon gets into trouble in the same way that the occasional cardiac surgeon does. It is a very personalized thing. Some groups explore only one side.

J. COLBERT: This is addressed to Dr. Neer who said that he does not see bone changes in his primary hyperparathyroid patients. Is the bone disease in secondary hyperparathyroidism different from that in the primary disease?

R. NEER: I didn't mean to say I didn't see any bone changes, because the most frequent reason for surgery in our study was the existence of premature osteopenia. We don't see rapid loss of bone over time in the patients as a group. There are individuals within that group who are losing bone more rapidly than normal. But as a total group they do not.

J. COLBERT: I'm talking about postsurgery.

R. NEER: We have seen an increase in bone mass following parathyroid surgery in people who had severe hyperparathyroid bone disease, but not in these individuals with mild hyperparathyroidism.

J. COLBERT: In our experience surgery for secondary hyperparathyroidism results in a dramatic increase in phalangeal bone density.

R. NEER: Yes, I agree that if one has severe hyperparathyroidism, as I'm sure most of your patients did, parathyroidectomy can cause dramatic improvement in bone mass, but that doesn't happen in patients who have mild hyperparathyroidism.

G. SEGRE: Some experience that we have recently had replicates previously reported experience from the Mayo Clinic. In the postoperative period, if you track patients long enough, a significant number will remain normocalcemic but still have an excess concentration of parathyroid hormone in the plasma. I wonder, how do you view this? How do you establish a cure and how do you think that such results influence the data that you are collecting with regards a postoperative cure?

S. POSEN: Dr. Segre, if I understand your question, you said that even after a successful parathyroidectomy, immunoreactive parathyroid hormone remains elevated although serum calcium remains normal. Is that right?

G. SEGRE: Right. I think there is a very significant percent of patients, somewhere around a third, who, following surgery, continue to have increased parathyroid hormone levels with normal serum calcium levels. Some of the studies are with ionized calcium, but most have been done with total calcium determinations which are in the normal range. One wonders about the direct effect of this elevated parathyroid hormone concentration on bone; how do you evaluate this in your considerations of who is cured?

S. POSEN: Perhaps I'm the wrong person to answer this because I wouldn't recommend surgery for these people even if they were hypercalcemic, so an elevated PTH, in the absence of hypercalcemia wouldn't bother me terribly much. However, I don't think elevated PTH levels in this situation are as common as you say. I would say no more than 10% of our operated patients fall into this category with our immunoassay, which perhaps is not as refined as yours. I'd like to hear what Dr. Bilezikian has to say about this.

J. BILEZIKIAN: Dr. Segre, I'd be interested to know more about your experience. What percentage of patients are you referring to? In my experience that's very uncommon, but I don't have your antibody.

G. SEGRE: I don't think it's necessarily a function of a magical antibody. We have a good antisera but it doesn't make results. In using our antisera we have found that there is roughly between 25 and 30 percent of people who were studied five years after surgery for parathyroid adenoma who seemed to have elevated levels of parathyroid hormone in circulation and with one exception, they're normocalcemic. A similar experience was found in the Mayo Clinic series using an antisera that had characteristics very different from ours. I don't remember the precise percent, but there was a very significant incidence of increased postoperative parathyroid hormone levels in the presence of normocalcemia.

M. KLEEREKOPER: I think it is appropriate to finish this session with an unanswered question about what really constitutes "cure" of mild primary hyperparathyroidism.

VII RECENT DEVELOPMENTS IN BONE PHYSIOLOGY

RECENT DEVELOPMENTS IN BONE PHYSIOLOGY - INTRODUCTION

A. M. Parfitt

Bone and Mineral Division, Henry Ford Hospital, Detroit, Michigan, U.S.A.

According to the quantum concept of bone remodelling proposed by Frost, bone formation in the adult human normally occurs only at sites where bone resorption has recently been completed. As a result, whole body rates of bone resorption and formation and their biochemical and kinetic markers depend mainly on the frequency with which new cycles of erosion and repair are iniated by the fusion of precursors into new osteoclasts, referred to as activation, but is largely independent of the function of differentiated cells. By contrast, whole body bone balance is critically dependent on the focal matching of microscopic volumes of bone resorbed and formed by individual teams of osteoclasts and osteoblasts and so on the number and lifetime work capacity of these cells.

When first proposed, this concept aroused a great deal of opposition, and even hostility, and its proponents have been so busy defending it and expounding its clinical implications that they have given little attention to the mechanisms involved. Yet the deceptively simple description just given conceals a host of unsolved problems in cell biology. What determines the occurrence of activation at a particular location at a particular time? Do the newly formed osteoclasts arise only from distant precursors or are local precursors also involved? Do macrophages and other mononuclear cells participate in normal as well as pathologic bone resorption? How do osteoclasts gain access to the bone beneath its cellular membrane? Why do osteoclasts normally avoid unmineralized bone matrix? What regulates the size, shape and depth of individual resorption cavities? What is the three dimensional path of individual osteoclasts? Does termination of resorption depend on cessation of osteoclast recruitment or on cessation of activity of osteoclasts in response to some unknown signal? What is the fate of the osteoclasts after they have completed their work?

Most crucial is the mechanism of spatial and temporal coupling of formation to resorption. The term "coupling" is often used imprecisely, but logically it encompasses all the mechanisms that ensure that osteoblasts assemble in the right place at the right time and in the right number, to ensure adequate replacement of the resorbed bone. What role, if any, is played by the various types of mononuclear cell that can be observed during the reversal phase between the disappearance of osteoclasts and the arrival of osteoblasts? Which of these cells is responsible for synthesizing the cement substance that joins the new bone to the old? What is the signal to osteoblast precursors to proliferate? Does the need for osteoblast recruitment continue until the new bone structural unit is completed or are all the osteoblasts in place at the outset? Does some constituent of the resorbed bone or of cement substance exert chemotaxis for osteoblasts? To what extent does adequate bone formation depend on the availability of precursor cells, on the genesis and effectiveness of mitogenic stimuli, or on the capacity of individual osteoblasts to form bone matrix? What is the relationship between the functional and structural changes that occur in osteoblasts during their life span? What determines which osteoblasts will become osteocytes, which will become lining cells and which will disintegrate? Is apoptosis involved in osteoblast disappearance? Why is the net effect of all these processes normally to add bone at the periosteum and subtract bone at the endosteum?

Many advances have been made in the study of isolated bone cells and some investigators believe that this approach will answer all the questions just posed, but it is clear that messages to and between cells are modulated by the local micro-environment, which may encompass different types of contact with other cells, different methods of attachment to connective tissue matrices, and different concentration profiles of ions and macromolecules in the local extracellular fluid. Furthermore, cell activity can be altered by mechanical stimuli and by bioelectric signals that can arise only at higher levels of organization. Fortunately, an increasing number of investigators are accepting the quantum concept as a framework for their experimental approach and for integrating in vitro and in vivo observations. In this spirit, Peck described the many new constituents of bone matrix and new factors that are synthesized by bone cells, and the possible roles of these substances in the local regulation of the remodeling cycle and eventually in the treatment of metabolic bone disease. Baylink concentrated on the discovery, purification and characterization of just one of these substances - human skeletal growth factor, a mitogen for bone cells that is present in bone matrix and may be released during bone resorption and so function as a coupling signal that could be disturbed in osteoporosis. Finally, Lanyon demonstrated the crucial importance of the strain induced in bone by functional load bearing as a regulation of bone remodelling. Functional strain could play a major part in orchestrating bone remodelling units and in determining the balance within each unit, effects of obvious relevance to the control of bone mass and the liability to fracture.

STUDIES ON HUMAN SKELETAL GROWTH FACTOR: INTERACTION WITH KNOWN MITOGENS AND CALCIUM REGULATING HORMONES

Subburaman Mohan, John R. Farley, Thomas A. Linkhart, Lee A. Murphy and David J. Baylink

Departments of Biochemistry, Physiology, Pediatrics and Medicine, Loma Linda University School of Medicine, and Mineral Metabolsim Laboratory, Jerry L. Pettis Memorial Veterans Hospital, Loma Linda, California 92357

Osteoporosis, which affects one fourth of North American postmenopausal women, is characterized by accelerated net loss of bone mass which results in increased susceptibility to fractures (1). We have proposed (2) that the failure of bone formation to balance bone resorption in osteoporosis (thus resulting in net bone loss) may be due to a progressive defect in skeletal coupling - a regulatory mechanism by which bone formation is stimulated in proportion to bone resorption. Our laboratory has observed that stimulation of resorption *in vivo* and *in vitro* by parathyroid hormone (PTH) or 1,25-dihydroxyvitamin D_3 (1,25-D_3) is accompanied by a proportional increase in bone formation. Furthermore, chick embryo tibiae in culture, stimulated by PTH or 1,25-D_3 to resorb, release a factor in the serum-free culture medium that stimulates bone cell proliferation and bone matrix formation *in vitro* (3). These results suggest that the coupling of bone formation to resorption is mediated by a factor that is released from bone matrix or from bone cells during resorption and acts to stimulate formation. In subsequent work, a factor which stimulates bone cell proliferation, collagen synthesis and bone formation *in vitro* has been extracted from embryonic and adult bone (4, 5). The factor partially purified from human bone, designated as human skeletal growth factor (hSGF) has molecular weight, heat sensitivity and biological activity similar to the factor in bone conditioned medium (6). In this paper, we describe some biological properties of hSGF and compare its mitogenic activity to other polypeptide growth factors, serum and trypsin. In addition, we describe the effects of bone resorbing agents on hSGF mitogenic activity.

CHEMICAL PROPERTIES

Our studies indicate that hSGF extracted from demineralized human bone matrix is a high molecular weight protein (>80,000 daltons). hSGF activity is sensitive to trypsin and resistant to inactivation by heat, extremes of pH, collagenase (6), 9 M urea, and 4 M guanidine HCl (unpublished). Similar to other mitogens, hSGF stimulates DNA synthesis several hours after addition to quiescent cells.

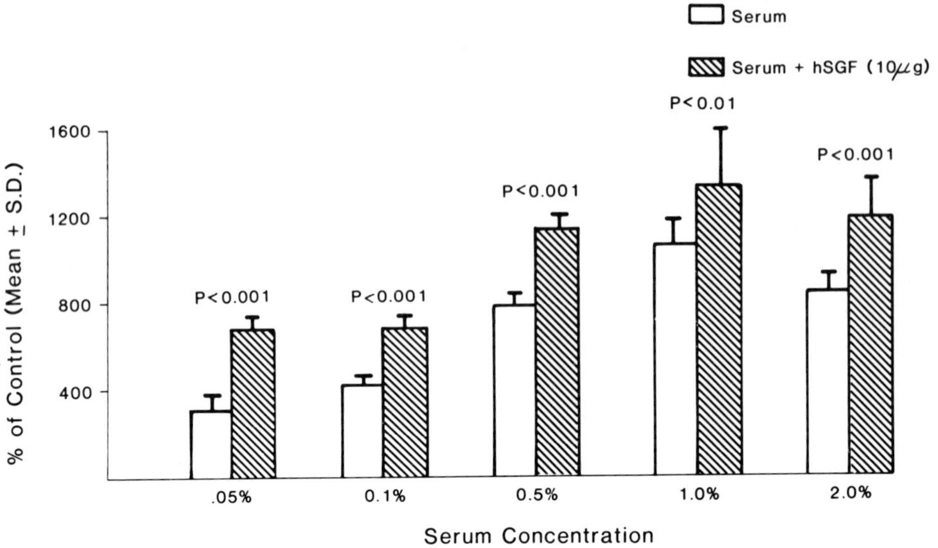

Figure 1: hSGF effect in the presence of fetal calf serum on chick embryo calvarial cells. Values are % stimulation (^{3}H-TdR incorporation into DNA) of unstimulated control and are averages +/- S.D. of 6 replicates except for 1% and 2% which are averages of 12 replicates pooled from 2 separate experiments.

INTERACTION WITH KNOWN MITOGENS AND SERUM

To determine whether hSGF stimulates cell proliferation by a mechanism common to other polypeptide growth factors, we examined the effects on DNA synthesis of known mitogens in combination with hSGF. Mitogenic activities of epidermal growth factor (EGF), fibroblast growth factor (FGF), platelet-derived growth factor (PDGF) and insulin-like growth factor-I (IGF-I) were determined with and without added hSGF using quiescent Balb/c 3T3 fibroblasts. At concentrations which produced maximal stimulatory effects, hSGF-stimulated ^{3}H-Thymidine (^{3}H-TdR) incorporation into TCA insoluble DNA was seven-fold greater than EGF, three-fold greater than IGF-I and PDGF and 1.4 times greater than FGF. Maximum stimulation by these four mitogens was significantly elevated by the addition of hSGF indicating that hSGF stimulates cell proliferation by a rate limiting mechanism different than that of the other mitogens tested (Table 1).

In a similar experiment, stimulation of chick embryo calvarial cell proliferation by fetal calf serum at different concentrations (0.05%, 0.1%, 0.5%, 1.0%, 2.0%) was significantly elevated by the addition of hSGF. The maximal stimulatory effect of serum (1050 +/- 133% of control with 1% added serum) increased by 27% ($p<0.01$) in the presence of hSGF (Figure 1). The results presented in Table 1 and Fig. 1 suggest that hSGF is distinct from the other known growth factors that were tested and from the growth promoting agents present in the serum (polypeptide growth factors as well as agents such as fibronectin and transferin).

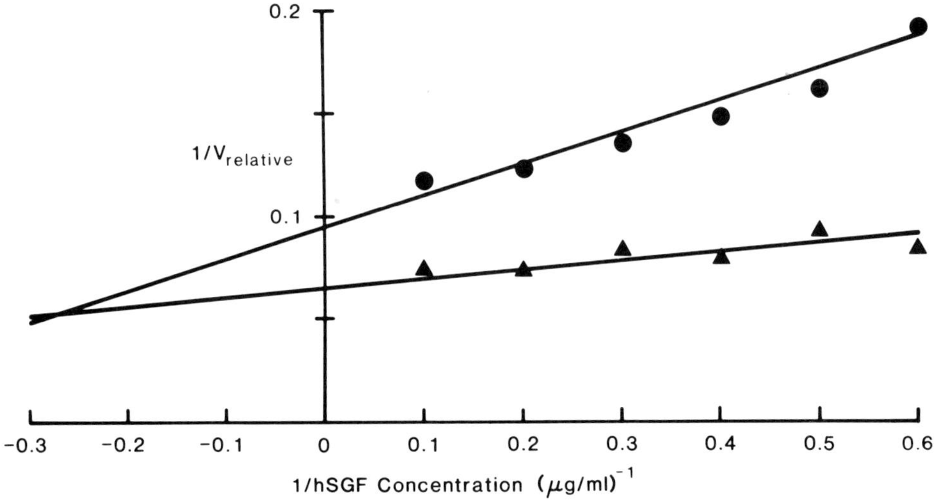

Figure 2: Interactions of PTE and hSGF on chick embryo calvarial cells. Reciprocal plots of percent stimulation (^{3}H-TdR incorporation) vs concentration of hSGF with (▲) and without (●) PTE (InM) added.

hSGF IS NOT A TRYPSIN LIKE PROTEASE

The ability of certain proteolytic enzymes to initiate DNA synthesis and cell division has been known since 1970 (7). Later studies with protease inhibitors indicated that the enzymatic activity of the proteases was necessary for initiation of cell division. To determine whether the growth promoting activity of hSGF is mediated by proteolytic activity, we examined the action of hSGF in the presence of protease inhibitors, phenylmethylsulfonylfluoride (PMSF) and soybean trypsin inhibitor (SBTI). DNA synthesis in calvarial cells was stimulated by trypsin, and this stimulation was inhibited by the protease inhibitors while the hSGF stimulation was not (Table 2). These results suggest that the action of hSGF is not mediated by a serine active protease.

Factor	% of hSGF activity -hSGF	+hSGF	Significance
Control	9.4 + 2.4	100.0 + 19	p<0.001
EGF (10 ng/ml)	13.7 + 3.0	92.0 + 27	p<0.001
FGF (10 ng/ml)	70.9 + 13.2	136.6 + 46.6	p<0.01
IGF (25 ng/ml)	30.2 + 4.6	84.3 + 13.7	p<0.001
PDGF(20 ng/ml)	34.8 + 2.3	75.3 + 9.9	p<0.001

Table 1: Effects of combination of hSGF with other polypeptide growth factors. 3T3 cells were plated at 70,000 cells/well in DMEM in 24 well culture dishes. 24 hrs after plating, the factors were added and incubated for an additional 22 hrs. The cells were then pulse labeled for 2 hrs with 2 µCi of ^{3}H-TdR and TCA precipitable radioactivity was quantitated. Incorporation is expressed as % of maximum incorporation stimulated by hSGF alone and is the average of 6 replicates.

Factor	% of unstimulated control (Mean + S.D.)
hSGF	1199 + 215
hSGF + PMSF + SBTI	1341 + 169
Trypsin	409 + 138
hSGF + Trypsin	653 + 139 *
hSGF + Trypsin + PMSF + SBTI	977 + 204
Trypsin + PMSF + SBTI	115 + 26 **

Table 2: Effects of protease inhibitors and trypsin on hSGF stimulated calvarial cell proliferation. Activity of hSGF was assayed by the incorporation of ^{3}H-TdR into TCA precipitable material in embryonic chick calvarial cells as described earlier (8). The cells were plated overnight in a serum-free medium (DMEM) and were then incubated with the test factor(s) for 18 hrs and pulse labeled with 2 µCi of ^{3}H-TdR for 2 hrs. In this experiment hSGF (12.5 mg/ml) and/or trypsin (5 mg/ml) were preincubated with or without protease inhibitors (phenylmethylsulfonylfluoride, PMSF and soybean trypsin inhibitor, SBTI, 1 mg/ml) for 3 hrs at room temperature. Final concentrations of hSGF, trypsin and protease inhibitors in the culture medium were 10, 4 and 1.6 µg/ml respectively. PMSF & SBTI by themselves did not influence ^{3}H-TdR incorporation. Data are average of 6 replicates.

*Significantly different from hSGF alone (p<0.001).

** Signficantly different from Trypsin (p<0.001).

INTERACTION WITH CALCIUM REGULATING HORMONES:

Because our interest in hSGF arose from _in vivo_ and _in vitro_ studies of the coupling of bone formation to bone resorption, we sought to determine if hormones which stimulate bone resorption affected hSGF activity _in vitro_. We examined the effects of PTH on hSGF mitogenic activity in the calvarial cell culture assay. PTH alone (0.1 nM from bovine parathyroid extract) increased ^{3}H-TdR incorporation to 138% of unstimulated controls, ($p<0.001$) while the stimulation by hSGF alone was several-fold greater than PTH. The addition of PTH to hSGF increased the stimulation of ^{3}H-TdR incorporation above the level observed for hSGF alone suggesting that hSGF is not a PTH-like substance. Reciprocal analysis suggests a mixed type interaction (Fig.2) with PTH increasing the maximal response (V_{max}) to hSGF and decreasing the apparent K_m for hSGF. In separate studies, 1,25-D_3 was also observed to interact with hSGF. Mitogenic activity of hSGF was increased at 1 nM 1,25-D_3 and decreased at 1 uM 1,25-D_3 (unpublished data).

SUMMARY

Evidence based on the molecular weight, purification methods, chemical and biological properties of hSGF suggests that hSGF is different from the other known mitogens tested. From these studies it seems that calcium regulating hormones such as PTH and 1,25-D_3 may modulate the mitogenic activity of hSGF. This interaction between the bone resorbing agents and hSGF may be an important factor in the regulation of bone volume.

ACKNOWLEDGEMENTS

This work was supported by NIH Grants (AM 31061, AM 31062) and by Veterans Administration Research Support. We thank Malcolm Ghazal and Rich Widstrom for technical assistance and Peggy Duane and Penny Nasabal for their help with the manuscript.

REFERENCES

1. Gruber, H.E. and Baylink, D.J. (1981): J. Amer. Geriat. Soc., 29(11), 490
2. Ivey, J.L. and Baylink, D.J. (1981): Metab. Bone Dis. and Rel. Res., 3, 3
3. Howard, H.A., Bottemiller, R.P., Turner, R.J., Rader, J.I. and Baylink, D.J. (1981): Proc. Natl. Acad. Sci., 78(5), 3204
4. Drivdahl, R.H., Howard, G.A. and Baylink, D.J. (1980) Calcif. Tiss. Res., 31, 52
5. Farley, J.R. and Baylink, D.J. (1982): Biochemistry, 21, 3502
6. Farley, J.R., Masuda, T., Wergedal, J.E. and Baylink, D.J. (1982): Biochemsitry, 21, 3502
7. Cunningham, D.D. (1981) In: Tissue Growth Factors, ed. Baserga, R. Springer Verlag, New York
8. Puzas, J.E., Drivdahl, R.H., Howard, G.A., and Baylink, D.J. (1981): Proc. Soc. Exp. Biol. Med., 166, 113

Discussion of paper by Dr. Baylink:

DR. GRAY: David, initially you isolated this factor only from diaphyseal bone. Has that observation held up, and if so, what does it mean in terms of local effects? Second, what cell do you think makes this material?

DR. BAYLINK: On the basis of hydroxyproline content, there's about twice as much of this factor in trabecular bone as in cortical bone. We do not know its cellular origin or even whether it is synthesized in bone.

DR. RAISZ: It is hard to understand how a 70,000 MW material could survive the resorptive factors released by osteoclasts. Could it be secreted by the cells?

DR. BAYLINK: Our factor survives a pH of 3 and heating to 70°C.

DR. RAISZ: But the lysosomal enzymes released by osteoclasts could digest almost any protein.

DR. BAYLINK: Some of our other chromotographic fractions have proteolytic activity and may break down the skeletal growth factor into a smaller molecule, but mitogenic activity is retained and even increased.

DR. NORDIN: What is the relationship between your compound and Marshall Urist's bone morphogenetic protein?

DR. BAYLINK: Urist's protein is of smaller molecular weight (17,000-23,000) and is insoluable in aqueous solution, so the two are chemically distinct. Whether they are functionally related is unknown.

DR. NORDIN: If you put yourself on a low calcium diet, your bone would be uncoupled and your resorption would be too high for your formation, or if you put it the other way around, your formation would be too low for your resorption. How does this differ from the situation in patients with osteoporosis?

DR. BAYLINK: Normal subjects are able to adjust to a moderately low calcium diet without going into negative calcium balance by conserving urine calcium, and by increasing fractional calcium absorption in the gut. These changes are mediated by increases in serum PTH and calcitriol. During this adjustment, there is an increase in bone resorption (also PTH and calcitriol mediated) and subsequently, a coupled increase in bone formation, so that bone is turning over faster but net bone loss is zero. When dietary calcium deficiency is severe, the gut and kidney can no longer compensate, and unbalanced coupling, (i.e., an increase in bone resorption without a further increase in bone formation) may lead to loss of bone from the skeletal mineral reservoir. The unbalanced coupling in the latter situation is a normal physiological response. In contrast, in postmenopausal osteoporotic patients, there is unbalanced coupling, (perhaps due to a faulty coupling mechanism), where resorption exceeds formation even when calcium intake is normal, and when there is a further increase in bone resorption from a moderately low calcium diet or from other causes, the result can be a further disparity between the two rates. Accordingly, in the kinetic data I showed on postmenopausal osteoporotics, the slope for bone formation as a function of bone resorption was less than 1 and as a result, the higher the bone resorption rate, the greater the absolute difference between bone resorption and bone formation and the greater the bone loss.

LOCALLY ELABORATED FACTORS IN THE COORDINATION OF BONE CELL ACTIVITY

W.A. Peck, Victor Shen, and Leonard Rifas

Department of Medicine, The Jewish Hospital of St. Louis and Washington University School of Medicine, St. Louis, MO, U.S.A.

Skeletal remodeling is the orderly removal and replacement of bone that occurs at local sites along the spicules of medullary bone, on the endosteal surfaces and in the Haversian systems of cortical bone, and, in some circumstances, at periosteal surfaces as well. As the pioneering observations of Frost have demonstrated, it is a local process involving multiple complex cellular events (1). Following activation, which may be initiated by mechanical stress, hormones, and other as yet unknown factors, cells of the monocyte-macrophage series are attracted to the activation site and fuse to form mature osteoclasts (2-6). The osteoclasts then proceed to resorb a quantum of bone, creating a resorption cavity of microscopic dimensions. The signal for termination of osteoclast activity, one important limiting determinant of the size of the resorption cavity, has not been defined. After an interval period during which mononucleated cells have been identified in the vicinity of the resorption cavity (7) osteoblasts are recruited from bone marrow mesenchyme (8,9) to the newly resorbed surface, and secrete a sufficient amount of osteoid to repair the resorption defect. The mechanism of replenishment of osteoclast precursors is unknown; in animal systems, macrophage-like osteoclast precursors may derive from nonskeletal reticuloendothelial organs (e.g., spleen) (6). The mesenchymal cells that are osteoblast precursors are capable of division, and thus the mitotic process tends to ensure maintenance of a stable pool of osteoblasts (8,9). It is evident that resorption and formation are closely regulated processes. In addition, they are in close quantitative and temporal linkage, so that the mass of bone in a given location, and, hence, the mass of the skeleton, do not change in the short term. Consequently, there may well be factors that facilitate the transition between resorption and formation. Controls may act at one or more levels: termination of resorption, initiation of osteoblast recruitment, and perhaps proliferation of osteoblast precursors.

Hormones are known to influence the number of remodeling sites, and perhaps the rate of remodeling as well. Not surprisingly, in view of the resorption-formation sequence, it is the resorptive process that manifests the principal responses to these systemic factors. The major stimulators of resorption are parathyroid hormone and $1\alpha,25\text{-}(OH)_2$ vitamin D_3, and the major inhibitor is calcitonin, although cortisol may act as a resorption inhibitor at physiological concentrations. Locally elaborated factors may affect remodeling, acting in several possible ways: transduction of mechanically triggered activation, attraction and attachment of cells to bone surfaces, stimulation of precursor cell migration and (where appropriate) proliferation, termination of osteoclast and osteoblast activity, and, importantly, linkage of resorption and formation.

Three types of local factors may contribute to the regulation of remodeling: first, biophysical (bioelectric and biomechanical) factors that influence bone cell behavior; second, chemical factors that mediate cell-cell communication; and third, components of the skeletal matrix which are capable of modifying bone cell activity, with or without prior release from the matrix during resorption. A single factor may serve multiple functions; for example, the transduction of biomechanical stimulation to bone cell activity and the promotion of precursor cell growth.

A variety of substances have now been identified that might serve as local mediators (stimulators and inhibitors) of bone cell activity; a) components of the organic matrix [bone morphogenetic protein (10,11), putative skeletal coupling factor (12,13), and osteocalcin (14,15)]; b) factors that have been identified in the incubation medium bathing organ-cultured bones and bone cells [bone-derived and bone cell-derived growth factors (16) and putative coupling factors (12,13)]; and, c) most recently, a factor elaborated by cells of the monocyte-macrophage series that stimulates osteoblast growth (macrophage-derived growth factor) (Rifas, L., Mitchell, K., and Peck, W.A., unpublished observations). In addition, many growth factors of non-skeletal origin have been found to modify bone cell mitosis, function, or both, including epidermal growth factor (17), fibroblast growth factor (18), and the somatomedins (19).

Of particular importance in the remodeling scenario are the factors that might link resorption and formation. Due to the pioneering work of Dr. David Baylink and his co-workers, we now know that organ-cultured bones undergoing hormone-stimulated resorption <u>in vitro</u> release a factor that has the capacity to engender subsequent bone formation (20). This activity may or may not be similar to the large peptide which has been extracted from human and animal bone that appears to be an osteoblast growth-stimulating factor (13,21). It is intriguing to speculate that components of the organic matrix, released during resorption, are the so-called "coupling mediators," engendering a proliferative response on the part of osteoblast precursors, osteoblast maturation, and perhaps initiation of bone formation. In addition to the "coupling factor," described by Baylink, and osteocalcin, the bone matrix is a storehouse of proteins, many of which are unidentified, that may serve important roles in the cell biology of bone.

Direct chemical mediation of cell-to-cell communication would seem to be a more efficacious mechanism of resorption-formation linkage than mediation by newly released matrix components in light of the greater potential for close regulation of their biosynthesis and release. Since macrophages participate in remodeling as osteoclast precursors and as elaborators of prostaglandins, we explored the possibility that they may also be responsible for synthesizing a factor that promotes osteoblast growth. In fact, we found that the conditioned medium from cultured rodent macrophages contains a heat-stable, trypsin-inhibitable, non-dialyzable factor that has the capacity to stimulate DNA synthesis and proliferation in isolated rat osteoblasts (Rifas, L., Mitchell, K., and Peck, W.A., unpublished observations). Moreover, we have obtained evidence that this factor is neither a prostaglandin, nor does it act on osteoblast-like cells by stimulating prostaglandin release. Although macrophage-derived growth factor also stimulates the growth of chondroblasts, it has no stimulatory effect on the proliferation of fibroblasts.

Local regulatory substances are likely to be important purveyors of biological information in skeletal remodeling. These factors, when identified, purified to homogeneity, and completely characterized, may have substantive clinical relevance. It may be possible to synthesize them in sufficient quantity, using recombinant techniques, to modify remodeling in patients with skeletal diseases. In addition, their assay in biological fluids may provide hitherto unavailable information concerning the status of skeletal remodeling in humans. The next five years will be an exciting period in the investigation of local regulation of bone metabolism.

REFERENCES

1. Frost, H.M. (1964): Mathematical Elements of Bone Remodeling. Charles C. Thomas, Springfield, Illinois.
2. Fischman, D.A. and Hay, E.D. (1962): Anat. Record, 143, 329.
3. Jee, W.S.S. and Nolan, P.D. (1963): Nature, 200, 225.
4. Gothlin, G. and Ericsson, J.L.E. (1973): Virch. Arch. Cell. Path., 12, 318.
5. Kahn, A.J. and Simmons, D.J. (1975): Nature, 258, 325.
6. Walker, D.G. (1975): Science, 190,784.
7. Tran Van, P., Vignery, A. and Baron, R. (1982): Cell Tiss. Res., 225, 283
8. Young, R.W. (1962): J. Cell Biol., 14, 357.
9. Owen, M. (1963): J. Cell Biol., 19, 19.
10. Urist, M.R. (1965): Science, 150, 893.
11. Huggins, C., Wiseman, S. and Reddi, H. (1970): J. Exp. Med., 132, 1250.
12. Drivdahl, R.H., Howard, G.A. and Baylink, D.J. (1982): Biochim. Biophys. Acta, 714, 26.
13. Farley, J.R. and Baylink, D.J. (1982): Biochemistry, 21, 3502.
14. Malone, J.D., Teitelbaum, S.L., Griffin, G.L, Senior, R.M. and Kahn, A.J. (1982): J. Cell Biology, 92, 227.
15. Mundy, G.R. and Poser, J.W. (1983): Calcif. Tiss. Int., 35, 164.
16. Canalis, E., Peck, W.A., and Raisz, L.G. (1980): Science, 210, 1021.
17. Canalis, E. and Raisz, L.G. (1979): Endocrinology, 104, 862.
18. Canalis, E. and Raisz, L.G. (1980): Metabolism, 29, 108.
19. Canalis, E. (1980): J. Clin. Invest, 66, 709.
20. Howard, G.A., Bottemiller, B.L., Turner, R.T., Rader, J.I. and Baylink, D.J. (1981): Proc. Natl. Acad. Sci. USA, 78, 3204.
21. Farley, J.R., Masuda, T., Wergedal, J.E. and Baylink, D.J. (1982): Biochemistry, 21, 3508.

Discussion of paper by Dr. Peck:

DR. MING CAI QIU: If bone matrix components attract osteoclasts, why are these cells seen predominantly on mineralized bone rather than osteoid?

DR. PECK: We know that mineralized bone surfaces are chemotactic for macrophages in <u>in vitro</u> systems, but the role of the mineral in modulating the signal is unknown. Also, there is a notion that activation of the remodeling cycle involves some change in the mineralized bone surface, such as contraction of the previously flattened osteoblast-derived lining cells, which exposes cell-free surfaces to surrounding macrophages. Perhaps this morphologic change in the lining cells requires mineral in the underlying matrix.

DR. RAISZ: Prostaglandin E_2 (PGE_2) is one of the few substances which is produced by bone cells and which can increase bone mass in vivo. Could PGE_2 function as a co-factor in cell replication and/or differentiation?

DR. PECK: This hasn't been tested systematically in any bone cell system. Indomethacin, which is a blocker of cyclo-oxygenase, does not impair bone formation in an organ culture system. In your system did it enhance the response to macrophages?

DR. RAISZ: No, there was no effect.

FUNCTIONAL LOAD BEARING AS A DETERMINANT FOR BONE REMODELLING[1]

Lance E. Lanyon and Clinton T. Rubin

Department of Anatomy and Cellular Biology, Tufts University Schools of Medicine and Veterinary Medicine, and Human Nutrition Research Center on Aging, Boston, MA, U.S.A.

Following growth, the need for bone remodelling is both structural and metabolic. "Metabolic remodelling" is required to provide a supply of mineral to maintain serum Ca. This objective could be accomplished by turnover in a small volume of mineralized tissue whose shape would be immaterial. The requirements for "structural remodelling" are more stringent. Each element of the skeleton must not only be made to conform to a certain anatomical shape, but must also be sufficiently robust to withstand functional load bearing. Such structural competence is only achieved and maintained as a continuing response to load bearing.

In any structure, the product of load, mass, geometry and material properties is the strain engendered within the tissue. Functionally induced strain is not only the most important parameter to control, but it also seems the most likely variable to which the cell population could respond. We propose therefore that the objective of mechanically related bone remodelling is to influence the architecture, and adjust the mass of the structure, in order to produce an acceptable (optimum?) level of functional strain within its tissue. Apart from the anabolic effect of steroids, the hormonal and metabolic influences commonly associated with bone metabolism either cause resorption or facilitate the progress of remodelling events without influencing their objective. We speculate therefore that the principal stimulus responsible for the achievement and maintenance of functional levels of bone mass is that generated by functional strain.[5] Only the absence of this stimulus is necessary to permit negatively balanced remodelling which will continue under hormonal control until a basic minimum mass is reached. It is not known to what extent load bearing can influence metabolically engendered remodelling or vice versa. However, it is as a result of these two often conflicting influences that the remodelling activity of the adult skeleton is controlled. In addition to providing the stimulus responsible for determining bone mass, functional strain is itself a cause of internal remodelling since customary strain levels are sufficiently high to cause a certain amount of fatigue damage within the tissue. Such damage can only be repaired by trabecular and intracortical remodelling which is structurally indistinguishable from that engendered by hormonal stimulation.

A number of animal experiments involving manipulation of a bone's functional strain environment have demonstrated that bone mass can be influenced by a very few load applications per day, and that the remodelling process is sensitive at least to the peak magnitude, rate, and distribution of strain.

---

[1]This work has been supported by MRC(UK), Arth. & Rheum. Council, Wellcome Trust, and NASA Grant #NAG 9-25.

1. Number of strain cycles. (1)

A preparation has been developed in which the ulna shaft in the wings of birds is isolated from normal functional load bearing by subarticular osteotomy. The cut ends of the isolated diaphysis are covered with stainless steel caps and pierced with Steinman pins which emerge through the skin on the dorsal and ventral surfaces of the wing. These pins are held together by external clamps so that wing movement cannot engender strains in the bone's shaft. Once a day, the fixators are removed and the pins engaged in a compressive loading device.

The effect of different numbers of load cycles was investigated in the rooster ulna by producing peak strain levels similar to those engendered in the intact bone during vigorous wing flapping. Bone Mineral Content at the midshaft was substantially increased (33%) by as few as 36 consecutive 0.5 Hz load cycles per day, and no additional new bone formation resulted from increasing this number from 36 to 360 or 1800. Furthermore, only 4 cycles per day of this potentially osteogenic stimulus prevented the resorptive remodelling which in the absence of loading leads to disuse osteoporosis.

2. Peak strain magnitude. (2)

Using a similar preparation in the turkey ulna, the number of cycles per day and the strain rate were kept constant (100 cycles at 0.01 sec^{-1}), and the peak strain magnitude altered. Functional isolation alone resulted in a reduction of cross-sectional area at the midshaft which 100 load cycles per day engendering peak strains of 500 microstrain were insufficient to prevent. However, at 1000 microstrain, bone area was maintained and strains above this level were associated with a proportional increase in new bone formation on both periosteal and endosteal surfaces. Both in this experiment and the preceding one, substantial endosteal and periosteal new bone formation occurred practically unaccompanied by intracortical remodelling. In both these experiments also it seemed that small amounts of strain generated stimulation produced either by the first few strain reversals, or by low strain levels, appeared to prevent the onset of resorptive remodelling whereas further reversals or higher strain levels resulted in osteogenesis.

3. Strain rate. (3)

The effect of the rate of change of strain was investigated by applying artificial loads to the sheep radius. In this preparation the peak strains and strain rates engendered could not be varied independently. Furthermore, during the period when not in the loading machine, the bone was used for weight bearing. Analysis between the remodelling and mechanical variables (change in area, thickness of new periosteal bone deposited, number of secondary osteones and peak strain, strain rate, etc.) showed that peak strain rate consistently produced the highest correlations. High strain rates were associated with greater amounts of new bone formation and low strain rates either with less osteogenesis or (in one case, at least) with resorption.

4. Strain distribution. (4)

In this experiment, the customary strain in the sheep radius was engendered by normal locomotion, but the strain distribution was altered slightly by removal of the small supporting ulna. Although the increase in strain at the bone surface during walking was less than 20%, the remodelling which resulted produced sufficient new bone, appropriately placed, to compensate for the structural loss of the ulna. This demonstrates not only the sensitivity of the remodelling response to small changes in strain distribution, but also that structural adaptation can occur without exceeding customary (rather than maximum) functional strain levels.

The most widespread cause of structural failure within the skeleton is that associated with post-menopausal osteoporosis. That bone loss in this condition should continue to the extent of structural collapse indicates that the mechanically adaptive control previously responsible for ensuring such competence has become ineffective. This probably reflects a change in both the "structurally" and "hormonally" engendered influences on bone remodelling. Reduction in the potentially osteogenic effect of load bearing may result from a decreased mechanical stimulus per se, a decreased ability of the bone cell population to respond to an appropriate mechanical stimulus, or a decreased perceived mechanical stimulus resulting from a strain regime which is inappropriate as a stimulus but nevertheless still causes tissue damage. Coincident with a decrease in the effectiveness of this potentially osteogenic strain generated effect is an increase in the hormonally mediated demand for resorption. This results from decreased Ca intake, reduced Ca absorption, reduced vit. D, and by removal of sex hormones which probably have a protective effect on remodelling.

Smith et al.'s demonstration that even in older women age-related bone loss can be modulated by exercise, underlines the continued importance of appropriate physical activity in maintaining bone mass. Current studies in our laboratory using calcium deficiency and artificial loading suggest that mechanical function can provide some protection from hormonally mediated demands for resorption. We hope that studies such as those reported here will eventually reveal the mechanism by which mechanical events are transduced into appropriate cellular responses. Until that time these results should provide immediate clinical benefit by defining those aspects of a bone's loading regime which are important in controlling bone mass, and thus indicating those aspects of exercise or physical therapy likely to be most beneficial for people at risk from deleterious bone loss.

REFERENCES

1. Rubin, C.T. and Lanyon, L.E. (1981): Orthopaedic Transactions, 5, 2, 237.
2. Rubin, C.T. and Lanyon, L.E. (1983): Transactions of Orthopaedic Research Society, 8, 70.
3. O'Connor, J.A., Lanyon, L.E. and MacFie, H. (1982): Journal of Biomechanics, 15, 767.
4. Lanyon, L.E., Goodship, A.E., Pye, C.J. and MacFie, H. (1982): Journal of Biomechanics, 15, 141.
5. Lanyon, L.E. (1980): In: Osteoporosis: Recent Advances in Pathogenesis and Treatment. Editors: De Luca et al., University Park Press.
6. Smith, E.L., Reddan, W. and Smith, P.E. (1981): Medicine and Science in Sports and Exercise, 13, 60.

Discussion of paper by Dr. Lanyon:

DR. FROST: In your experiments the bone loss occurred on the endosteal surface, and the gain on periosteal surface is so the effect of mechanical strain is modified by local factors.

DR. LANYON: Mechanical loading stimulated bone formation endosteally as well as periosteally. The location of bone deposition is governed by some mechanical rationale that we don't understand. It does not appear to be a random response to a general need for increased strength.

DR. BOHR: I agree that exercise is very important for bone formation. Do you think the stimulus is mechanical or electrical?

DR. LANYON: I don't know. Rather than responding to the mechanical stimulus themselves, the cells may be responding to the electrical environment that mechanical strain will cause within bone tissue, but the literature is confused.

DR. ARNAUD: Does removal of any endocrine gland alter the response to strain?

DR. LANYON: We have not done those experiments, but mechanical stimulation does protect the skeleton to a certain extent from the effects of calcium deprivation.

DR. KORKOR: Could changes in bone blood flow account for your results?

DR. LANYON: I think not, because of the graded response to differing amounts of strain. I do not think we would have been able to demonstrate a nice dose-response curve going through zero if blood flow had been involved. We also take great care to ensure that the nutrient artery and vein are undisturbed and can check their patency on post-mortem histology.

DR. PARFITT: In some tissues, such as the liver, the regulation of mass is partly achieved by inhibitors of mitosis called chalones. Is it possible that part of the increase in bone mass that you observed is related to a chalone from bone, rather than directly to mechanical strain?

DR. LANYON: It is certainly possible that rather than stimulating osteogenesis directly, mechanical strain, or something engendered by it, suppresses an inhibitory factor, allowing an increase in bone mass.

DR. AKERSTROM: Using the electron-probe we find that after trauma to the tibia in patients there is much greater loss of mineral than loss of bone volume.

DR. LANYON: We have not looked at mineral separately. I don't think our results are due to trauma, however, since the surgical intervention is the same for all groups and the strains are all within the physiological range.

VIII SECONDARY HYPERPARATHYROIDISM AND PTH-MEDIATED BONE LOSS

PTH-MEDIATED BONE LOSS: An Overview

Sudhaker D. Rao

Bone and Mineral Research Laboratory, Henry Ford Hospital, Detroit, Michigan, U.S.A.

Among the many causes of diminished skeletal mass, parathyroid hormone (PTH) mediated bone resorption has been the most widely studied experimentally and age-related osteoporosis the least understood. Because of histologic heterogeneity, it has been assumed that the etiology of osteoporosis, whether postmenopausal (Type I) or senile (Type II), is multifactorial (1). This session examined the possible contribution of PTH-mediated bone loss to the pathogenesis of osteoporosis.

Dr. Raisz reviewed the actions of PTH on bone that might cause bone loss. Bone resorption is stimulated acutely, with an increase in both the activity and the number of osteoclasts. These cells lack PTH receptors, and the effect may be mediated by an action on the bone lining cells (2). These and other cells of osteoblast lineage possess PTH receptors, and PTH acutely inhibits collagen synthesis. The longer term effect to increase bone formation is probably brought about by the coupling mechanism (3). Whether the summation of these short- and long-term effects is catabolic or anabolic may depend on the intake and absorption of dietary calcium and on the plasma phosphate level.

Dr. Baron reviewed the histologic assessment of bone resorption. Osteoclasts occupy only a small fraction of the total crenated or Howship's lacunar surface, the remainder being covered by various kinds of mononuclear cells that appear in the time interval between the end of resorption and the beginning of formation, and identify the so-called reversal surface. In hyperparathyroidism and other states of increased bone turnover the increase in total resorption surface reflects an increase in osteoclast surface. But in postmenopausal and other types of osteoporosis the increase in total resorption surface reflects only an increase in reversal surface, so that increased total resorption surface is not a valid index of increased resorption rate in osteoporosis. Looking at another facet of the histologic assessment of bone resorption, Dr. Qiu found that osteoclasts normally avoid osteoid and resorb only unmineralized bone, but that osteoclastic resorption of osteoid may occur with the stimulus of severe hyperparathyroidism (4).

Dr. Kleerekoper demonstrated that chronic hyperparathyroidism, whether primary or secondary, accelerates age-related loss of cortical bone. Loss of trabecular bone was observed only in a small subset of patients with primary hyperparathyroidism, but was more substantial in patients with secondary hyperparathyroidism due to gastrointestinal malabsorption of calcium. However, even in these patients the relative deficit was significantly greater for cortical than for trabecular bone. This conclusion differs from that of other investigators, partly because of a different interpretation of measurements by single photon absorptiometry at the distal radius. This is normally believed to be relatively more sensitive to loss of trabecular bone, but our studies have indicated that any trabecular bone at this site is metabolically inert and that, as at the proximal site, losses are due predominantly to cortical thinning. To avoid selection bias, none of the patients had sustained a fracture, but in another session Rao showed a significant increase in fracture risk in patients with secondary hyperparathyroidism without osteomalacia (5).

Dr. Lips examined the relationship between subclinical vitamin D deficiency in the elderly and hip fractures. Iliac histomorphometry of the patients with hip fracture could be divided into three groups: those with increased turnover (increased resorption and formation), impaired coupling (increased resorption and normal formation), and low turnover (depression of both resorption and formation). This analysis was based purely on static measurements, not on kinetic studies with tetracycline labeling. In the high turnover group the plasma 25OHD level was low and cortical thickness in the ilium significantly reduced. None of the patients had osteomalacia as defined elsewhere (5). The data were consistent with the view that the early osseous effects of vitamin D deficiency are mainly those of secondary hyperparathyroidism leading to accelerated loss of cortical bone. More generally, PTH-mediated bone loss probably makes little contribution to postmenopausal (Type I) osteoporosis with vertebral compression fractures, but may make a significant contribution to senile (Type II) osteoporosis leading to hip fractures.

REFERENCES

1. Riggs, B.L., L.J. Melton III, H.W. Wahner: Heterogeneity of involutional osteoporosis: evidence for two distinct osteoporosis syndromes. Clinical Disorders of Bone and Mineral Metabolism, this volume.
2. Parfitt, A.M., C.H.E. Mathews, A.R. Villanueva, D.S. Rao, M. Rogers, M. Kleerekoper, and B. Frame: Microstructural and cellular basis of age related bone loss and osteoporosis. Clinical Disorders of Bone and Mineral Metabolism, this volume.
3. Mohan, S., J.R. Farley, T.A. Linkhart, L.A. Murphy and D.J. Baylink: Studies on human skeletal growth factor: interaction with known mitogens and calcium regulating hormones. Clinical Disorders of Bone and Mineral Metabolism, this volume.
4. Qiu, Ming Cai, C. Mathews, A.M. Parfitt: Osteoclastic resorption of osteoid in secondary hyperparathyroidism. Clinical Disorders of Bone and Mineral Metabolism, this volume.
5. Rao, D. Sudhaker, A. Villanueva, M. Mathews, B. Pumo, B. Frame, M. Kleerekoper, and A.M. Parfitt: Histologic evolution of vitamin-D depletion in patients with intestinal malabsorption or dietary deficiency. Clinical Disorders of Bone and Mineral Metabolism, this volume.

ESTIMATION OF TRABECULAR BONE RESORPTION BY HISTOMORPHOMETRY: EVIDENCE FOR A PROLONGED REVERSAL PHASE WITH NORMAL RESORPTION IN POST-MENOPAUSAL OSTEOPOROSIS AND COUPLED INCREASED RESORPTION IN PRIMARY HYPERPARATHYROIDISM

Roland Baron, Sam Magee, Ann Silverglate, Arthur Broadus and Robert Lang

Yale University School of Medicine, Department of Internal Medicine, Endocrine Section, 333 Cedar Street, New Haven, Connecticut 06510, U.S.A.

INTRODUCTION

The pathogenesis of trabecular bone loss in post-menopausal osteoporosis (PMOP) is still the subject of numerous controversies. Although it is now recognized that the bone remodeling activity in such patients is heterogeneous (1-3) the mechanisms leading to bone loss have been successively attributed to an increased bone resorption (4,5) or to a decreased formation (2). On the other hand, patients with primary hyperparathyroidism (1°HPT) are usually found to have, as a group, a normal amount of trabecular bone, despite an increased resorption (6).

Our experimental studies on the bone remodeling sequence in the rat allowed us to describe an intermediate phase between resorption and formation, termed the reversal phase (7,8). During this reversal phase, cells that are neither osteoclasts nor osteoblasts were observed within recently created Howship's lacunae. Further studies have recently allowed us to demonstrate that 1) reversal really occurs after resorption and before formation (9); 2) the cells present during the reversal phase are mononuclear phagocytes (10) and 3) the cement line is formed during this phase (10). These observations therefore led us to consider the possibility that the reversal phase was, in fact, the morphological counterpart for the coupling mechanism between R and F.

It is of importance to make a distinction between two pathways that would both lead to bone loss (11): 1) uncoupling, a situation in which the coupling message is not functioning and where osteoblasts do not appear in the remodeling focus, therefore leading to an accumulation of Howship's lacunae without osteoclasts and 2) imbalance, a situation in which the coupling occurs but where the osteoblasts do not synthesize as much matrix as was previously resorbed by the osteoclasts.

As previously discussed in a comparison between osteopenic patients and patients with a normal or high trabecular bone volume (11) our morphometric approach to the evaluation of coupling in bone biopsies has been based upon the fact that, under normal circumstances, bone formation occurs in each Howship's lacuna after a constant delay, the reversal phase, the osteoblasts filling the lacunae at the same rate that osteoclasts are creating them. Consequently, the ratio of reversal to osteoclastic lacunae should remain constant when coupling is occurring normally even when osteoclastic resorption is increased.

We have, in the present study, analyzed by histomorphometry of iliac crest biopsies the coupling status of 19 post-menopausal osteoporotic women and compared the results to 29 patients with primary hyperparathyroidism (5 males and 24 females, of which 17 were post-menopausal at the time of the biopsy).

PATIENTS AND METHODS

The group with PMOP was selected according to the following criteria: 1) presence of more than one non-traumatic vertebral compression fracture and osteoporosis by X-rays; 2) women older than 50 and with natural or surgical menopause; 3) normal serum and urine biochemistry (PTH, Ca, P, Mg, Alkaline Phosphatase, Creatinine, Urinary Calcium, NcAMP); 4) no osteomalacia on biopsy; 5) no other disease and no medication interfering with calcium metabolism. The 1°HPT group was selected according to the usual criteria for this endocrine disorder: they all had surgically and/or biochemically proven HPT (increased PTH, NcAMP, $1,25(OH)_2D_3$ and serum Ca).

Iliac crest biopsies were obtained in all patients after double fluorescent labelings, processed undecalcified and analyzed histomorphometrically for the trabecular bone area.

RESULTS AND DISCUSSION

The results showed that, when considering only the total Howship's lacunae surface, i.e. without making the distinction between osteoclastic resorption and reversal surfaces, no difference was found between the two groups. Although this observation has led others to conclude at an increased bone resorption in PMOP (4,5), this interpretation cannot be made on the basis of total lacunae surface (8,11). When osteoclastic surface is taken into account separately, it becomes clear that this parameter is increased in 1°HPT and not in PMOP taken as a group. Three PMOP patients had, however, an increased osteoclastic surface. Further analysis of the relationships between osteoclastic surface and total Howship's lacunae allowed a very good separation of the two groups of patients. In the 1°HPT group, osteoclastic surface was linearly correlated both with total lacunae and with reversal lacunae, so that the reversal to osteoclastic surface ratio was actually lower than normal; as expected in such a situation, there was also a good correlation between osteoclasts and the bone formation rate derived from the analysis of fluorescent labels. This indicated a normal coupling with a high turnover in 1°HPT patients.

In the PMOP group, on the other hand, the osteoclastic surface was correlated neither with the total lacunae, nor with the reversal lacunae or the bone formation rate. As a group, they presented with a low bone formation rate for their osteoclastic surface, including the 3 patients with increased resorption.

Most of the patients in this group, the 3 high resorption patients set aside, had a marked accumulation of Howship's lacunae despite a normal osteoclastic surface. Consequently, the reversal to osteoclastic surface ratio was very high in the PMOP group. The 3 high resorption patients had, however, a decreased ratio as observed in the 1°HPT group.

It is concluded from this study that 16 out of 19 patients with PMOP had normal bone resorption and an uncoupling of resorption to formation, leading to a low bone formation rate, an accumulation of Howship's lacunae and therefore to bone loss. Three patients, on the other hand, had an increased and coupled turnover as demonstrated by the lack of accumulation of Howship's lacunae but a slight imbalance between R and F with a proportionally low bone formation rate, given their increased resorption.

The 1°HPT group, on the other hand, demonstrated a coupled and balanced increased bone turnover with the exception of 2 post-menopausal women who were also osteopenic and demonstrated the same bone morphometric abnormalities than the high turnover PMOP patients.

Both groups of patients, despite a relative clinical and biochemical homogeneity, demonstrated some heterogeneity in terms of their bone histomorphometry. They also overlapped in some respects since some 1°HPT patients had low bone volume and a relative decrease in bone formation rates and some PMOP patients had increased resorption. Very interestingly, these latter also had circulating PTH levels which were at the upper limit of normal and elevated hydroxyprolinuria.

In conclusion, these results demonstrate that 1) the increased extent of Howship's lacunae in most PMOP patients is not related with an increased resorption but with a prolonged or aborted reversal phase (uncoupling); 2) the same increase in lacunae observed in 1°HPT patients is due to an increased resorption but with a normal coupling and 3) a subgroup of patients (3/19 PMOP and 2/17 PM 1°HPT) show high turnover OP with a normal coupling but an imbalance between resorption and formation.

This study reemphasizes the need to measure the osteoclastic and reversal surfaces separately to analyze bone resorption and the coupling process in patients with metabolic bone diseases.

ACKNOWLEDGEMENT

This work has been supported in part by the GCRC Grant RR125 and by Grants DE04724 and AM29789 from the National Institute of Health.

REFERENCES

1. Whyte, M.P., Bergfeld, M.A., Murphy, W.A., Avioli, L.V. and Teitelbaum, S.L. (1982): Am. J. Med., 72, 193.
2. Parfitt, A.M., Mathews, C., Rao, D., Frame, B., Kleerekoper, M., Villanueva, A.R. (1981): In: Osteoporosis: Recent Advances in Pathogenesis and Treatment, pp. 321-330. Editors: H.F. DeLuca, H.M. Frost, W.S.S. Jee, C.C. Johnston, Jr., A.M. Parfitt. University Park Press, Baltimore, MD.
3. Meunier, P.J., Sellami, S., Briancon, D., Edouard, C. (1981): In: Osteoporosis: Recent Advances in Pathogenesis and Treatment, pp. 293-301. Editors: H.F. DeLuca, H.M. Frost, W.S.S. Jee, C.C. Johnston, Jr., A.M. Parfitt, University Park Press, Baltimore, MD.
4. Jowsey, J., Kelly, P.J., Riggs, B.L., Bianco, A.J., Scholz, D.A. and Gershon-Cohen, J. (1965): J. Bone Joint Surg., 47-A, 785.
5. Nordin, B.E.C., Aaron, J., Speed, R., Crilly, R.G. (1981): Lancet, 11, 277.
6. Mosekilde, L., Melsen, F. (1978): Acta Med. Scand., 204, 97.
7. Baron, R. (1973): J. Biol. Buccale, 1, 151.
8. Baron, R. (1977): In: Bone Histomorphometry, pp. 179-183. Editor: P.J. Meunier. Lab. Armour Montagu, Paris.
9. Tran Van, P., Vignery, A. and Baron, R. (1982): Anat. Rec., 202, 445.
10. Tran Van, P., Vignery, A. and Baron, R. (1982): Cell Tiss. Res., 225, 283.
11. Baron, R., Vignery, A. and Lang, R. (1980): In: Osteoporosis: Recent Advances in Pathogenesis and Treatment, pp. 311-320. Editors: H.F. Deluca, H.M. Frost, W.S.S. Jee, C.C. Johnston, Jr., A.M. Parfitt. University Park Press, Baltimore, MD.

Discussion following paper by: R. BARON

L. RAISZ: Dr. Meunier showed that the matrix apposition rate was decreased in hyperparathyroidism. Is that true in your study as well?

R. BARON: Yes, it is true. In both groups, the linear appositional rate is decreased, more in the osteoporotics. What I showed is bone formation rate at the tissue level which takes into account the extent of the double and half the single labeled surfaces.

M. PARFITT: You showed an acid phosphatase staining cell and stated that it was not an osteoclast. Dr. Evans, who I believe is in the audience, adapted a method previously developed in Dr. Baylink's laboratory which defines an osteoclast as an acid phosphatase-containing cell. Would you comment?

R. BARON: Acid phosphatase is not a privilege of osteoclasts. Any cell that is involved in phagocytosis will have a large number of lysosomes and, therefore, acid phosphatase will be present. My definition of an osteoclast is that it first has to be in a lacuna; second, it has to be multinucleated; and, third, it has to have a ruffled border.

M. PARFITT: Do you rule out the possibility that a mononuclear cell might engage in bone resorption?

R. BARON: I do not, but to demonstrate that, you would have to have electron microscopic evidence of a ruffled border.

J. KANIS: It seems important from the point of view of the pathophysiology of osteoporosis to distinguish between imbalance and uncoupling in describing an increase in the extent of the reversal phase which will lead to an imbalance. How do you conclude that it is an uncoupling, rather than an absence of recruitment at previous resorption sites?

R. BARON: This is an important question. At the systemic level, and also actually at the tissue level, both mechanisms lead to what can be called imbalance, where the amount of bone that is formed does not equal to the amount of bone that is resorbed. However, I believe that our data show there are two ways to arrive at this systemic imbalance. One is a failure of osteoblasts recruitment; and therefore an accumulation of aborted reversal lacunae.

J. KANIS: The question is really how do you distinguish between the two?

R. BARON: In one case you have a disproportional accumulation of reversal lacunae, and in the other you have a decreased bone formation rate without an accumulation of lacunae.

M. FALLON: I am not sure the audience appreciated how difficult it is to cut undecalcified sections of bone for study by electron microscopy. My question is how sure are you that the inactive lacunae or reversal phases do not require another round of bone resorption before they initiate a bone-forming sequence?

R. BARON: I have no data, but I would like to know that. Let me put it another way. We know that once osteoblast formation is initiated, resorption is inhibited for a while for one reason or another. I do not know whether the cement line that is formed during the reversal phase is also inhibitory for resorption. I believe it is, but I do not have any direct evidence for it.

M. FALLON: The inactive cells that are present, when stained histochemically for alkaline phosphatase, in my experience, are positive even though they are extremely thin and attenuated. My experience with sodium fluoride-treated patients would indicate that they deposit bone at these inactive sites without a previous round of bone resorption.

J. REEVE: I wonder whether the abnormality might not be in the hyperparathyroid patients rather than in the osteoporotic patients? In collaboration with Dr. Meunier's group, we have done a study in which we looked at calcium balances performed simultaneously with bone biopsies. We were attracted by the hypothesis that the arrest during the reversal phase might be associated with a significant negative calcium balance in some of our patients. By means of a bi-variable regression, we looked independently for a bone-forming contribution to the calcium balance with second independent variable being active osteoclasts or the total resorption surfaces. Both osteoclast numbers and total resorption surfaces correlated similarly, which led me to the thought that perhaps the difference between the two groups might be that the hyperparathyroid patients are going through a very short reversal phase in contrast to a longer reversal phase in the osteoporotic patients. Perhaps the osteoporotic patients do "reverse" in the end, but the negative balance seen sometimes may be because osteoblasts fail prematurely.

R. BARON: That is an interesting comment, and it is true that in hyperparathyroid patients there is a shortening of this intermediate phase. Let us state it in this way; the coupling is faster in hyperparathyroid patients.

Clearly in the osteoporotic patients it occurs slower than normal. Now about your correlations. I think if you make statistical analyses of these patients, and especially since you have more patients than we do, the number of patients in what I call a coupled situation, will increase proportionately. If you make a correlation, you will find it positive; however, I think you are dealing with two separate groups with an overlap.

MECHANISMS OF PARATHYROID HORMONE MEDIATED BONE LOSS

Lawrence G. Raisz

Division of Endocrinology and Metabolism, University of Connecticut School of Medicine, Farmington, CT, U.S.A.

Parathyroid hormone (PTH) carries out it physiologic function of maintaining extracellular (and probably also intracellular) calcium concentration by affecting multiple organ systems (1). When the calcium supply is ample, stimulation of renal tubular reabsorption of calcium and inhibition of tubular reabsorption of phosphate, together with stimulation of renal 1,25 dihydroxyvitamin D synthesis and consequent enhancement of intestinal calcium absorption, are probably sufficient. However, the appearance of parathyroid glands in evolution is closely related to the need to maintain calcium concentration in the absence of exogenous calcium. Under these circumstances, PTH can only maintain extracellular calcium concentration by stimulating bone resorption and inhibiting its formation (2). Stimulation of bone resorption by PTH was demonstrated many years ago, but we know less about its precise mechanism than we do about the inhibitory effect of PTH on bone formation. These effects of PTH are catabolic and result in bone loss. Thus in calcium deficiency the structural functions of the skeleton may be impaired to fulfill its metabolic function as a storehouse of mineral.

PTH can produce an anabolic effect on the skeleton under certain circumstances. This is best demonstrated when PTH is administered intermittently and there is an adequate supply of mineral (3). It is probably an indirect effect of PTH, perhaps mediated by the release of a skeletal growth factor during the resorptive process. Both the catabolic and anabolic effects of PTH can be observed clinically. The former is presumably largely responsible for the diminished bone mass seen in patients with primary hyperparathyroidism (4). On the other hand, some patients treated intermittently with small doses of PTH show positive calcium balance and some increase in trabecular bone mass.

Many experiments have demonstrated an increase in the activity and number of osteoclasts in response to PTH, both in vivo and in vitro. In quantitative electron microscopic studies, the ruffled border area can increase 30 minutes after PTH administration (5). Osteoclast number can increase within a few hours. Thymidine incorporation may also increase, suggesting that PTH has an effect on cell replication. However, this does not appear to be essential for the PTH response since in organ cultures of fetal rat long bones the PTH response is not inhibited by concentrations of hydroxyurea which block thymidine incorporation into DNA (6). Since the increase in osteoclast numbers is still observed in the presence of hydroxyurea we conclude that PTH can stimulate an existing population of local preosteoclasts which coalesce and form active osteoclasts. In vivo, blood-borne precursors may form osteoclasts in response to PTH (7). Although these effects of PTH are direct in the sense that they occur in isolated bone in organ culture, they may not be exerted directly on the osteoclasts and preosteoclasts. It has not been possible to demonstrate PTH receptors on osteoclasts. Moreover, isolated osteoclasts which respond morphologically to calcitonin show no morphologic change in response to PTH (8,9). However, these methods are of limited sensitivity and certainly do not rule out a direct action of PTH. Effects of PTH on the osteoclast precursor are even more difficult to study since we cannot identify this cell.

An alternative hypothesis, suggested by Rodan and Martin (10), is that PTH exerts its direct effects on osteoblasts. This could result in secondary effects on bone resorption and would not require PTH receptors on the osteoclast. The secondary effect might be mediated by alterations in bone surface morphology, since PTH alters the shape of osteoblasts. Alternatively, a local osteoclast stimulating factor could be secreted in response to PTH. One local bone resorber, prostaglandin E_2, can be ruled out as the mediator since PTH-stimulated bone resorption is not abrogated by maneuvers which block endogenous prostaglandin synthesis.

Although the inhibitory effect of PTH on osteoblasts was discovered later than stimulation of resorption, we know more about its mechanism. Osteoblasts have PTH receptors (11). Cultured cells having an osteoblastic phenotype, including both normal cells and clonal lines derived from osteosarcomas, show activation of adenyl cyclase and cyclic AMP dependent protein kinase in response to PTH (12). These effects occur in a few minutes, but it takes much longer to see morphologic alterations, decreased collagen synthesis and decreased alkaline phosphatase activity (13,14). The decrease in collagen synthesis has been carefully studied in organ cultures of fetal rat calvaria. On the basis of measurements of procollagen mRNA activity using a cell-free translation system and more recently using a cDNA probe, the decrease is probably due to a transcriptional effect.

Cyclic AMP and calcium appear to be likely candidates as intracellular messengers which might link the binding of PTH on its surface receptor to a nuclear event. Agents which increase cyclic AMP such as dibutyryl cyclic AMP and isobutyl methylxanthine can mimic the effect of PTH on osteoblast collagen synthesis (2). The calcium ionophore, A23187, also inhibits collagen synthesis, but the mechanism may be different because it is a potent inhibitor of DNA synthesis as well (15).

The anabolic effect of PTH has been studied largely in vivo. It has been demonstrated in organ cultures with limited exposure to PTH and ascribed to release of a local growth factor during the resorption (16). Recently we have examined trabecular and cortical bone separately in rats and found that both show an increase in mass (M. Gunness-Hey and J. Hock, unpublished observations). Hypercalcemia does not appear to be essential for the effect on bone mass.

The most striking decreases in bone mass in hyperparathyroidism are seen in postmenopausal women. Estrogen reverses some of the manifestations of hyperparathyroidism and appears to be effective in reducing PTH-mediated bone resorption in vivo. While the effect of estrogen appears to be on bone resorption as assessed from microradiographic and chemical studies (17), the possibility that estrogen also opposes the inhibitory effect of PTH on bone formation has not been ruled out. Since it has been impossible to demonstrate estrogen receptors or in vitro effects in bone (18,19), indirect mechanisms have been proposed. The synthesis of 1,25-dihydroxyvitamin D may be increased (20). This could result in increased calcium absorption, which would in turn decrease PTH and increase calcitonin secretion (21). However, this would not explain the observation that estrogen-treated hyperparathyroid patients show a decrease in serum calcium concentration, unless intermittent increases in calcitonin secretion could decrease bone resorption and oppose the action of PTH.

In conclusion, PTH has been shown to stimulate bone resorption and inhibit bone formation in organ culture. The effect on bone formation appears to be direct and due at least in part to decreased transcription of procollagen mRNA. The effect on bone resorption could be mediated by effects on osteoblasts, but direct effects on preosteoclasts or osteoclasts have not been ruled out. In vivo, the catabolic effects result in decreased bone mass in hyperparathyroidism, but when PTH is administered intermittently with adequate supplies of calcium and phosphate in the diets, there is an increase in bone mass. PTH-mediated bone loss appears to be enhanced in the absence of estrogen, but the mechanism is unknown.

REFERENCES

1. Parsons, J.A. (1976): In: The Biochemistry and Physiology of Bone, Vol. 4, p. 159. Editor: G.H. Bourne. Academic Press, New York.
2. Dietrich, J.W., Canalis, E.M., Maina D.M. and Raisz, L.G. (1976): Endocrinology, 98, 943.
3. Podbesek, R.D., Stevenson, R., Zanelli, G.D., Edouard, C., Meunier, P.J., Reeve, J. and Parsons, J.A. (1981): In: Hormonal Control of Calcium Metabolism, Intl. Cong. Ser. 511, p 118. Excerpta Medica, Amsterdam.
4. Seeman, E., Wahner, H.W., Offord, K.P., Kumar, R., Johnson, W.J. and Riggs, B.L. (1982): J. Clin. Invest. 69, 1302.
5. Holtrop, M.E., King, G.J., Cox, K.A. and Reit, B. (1979): Calcif. Tissue Int. 27, 129.
6. Lorenzo, J.A. and Raisz, L.G. (1981): Calcif. Tissue Int. 33, 296.
7. Owen, M. (1978): Calcif. Tissue Int. 25, 205.
8. Chambers, T.J. and Magnus, C.J. (1982): J. Pathol. 136, 27.
9. Chambers, T.J. and Dunn, C.J. (1982): J. Pathol. 137, 193.
10. Rodan, G.A. and Martin, T.J. (1981): Calcif. Tissue Int. 33, 349.
11. Silve, C.M., Hradik, G., Jones, A. and Arnaud, C.D. (1981): Calcif. Tissue Int. 33, 325.
12. Partridge, N.C., Kemp, B.E., Veroni, M.C. and Martin, T.J. (1981): Endocrinology 108, 220.
13. Kream, B.E., Rowe, D.W., Gworek, S.C. and Raisz, L.G. (1980): Proc. Natl. Acad. Sci. USA 77:5654.
14. Majeska, R.J., Rodan, S.B. and Rodan, G.A. (1980): Endocrinology 107:1494.
15. Dietrich, J.W. and Paddock, D.N. (1979): Endocrinology 104, 493.
16. Howard, G.A., Bottemiller, B.L., Turner, R.T., Rader, J.I. and Baylink, D.J. (1981): Proc. Natl. Acad. Sci. USA 78, 3204.
17. Riggs, B.L., Jowsey, J., Goldsmith, R.S., Kelly, P.J., Hoffman, D.L. and Arnaud, C.D. (1972): J. Clin. Invest. 51, 1659.
18. Caputo, B.C., Meadows, D. and Raisz, L.G. (1976): Endocrinology 98, 1065.
19. Chen, T.L. and Feldman, D. (1978): Endocrinology 102, 236.
20. Gallagher, J.C., Riggs, B.L. and DeLuca, H.F. (1980): J. Clin. Endocrinol. Metab. 51, 1359.

Discussion following paper by L. RAISZ:

H. MALLUCHE: We conducted an experiment to study the in vivo effects of parathyroid hormone on bone. Parathyroid hormone was infused in physiologic doses over nine months to beagle dogs. We found an increase in bone resorption and an increase in bone formation but there was no net bone gain or loss. In addition, several years ago we published a study which found that patients on dialysis having high parathyroid hormone levels do not experience changes in bone mass, at least not in trabecular bone volume, if factors such as immobilization are avoided. Thus, it appears to me that parathyroid hormone, at least in these in vivo studies, does not affect bone mass.

L. RAISZ. I think that physiologic concentrations of parathyroid hormone almost by definition do not effect net bone mass. In other words, if you had an adverse effect from a physiological amount of PTH, then it would not be physiologic. Perhaps you are implying that in renal osteodystrophy there may be some protection from net bone loss by the high ambient phosphate. I do not know if that is one of the possibilities you considered. We would love to know more about that. Of course, when the plasma phosphate is lowered too much, a new problem of osteomalacia may arise.

M. PARFITT: You speculated that the low serum phosphate of hyperparathyroidism might be important. At the phosphate meeting in New York we reported a significant correlation between the serum phosphate level and the mineral apposition rate corrected for fractional labelling in states of primary and secondary hyperparathyroidism. In Dr. Malluche's study of experimental hyperparathyroidism, both the mineral appositional rate and the serum phosphate remained normal.

L. RAISZ: I think we should continue to emphasize the importance of phosphate almost as a hormone instead of an ion. Remember that phosphate, unlike other mineral ions, does increase or decrease with changes in growth. High phosphate levles are generally associated with greater proportional growth rates, both within and between different species. We cannot look at any hormone by itself without considering the concurrent effects of phosphate.

L. DEFTOS: In reference to estrogen's effect on bone or lack thereof, let me remind you that estrogens in a number of animal systems and also in humans have been shown to increase calcitonin secretion. Although I do not think that this is the whole explanation, it might be part of the explanation for the estrogen effect on bone; since calcitonin does have a direct effect on inhibiting bone resorption.

L. RAISZ: Of all of the ways that estrogen might work, the most attractive one at the moment seems to be the concept that calcitonin might be the mediator. Certainly, if increased calcitonin production occurs with estrogen administration, and is intermittent, it could act as an intermittent break on the bone resorption. One of the problems we have is that continuous high levels of calcitonin do not produce a prolonged and effective inhibition of bone resorption. We all are aware of the escape phenomenon. The escape phenomenon, of course, is associated with continuous high levels of calcitonin. We do not know what intermittent physiologic changes mean that occur in postmenopausal women. They may be more important in regulating bone resorption.

PTH MEDIATED BONE LOSS IN PRIMARY AND SECONDARY HYPERPARATHYROIDISM

M. Kleerekoper, A.R. Villanueva, C.H.E. Mathews, D.S. Rao, B. Pumo and A.M. Parfitt

Bone and Mineral Division, Henry Ford Hospital, Detroit, MI, U.S.A.

The precise pathogenesis of age-related bone loss is uncertain, but it is clearly multifactorial. A role for chronic parathyroid hormone excess in the pathogenesis of age-related bone loss can be inferred from the changes in mineral homeostasis that accompany the aging process. Intestinal absorption of calcium and glomerular filtration rate, both stimuli to parathyroid hormone secretion, decline with age, and direct measurement of either serum immunoreactive parathyroid hormone or nephrogenous cyclic AMP indicate that there is indeed a "physiologic" increase in parathyroid hormone secretion that accompanies the aging process (1-3). However, most patients with clinical manifestations of age-related bone loss i.e., osteoporosis or, more precisely, vertebral and hip fractures, have no biochemical or histologic evidence of hyperparathyroidism at the time of fracture (4). Either chronic parathyroid hormone excess does not contribute significantly to age-related bone loss or its effect has passed by the time the patient presents with fracture, or our techniques are too insensitive to detect the effects of the very mild "physiologic" hyperparathyroidism of aging.

The role of chronic parathyroid hormone excess in the pathogenesis of age-related bone loss may be clarified by examining bone in primary and secondary hyperparathyroidism, two conditions where the effects of parathyroid hormone on bone loss may be magnified. In parathyroid hormone excess relative loss of trabecular bone has been inferred from photon absorptiometry of the proximal and distal radius and the spine (5) and from the increased frequency of vertebral fractures (6).

Single beam photon absorptiometry of the radius was performed on 115 white females with primary hyperparathyroidism and results compared to 284 white female control subjects. There was no difference in mean age (57 ± 14 yrs vs 55 ± 14 yrs), height (162 ± 6 cm vs 163 ± 6 cm) or weight (69 ± 18 Kg vs 68 ± 15 Kg) between the two groups. Bone mineral density at the radial mid-shaft was 14.6% lower in the patients with hyperparathyroidism and at the distal radius the deficit in bone mineral was 16.5%. A similar study was performed on 24 patients with hyperparathyroidism secondary to intestinal malabsorption of calcium. This group, in whom there was biochemical evidence of hyperparathyroidism (elevated serum immunoreactive parathyroid hormone and/or elevated nephrogenous cyclic AMP), was selected from a larger group of patients with malabsorption on the basis of absence of skeletal fractures and absence of histologic evidence of osteomalacia. The bone mineral deficit at the radial mid-shaft in secondary hyperparathyroidism was 23.8% and the deficit at the distal radius was 25.2%. There is general agreement that photon absorptiometry at the radial mid-shaft is a measure of cortical bone mass, but the relative contribution of cortical and trabecular bone to the measurements made by photon absorptiometry at the distal radius is uncertain. We have previously established that any trabecular bone at this latter site is metabolically inert and that deficits at both sites are due mainly to cortical thinning.

Iliac crest bone histomorphometry was performed on a separate group of 42 patients with primary hyperparathyroidism and the 24 patients with secondary hyperparathyroidism described above. Results were compared to normal controls.

Comparisons were also made between groups. In primary hyperparathyroidism there was no deficit in trabecular bone volume or its components - mean trabecular plate thickness and mean trabecular plate density - but in 5 cases (12%) trabecular bone volume was below the 95% confidence limits of the regression on age in normals. Trabecular bone volume was 20% lower in secondary hyperparathyroidism than in primary hyperparathyroidism (17.1% vs 21.4%) with a 9% reduction in mean trabecular plate thickness and a 15% reduction in mean trabecular plate density. An increase in relative osteoid volume of similar magnitude was seen in both primary and secondary hyperparathyroidism. In both cases this resulted from an increase in extent of the trabecular surface covered by osteoid rather than in mean osteoid seam width, which was normal in both groups. Likewise, the extent of non-osteoid surface covered by osteoclasts was increased to the same extent in primary and secondary hyperparathyroidism. Because of the selection criteria, none of the patients with secondary hyperparathyroidism in this study had histologic evidence of osteomalacia (defined for this study as a mean osteoid seam width >15 μm and a mineralization lag time >100 days). However, there was a short delay in mineralization of newly formed osteoid seen in secondary hyperparathyroidism that was not apparent in primary hyperparathyroidism. Thus the greater deficit in trabecular bone volume in secondary hyperparathyroidism may reflect an additional deleterious effect on the skeleton of factors other than chronic parathyroid hormone excess, such as malabsorption of calcium.

CONCLUSIONS

These data demonstrate that: 1) A chronic increase in parathyroid hormone secretion, whether it be a primary phenomenon or secondary to known abnormalities in mineral homeostasis, accelerates age-related loss of cortical bone from the extremities. In some cases there may also be an accelerated loss of trabecular bone from the axial skeleton. Both losses are augmented by calcium malabsorption. 2) Parathyroid hormone excess may contribute modestly to the pathogenesis of vertebral fractures, in which the trabecular bone deficit averages 40% and is relatively greater than the cortical bone deficit. 3) Parathyroid hormone excess is probably more important in the pathogenesis of hip fractures, in which loss of cortical bone is relatively greater and loss of trabecular bone relatively less than in vertebral fracture. 4) Use of human parathyroid hormone in the treatment of patients with vertebral fracture should be tempered by caution concerning a possible increase in the risk of hip fracture.

REFERENCES

1. Gallagher, J.C., Riggs, B.L., Eisman, J., Hanistra, A., Arnaud, S.B. and DeLuca, H.F. (1979): J. Clin. Invest. 64, 729.
2. Davies, D.G. and Shock, N.W. (1950): J. Clin. Invest. 29, 496.
3. Insogna, K.L., Lewis, A.M., Lipinski, B.A., Bryant, C. and Baran, P.T. (1981): J. Clin. Invest. 53, 1072.
4. Kleerekoper, M., Frame, B., Villanueva, A.R., Oliver, I., Rao, D.S., Matkovic, V. and Parfitt, A.M. (1981). In: Osteoporosis. Recent Advances in Pathogenesis and Treatment, p. 441. Editors: H.F. DeLuca et al. University Park Press, Baltimore.
5. Seeman, E., Wahner, H.W., Offerek, T.P., Kumar, R., Johnson, W.J. and Riggs, B.C. (1982). J. Clin. Invest. 69, 1302.
6. Dauphine, R.T., Riggs, B.L. and Scholz, D.A. (1975). Ann. Intern. Med. 83, 365.

Discussion following paper by M. KLEEREKOPER

L. AVIOLI: Dr. Nordin in the audience, and others have for some time been equating vitamin D deficiency with hip and femoral neck fractures. We heard yesterday that a tendency for PTH excess, if anything is related to hip fractures rather than vertebral fractures. We heard Dr. DeLuca tell us that in order to get a maximal effect of PTH on bone, you need vitamin D. How do you put this together? If there is a tendency for vitamin D deficiency to result in a hip fracture, and if there is a tendency for hip fracture to be related to so called "senecent" mild hyperparathyroidsim, one could reason that with less vitamin D the same amount of parathyroidhormone would cause less bone resorption. I am sure you have thought about this potential "Catch 22".

M. KLEEREKOPER: We have thought about it a great deal. I am not going to answer that now because Dr. Rao is going to talk about that at length this afternoon.

G. PALMIERI: Dr. Kleerekoper, just a question about the young women with hyperparathyroidism who showed more loss than postmenopausal women. Although, estrogen may still be playing a role, what happened with this first group which is more severely hyperparathyroid than the second group which did not manifest the disease until there was lack of estrogen. Since bone loss is very difficult to regain after it is gone, this situation is similar to what is observed in Cushing's syndrome. We have to take a more serious look of treatment at a time before the bone loss begins to occur.

M. KLEEREKOPER: I agree.

P. MEUNIER: I have no explanation for this special bone loss in premenopausal females as compared to the postmenopausal females. Maybe estrogens are bad for bone in the presence of PTH. It is a provocative question.

J. COBURN: Did you correlate the differences between your primary and secondary hyperparathyroid patients with regards to serum $1,25(OH)_2D$ levels and serum calcium?

M. KLEEREKOPER: This group of patients had normal serum 25(OH)D, $1,25(OH)_2D$, calcium and phosphate levels.

C. ARNUAD: Another factor that is missing in these individuals is estrogen, or at least an estrogen-like action. It is conceivable that the degree to which estrogen protects the bone against parathyroid hormone is considerably more diminished in these individuals than if they have vitamin D deficiency. We have a very complex situation with respect to the ultimate effect of parathyroid hormone on bone because it could be much greater than we might anticipate in estrogen deficient individuals.

M. KLEEREKOPER: Looking at the effects of individual hormones and trophic agents independently is hard enough, but when you try to combine the effects of vitamin D, estrogen, parathyroid hormone all together it becomes very complex.

H. GENANT: Dr. Schlenker published a study in Calcified Tissue Research in 1976 which clearly demonstrates that the ratio of cancellous to cortical bone in the radius is a function of the distance from the articular surface. The controversy that exists with single photon absorptiometry relates to where one actually measures. At the distal radial site generally measured (3cm proximal to the styloid) the percentage trabecular bone is 10 to 20 percent. In studies with Dr. Kolb we have measured approximately thirty primary hyperparathyroid patients using quantitative CT of the spine and photon absorptiometry of the radius, with results similar to yours. In the group there is an approximate 15% decrement in the spine and approximately the same decrement in the peripheral cortex. But interestingly, in some patients with secondary hyperparathyroidism due to renal failure, we have found an elevated spinal bone mineral content in the setting of the rugger-jersey spine. I was interested to see that you found only a mineral decrement in the secondary hyperparathyroid group, yet we know clinically that up to 20-30% of secondary hyperparathyroid patients may have osteosclerosis in the setting of chronic renal failure.

M. KLEEREKOPER: This is a select group of patients with secondary hyperparathyroidism, as are the patients with the rugger-jersey spine.

H. GENANT: Yes, with much more severe bone disease.

M. PARFITT: It is an entirely different situation. These are patients with normal renal function, and we never see vertebral osteosclerosis in patients with intestinal malabsorption. You are talking about renal failure and secondary hyperparathyroidism lumped together regardless of the etiology. We are talking about secondary hyperparathyroidism occurring in the context of either dietary deficiency of vitamin D or intestinal malabsorption of calcium and/or vitamin D.

VITAMIN D DEFICIENCY AND HIP FRACTURES: CAUSE OR COINCIDENCE ?

P. Lips, M.J.M. Jongen, F.C. van Ginkel, W.J.F. van der Vijgh, R. Bouillon*, W.H.L. Hackeng**, J.C. Netelenbos

Department of Internal Medicine, Academisch Ziekenhuis der Vrije Universiteit, P.B. 7057, 1007 MB Amsterdam, The Netherlands
*) Rega Instituut, Leuven, Belgium
**) Bergwegziekenhuis, Rotterdam, The Netherlands

Hip fractures are provoked by a trauma in patients with a fragile skeleton. Osteopenia is usually observed, but it is not necessarily more severe than in controls of similar age and sex. Osteomalacia and vitamin D deficiency have been described with varying incidence in patients with hip fracture (3). A causal link would have important implications for prevention. We studied patients with hip fracture in order to assess the incidence of metabolic bone disease with special emphasis on vitamin D deficiency and its consequences.

SUBJECTS AND METHODS

The study included 125 consecutive patients with hip fracture admitted to the Onze Lieve Vrouwe Gasthuis in Amsterdam during a 15 months period. Forty-one were men and 84 were women and their mean age ± SD was 75.9 ± 11.0 yr. Control subjects were healthy volunteers without a history of hip fracture. They lived independently in an apartment-house for aged people and prepared their own meals. The control group consisted of 20 men and 54 women with a mean age of 75.6 ± 4.2 yr. The examination of controls was spread over the year. Creatinine, serum proteins, calcium, phosphate, and alkaline phosphatase were measured in serum samples according to methods described in detail (3). The serum concentration of parathyroid hormone (PTH) was measured by radioimmunoassay using an antibody specific for the midregion (4). The vitamin D metabolites 25(OH)D, $24,25(OH)_2D$ and $1,25(OH)_2D$ were measured by competitive protein binding assay after purification by gradient HPLC (2). Vitamin D binding protein (DBP) was measured in serum samples by single radial immunodiffusion (1). Transilial biopsies, obtained from 89 patients within one week of the fracture, were included in methylmethacrylate without decalcification. Goldner stained sections were evaluated using histomorphometric techniques described in detail (3). The following bone mass parameters were measured: mean cortical thickness (CT), cortical porosity (POR), and trabecular bone volume (TBV). The following remodeling parameters were measured in trabecular bone: relative osteoid volume (ROV), relative osteoid surface (ROS), thickness index of osteoid seams (TIOS), i.e. 100 x ROV/ROS (an estimate of osteoid thickness), mean width of osteoid seams (WOS), relative resorption surface (RRS), and the number of osteoclasts per mm^2 of section (OC). Statistical evaluation was by analysis of variance with age and sex as covariates (ANOVA).

This study was supported by the Praeventiefonds, The Hague.

RESULTS

Biochemical data of patients and controls are presented in Table 1. Serum concentrations of total protein, albumin, DBP, and the vitamin D metabolites were lower in the patients than in the controls. Serum vitamin D metabolite concentrations correlated with serum DBP in the patients (for 25(OH)D, $24,25(OH)_2D$ and $1,25(OH)_2D$: r= 0.34, 0.28 and 0.46 respectively; $P < 0.005$), but

Table 1. Biochemical data of patients with hip fracture and aged control subjects with results of ANOVA.

	controls		patients			sign.
	n	mean±SD	n	mean±SD		P
creatinine	74	85±16	125	86±26	µmol/l	n.s.
total protein	74	73.5±3.8	125	61.6±7.5	g/l	<0.001
albumin	74	41.9±2.8	125	32.5±4.8	g/l	<0.001
DBP	71	371±44	118	315±60	mg/l	<0.001
calcium	74	2.35±0.12	125	2.13±0.16	mmol/l	n.s. [a]
phosphate	74	1.09±0.15	125	1.11±0.26	mmol/l	n.s.
alk.phosph.	74	2.1±0.5	125	2.0±0.7	Bessey U	n.s.
PTH	74	0.12±0.05	125	0.11±0.05	µgeq/l	n.s.
25(OH)D	74	32.9±13.6	124	18.5±10.6	nmol/l	<0.001 [b]
$24,25(OH)_2D$	74	2.3±1.9	124	1.0±1.4	nmol/l	<0.001 [b]
$1,25(OH)_2D$	73	105±31	124	79±46	pmol/l	<0.001 [b]

[a] serum proteins were included as covariates in ANOVA (3)

[b] when including serum DBP as covariate in ANOVA, the result was for 25(OH)D and $24,25(OH)_2D$ $P < 0.001$, and for $1,25(OH)_2D$ $P=0.07$

such correlations were absent in the control group. When correcting for differences in serum DBP (by including DBP as covariate in ANOVA), the difference in serum $1,25(OH)_2D$ between the two groups was not significant. The vitamin D status of patients and controls is compared with that of 217 young controls (spread over the year) in Table 2. In patients and controls a seasonal variation was observed in the serum concentrations of 25(OH)D, $24,25(OH)_2D$ and PTH. Serum PTH was maximal in winter when the vitamin D metabolites were minimal (4).

Table 2. Vitamin D status in patients with hip fracture, aged controls and young control subjects living in Amsterdam (n = 217, mean age 38.5 ± 11.4 yr).

	young contr.	aged contr.	patients
25(OH)D,mean±SD	52.5±21.9	32.9±13.6	18.5±10.6 nmol/l
25(OH)D <30 nmol/l	18 %	46 %	87 %
25(OH)D <15 nmol/l	0.5 %	4 %	38 %

Histomorphometric results have been reported in detail (3). Whereas the relative osteoid volume and surface were moderately increased in some patients, the thickness index of osteoid seams was lower than control values (3). The mean width of osteoid seams was not increased in any biopsy (highest value 12.1 µm). The biopsies were arranged into three subgroups using remodeling parameters: "high turnover", characterized by increased resorption parameters and normal to increased osteoid surface (n=19), "uncoupling", with increased resorption and low osteoid surfaces (n=9), and a "rest" group with normal or low remodeling parameters (n=61). Remodeling and bone mass parameters in the three subgroups are compared in Table 3. "High turnover" was associated with

Table 3. Histomorphometric data in 3 subgroups, classified using remodeling parameters, with results of ANOVA.

	"high turnover"		"uncoupling"		"rest"			sign.
	n	mean±SD	n	mean±SD	n	mean±SD		P
CT	14	507±138	9	798±333	48	740±353	μm	<0.05 a)
POR	15	7.5±2.4	9	7.9±4.5	32	7.7±3.9	%	n.s.
TBV	18	15.1±6.0	9	14.6±5.5	54	12.7±5.0	%	n.s.
ROV	19	4.8±2.0	9	1.5±0.8	60	1.9±1.1	%	<0.001 a)
ROS	19	31.1±12.4	9	11.4±5.5	60	12.7±7.2	%	<0.001 a)
TIOS	19	15.7±4.4	9	13.6±4.7	60	15.6±6.7		n.s.
RRS	19	8.0±2.7	9	9.1±2.6	59	3.3±1.3	%	<0.001 b)
OC	19	0.60±0.41	7	0.49±0.26	20	0.22±0.18	mm^{-2}	<0.01 b)

a) "high turnover" different from "uncoupling" and "rest"
b) "high turnover" and "uncoupling" different from "rest"

significant cortical thinning.

Histomorphometric parameters did not correlate with the vitamin D metabolite concentrations. Increased values of relative osteoid volume (⩾5%, max. 9.9%, n=9) and relative osteoid surface (⩾25%, n=15) were always associated with a serum 25(OH)D level below 30 nmol/l. A correlation was observed between relative osteoid surface and serum PTH (r=0.25, P<0.05). Serum PTH tended to be higher in the "high turnover" and "uncoupling" groups than in the "rest" group (0.13±0.04 vs 0.11±0.05 μgeq/l, 0.05<P<0.10).

DISCUSSION

The low serum 25(OH)D concentrations indicate vitamin D deficiency in many patients, as observed in other studies (7). The low serum 1,25(OH)$_2$D in the patients, however, corresponds to the decrease in serum DBP and albumin, which is probably induced by the fracture (3). The "free" serum 1,25(OH)$_2$D concentration probably is almost similar in patients and controls. Osteomalacia occurs in patients with hip fracture, but its incidence has been overestimated (7). In our study overt osteomalacia was not observed, as osteoid seam thickness was not increased. However, "high turnover" may be the histological expression of early vitamin D deficiency (6). Evidence in support of an intermediary role of PTH is given by the borderline increased serum PTH and the correlation with osteoid surface. The seasonal variation of serum PTH, inverse to that of serum 25(OH)D, also suggests secondary hyperparathyroidism (4). "High turnover" leads to cortical osteopenia. Along this way vitamin D deficiency may be the cause of the fracture in 20 % of the patients. However, in other patients vitamin D deficiency does not induce a clear histological reaction. This could be due to a decreased vitality of the osteoblasts in old age.

Another consequence of vitamin D deficiency could be muscle weakness predisposing to falls (7). However, low serum 25(OH)D concentrations may also be coincidental and relate to the poor general health of many aged people (7). In our study the lowest serum 25(OH)D levels were observed in patients which were institutionalized prior to fracture (n=38, 14.3±6.2 nmol/l)(5). They were chronically ill, did not go outside and had the lowest vitamin D intake (75 IU/day).

In conclusion , evidence for a causal relationship between vitamin D deficiency and hip fractures at best exists in 20 % of the patients. The ultimate proof should be furnished by a decreasing incidence of hip fractures after long term vitamin D supplementation in the aged.

ACKNOWLEDGEMENT

We are grateful to Dr.B.Veraart, Dr.J. Borggreve, Dr. C.L. van Schaik and Dr.H. Kruyswijk from the Onze Lieve Vrouwe Gasthuis for their cooperation in the study. Prof.C. van der Meer and Prof. P. Meunier gave invaluable advice. Mrs. J. van der Hooft and Mrs. M.Stevens provided secretarial assistance.

REFERENCES

1. Bouillon R, van Assche FA, van Baelen H, Heyns W, de Moor P (1981): J.Clin.Invest. 67, 589.
2. Jongen MJM, van der Vijgh WJF, Willems HJJ, Netelenbos JC, Lips P (1981): Clin. Chem. 27, 1757.
3. Lips P, Netelenbos JC, Jongen MJM, van Ginkel FC, Althuis AL, van Schaik CL, van der Vijgh WJF, Vermeiden JPW,van der Meer C (1982): Metab. Bone Dis. Rel. Res. 4, 85
4. Lips P, Hackeng WHL, Jongen MJM, van Ginkel FC, Netelenbos JC (1983): J. Clin. Endocrinol. Metab. 57 (in press).
5. Lips P (1982) Metabolic causes and prevention of femoral neck fractures. PhD Thesis, Vrije Universiteit, Amsterdam.
6. Parfitt AM, Mathews C, Rao D, Frame B, Kleerekoper M, Villanueva AR (1981): in: Osteoporosis: recent advances in pathogenesis and treatment p. 321. Editor: H.F. DeLuca et al. University Park Press, Baltimore.
7. Parfitt AM, Gallagher JC, Heaney RP, Johnston CC, Neer R, Whedon GD (1982): Am. J. Clin. Nutr. 36, 1014

Discussion following paper by: P. LIPS

R. MARCUS: I once was admonished by an orthopedic surgeon for not drawing a distinction between femoral neck and intertrochanteric fractures. He was certain that the pathophysiology of these two events was different, yet I have heard the term hip fractures used both by you and others without drawing that distinction. I want to ask you whether you think that it is an important distinction to make; and, whether you separated your patient population into groups with the two different types of fractures?

P. LIPS: In our study there were 70 intertrochanteric and 55 transcervical fractures. I did not present the bone mass parameters, but there was a striking difference between the two types with the trabecular bone volume much lower in the intertrochanteric fractures.

C. JOHNSTON: One point that has not been mentioned today has to do with the graded response of parathyroid hormone. As you know Dr. Parsons started studies which suggested that with a low or intermittent dose of PTH, you could increase trabecular bone volume with parathyroid hormone. Perhaps with larger doses both trabecular and cortical bone is lost. I wonder if the dose response of the hormone has any effect on the difference in trabecular and cortical bone loss.

P. LIPS: It could be. It was disappointing to us that there was no difference in serum PTH levels between controls and patients. I do not know how much and to what extent serum PTH is influenced by the fractures as such.

J. PETTIFOR: You mentioned a number of your patients with high bone turnover were vitamin D deficient. Vitamin D deficiency may be a manifestation of poor nutritional status; but in fact, there may be calcium deficiency in addition to vitamin D deficiency. Your $1,25(OH)_2D$ levels were no different in patients and controls; yet the 25(OH)D levels were lower while the $1,25(OH)_2D$ levels were fairly constant. One wonders whether, infact, you have a combination of both calcium and vitamin D deficiency.

P. LIPS: The average level of $1,25(OH)_2D$ in the two groups was no different, but the dispersion of values is quite high. For instance, there is a group with slightly increased creatinine levels, and they have low $1,25(OH)_2D$ levels. I think there are slight differences in $1,25(OH)_2D$ concentrations that can explain some of the observations.

J. COBRUN: Why do you think the D-binding protein and albumin levels are low? Do these patients have malabsorption, malnutrition, or some other problem that may be a factor?

P. LIPS. There are extensive studies on this subject. For instance, patients operated for gallstones or total hip replacement have the same fall in serum albumin on the first day after the operation; sometimes as much as 25%. We suspect that in most patients it is an effect of the fracture, but of course there are some patients who do have malabsorption or who are in poor general health.

J. KANIS: This relates to whether the abnormalities that you see in vitamin D levels are a cause of the fracture. You rightly described the changes that occur postoperatively in the vitamin D-binding protein. I understand though, that Dr. R. Bouillon has also measured DBP after hip fractures. According to his observations, all the changes in vitamin D metabolites that have been described are accountable for by changes in DBP. My question relates to the interval after operation that you studied your patients. How do the metabolites change postoperatively in relation to changes in DBP?

P. LIPS: I think the decrease of albumin and vitamin D binding protein is partly explained by the large blood loss that occurs after a hip fracture. The loss averages about one liter. Part of it may also be a synthesis problem in the liver, just as after major operations. Dr. Bouillon did the DBP measurements in our study. Only the difference in $1,25(OH)_2D$ between patients and controls is accountable for changes in DBP.

OSTEOCLASTIC RESORPTION OF OSTEOID IN SECONDARY HYPERPARATHYROIDISM

Ming Cai Qiu*, C. Mathews, A.M. Parfitt

Bone and Mineral Research Laboratory, Henry Ford Hospital, Detroit, Michigan, 48202, U.S.A.

*On leave from Tianjin Medical College, Tianjin, the People's Republic of China

INTRODUCTION

It is commonly believed that osteoclastic resorption takes place only on mineralized bone (1,2), but casual observations of osteoclasts apparently resorbing osteoid have been reported, especially in severe hyperparathyroidism (3). Because of possible relevance to the mechanisms of bone resorption, a systematic quantitative study of this phenomenon was undertaken.

MATERIALS AND METHODS

We studied 48 patients with secondary hyperparathyroidism including 29 with intestinal malabsorption or dietary deficiency of vitamin D, of whom 18 had osteomalacia, and 19 with renal osteodystrophy, of whom 10 had osteomalacia. Transiliac bone biopsies were performed after double tetracycline labeling, prestained by the Villanueva method, plastic embedded, sectioned and stained with toluidine blue. Criteria for osteomalacia were mean osteoid seam width >15.0 μm, and mean mineralization lag time >100 days (4). Using the Zeiss MOP-3 digitizing system we measured the surface extent of resorption lacunae with or without osteoclasts, on mineralized bone and on osteoid. In addition, we counted the number of osteoclast profiles and the number of nuclei in each profile adjacent to mineralized bone and to osteoid.

TABLE 1 - Osteoclast Surface (mean ± SD). TS=total surface, HPT=hyperparathyroidism, OM=osteomalacia, MBS=mineralized bone surface, OS=osteoid surface, Ocl=osteoclasts.

	Vitamin D deficiency		Renal osteodystrophy	
	HPT	OM	HPT	OM
Mineralized bone surface (% TS)	56.6±24.8	24.8±15.2	29.5±25.2	16.0±19.9
Osteoclasts (% MBS)	1.8±1.7	10.4±14.2	18.3±20.6	4.7±6.6
Osteoclasts on MB (% TS)	1.0±0.9	1.2±1.5	3.3±2.5	0.6±1.1
Osteoid surface (% TS)	43.3±24.7	85.2±15.2	70.5±25.2	84.0±20.0
Osteoclasts (% OS)	0.4±0.8	1.7±2.1	2.1±1.7	1.0±1.4
Osteoclasts on osteoid (% TS)	1.2	2.7	4.9	1.3
Osteoid osteoclasts (% total Ocl)	15.0	56.1	32.6	53.7

RESULTS AND DISCUSSION

The proportion of surface covered by osteoclasts was substantially higher for mineralized bone than for osteoid in each diagnostic category (Table 1), with relative increases ranging from 4-10 fold; for the pooled data the

Figure 1. (Opposite page) Photomicrograph of iliac trabecular bone of patient with osteomalacia and secondary hyperparathyroidism. Upper Panel (A) - low power view; Lower Panel (B) - higher power view of region shown by circle. MB=mineralized bone, OST=osteoid, Ocl=osteoclasts.

A

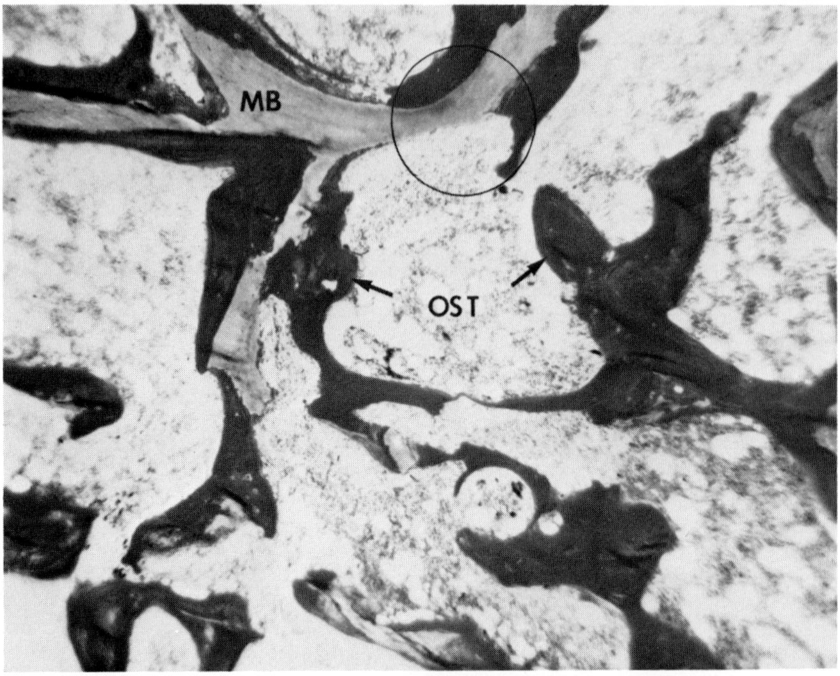

B

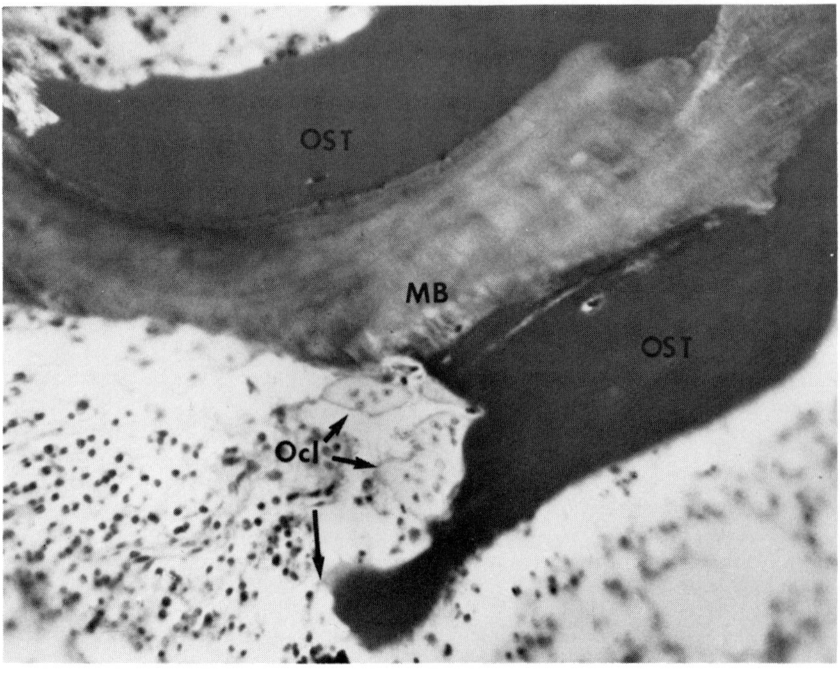

difference was highly significant ($t=4.047$, $p<0.001$). Nevertheless, osteoclasts apparently eroding osteoid, closely justaposed to scalloped resorption lacunae, were observed in the majority of patients; the morphologic evidence for resorption of osteoid is as strong as the morphologic evidence for resorption of mineralized bone (Figure 1). In both types of osteomalacia, because of the much greater extent of osteoid than of mineralized bone, the osteoid osteoclast surface represented more than half of the total osteoclast surface; osteoid (Table 1) resorption probably increases in response to the reduced extent of mineralized bone.

In vitamin D deficiency, the transition from secondary hyperparathyroidism alone to osteomalacia (4) was accompanied by a substantial increase in osteoid resorption, relative both to osteoid surface and to total surface. Mineralized bone osteoclast surface did not change significantly in relation to total surface but increased substantially in relation to mineralized bone surface. By contrast, in renal osteodystrophy the transition to osteomalacia was accompanied by a *fall* in osteoid resorption and an even greater fall in mineralized bone resorption. This is in keeping with the high frequency of relative hypoparathyroidism in these patients, either spontaneous or resulting from parathyroid surgery (5).

TABLE 2 - Osteoclast nuclei (per profile, mean ± SD). MB=mineralized bone.

	Vitamin D deficiency		Renal osteodystrophy		Combined
	HPT	OM	HPT	OM	(SE)
Osteoid osteoclasts	3.4±0.8	4.3±1.2	5.0±0.7	5.6±1.8	4.29±0.23
MB osteoclasts	2.4±1.0	2.8±1.0	3.2±0.8	2.8±0.4	2.79±0.14

For each diagnostic category, osteoclasts resorbing osteoid had more nuclei per profile than osteoclasts resorbing mineralized bone (Table 2); for the pooled data this difference was highly significant ($t=10.04$, $p<0.001$). As in Paget's disease, a larger number of nuclei may indicate increased osteoclast vigor; possibly such osteoclasts are able to release collagenolytic enzymes in higher concentration. Also, in vitamin D deficiency, the transition to osteomalacia was accompanied by a significant increase in the number of nuclei per profile in osteoid osteoclasts ($t=2.407$, $p<0.025$), which may be yet another manifestation of more severe hyperparathyroidism.

SUMMARY

We made a quantitative study of osteoid resorption in 48 patients with secondary hyperparathyroidism, with or without osteomalacia, due to vitamin D deficiency or renal osteodystrophy. In these patients the morphologic evidence for resorption of osteoid by osteoclasts is as strong as the morphologic evidence for resorption of mineralized bone. The proportion of surface covered by osteoclasts is substantially higher for mineralized bone than for osteoid, but in osteomalacia the osteoid surface is so high that the osteoid osteoclast surface represented more than half the total osteoclast surface. Osteoclasts resorbing osteoid have more nuclei than osteoclast resorbing mineralized bone, possibly indicating increased cellular vigor and ability to digest collagen without prior demineralization. Osteoid resorption is a response to severe hyperparathyroidism and reduced availability of mineralized bone surface.

REFERENCES

1. Bordier P., and S. Tun Chot: Histological aspects of bone remodelling, with special reference to the effects of parathyroid hormone and vitamin D. In: Clinical Aspects of Metabolic Bone Disease. B. Frame, A.M.

Parfitt, H. Duncan (eds), Excerpta Medica, pp. 95-102, 1972.
2. Aaron, J.E.: Histology and Micro-anatomy of Bone. In: Calcium, Phosphate and Magnesium Metabolism. B.E.C. Nordin (ed), Churchill Livingstone, pp. 298-356, 1976.
3. Parfitt, A.M.: The actions of parathyroid hormone on bone. Relation to bone remodelling and turnover, calcium homeostasis and metabolic bone disease. III. PTH and osteoblasts, the relationship between bone turnover and bone loss, and the state of the bones in primary hyperparathyroidism. Metabolism 25:1033-1069, 1976.
4. Rao, D.S., A. Villanueva, M. Mathews, B. Pumo, B. Frame, and A.M. Parfitt: Histologic evolution of vitamin D depletion in patients with intestinal malabsorption or dietary deficiency. Clinical Disorders of Bone and Mineral Metabolism, this volume.
5. Sherrard D., S. Ott, N. Maloney, D. Andrery: Uremic osteodystrophy. Classification, Cause and Treatment. Clinical Disorders of Bone and Mineral Metabolism, this volume.

IX OSTEOMALACIA AND NUTRITIONAL BONE DISEASE

OSTEOMALACIA - OVERVIEW

Boy Frame, M.D.

Recent advances in laboratory methods and techniques that relate to bone and mineral metabolism have allowed a detailed study of factors that are of importance in bone formation. Osteomalacia results from a disturbance in mineralization of bone matrix. Theoretically, bone matrix may fail to mineralize because of abnormalities in collagen and matrix proteins, or because of an alteration in mineral metabolism occurring at the mineralization front. The result is an accumulation of increased quantities of unmineralized bone matrix or osteoid over bone surfaces.

Rickets is more apparent in children who have otherwise normal growth pattern including that of cartilage present in the growth plates of long bones. Likewise, osteomalacia is perhaps less apt to occur when there is a deficit in normal bone matrix formation. In order for a defect in bone mineralization to be fully expressed, adequate bone matrix first has to be deposited.

The table lists some of the factors that are currently considered to be of possible significance in the formation of bone matrix and mineralization.

TABLE

Factors that may influence bone matrix formation and mineralization

1. Bone resorption in bone remodelling units (BRUs)
    a) release of a coupling factor that stimulates osteoblasts
2. Osteoblast function
    a) collagen formation and maturation
        1) chronologic age of person
        2) insulin
        3) growth hormone (via somatomedin)
    b) bone matrix proteins
        1) osteocalcin (gla protein)
        2) osteonectin
        3) proteoglycans
3. Mineralization at the mineralization front
    a) ambient Ca, PO_4 concentrations
    b) pH at mineralization front
    c) amorphous Ca, PO_4 (ACP) preceding hydroxyapatite formation (?)
    d) vitamin D metabolites
        1) maintain adequate ambient Ca, PO_4 levels
        2) ? direct effect on osteoblasts and/or mineralization front
    e) parathyroid hormone
    f) piezoelectric fields (exercise and stress)

g) inhibitors of mineralization
   1) pyrophosphates } destroyed by phosphatases
   2) ATP } and ATPases
   3) foreign ions, such as aluminum
h) matrix vesicles
   1) facilitates mineral and enzyme concentration at the mineralization front

---

Recent studies noted elsewhere in this volume suggest that bone resorption itself may be important as an initiating event for osteoblast formation and function in the bone remodelling unit (BMU). A high molecular weight polypeptide from tissue cultures and demineralized human bone matrix has been isolated which stimulates osteoblast proliferation and matrix formation. An alteration in the release or a defect in this coupling or skeletal growth factor could theoretically influence subsequent osteoblast vigor and function.

Collagen synthesis is the initial and major component of bone matrix formation. Maturation of collagen, which appears to be important for mineralization is characterized by increasing intra-and extrafibullar cross-linking of collagen fibers. Some defects in mineralization appear to result from an abnormality in collagen structure. For instance, in the rare skeletal disorder known as fibrogenesis imperfecta ossium a marked distortion of the normally polarized collagen fibers is observed which appears to result in impaired mineralization and increased number of widened osteoid seams.

The chronologic age of the person and the age of the osteoblasts appear to be factors that influence the rate and extent of matrix formation, since the matrix appositional rate decreases with age and as the distance from the cement line in individual BMUs increases in extent. Somewhat surprising perhaps is the fact that only insulin and growth hormone, the latter via somatomedin, have been found to directly stimulate bone collagen synthesis. Other hormones appear to play primarily a modulating role in collagen formation.

Recently, more attention has been given to the role of non-collagenous bone matrix proteins as a possible cause of defective mineralization. Osteocalcin (gla protein) has been extensively studied, but its primary role in bone metabolism is still to be determined. It appears to have an affinity for binding to hydroxyapatite, but only after the latter's maturation from an initial amorphous mineral phase. Another bone matrix protein osteonectin appears to facilitate the nucleation of calcium phosphate mineral onto the surface of type I collagen.

Proteoglycans and glycoproteins are additionally important extracollagenous proteins in bone matrix. While their role in mineralization needs further clarification, they do have a high binding affinity for calcium, which is thought to be related to the presence of a large number of free acidic groups. Theoretically, an excess of calcium binding to proteoglycans might interfere with normal mineral deposition at the mineralization front. It is possible that certain rare forms of osteomalacia may be related to a defect in concentration or function of one or more of the matrix proteins. One such form of osteomalacia may be that of axial osteomalacia. In this skeletal affliction, osteomalacia of the axial skeleton exhibiting a coarsened trabecular pattern on skeletal x-rays develops which does not appear to be associated with any obvious disturbance in mineral or vitamin D metabolism. Perhaps an abnormality in one of the extracollagenous matrix proteins might account for a mineralization defect under these circumstances.

Because methods of study have been easier, most identified form of osteomalacia so far have been related to disturbances in mineral and vitamin D metabolism. After appropriate maturation of bone matrix over a period of 10 to 15 days, primary mineralization occurs at the mineralization front when about 80% of the mineral is deposited in the first few days. This primary mineralization is thought be be largely under the control of the osteoblasts and nearby osteoid osteocytes. The remainder of the mineral is deposited at a slower rate over a period of six months or more and is known as secondary mineralization. Osteoblast influence appears to be less important in this latter phase of mineral deposition.

A number of chemical and physiological factors must interact at just the right time for mineralization to proceed normally at the mineralization front. Ambient concentrations of calcium and phosphate undoubtedly are important, particularly the latter. It is well known that osteomalacia occurs in many patients with chronic hypophosphatemia. However, osteomalacia does not always appear in patients with chronic hypophosphatemia, so other modulating factors undoubtedly are important. In this section, M.C. deVernejoul and Associates report findings in 19 male patients with chronic hypophosphatemia due to a renal phosphate leak, independent of PTH. While there was no osteoid accumulation in these patients, a decreased osteoblast appositional rate was nevertheless present. As is the case in rickets, it is possible that a normal growth of bone matrix has to be present before a mineralization defect can become fully expressed.

Relatives of patients with X-linked hypophosphatemic rickets and osteomalacia may exhibit hypophosphatemia without apparent bone involvement. However, not many of these patients have had careful study of bone biopsy specimens using current histomorphometric techniques to exclude a defect in mineralization. Chronic hypocalcemia only rarely appears to result in rickets and osteomalacia and then primarily in rapidly growing children, who have subsisted on a calcium deficient diet.

H^+ concentration appears an important factor in the clinical events that occur at the mineralization front. Chronic systemic acidosis as occurs in patients who have undergone ureterosigmoidostomy can result in osteomalacia, even in the presence of normal serum levels of calcium and phosphorus.

Most theories of calcification suggest that crystalline hydroxyapatite is preceded by an amorphous noncrystalline calcium phosphate complex, but recent studies question the validity of this concept.

The role of several vitamin D metabolites in bone mineralization is discussed extensively elsewhere in this Proceedings. The importance of these metabolites in maintaining adequate serum concentrations of calcium and phosphorus is unquestioned. Whether they have an additional direct effect on osteoblasts or on the events occurring at the mineralization front is hotly debated. The evidence would seem to suggest that they do, at least under some circumstances.

Parathyroid hormone appears to have a direct effect or in some other way enhances the availability of minerals at the mineralization front. Decreased parathyroid function in some patients with renal osteodystrophy appears to increase the tendency towards the development of a form of osteomalacia that is resistant to the usual treatment.

Exercise by initiating shearing forces on mineral crystals induces electrical fields (piezoelectrical) which appears to influence bone formation. Fracture non-union is now being successfully treated in some instances by application of low-grade pulsed electrical currents. The importance of such electrical fields in the process of normal matrix formation and mineralization is probably important but difficult to prove.

Perhaps just as important as the factors that enhance mineralization of bone matrix are the inhibitors of mineralization that have been identified in bone. Both pyrophosphates and ATP are known to impede different phases of mineral formation and deposition. Removal of these inhibitors by endogenous pyrophosphates (phosphatases) and ATPases favor mineralization. Hypophosphatasia, where there is a deficiency of alkaline phosphatase and an increase in the inhibitor phosphoethanolamine may be an example where the importance of mineralization inhibitors play a role in the development of rickets and osteomalacia.

Much current investigation is centered on the place of matrix vesicles in mineralization of cartilage and bone matrix. These structures are detected by ultrastructural examination at mineralizing sites in cartilage and bone. They consist of membrane-bound concentrations of mineral and enzymes, which appear at the initial site of mineral deposition. The role of these matrix vesicles in different forms of osteomalacia needs further study.

It is obvious that bone matrix formation and its mineralization is complex and that many possibilities exist for the occurrence of metabolic defects which may lead to impaired mineralization. Further utilization of electronspectroscopic imaging, as described by Arsenault and associates, should help define the multiple factors at the mineralization front which are important for mineral deposition. These authors were able to demonstrate that an increased concentration of aluminum at the zone of calcification in the growth plate retards normal mineralization in aluminum treated rats. Other studies have demonstrated the importance of aluminum in inhibiting mineralization, both in the treatment resistant osteomalacia observed in hemodialysis patients with renal osteodystrophy and also in patients who have been maintained on total parenteral nutrition. The use of electron probes in association with histochemical techniques offer promise for the future in the study of the mineralization process. One day we may well have a detailed map of the osteoid seam, where the concentrations of all important factors needed for normal mineralization can be measured and variations from normal detected.

Bone histomorphometry with the use of double tetracycline labeling techniques and undecalcified bone sections has come of age. An absence of osteomalacia, or at the other extreme, florid osteomalacia, can readily be identified in most established calcified tissue laboratories. However, there is less agreement on criteria for the earliest histomorphometric signs of osteomalacia, especially when accompanied by secondary hyperparathyroidism. International agreement should be sought in establishing histodynamic criteria for all stages of osteomalacia. Studies from different clinical research centers can then be more readily compared. D. Rao and others in Dr. Parfitt's laboratory address the problem. For kinetic criteria in making the diagnosis of osteomalacia, these investigators use a mean osteoid seam width of greater than 15.0 μm and a mineralization lag time of greater than 100 days. They stress that the early effects of hypovitaminosis D are mainly those of secondary hyperparathyroidism. As vitamin D deficient osteopathy progresses, the mineralization defect becomes more apparent with a progressive accumulation of osteoid.

Metabolic bone disease is a common problem in patients with chronic liver disease. It is commonly taught that patients with chronic biliary tract obstruction are more likely to have osteomalacia and that patients with chronic diffuse hepatocellular disease to have osteoporosis. Etiologic factors thought to be important are defective vitamin D and 25 hydroxyvitamin D absorption, impaired synthesis of 25 hydroxyvitamin D, the deleterious effects of chronic alcoholism on the skeleton, hypoproteinemia, and other ill-defined nutritional deficiencies. In view of this, the findings of Recker and associates in patients with primary biliary and alcoholic cirrhosis are somewhat surprising. They found no evidence of vitamin D deficiency or osteomalacia and bone histologic changes in both groups of patients were indistinguishable from those patients with postmenopausal osteoporosis. Much work still needs to be done in trying to determine the pathogenesis of the bone disease in patients with a variety of chronic liver disorders. The type, degree, and duration of liver disease needs to be correlated with defects in mineral and vitamin D metabolism as well as with skeletal histomorphometric changes in the skeleton. The results of Recker and associates are discouraging with respect to the possibility of effective treatment in patients with metabolic bone disease due to chronic liver failure no matter what the underlying etiology.

Many are of the opinion that sporadic hypophosphatemic osteomalacia in the adult is almost always related to an underlying tumor, usually mesenchymal in nature. Such tumors may be quite small and difficult to detect. The effort to find such tumors is well worthwhile, however, since successful removal often leads to an improvement or cure of the underlying osteomalacia. Renal phosphate wastage and hypophosphatemia appear to be the cause of the osteomalacia in such patients.

Studies reported by Drezner and associates shed further light on this paraneoplastic syndrome of tumor-induced osteomalacia. Their studies suggest further evidence of a tumor-induced alteration of vitamin D metabolism which may cause a urinary phosphate leak. The agent produced by tumors which interferes with renal 1-hydroxylation of 25 hydroxyvitamin D has so far eluded identification. Further efforts in its identification need to be made.

The number of identifiable causes of osteomalacia continue to increase. It appears that foreign ions deposited at the mineralization front can interfere with normal mineralization. This is perhaps not surprising. S.M. Ott and associates present evidence that the etiology of the metabolic bone disease observed in patients receiving total parenteral nutrition (TPN) is somewhat similar to the resistant form of osteomalacia observed in some patients with renal osteodystrophy who have been maintained on hemodialysis. In both conditions aluminum from exogenous sources is deposited at the mineralization front and appears to interfere with normal mineral deposition. Removal of the aluminum with the passage of time or after the use of desferrioxamine allows normal matrix mineralization to recover. In the case of bone disease associated with total parenteral nutrition, aluminum contamination of the casein used in the TPN solution is the possible culprit. Now that the problem appears to have been identified, correction should be possible. Steps should be taken to make sure that TPN solutions do not contain aluminum or other potentially toxic trace elements that can impair normal mineralization. If this approach is effective, perhaps the painful disabling bone disease seen in these patients will no longer be observed. It should be remembered that not all workers have had a similar experience with regards aluminum as an etiologic agent in TPN bone disease. Perhaps this crippling bone disorder is multifactoral.

SPATIAL DISTRIBUTIONS OF ALUMINUM, PHOSPHORUS AND CALCIUM IN MINERALIZING EPIPHYSEAL GROWTH PLATES OF ALUMINUM-TREATED RATS BY ELECTRON SPECTROSCOPIC IMAGING

A.L. Arsenault, F.P. Ottensmeyer and A.B. Hodsman*

Department of Medical Biophysics, Ontario Cancer Institute, Toronto, Ontario and *Department of Medicine, St. Joseph's Hospital, London, Ontario, Canada

A severe osteomalacic syndrome affects some 2% of the hemodialysis population in North America. This figure is substantially higher in Europe (1). Several studies have associated this syndrome, dialysis osteomalacia, with the accumulation of aluminum (Al) in bone from the Al-containing dialysate water and from aluminum hydroxide administration. Biopsies from dialysis osteomalacic patients reveal a positive correlation of stainable Al in trabecular bone with the presence of Al measured by atomic absorption and a corresponding reduction in the degree of mineralization (2). Similarly, rats receiving repeated parenteral Al accumulate Al in bone (3). However, this accumulation occurs at a signficantly lower level in animals on Vitamin D-supplemented diets than those on Vitamin D-deficient diets (4). In that experimental model osteomalacia was observed in metaphyseal trabecular bone (3) but not in Vitamin D-supplemented rats (4). In the latter rats only the occasional area of interface Al-staining was observed along the subepiphyseal trabeculae.

In order to achieve a better understanding of Al's toxicity and distribution within such calcifying matrices we have applied electron spectroscopic imaging to the epiphyseal growth plate of Al-treated rats. This technique enables the direct visualization of chemical and morphological information with a spatial resolution of 0.3 - 0.5 nm at a detection sensitivity of 2×10^{-21}g (5,6). These capabilities coupled to computer-assisted image processing allow quantitative analysis of atomic elements and the visualization of their spatial distributions individually or relative to each other (7,8). Using this technique we have directly visualized aluminum, phosphorus and calcium within early mineral deposits of the epiphyseal zone of provisional calcification in Al-treated rats.

MATERIALS AND METHODS

Twenty day old rats (Holtzman strain) were equilibrated on a Vitamin D-deficient diet (Teklad #TD79180, Madison, Wi; 0.6% Ca, 0.2% P) for 2wk, after which Vitamin D_3 supplement was provided in a dose of 5 µg/wk to insure normal bone development. Half of these rats received parenteral $AlCl_3$ in 0.9% saline at an average dose of 0.75 mg/day over 55 days. The remaining rats were not given Al supplements nor injections of saline. At sacrifice each rat weighed from 250 - 280 g.

Small slices of proximal tibial heads were placed in 5% glutaraldehyde (pH 7.3) buffered in 0.2 M sodium cacodylate containing 5% sucrose for 2hr at 1 C. Tissues were osmicated for 2 hr at 1 C, dehydrated through a graded series of ethanols to propylene oxide and flat embedded in Spurr resin. Ultrathin sections (30-40 nm) were placed on grids and examined at 80 kV in a

Siemens Elmiskop 102 electron microscope fitted with a modified imaging electron energy energy loss analyser (5). Excitations from the $L_{2,3}$-absorption edge of Al, P and Ca have been used to localize the distribution of these elements. Elemental maps were made by bracketing the absorption edges of 72 eV (electron volts) for Al at 50 and 90 eV, 132 eV for P at 110 and 150 eV and 349 eV for Ca at 320 and 360 eV. Areas of interest on these sets of electron spectroscopic images (ESI's) were digitized in 512x512 arrays on a Perkin-Elmer Microdensitometer Model 1010A. These matrices were processed by computer (Digital Equipment Corp., VAX 11/780, Maynard, Ma) and displayed in black and white on a video display system (Genisco Computers GCT-300, Costa Mesa, Ca) and photographed.

RESULTS

Composite diagrams along the longitudinal axis of epiphyseal zones of hypertrophy in control and Al-treated rats are shown in Figs. 1a and 1b respectively. These figures were drawn from ESI's and serve to illustrate the fine structural details of the cartilage matrix along the longitudinal septum and the contained zone of provisional calcification (PC). In contrast to the control animals, Al-treated rats exhibit a spatially reduced zone of provisional calcification. This reduction occurs consistently at the mineralization front of this zone and is characterized by a reduced number of early mineral deposits as indicated in Fig. 1b. Aluminum treatment produces a more abrupt transition from a non-calcified matrix to a calcified matrix. The area indicated by arrows in Fig. 1b is comparable to the ESI (electron spectroscopic image) shown in Fig. 2. From an Al-loaded animal an aggregate of early mineral deposits (MD) within the zone of provisional calcification is shown in an unstained ESI at 180 eV (Fig. 2). ESI's appear in reverse contrast to conventional electron micrographs due to image formation by only scattered electrons which even in unstained thin sections reveal high contrast structural details produced by density differences within the specimen. Individual mineral deposits are composed of clustered, elongated plate-like structures (apatite?). Surrounding these deposits is the lucent cartilage matrix containing proteoglycan aggregates and collagen fibers. The enclosed area of Fig. 2 has been digitized and displayed as high spatial resolution maps of Al, P and Ca in Figs. 3a, b and c respectively. It is evident that Al is superimposed directly over the distributions of P and Ca within these mineral deposits. In these deposits the Al content does not appear to alter the normal distribution and spatial inter-relationships of P and Ca as observed in the control animals in which Al was not detected. Later stages of mineralization in the zone of provisional calcification and subepiphyseal trabeculae have been analyzed and exhibit the same spatial relationships of Al, P and Ca as those in Fig. 3.

DISCUSSION

The application of electron spectroscopic imaging to the study of aluminum in calcifying matrices has confirmed and extended earlier observations in dialysis osteomalacic patients (1,2,3) and in Al-loaded experimental animals (3,4) that bone tissue accumulates aluminum within mineral deposits. The capabilities of high spatial resolution and direct visualization of atomic distributions over entire micrographs permit the detailed

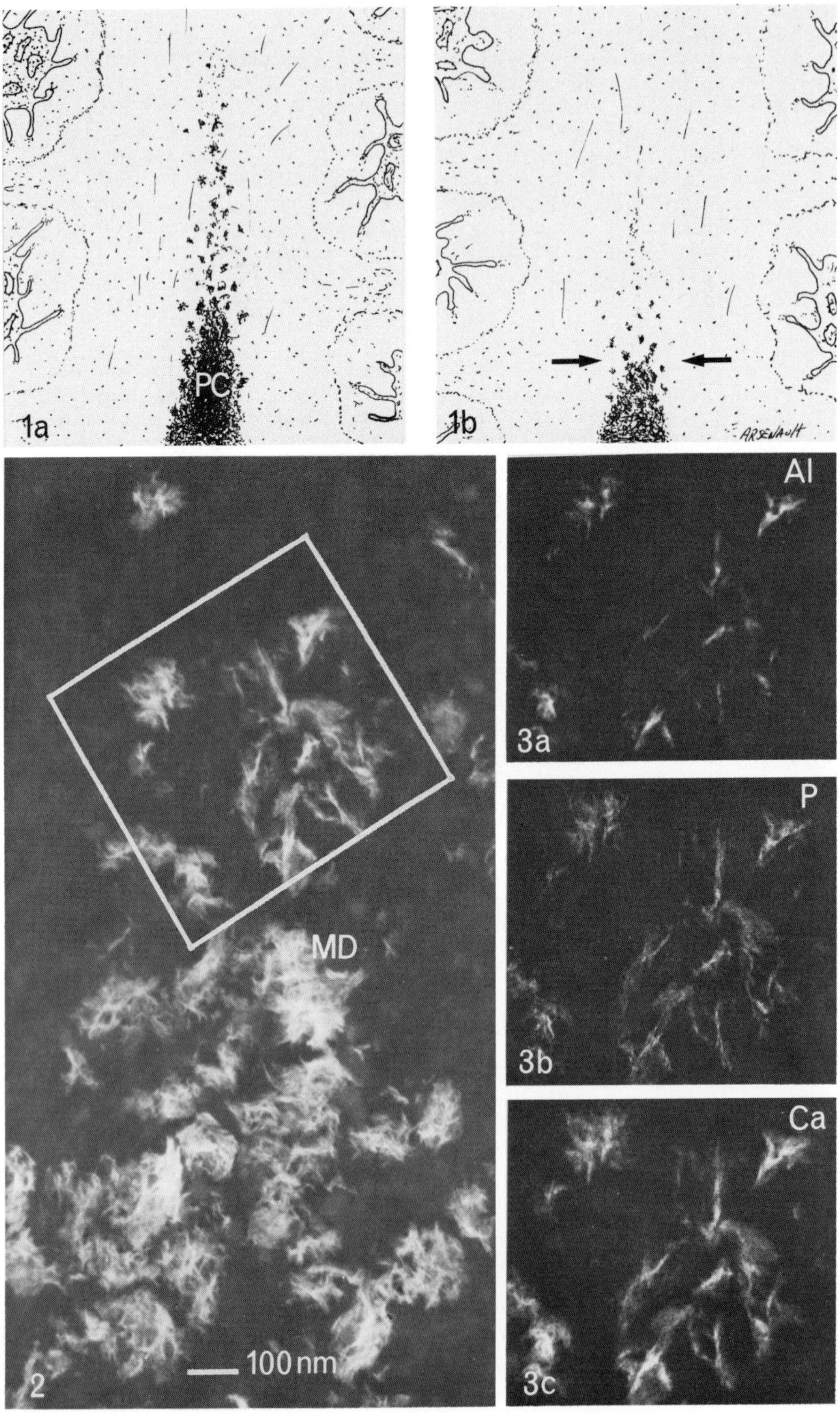
PC
1a
1b
ARSENAULT
MD
100 nm
2
Al
3a
P
3b
Ca
3c

analysis of the chemistry associated with fine structural morphology which is found in such biological prossesses as mineralization. In this study Al is superimposed over both P and Ca indicating the homogeneous incorporation of this element into mineral deposits. Comparisons made between Ca/P within mineral deposits of control and Al-loaded animals reveal unaltered distributions and quantities. This suggests that although Al is present in these areas it does not interfere with the 'normal' Ca/P composition.

The exact mechanism by which Al illicits its pathogenic affect of bone mineralization impairment, as in the case of dialysis osteomalacia, is currently not understood. In the present study, we have noticed a reduction in the mineralization front in the zone of provisional calcification induced by Al treatment. This front represents the area in which Ca/P compounds are formed -- the nucleation site. From this preliminary study it appears that the presence of Al within the cartilage matrix delays the process of nucleation to a particular threshold level after which nucleation and subsequent mineralization proceeds incorporating the Al into solid phase mineral deposits.

REFERENCES

1. Hodsman, A.B., Sherrard, D.J., Alfrey, A.C., Ott, S., Brickman, A.S., Miller, N.L., Maloney, N.A. and Coburn, J.W. (1982): J. Clin. Endocrinol. Metab. 54, 539.
2. Maloney, N.A., Ott, S., Alfrey, A.C., Miller, N.L., Coburn, J.W. and Sharrard, D.J. (1982): J. Lab. Clin. Med. 99, 206.
3. Ellis, H.A., McCarthy, J.H. and Herrington, J. (1979): J. Clin. Pathol. 32, 832.
4. Hodsman, A.B., Anderson, C. and Leung, F.Y. (1983): Min. Electrolyte Metab. (in press).
5. Ottensmeyer, F.P. and Andrew, J.W. (1980): J. Ultrastruct. Res. 72, 336.
6. Adamson-Sharpe, K.M. and Ottensmeyer, F.P. (1981): J. Microsc. (Oxford) 122, 309.
7. Arsenault, A.L. and Ottensmeyer, F.P. (1983): Proc. Natl. Acad. Sci. USA 80, 1322.
8. Arsenault, A.L. and Ottensmeyer, F.P. (1983): J. Microsc. (Oxford) (in press).

Discussion following paper by L. Arsenault:

H. KRONENBER: Can you tell us anything about the mineral distribution along collagen fibers?

L. ARSENAULT: Yes, I have looked at collagen fibers in the early stages of mineralization in two different systems; one is a tissue culture system in calvaria of chickens and the other is in the periosteal bone of mice. I find that there are deposits of granules within the entire region of these collagen fibers and on analysis I've determined that there is phosphorus and sulfur in these granules. I must say that I was surprised at the results, but there was no calcium in the granules.

HISTOLOGIC EVOLUTION OF VITAMIN-D DEPLETION IN PATIENTS WITH INTESTINAL MALABSORPTION OR DIETARY DEFICIENCY

D. Sudhaker Rao, A. Villanueva, M. Mathews, B. Pumo, B. Frame, M. Kleerekoper and A.M. Parfitt

Division of Bone and Mineral Metabolism, Department of Medicine, Henry Ford Hospital, Detroit, Michigan, U.S.A.

Advanced osteomalacia is well characterized but its early histologic identification is controversial. Accordingly, we examined iliac bone biopsies after in vivo double tetracycline labeling in patients with varying degrees of vitamin D depletion due either to intestinal malabsorption or to dietary deficiency.

PATIENTS AND METHODS

65 patients with vitamin D depletion (plasma calcidiol <10 ng/ml), secondary hyperparathyroidism (HPT) and osteopenia (hypovitaminosis D osteopathy-HVO) were compared with 10 patients with secondary HPT alone (plasma calcidiol ≥ 10 ng/ml) and with 22 normal postmenopausal white females. Iliac bone biopsies were examined by established methods (1). Corrected mineral apposition rate (cMAR) was calculated as cMAR=MAR x fL where fL is the fraction of labeled osteoid. In patients without osteomalacia, cMAR is an index of the mean rate of matrix apposition.

RESULTS - CLASSIFICATION OF PATIENTS

In the entire patient group there was a hyperbolic relationship between osteoid seam width and osteoid surface, such that seam width remained close to normal until osteoid surface exceeded 70%, but increased markedly thereafter as osteoid surface increased toward 100%. Patients in whom osteomalacia would be diagnosed according to conventional criteria (based on osteoid volume or osteoid width) all had a greatly prolonged mineralization lag time (MLT= osteoid seam width/cMAR). Accordingly, we chose a combination of osteoid seam width >15 μm and MLT >100 days as histologic and kinetic criteria for osteomalacia; these were fulfilled by 39 patients and the remaining 26 patients were classified as HVOi.

In normal subjects and in patients with secondary HPT but without osteomalacia (with or without vitamin D deficiency) there was no correlation between osteoid seam width and osteoid surface, but a significant positive correlation between osteoid seam width and corrected mineral apposition rate. Conversely, in patients with osteomalacia there was a significant positive correlation between osteoid seam width and osteoid surface, and a significant negative correlation between osteoid seam width and corrected mineral apposition rate, reversing the normal relationship. Patients with osteomalacia were further subdivided into those with double tetracycline labels in the biopsy (HVOii-11 cases) and those with no double labels (HVOiii-28 cases).

RESULTS - CHARACTERIZATION OF SUBGROUPS

a. Comparison between secondary HPT alone and HVOi. Both groups had normal values for plasma calcium (Ca), phosphate (P) and Ca x P product, and increased values for serum alkaline phosphatase (AP) and nephrogenous cyclic AMP. Bone histomorphometry in both groups showed increased osteoid surface, relative osteoid volume, osteoclast surface as % of nonosteoid surface and bone formation rate, and an approximate 25% reduction in trabecular bone volume. There were no significant differences in any of these measurements between the groups with or without vitamin D deficiency. However, in HVOi cMAR was slightly but significantly depressed and MLT significantly prolonged.

b. Evolution of HVO. The transition from HVOi to HVOiii was marked by progressively more abnormal values for osteoid indices and osteoclast surface, plasma Ca, P, and AP, Nc'AMP and plasma D-metabolite levels. Bone formation rate, which was increased in HVOi, declined progressively, reaching zero (by definition) in HVOiii. Patients with osteomalacia had similarly depressed values for TBV but had fewer fractures than patients with HVOi. Conversely, bone pain and muscle weakness were rare in patients with HVOi but common in those with osteomalacia. Looser's zones were rare but occurred only in HVOiii.

DISCUSSION

We have identified a stage in the evolution of vitamin D depletion characterized by lack of symptoms, biochemical and histologic evidence of secondary HPT, and significant osteopenia, both trabecular (biopsy data) and cortical (2). This state appears to increase fracture risk, and therefore requires recognition and treatment with vitamin D (or a metabolite thereof) in order to suppress secondary HPT. The most useful non-invasive clues to the diagnosis were an appropriate clinical context and a raised alkaline phosphatase.

Our histologic and kinetic criteria for osteomalacia largely preserve the clinical, biochemical and radiographic features of this disorder. No patient with osteomalacia as we define it had completely normal values for plasma Ca, P, and AP. Many patients with HVOi would fulfill the criteria for osteomalacia proposed by other investigators, based on increased osteoid surface and reduced fractional labeling. Designating such patients as having osteomalacia emphasizes the need for treatment with vitamin D, but undermines the histologic distinction between osteomalacia and hyperparathyroid bone disease, so that the term osteomalacia ceases to have any useful meaning.

CONCLUSIONS

1. In early vitamin D depletion the effects on bone are primarily those of secondary HPT. With increasing severity and/or duration, mineralization becomes progressively more defective, bone formation rate declines, osteoid increases in thickness as well as surface, and osteitis fibrosa becomes more severe.
2. Based on the interrelationships between the data, we propose as kinetic criteria for osteomalacia mean osteoid seam width >15 μm and mineralization lag time >100 days. Osteomalacia defined in this way retains its traditional clinical, biochemical and radiographic connotations.
3. There is a stage in the evolution of vitamin D depletion characterized by lack of symptoms, histologic evidence of HPT, osteopenia, and increased fracture risk; withholding the diagnosis of osteomalacia from such patients in no way reduces their need for treatment with vitamin D.

REFERENCES

1. Recker, R. (ed). Bone Histomorphometry: Techniques and Interpretation. CRC Press, Boca Raton, 1983.
2. Kleerekoper, M., et al: PTH Mediated Bone Loss in Primary and Secondary Hyperparathyroidism, this volume.

Discussion following paper by S. Rao:

B. FRAME: Dr. Rao, you make the histologic diagnosis of osteomalacia look very easy. I am sure there must be disagreement somewhere in the audience.

J. M. PETTIFOR: You showed normal plasma 1,25$(OH)_2$D values in the first two stages with decreasing 25(OH)D levels. Do you think that 25(OH)D or another metabolite besides 1,25$(OH)_2$D is important for calcium absorption? Is it possible that your patients with intestinal disease have concurrent malabsorption of vitamin D and calcium and that the initial stages are related to calcium deficiency? Once the 1,25$(OH)_2$D values fall, then you may have true nutritional vitamin D deficiency.

S. RAO: The development of osteomalacia in the presence of normal 1,25 $(OH)_2$D levels, that is in Stage II, is unexplained, but all cases had a reduction in the calcium phosphate product. The 1,25$(OH)_2$D level is probably subnormal for the levels of serum phosphate and PTH and may be unable to promote normal calcium and phosphate absorption in the presence of intestinal disease, which our patients had.

P. LIPS: Your hypovitaminosis D Type I resembles very much our "high turnover" group with the exception that the alkaline phosphatase was not elevated in our patients.

S. RAO: I can't explain the difference; perhaps elderly patients are less able to have an appropriate osteoblast response.

J. O'RIORDAN: I don't think many of your patients were truly vitamin D deficient. If you take a lower limit of normal at 10 ng/ml, then half of the British population is vitamin D deficient.

S. RAO: The mean level of plasma calcidiol was 5.25 ng/ml.

J. O'RIORDAN: I don't think you get clinical deficiency unless the serum level of 25(OH)D is below 2 ng/ml. Moreover, the 1,25$(OH)_2$D level has to be below 22 pg/ml before you are D deficient. Perhaps the situation is different in patients with intestinal disease.

H. MALLUCHE: You showed us patient groups with and without vitamin D deficiency, and groups with and without tetracycline labeling. Apparently your main criterion for diagnosis of osteomalacia is an increased mineralization lag time. Doesn't tetracycline labeling enter into your calculation of mineralization lag time?

M. PARFITT: Yes, of course the fractional labeling enters into the calculation of the mineralization lag time. We subdivided the groups purely on morphologic criteria, and the criterion for dividing the patients with osteomalacia into mild and severe groups was whether they had double tetracycline lables, however short in extent, or had no double labels. It turns out that when you subdivide the patients according to these morphologic criteria there are biochemical, clinical and radiographic differences between the groups.

PRIMARY BILIARY CIRRHOSIS AND ALCOHOLIC CIRRHOSIS AS EXAMPLES OF CHRONIC LIVER DISEASE ASSOCIATED WITH BONE DISEASE

Robert R. Recker, Willis Maddrey, Frank Herlong, Michael Sorrell and Robert Russell

Creighton University, Omaha, NE, Johns Hopkins University, Baltimore, MD and University of Nebraska, Omaha, NE, U.S.A.

INTRODUCTION

Patients with chronic liver disease often suffer from bone pain and tenderness and pathological fractures. Since the liver is heavily involved in vitamin D metabolism being the site of 25 hydroxylation of calciferol resulting in the formation of 25 hydroxyvitamin D, it is widely assumed that chronic liver disease results in impaired production of 25OHD and consequent bone disease. We undertook to study the efficacy of oral administration of 25OHD in primary biliary cirrhosis (PBC) and alcoholic cirrhosis (AC), both of which are prototypes of chronic liver disease which lead to the development of hepatic osteodystrophy. In the course of this study we found that hepatic osteodystrophy is fundamentally a problem of bone loss apparently not due to vitamin D deficiency and not reversed by treatment with vitamin D or its active metabolite, 25 hydroxyvitamin D.

METHODS

This report describes findings in 15 patients with primary biliary cirrhosis from Baltimore and 12 from Omaha. All were women between ages 32 and 61 and had liver biopsies, positive serum antimitochondrial antibodies and patent biliary tracts. Eighteen patients with alcoholic cirrhosis were males from Baltimore between ages 45 and 57. They were selected from a group of 56 patients with advanced cirrhosis on the basis of a serum 25OHD level less than 20 ng/ml. They were divided into three groups of six each, with one group receiving placebo, one receiving vitamin D2 and one receiving 25OHD. Nine patients had pretreatment bone biopsies and five of these had posttreatment bone biopsies. None of the placebo patients had posttreatment bone biopsies, three of the vitamin D2 group did along with two of the 25OHD group. Serum iPTH and 25OHD levels were measured at the Upjohn Laboratory (Kalamazoo). Transilial bone biopsies were obtained with a Bordier trephine of 8 mm inner diameter. The bone specimens were fixed, dehydrated and defatted in ethanol and embedded in methylmethacrylate. Thin sections were made (undecalcified) with a Jung sledge microtome and mounted unstained for fluorescent microscopy or stained with Goldners or toluidine blue for light microscopy. Histomorphometry was performed with light and fluorescent microscopy using an integrating eyepiece with a hemispherical line grid and micrometer (1).

RESULTS

Baseline and treatment biochemical data are presented in

Table I for the Baltimore PBC patients only. Baseline serum 25OHD levels were low but there was considerable scatter among the data. Eleven patients had values below 15 ng/dl. There was

TABLE I

Biochemical Data

Serum Levels	Normal	Primary Biliary Cirrhosis Baseline			Treatment		
		$\bar{x}$	SD	N	$\bar{x}$	SD	N
Ionized Calcium	4.3-5.0 mg/dl	4.63	.27	15	4.46	.25	8
Phosphorus	3.5-5.0 mg/dl	3.56	.31	15	3.65	.35	12
25OHD	15-40 ng/dl	11.92	7.78	15	31.62[a]	17.85	15
IPTH	3-10 mμ mEq/ml	3.1	.04	15	3.2	.05	12
24 hr urine calcium	mg/24 hr	73	65	15	240[a]	169	12

Data are modified from reference (2) with permission. a - Significantly different from baseline, $p < .05$, t-test of pairs.

no correlation between 25OHD levels and any of the biochemical or histologic variables. Treatment resulted in a significant rise to an average level of 31.62 ng/dl. The remaining biochemical parameters were not abnormal at baseline and the only change during treatment was a rise in urine calcium from 73 mg/24 hours to 240 mg/24 hours. Serum calcium, phosphorus and iPTH levels did not suggest a vitamin D deficient state.

TABLE II

Histomorphometric Data

	Normal[a]		Primary Biliary Cirrhosis Baseline			Treatment		
	$\bar{x}$	SD	$\bar{x}$	SD	N	$\bar{x}$	SD	N
V^b	.210	.034	.241	.067	27	.176[c]	.048	22
V_{osf}	.018	.010	.015	.023	27	.014	.014	21
osw	6.860	4.20	10.000	5.000	27	7.000[c]	5.000	22
S_f	.179	.096	.064	.070	27	.064	.063	22
S_r	.042	.050	.082	.066	27	.035[c]	.033	22
$\bar{M}$	.206	.037	.210	.048	23	.179	.039	16
S_{fa}	.123	.015	.062	.052	23	.032	.036	18

a - Composite normal adapted from the literature; b - key to symbols, v = trabecular bone volume, V_{osf} = osteoid volume, osw = osteoid seam width in microns, S_f = fractional osteoid surface, S_r = fractional resorption surface, $\bar{M}$ = appositional rate in mm/yr and S_{fa} = fractional double label surface; c - significantly different from baseline, $p < .05$.

A selected portion of bone histomorphometric data from the entire group of PBC patients is presented in Table II. The baseline data showed few abnormalities, the principal ones being reduced S_f, increased S_r, and reduced S_{fa}. Trabecular bone volume and V_{osf} were normal and osw was slightly increased. The $\bar{M}$ was normal. Rigorous comparisons with normal are not possible here because the normal data in Tables II and III are a composite

TABLE III

Histomorphometric Data

	Normal[a]		Alcoholic Cirrhosis Baseline			Treatment[b]		
	$\bar{x}$	SD	$\bar{x}$	SD	N	$\bar{x}$	SD	N
V^c	.210	.034	.166	.054	9	.201	.063	5
V_{osf}	.018	.010	.012	.009	9	.019	.015	5
osw	6.860	4.20	9.600	3.800	8	9.600	5.000	5
S_f	.179	.096	.048	.020	9	.088	.052	5
S_r	.042	.050	.026	.020	9	.108	.148	5
$\bar{M}$	.206	.037	.227	.062	7	.246	-	1
S_{fa}	.123	.015	.018	.009	7	.101	-	1

a - Composite normal adapted from the literature; b - 6 to 8 months passed before the treatment biopsy was done. Of the 5 treatment biopsies, 3 received vitamin D2 and 2 received 25OHD; c - key to symbols as in Table I.

adapted from the world's literature. Nevertheless, the baseline data are compatible with reduced bone remodeling rates. The changes noted on the second biopsies were a reduction in V, osw, S_r and S_{fa}, the latter not reaching statistical significance.

Biochemical data from the AC patients were all normal and with the possible exception of serum 25OHD levels did not reflect a state of vitamin D deficiency. Bone density of the distal radius by single photon absorptiometry went from .65 to .78 gm/cm in the two treatment groups combined. There was a striking rise in serum 25OHD levels in both treatment groups and the change was similar whether treatment was vitamin D2 or 25OHD. The histomorphometric results for the AC patients are shown in Table III. Again, rigorous comparisons with the normal data are not valid because of the need to use a composite normal taken from the literature. However, the results seem to show reductions in V, S_f, S_r and S_{fa} and no abnormality in V_{osf} or osw. Neither the biochemical or histomorphometric findings suggest a vitamin D deficient state.

DISCUSSION

Bone disease is a serious clinical problem in patients with PBC, manifest chiefly by bone pain and tenderness in most patients coupled with multiple fractures usually of the spine in some. In a few patients with PBC, massive skeletal collapse occurs with disastrous consequences. While bone loss is common in AC patients, fractures are not as frequent as in PBC. In both of these diseases, there seems to be widespread agreement that the most prominent and frequent bone lesion is osteoporosis, defined as bone loss with skeletal fragility and high risk of pathological fracture. However, there is uncertainty regarding the incidence of coexisting osteomalacia in both cases (3). In PBC some authors have reported an incidence of osteomalacia as high as 50 percent (4). None of our patients had bone biopsy evidence of osteomalacia, and most did not even have the reduced trabecular bone volume of osteoporosis. Nevertheless, there was a striking reduction in bone volume during followup, and bone loss was corroborated by the forearm densitometry measurements done in Baltimore.

Much of the attention given to the cause of bone disease in PBC has focused on alterations in vitamin D metabolism and decreased gut absorption of calcium. If defective calcium absorption efficiency is the primary cause of bone loss then the plasma homeostatic system for calcium economy should respond by revealing decreased serum calcium levels, increased serum iPTH levels, decreased urine calcium excretion and reduction in serum phosphorus concentration. In fact, none of these were found in this study nor have they been found in most of the patients reported in the literature.

It should be pointed out that vitamin D deficient osteomalacia does occur occasionally in PBC patients (5). Certainly these patients should be screened for this possibility by periodic measurements of serum 25OHD levels. Any level less than 20 ng/ml should result in treatment with oral 25OHD (Calderol, Upjohn) at a starting dose of 50 mcg daily, adjusting upward if necessary until the serum level is greater than 20 ng/ml. This should assure that no patient unnecessarily suffer osteomalacia along with osteoporosis.

The conclusions from this study are as follows: 1) the principal bone lesion in the PBC and AC is osteoporosis; 2) osteomalacia is infrequent though it may occur in a few cases of PBC; 3) biochemical measurements associated with calcium homeostasis are normal and do not suggest a deficiency in vitamin D.

Since the remodeling defect appears to be a shortened osteoblast life span, real progress in treatment awaits research into the mechanisms controlling the remodeling process. There is very little known about the control of differentiation of osteoclast and osteoblast precursors or about the control of 'blast and 'clast work efficiency or life span; and nothing is known about how the bone cells are directed to function at a given bone surface. While present research suggests that vitamin D or its metabolites do not play a major role in hepatic osteodystrophy, patients with chronic liver disease should not be allowed to become vitamin D deficient; and it is still possible that one of the vitamin D metabolites directly influences osteoblast life span and this metabolite could be deficient in these patients.

REFERENCES

1. Recker, R.R., Editor, (1983): Bone Histomorphometry: Techniques and Interpretation. CRC Press, Boca Raton, Florida.
2. Herlong, H.F., Recker, R.R. and Maddrey, W.C. (1982): Gastroenterology, 83, 103.
3. Long, R.G., Meinhard, E., Skinner, R.K., Varghese, Z., Wills, M.R. and Sherlock, S. (1978): Gut, 19, 85.
4. Compston, J.E., Horton, W.L. and Thompson, R.P.H. (1979): Gut, 20, 133.
5. Kehayoglou, A.K., Holdsworth, C.D., Agnew, J.E., Whelton, M.J. and Sherlock, S. (1968): Lancet, April 6, 715.

Discussion following paper by R. Recker:

L. DEFTOS: What were the $1,25(OH)_2D$ levels in your patients?

R. RECKER: We did not measure them.

L. DEFTOS: One could question whether osteomalacia was likely to be present if $1,25(OH)_2D$ levels were not below normal.

R. RECKER: I would have thought so before, but at this meeting we have heard osteomalacia reported in the presence of low, normal and high $1,25(OH)_2D$ levels.

J. COMPSTON: We have data which is in agreement with yours. Recently we studied in collaboration with colleagues at Kings' College Hospital, 70 patients with either chronic alcoholic liver disease or primary biliary cirrhosis. All had received double tetracycline labeling, and none had histological osteomalacia.

O. SCHAADT: In female patients with chronic nonalcoholic liver disease, we measured the bone mineral content in the lumbar spine, femoral neck and femoral shaft with the dual-photon technique. We found a significant average reduction in the lumbar spine of 15%, but in the femoral shaft, which is predominantly cortical bone, the bone mineral loss was only 5%, which was not significant.

CHRONIC HYPOPHOSPHATEMIA WITHOUT OSTEOMALACIA

M.C. de Vernejoul, P.J. Marie, L. Miravet and A. Ryckewaert

Clinique de Rhumatologie, INSERM U.18, Hôpital Lariboisière, 6 rue Guy Patin 75010 PARIS

The role of phosphate on bone remodelling has been studied experimentally in vitro and in vivo. In bone culture the decrease in phosphate concentration in the medium induces an increase in bone resorption and a decrease of collagen synthesis (1). In young rats phosphate deficiency induces in the same manner an increase in bone resorption and a decrease in bone formation associated with a mineralization defect (2). In man phosphate deficiency whether due to decrease in digestive absorption or to a renal phosphate wasting is usually associated with osteomalacia. However we observed that some patients with chronic hypophosphatemia had no detectable osteomalacia and we then decided to carry out a study of these cases.

PATIENTS AND METHODS

Patients were selected on two criteria. All of them had serum phosphate lower than 2.8mg/dl on repeated fasting blood samples. All of them had a non decalcified bone biopsy with no evidence of osteomalacia. 19 male patients aged from 19 to 63 years filled these criteria. Clinical presentation was heterogeneous. Nine patients had renal lithiasis, three patients had osteoporosis with crushed vertebrae, seven patients were lumbalgic and hypophosphatemia was recorded on systematic check up. Patients were divided in three groups according to the clinical presentation. For any patient, no concomittant disease or medication could be responsible for the low serum phosphate.

Bone histomorphometry was performed after single tetracycline labelling. Normal values were obtained from Bordier's data.

RESULTS

Biochemical data were recorded separately for each clinical group (Table 1) For all the hypophosphatemic patients serum creatinine (0.89 $\pm$ 0.09mg/dl) and calcium levels (9.4 $\pm$ 0.3mg/dl) were in the normal range. Alkaline phosphatase was normal in all patients. The average level of serum phosphate was 2.49 $\pm$ 0.21mg/dl. In no patient serum phosphate level was below 2.1mg/dl. This decreased serum phosphate was related to a renal phosphate wasting as TmP/GFR was 2.0 $\pm$ 0.1mg/100ml. Serum iPTH was measured with a COOH terminal antibody. Results expressed in ng/pro/ml (Dr. Gueris) or in uEq/ml (Dr. Arnaud) were in all patients below the upper limit of the normal range. Mean level was 1.6ng/pro/ml (normal value between 4 and 8ng/pro/ml) and 17mEq/ml (normal value below 40mEq/ml). The average value of serum iPTH was low. 24 hours urinary calcium was increased in the three groups of patients whether or no they had renal lithiasis. Hydroxyprolinuria was in the normal range. Serum $1.25(OH)_2$ vitamin D level was measured in four patients. Results were 13,32,51 and 82pg/ml (control values : 37 $\pm$ 24pg/ml).

TABLE 1 Biochemical data (mean ± SD)

	Serum phosphate mg/dl	TmP/GFR mg/100ml	Urinary calcium mg/24 h	Urinary hydroxyproline mg/24 h
Lithiasis n = 9	2.51 ± 1.9	1.9 ± 0.2	461 ± 91	44 ± 7
Osteoporosis n = 3	2.57 ± 1.55	1.9 ± 0.1	367 ± 111	41 ± 18
Lombalgic n = 7	2.47 ± 2.7	2.1 ± 0.1	381 ± 119	33 ± 15
Pooled data n = 19	2.49 ± 2.1	2.0 ± 0.1	390 ± 100	39 ± 13
Control values	3.50 ± 0.7	3.3 ± 1.9	200 ± 100	35 ± 15

Bone histomorphometry (Table 2) revealed normal osteoid volume and increased osteoid surface ($p<0.01$). The osteoid thickness was in the normal range. The mineralization front was 58 ± 10% and was significantly decreased compared to controls but was still higher than in osteomalacia where the average value is 19 ± 8%.

TABLE 2 Bone histomorphometry (mean ± SD)

	Osteoid volume %	Osteoid surfaces %	Osteoid thickness um	Mineralization front %
Lithiasis n = 9	3.9 ± 1.8	22.0 ± 3.9	8.0 ± 2.0	60.8 ± 11.7
Osteoporosis n = 3	4.4 ± 1.7	23.3 ± 9.0	6.0 ± 1.1	62.0 ± 8.2
Lombalgic n = 7	5.5 ± 2.6	16.3 ± 6.6	7.8 ± 1.7	55.3 ± 10.5
Pooled data n = 19	4.6 ± 2.2	21.6 ± 6.7	7.7 ± 1.6	58.7 ± 10.6
Controls	5.5 ± 0.4	13.9 ± 1.3	9.5 ± 0.7	65.0 ± 3.1

The extent of osteoblastic surface was markedly decreased (p 0.01) as the mean wall thickness (p 0.01) indicating that the patients had decreased bone formation. Resorption was not significantly different from controls.

As a consequence of this decreased formation trabecular bone volume was slightly decreased in all the three groups whether of not clinical osteoporosis was present (Table 3).

There was no relation between fasting serum phosphate and any histological parameter. However the histological results were not significantly different in each of the three clinical groups which supports a role for hypophosphatemia in the patient's osteopathy.

TABLE 3 Bone histomorphometry mean ± SD

	Osteoblastic surface %	Mean wall thickness µm	Osteoclastic resorption surface %	Trabecular bone volume %
Lithiasis n = 9	2.8 ± 1.1	46 ± 9	0.76 ± 0.53	15.1 ± 2.7
Osteoporosis n = 3	3.1 ± 1.6	35 ± 1	0.53 ± 0.11	13.2 ± 0.1
Lombalgic n = 7	2.9 ± 0.9	39 ± 8	0.68 ± 0.50	13.1 ± 2.0
Pooled data n = 19	2.9 ± 1.0*	41 ± 8*	0.69 ± 0.48	14.0 ± 2.4*
Controls	5.4 ± 0.9	59 ± 9	0.51 ± 0.14	19.3 ± 1.3

COMMENTS

Ivey et al. (2) showed that in young rats, low serum phosphate levels resulted in defective mineralization, a decrease in matrix production and an increase in the osteoclastic resorption. These three anomalies do not occur together in human metabolic bone disorders due to primary hypophosphatemia. In man, primary hypophosphatemia occurs either as vitamin-resistant osteomalacia or as osteoporosis as in our patients. Since in both instances blood calcium levels are normal, we were interested in determining if other hypophosphatemia related factors were responsible for differences in the two groups and if certain anomalies could be traced to phosphorus activity proper.

The absence of osteomalacia in our patients suggests that the condition is not caused by phosphate depletion alone. The fact that the mean phosphate level in our patients was not very low may not explain why they did not develop osteomalacia since in some patients concentrations of 2.1mg/dl were recorded. Levels of this magnitude are often observed in hypophosphatemic osteomalacia. Therapeutic trials have also provided evidence that phosphate may not play a key role in the development of osteomalacia. Phosphate treatment does not have a healing effect on osteomalacia encountered in X-linked hypophosphatemia but does correct defective mineralization of the growth plate (3). Similarly, in osteomalacia due to mesenchymal tumors, phosphate alone or combined with vitamin D does not result in healing of the bone lesion.

This suggests that in hypophosphatemic osteomalacia, there is a hypophosphatemia-related factor promoting defective mineralization. In acquired hypophosphatemic osteomalacia (adult onset hypophosphatemia, mesenchymal cell tumors and some cases of Fanconi syndrome), serum $1.25(OH)_2D_3$ levels are always very low, whereas in our patients they were within the normal range. Although there has not been any experimental evidence pointing to the direct role of $1.25(OH)_2D_3$ in mineralization of the bone, low serum levels of both $1.25(OH)_2D_3$ and phosphate seem to have a determining effect in the development of osteomalacia. This key role of $1.25(OH)_2D_3$ has been supported by the observations of Drezner et al. (4) who found that physiologic doses of the compound had a markedly healing effect on hypophosphatemic osteomalacia.

Yet, in the case of X-linked hypophosphatemia, serum $1.25(OH)_2D_3$ levels are normal and supraphysiologic doses are needed to cure the existing osteomalacia. These findings seem to indicate abnormal osteoblast activity in this affection.

Contrary to findings in osteomalacia, reduced matrix formation may be considered a direct result of phosphate depletion. Raisz et al. (1) showed in in vitro studies that low phosphate concentrations in the medium reduced collagen synthesis. Low collagen production was demonstrated in all our hypophosphatemic patients by the decrease in the mean wall thickness. This may be due to a drop in the bone apposition rate and/or in the recruitment or the life span of the osteoblasts. The reduction in osteoblast surfaces in our patients argues in favour of the latter hypothesis. In 5 patients with a clinical profile identical to that of our patients, Parfitt (5) recorded a decrease in the bone apposition rate. It is likely that reduced collagen synthesis is due to both mechanisms combined.

The question arises whether decreased bone formation in our patients was directly related to phosphate depletion or rather to the low iPTH levels recorded. A number of experimental and clinical findings provide evidence that PTH decreases the apposition of bone matrix. It cannot therefore be held responsible for the reduced mean wall thickness observed. On the other hand, PTH increases osteoblast surfaces and the low serum PTH levels we recorded may explain why osteoblast surfaces in our patients were reduced.

In vitro, hypophosphatemia increases osteolysis and in vivo, it induces hyper-resorption in young rats due to an increase in serum 1.25(OH)2D3 levels. In our patients, there was no histological evidence of high resorption. The low circulating iPTH levels we observed suggest that in man, elevated concentrations of iPTH are needed for excessive osteoclast resorption related to elevated $1.25(OH)_2D_3$ levels to occur.

In conclusion, in our patients with hypophosphatemia, the existence of a bone disease characterized by a decrease in the bone matrix suggests that in adults, phosphate depletion does not necessarily induce osteomalacia but can result in defective matrix formation.

RAISZ L.G. Bone formation and resorption in tissue culture. Arch. Intern. Med. 1970, 126, 887-890.

IVEY J.L., MOREY F.R. & BAYLINK D.J. The effects of phosphate depletion on bone. In Homeostasis of phosphate and other minerals. Advances in experimental medicine and biology, vol. 103, 1977, S.G. Massry, Eritz Arapado, Eds. Plenum Press, 373-380.

GLORIEUX F.H., MARIE P.J., PETTIFOR J.M. & DELVIN E.E. Bone response to phosphate salts ergocalciferol and calcitriol in hypophosphatemic vitamin D resistant rickets. N. Engl. J. Med., 1980, 303, 1023-1031.

DREZNER M.K. & FEINGLOS M.N. Osteomalacia due to 1 alpha 25 hydroxycholecalciferol deficiency association with a geant cell tumor of bone. J. Clin. Invest., 1977, 60, 1046-1059.

PARFITT A.M. & VILLANUEVA A.R. Hypophosphatemia and osteoblast function in human bone disease. Advances in experimental medicine and biology, Vol. 105, 1981, S.G., Massry, J.M. Letteri Eritz Eds Plenum Press, 209-217.

Discussion following paper by M. deVernejoul:

A. M. PARFITT: You mentioned that you excluded patients who had osteomalacia. If you include all of your patients with unexplained hypophosphatemia, what proportion will have osteomalacia and what proportion will fall into the category that you have just described?

M. deVERNEJOUL: We have only 5 patients with adult onset hypophosphatemia and osteomalacia, but 25 patients with non-osteomalacic hypophosphatemia.

H. MALLUCHE: How can you discriminate passive uptake of tetracycline from active deposition if you use only a single label? Could you have missed a subtle mineralization defect?

M. deVERNEJOUL: Most of the patients were studied before we used the double tetracycline labeling technique.

U. LIBERMAN: Did you measure gastrointestinal calcium absorption?

M. deVERNEJOUL: Only in a few patients, where it was increased.

U. LIBERMAN: We have studied a group of patients with a similar syndrome, all with elevated levels of $1,25(OH)_2D$, which may explain the hypercalciuria.

F. GLORIEUX: There is another group of hypophosphatemic individuals who may not be suffering from osteomalacia, the so-called carriers of familial hypophosphatemia who are all females.

BONE DISEASE IN PATIENTS RECEIVING TOTAL PARENTERAL NUTRITION

Susan M. Ott, Norma A. Maloney, Gordon L. Klein, Allen C. Alfrey, Marvin E. Ament, Jack W. Coburn, and Donald J. Sherrard

Department of Medicine, VA Medical Center and University of Washington, Seattle, WA, VA Wadsworth and UCLA, Los Angeles, CA, and VA Medical Center and University of Colorado, Denver, CO, U.S.A.

Patients who have been receiving total parenteral nutrition may develop metabolic bone disease. This has been described in patients with a wide variety of bowel lesions, including radiation enteritis, Crohn's disease, intestinal vasculitis, pseudo-obstruction, and infarction.

We have observed that the bone symptoms appear when other signs of malnutrition are improving. The patients may complain of bone pain (in knees, ankles, back, ribs, elbows, and heels) and may sustain fractures.

Measurements of bone mass, using either photon densitometry or calcium by neutron activation analysis in trunk and thigh (bone calcium index) demonstrate low bone mass. As a group, patients in Shike's study showed no significant change in the bone calcium index over 6-28 months of TPN. A subsequent report showed a decrease in the calcium index in the patients who received vitamin D in TPN over 8-36 months.

The serum laboratory values in these patients show normal calcium, although serial tests may reveal intermittently high values. Phosphate, magnesium, and renal function tests are normal. Alkaline phosphatase is elevated. The parathyroid hormone (PTH) is usually low or normal. Although reported 25-OH-vitamin D levels have been normal, the 1,25 $(OH)_2$ vitamin D (1,25-D) levels are low. Urine collections show high 24 hour calcium values, which were greater than 300 mg in 11 of 16 in Shike's study, with some values above 1000 mg/day. The urine calcium values frequently exceed the calcium intake. When collections were separated into day and night, the average 12° day calcium was 84 $\pm$ 36 mg in a group of 11 patients who infused their TPN over night. The 12° night calicum values were 456 $\pm$ 72 mg.

Bone histological findings have been reported by Shike et al and by us. The total bone area is decreased compared to normals (see Figure 1). In some patients amount of osteoid is increased (see Figure 2). Most of those with excess osteoid have classical osteomalacia, since they also have low bone formation as measured by double tetracycline labels. We have, however, seen a patient with elevated bone formation and increased osteoid; she had hyperparathyroidism. (This emphasizes the importance of tetracycline labels) The patients with a normal amount of osteoid do not have normal formation. In fact, most of them also have low bone formation, as seen in Figure 3. In these bones there is abnormal formation as well as mineralization of the osteoid. This aplastic lesion is a physiological varient of classical osteomalacia. Both lesions demonstrate abnormal mineralization, and the accumulation of osteoid depends on the relative rate of matrix formation.

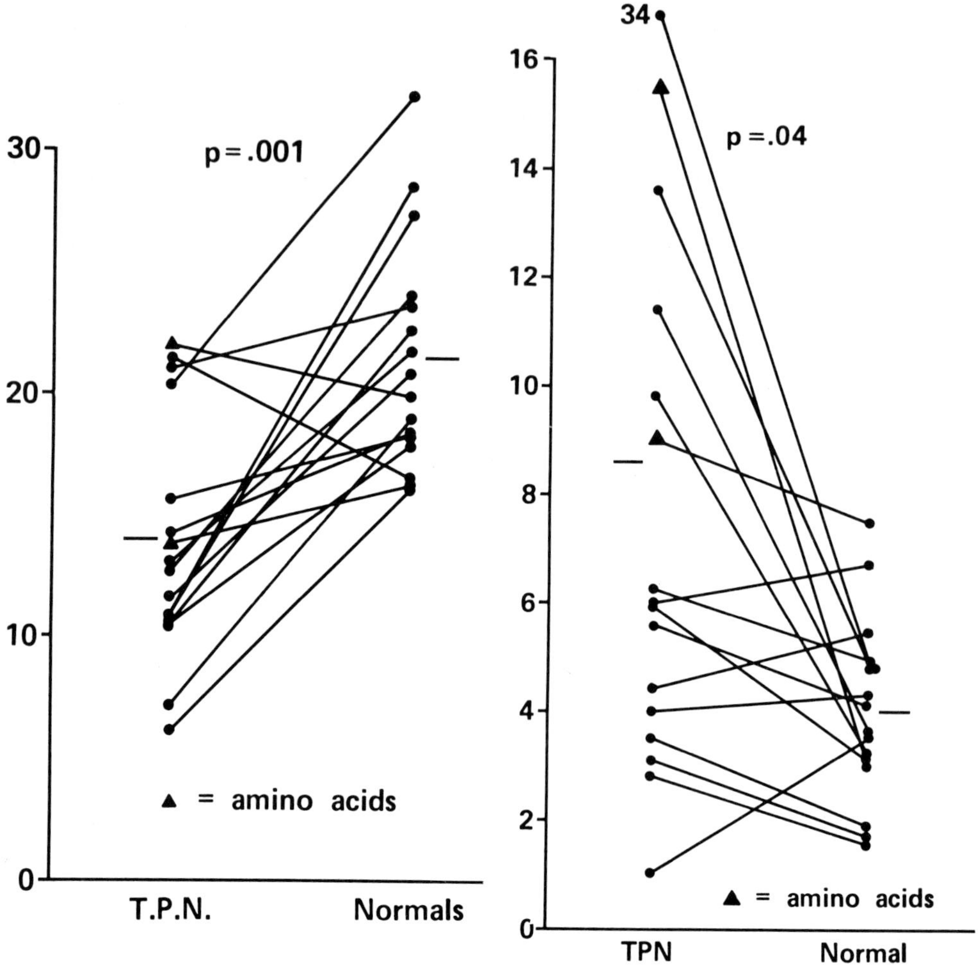

Figure 1 (left) Total bone area as % tissue area in patients receiving TPN. Each line connects the patient to his or her age- and sex matched control. Bars show mean values. Figure 2 (right) osteoid area as % total bone area.

What causes the low bone formation is these patients? We biopsied 16 patients with symptomatic bone disease, and found that all 14 who had received casein hydlrolysate as their protein source had positive histochemical stain for bone aluminum. This was confirmed by chemical analysis in 11 of the biopsies. The two patients who received amino acids did not have aluminum. The aluminum values were inversely correlated to the measured bone formation rates. We also stained sections from the patients described by Shike, et al and found positive bone aluminum stains in 4 patients.

The presence of aluminum in the bones of these patients does not necessarily mean aluminum caused the bone lesions.

However, recent epidemiological, clinical, and animal studies have suggested that aluminum is toxic. Rats and dogs develop osteomalacia after aluminum administration. Hemodialysis patients who have been exposed to aluminum via their dialysate water have a high incidence of osteomalacia or aplastic bone. We have found that 70% of patients with renal osteomalacia have high stainable bone aluminum, whereas no aluminum is seen in normals or in patients with osteoporosis or nutritional osteomalacia. It is interesting that both the TPN and renal patients have high bone aluminum, low bone formation rates, low 1,25-D levels, and inappropriately low serum PTH levels.

Aluminum kinetics have been studied in TPN patients. The source of aluminum was probably the casein, which contained 2.3 mg aluminum/liter. Thus, the patients received one to two mgs of aluminum daily. The urine alunimum values were increased, to 1264 $\pm$ 196 μgm/day (compared to 15 μgm/day in normal individuals). Fecal losses were small (5-70 μg/day) so that the patients are in positive aluminum balance. Studies of plasma levels during TPN infusion suggest that aluminum is highly tissue bound.

After our patients were changed to TPN solutions containing amino acids without aluminum contamination, the serum and urine aluminum values decreased. Bone aluminum decreased slowly. One patient had a second biopsy after 42 months. Stainable aluminum had diminished, and tetracycline labels showed separation in the cortex, but not in trabecular bone. A year later aluminum staining was no longer present, and bone formation was normal.

It is not clear if aluminum is a factor in the vitamin D or PTH abnormalities seen in the TPN patients. In vitro studies have shown that aluminum inhibits release of PTH. But in TPN patients, the transient hypercalcemia during infusions of TPN may inhibit the parathyroid. When calcium free solution was used in 3 patients, the serum calium fell slightly, and the PTH increased. The low serum 1,25-D levels might be a consequence of low PTH levels or of the infusion-induced calcium increase. However, in the patients whose PTH increased with the low-calcium TPN, the 1,25-D levels remained low. It is possible that aluminum inhibits renal 1 -hydroxylase. It is also possible that the bowel disease itself contributes to low 1,25-D levels. Lemann et al studied normals who developed low 1,25-D levels within several days of changing to liquid diets with normal mineral content (78 $\pm$ 19 pM to 48 $\pm$ 18 pM). No differences in serum calcium or PTH were seen. The 1,25-D returned to normal when fiber was added. Vitamin D in the TPN solution may also play a role in the development of bone disease. When Shike et al removed vitamin D from the TPN solution, the bone formation rates improved. The reasons for this are unknown.

In conclusion, patients receiving chronic TPN may develop bone disease. Some may have osteosporosis or osteomalacia from their pre-existing bowel disease. Abnormalities in urine calcium excretion, serum PTH, and vitamin D metabolism may play a role in the development of the bone disease. We have found that aluminum contamination of the TPN solution is associated with low bone formation in these patients. This factor is preventable, and parenteral solutions should be monitored to avoid aluminum infusion.

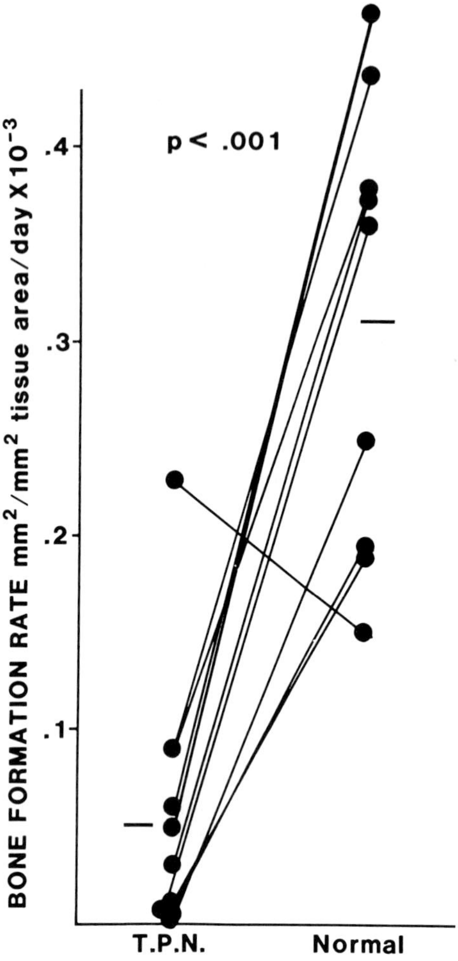

Figure 3 Bone formation rate measured by double tetracycline labels in TPN patients and normals. Lines connect each patient to his or her age and sex matched normal control. Bars show mean values for each group.

1. Shike M, Harrison JE, Sturtridge WC, et al. Metabolic bone disease in patients receiving long term total parenteral nutrition. Ann Intern Med. 1980; 92:343-350.
2. Klein GL, Targoff CM, Ament ME, et al. Bone disease associated with total parenteral nutrition. Lancet. 1980; 2:1041-4.
3. Klein GL, Horst RL, Norman AW. Reduced serum levels of 1,25-dihydroxyvitamin D during long term total parenteral nutrition. Ann Intern Med. 1981; 94:638-43.
4. Shike M, Sturtridge WC, Tam CS, et al. A possible role of vitamin D in the genesis of parenteral nutrition induced metabolic bone disease. Ann Intern Med. 1981; 95:560-8.
5. Klein GL, Alfrey AC, Miller NL, et al. Aluminum loading during total parenteral nutrition. Am J Clin Nutrit. 1982; 35:1425-9.
6. Lemann J, Adams ND, Gray RW. Liquid formula diets reduce serum 1,25-$(OH)_2$-vitamin D concentrations in humans. In: Norman AW, et al, eds. Vitamin D, Chemical, Biochemical, and Clinical Endocrinology of Calcium Metabolism. Berlin: Walter de Gruyter & Co., 1982:669-75.

Discussion following paper by S. Ott:

B. FRAME: Aluminum seems to be the popular metal these days. We have heard from Dr. Ott about this metal in a newly described variety of bone disease, occurring in patients who are receiving total parenteral nutrition. Others have had a different experience with the role of aluminum in this bone disease, so it seems that the question is still open.

Dr. Ott, were you able to determine which lot numbers of casein contained high concentrations of aluminum and if so, could you correlate these lots with the occurrence of osteomalacia in your patients?

J. COBURN: Every sample of casein that we used in our patients, including those in the laboratory, had substantial amounts of aluminum.

S. POSEN: Did any of your patients have neurological symptoms of dialysis dementia? If not, would you care to speculate why?

S. OTT: They didn't have any, and we would guess that they had not been exposed long enough or the levels were not high enough to cause the neurological symptoms that you see in dialysis patients, who have a much larger exposure.

PHYSICIAN: Do you know why casein contains aluminum?

S. OTT: I think it has to do with the way casein is processed.

G. WILLIE: Have you noticed the osteomalacic syndrome in any patients who were maintained throughout on just amino acid solutions; since there are reports where patients with TPN bone disease had never been exposed to casein hydrolysates?

S. OTT: We looked at two patients on amino acid solutions who did not have stainable aluminum in the bone. We have also found that aluminum can be found in albumin solutions.

C. NORDIN: Does the infusion raise the plasma phosphate? If so, perhaps you are switching off $1,25(OH)_2D$ synthesis.

J. COBURN: The serum phosphorus levels are generally normal before infusion and lower at the end of the infusion than before, probably related to the glucose in the solutions. The highest level was 4.5-4.6 mg/dl so I don't think hyperphosphatemia accounted for the low $1,25(OH)_2D$ levels.

J. HARRISON: In Toronto we have seen an osteomalacic bone disease associated with TPN, which does not seem to be related to aluminum. None of the patients who developed this disease were on casein hydrolysate or had ever been on it. Two patients who had been on casein hydrolysate for about 10 years do have high aluminum levels and never developed significant bone disease. In the paper we will present later at this meeting we will demonstrate that our patients improved after vitamin D was removed from the solutions.

R. NEER: This syndrome can occur in patients who are not receiving TPN and who are not on renal hemodialysis. In a personal case, aluminum intoxication causing osteomalacia was eventually traced to cooking utensils. Aluminum exposure should be sought whenever one has a patient with cryptogenic osteomalacia.

A. M. PARFITT: Do you have osteoid seam width and volume measurements in your patients?

S. OTT: Osteoid area in two dimensions is the same measurement as osteois volume. Osteoid seams are wide in the patients who have increased osteoid area, but normal otherwise.

THE PATHOGENESIS OF TUMOR-INDUCED OSTEOMALACIA: A NEW PERSPECTIVE[1]

Peter C. Brazy, Bruce Lobaugh, Kenneth W. Lyles and Marc K. Drezner

Departments of Medicine, Surgery, and Physiology, Duke University Medical Center, Durham, North Carolina, U.S.A.

The tumor-induced osteomalacia (TIO) syndrome is characterized by remission of unexplained osteomalacia and/or rickets after resection of a coexisting tumor. This disease, although apparently relatively rare, has been recognized with increasing frequency during the past 10 years. Indeed, in 1976 only eleven patients with this disorder had been described in the literature but by 1982 thirty-nine additional affected subjects were reported (1).

The spectrum of clinical findings in these patients includes bone pain and/or muscle weakness with occasional recurrent long bone fracture. In addition, affected youths often manifest fatigue, gait disturbance, slow growth and skeletal deformities, including bowing of the lower extremeties.

The tumors associated with this syndrome have been generally of mesenchymal origin (e.g. giant cell tumors of bone, sarcomas, hemangiomas). However, the frequent occurrence of Looser zones in the X-rays of moribund patients with carcinomas of epidermal and endodermal derivation indicates that this disease may be more widespread and prevalent than previously appreciated. The recent observation and documentation of TIO in association with breast carcinoma and prostate carcinoma support this conclusion (2,3).

The biochemical findings characterizing this disorder include hypophosphatemia and an abnormally low renal tubular maximum for the reabsorption of phosphorus per liter of glomerular filtrate, indicative of renal phosphate wasting. In addition, affected subjects generally manifest gastrointestinal malabsorption of phosphorus. The renal phosphorus wasting and gastrointestinal malabsorption result in a negative phosphorus balance.

The serum calcium concentration in patients with TIO is generally at a level marginally below normal, although values within the normal range have been reported. In spite of the subnormal serum calcium level, the serum parathyroid hormone concentration, when measured by assays with varying antigenic specificity, has been unexpectedly normal. The intestinal absorption of calcium in affected subjects is abnormally low but a positive calcium balance is maintained by virtue of renal conservation of calcium.

At present, the pathogenesis of TIO remains unknown. The apparent infrequent incidence of the disorder and its possible heterogeneous nature have precluded definitive study. Nevertheless, an increased understanding of vitamin D metabolism (and its relationship to calcium and phosphorus homeostasis), the development of assays of serum vitamin D metabolites, and the availability of vitamin D metabolites for therapeutic trials have permitted

[1]Grants from the NCI (CA-11265) and the NIAMDDK (AM-27032; AM-00643) supported studies performed in the authors' laboratory.

critical re-evaluation of the factors which underlie TIO.

Over the past several years investigations in our laboratory and several others have been designed to define the spectrum of biochemical abnormalities characteristic of TIO and to investigate both the pathophysiology and therapy of this disease. Affected patients have had mesenchymal tumors, prostatic carcinoma or Linear Nevus Sebaceous Syndrome (with vitamin D resistant rickets/ osteomalacia).

PATHOGENESIS OF TUMOR-INDUCED OSTEOMALACIA

Since the first recognition of TIO in 1947, several investigators have speculated that this form of vitamin D-refractory osteomalacia is caused by tumor secretion of a factor(s) which results in the development of abnormal bone mineralization. At present, however, it remains unclear whether the resultant osteomalacia is a consequence of the tumor factor(s) effecting phosphaturia directly, inhibiting vitamin D metabolism or both. Nevertheless, since the biochemical abnormailities of TIO are, for the most part, typical of the vitamin D deficiency state, several investigators have explored the possibility that abnormal vitamin D metabolism underlies the genesis of TIO.

The results of studies from several laboratories suggest that TIO is due, in part, to tumor mediated inhibition of $1,25(OH)_2D_3$ production. Observations that support this conclusion include: 1) the presence of a decreased circulating level of $1,25(OH)_2D$ in 13 of 13 reported patients who manifested the characteristic syndrome, in spite of a normal or elevated serum 25(OH)D concentration (1); 2) normalization of the serum $1,25(OH)_2D$ concentration promptly after surgical removal of the coincident tumor, and in association with resolution of the characteristic biochemical abnormalities of the syndrome (4-6); and 3) nearly complete or total return of the discrepant biochemistries to normal and/or healing of the attendant osteomalacia (as assessed by bone biopsy) in some, but not all, affected patients treated with $1,25(OH)_2D_3$ at presumed physiological doses (1).

Further amplification of these observations has become possible because heterotransplantation of tumor tissue from an affected subject into an athymic nude mouse has created an animal model of the TIO syndrome (1). The tumor bearing mice manifest many of the biochemical abnormalities characteristic of the TIO syndrome. The serum phosphorus concentration in host mice averages 4.5 ± 0.16 mg/dl, a value significantly less than that in normal athymic nude mice, 7.4 ± 0.19 mg/dl, and in mice bearing tumor from non-affected subjects, 7.2 ± 0.06 mg/dl. Moreover, renal phosphate excretion in the tumor-bearing mice is increased significantly above normal. Thus, host animals have a urine phosphate excretion index of 1.0 ± 0.18, while mice bearing tumors from non-affected subjects and normals have values of 0.5 ± 0.05 and 0.4 ± 0.02, respectively.

Most importantly, recent studies in the animal model indicate that a defect in vitamin D metabolism is part of the TIO syndrome. In these investigations we have found that the 25(OH)D-1-hydroxylase activity in the hypophosphatemic tumor-bearing mice is significantly less than that in either normals or (non-affected) tumor-bearing hosts. These data confirm the presence of abnormal vitamin D metabolism in patients with TIO and indicate that the apparent defect is due to an inhibition of 1,25(OH)D production.

More recently, we have also discovered that 25(OH)D-24R-hydroxylase activity is increased in affected tumor-bearing mice. Thus, it is likely that the abnormality in vitamin D metabolism characteristic of TIO is more complex than previously recognized. In any case, the sum of these observations are consistent with the supposition that in TIO the tumor produced factor(s) disrupts vitamin D metabolism which results in the osteomalacia and attendant biochemical abnormalities.

In spite of these observations, additional data indicate that alternate and/or ancillary abnormalities may play a roll in the pathogenesis of this syndrome. Thus, several recent osbervations indicate that $1,25(OH)_2D$ deficiency does not account for all aspects of TIO in each affected subject. First, there is no apparent explanation for the extreme degree of phosphaturia that occurs in affected subjects who manifest only $1,25(OH)_2D$ deficiency and not increased circulating levels of parathyroid hormone. And secondly, the recent demonstration (7,8) of phosphaturic activity in saline extracts of tumors (from two patients with TIO) is not easily explicable by $1,25(OH)_2D$ deficiency alone. Indeed, these data suggest that tumor production of a phosphaturic factor is a part of the TIO syndrome.

Although these observations suggest that the pathogenesis of TIO is incompletely understood, investigators have overlooked the possibility that the proposed defect in vitamin D metabolism and the phosphaturia may be interrelated abnormalities which coordinately result in the phenotypic expression of TIO. In recent studies, however, we have begun to explore this possibility. Employing isolated perfused renal tubules from normal mice, we examined the effects of vitamin D metabolites on phosphate transport (J-phos). In initial experiments, we observed that exposure of the proximal convoluted tubules to a combination of vitamin D metabolites (25(OH)D; $24,25(OH)_2D$; $1,25(OH)_2D$), in amounts equal to those circulating in normal mice, results in a significant enhancement of J-phos. A similar effect was manifest when circulating levels of "free" vitamin D metabolites were approximated by reducing the concentration of these compounds by 99%. In contrast, we observed no enhancement of J-phos when the tubules were exposed to vitamin D metabolites in concentrations (total and free) equivalent to those circulating in the athymic nude mouse model of TIO. In these hosts serum $1,25(OH)_2D$ levels are decreased and serum $24,25(OH)_2D$ increased in accord with the abnormal renal 25(OH)D-1α-(and 24R-) hydroxylase activity which we had discovered.

These data indicate that a "normal mixture" of vitamin D metabolites has a direct positive effect on renal phosphate transport. Moreover, the absence of such an effect in response to an "abnormal mixture" of vitamin D metabolites provides a possible explanation for the phosphaturia observed in TIO. Indeed these observations provide the first link between the two disparate abnormalities characteristic of TIO, abnormal vitamin D metabolism and phosphaturia. In addition, they further support the possibility that the tumor secreted factor(s) in TIO exerts its action through primary (and perhaps sole) effect on vitamin D metabolism.

Although further studies are necessary to confirm this hypothesis, it is important to note that previous observations suggest a possible mechanism by which alterations in vitamin D metabolism may result in commensurate changes in renal phosphate transport. In sum, a potpourri of studies indicate that: 1) variations in renal phosphate transport may result from alterations in mitochondrial oxidative metabolism (9); and 2) vitamin D metabolites exert profound and specific effects on mitochondrial oxidation (10). Further studies will be necessary to establish whether alterations in the ratio of $1,25(OH)_2D_3/24,25(OH)_2D_3$ results in the appropriate changes in mitochondrial function.

In any case, the studies from our laboratory and others have provided new insight into the possible pathogenesis of TIO. Although, ultimate understanding of the factors underlying this disease awaits additional investigation, rationale therapeutic interventions may soon be possible. Thus, effors may be directed not only at increasing the serum, $1,25(OH)_2D$ concentration but preventing a reciprocal elevation of serum $24,25(OH)_2D$ levels, in order to enhance phosphate transport. Such therapeutic trials are currently underway in animals and man.

REFERENCES

1. Lobaugh, B., Burch, W.M. Jr. and Drezner, M.K. (1983): In: Vitamin D Metabolism: Basic And Clinical Aspects, In press. Editor: R. Kumar. Martinus Nijhoff, The Hague, The Netherlands.

2. Bhattacharyya, M. and DeLuca, H.F. (1974): Arch. Biochem. Biophys., 160, 58.

3. Lyles, K.W., Berry, W.R., Haussler, M.R. and Harrelson, J.M. (1980): Ann. Inter. Med., 93, 275.

4. Parker, M.S., Klein, I., Haussler, M.R. and Mintz, D.H. (1981): JAMA, 245, 492.

5. Sweet, R.A., Males, J.L., Hamstra, A.J. and DeLuca, H.F. (1980): Ann. Inter. Med., 93, 279.

6. Fukumoto, Y., Tarui, S., Tsukiyama, K., Ichihara, K., Moriwaki, K., Nonaka, K., Mizushima, T., Kobayashi, Y., Dokah, S., Fukunagu, M. and Morita, R. (1979): J. Clin. Endocrinol. Metab., 49, 873.

7. Popovtzer, M.M. (1981): Clin. Res. 29, 418A.

8. Aschinberg, L.C., Solomon, L.M., Zeis, P.M., Justice, P. and Rosenthal, I.M. (1977): Pediatrics, 91, 56.

9. Brazy, P.C., Balaban, R.S., Gullans, S.R., Mandell, L.J. and Dennis, V.W. (1980): J. Clin. Invest., 66, 1211.

10. DeLuca, H.F., Gran., F.C., Steinbock, H. and Reiser, S. (1957): J. Biol. Chem., 228, 469.

Discussion following paper by M. Drezner:

B. FRAME: Have you had any patients who have tumor-related osteomalacia with concomitant tumor-related hypercalcemia?

M. DREZNER: No

A. HODGSON: You reported an apparent cure in one patient simply by giving 1,25$(OH)_2$D alone. I and others have found it necessary also to give supplemental phosphate.

M. DREZNER: The normal response to administered 1,25$(OH)_2$D is to increase 24,25$(OH)_2$D, which may preserve the adverse ratio of vitamin D metabolites in terms of effects on phosphate excretion.

L. SHERWOOD: Have you looked at the tumors in mice to see whether extracts have any phosphaturic activity?

M. DREZNER: Not yet. Others have found such a phosphaturic activity.

C. NORDIN: I recently treated a patient with this type of osteomalacia due to a hemangiopericytoma with 1,25$(OH)_2$D in a dose up to 2 μg per day for six months; her calcium absorption returned to normal, but her plasma phosphate and TMP/GFR did not change. The tumor was then removed and within one week her TMP/GFR was normal. I feel that there is more to it than just 1,25 $(OH)_2$D deficiency.

M. DREZNER: 1,25$(OH)_2$D deficiency is only one part of the vitamin D abnormality, and the increase in 24,25$(OH)_2$D that we observed in animals may contribute to the phosphaturia. Consequently, it does not surprise me that 1,25$(OH)_2$D therapy will not correct the TMP/GFR in some patients, because an increase in 24,25$(OH)_2$D will occur secondary to the therapy.

S. MARX: I have observed the evolution of increased PTH and Nc'AMP in one patient with this syndrome due to an unresectable tumor. Have you studied the parathyroids in the animal model? Do you know of any other patients who have developed secondary hyperparathyroidism?

M. DREZNER: One of our patients presented with what we thought was primary hyperparathyroidism. His non-parathyroid tumor had been present for some 20-odd years. He had successful parathyroid surgery which normalized the high serum calcium, but did not alter his low serum phosphorus level. In the athymic nude mice, it's difficult to keep the animals alive long enough to determine whether endogenous stimulation of parathyroid function might occur.

A. NORMAN: Two questions with respect to your nude mide data. What were the blood levels of the vitamin D metabolites? Have you assessed the biochemical performance of the 1-hydroxylase in the nude mice in terms of the K_M and V max for 25-hydroxyvitamin D?

M DREZNER: Serum 1,25$(OH)_2$D is somewhat low, and serum 24,25$(OH)_2$D is about five-fold increased over normal. With regard to the second question, we run the 1-hydroxylase assay to obtain a V max in the way DeLuca has reported with saturating concentrations of 25-hydroxy D. Calculations of the K_M could be done, but it would be relatively meangingless.

W. RYAN: I treated a patient with a hemangiopericytoma for about six years with fairly large doses of vitamin D and phosphate. On 250,000 units a day, the serum calcium increased to 11.5% and 1,25$(OH)_2$D, which was subnormal before therapy, increased to a high normal range of about 50 pg/ml. Despite this, the serum phosphate did not increase. When we removed the tumor, the serum phosphate promptly increased, as did the tubular reabsorption of phosphate. The 1,25$(OH)_2$D increased within a few days to about ten times normal. It is now slowly decreasing over the past several weeks, but it is still elevated despite the patient not receiving vitamin D for at least six months.

M. DREZNER: When you treat with vitamin D you are also going to increase the 24,25$(OH)_2$D, as much or more than the 1,25$(OH)_2$D. I wonder whether this might contribute to the lack of resolution of the phosphaturia. My proposal seems to explain what is happening in our colony of athymic nude mice, but may not be related to the human disease.

X RENAL OSTEODYSTROPHY

INTRODUCTION AND OVERVIEW OF BONE DISEASE IN UREMIA

Jack W. Coburn, M.D.

Medical and Research Services, V.A. Wadsworth Medical Center and Dept of Medicine, U.C.L.A. School of Medicine, Los Angeles, CA, U.S.A.

The following communications on mineral metabolism and bone disease in renal failure will focus on certain important and recent developments rather than attempt to be comprehensive. The reader is referred elsewhere for a more complete discussion of these problems (1,2). My review will summarize views on pathogenesis and management of the bone diseases encountered. Emphasis will be placed on the view that more than one process acts to distort mineral metabolism in renal failure. The use of the term, "renal osteodystrophy," to apply to abnormal calcium metabolism in a uremic patient provides little more insight into pathogenesis than might the term, "fever," aid in the evaluation of a patient with sepsis before the advent of clinical bacteriology.

Sherrard and colleagues will summarize a 15 year evaluation of patients with end-stage renal disease (ESRD), based on clinical findings, the histomorphometic study of bone, and staining of bone for aluminum. With nearly 10 years experience with the use of the active vitamin D sterols, there remains uncertainty regarding the indications for their use and the effects to be expected. Massry and colleagues present results of a controlled study of the use of calcitriol ($1,25(OH)_2$-vitamin D_3) in patients with moderate renal failure; I will summarize data on the use of calcitriol to treat and prevent bone disease in dialysis patients. Slatopolsky and colleagues have other new and rather different results with parenteral calcitriol.

Finally, growing evidence indicates that aluminum accumulation in bone plays a pathogenic role in causing osteomalacia in patients with end-stage uremia; Ackrill and coworkers will review this problem and the methods for chelation and removal of aluminum from the body.

PATHOGENESIS OF SECONDARY HYPERPARATHYROIDISM

Secondary hyperparathyroidism is nearly universal in those with renal insufficiency; it originates early in the course of progressive kidney disease, presumably because of transient hypocalcemia. The two prime candidates as causes of hypocalcemia are phosphate retention, developing because of a reduced renal capacity to excrete phosphate, and the reduction in the renal generation of the renal hormone, $1,25(OH)_2$-vitamin D_3. There is reduced skeletal responsiveness to the calcemic action of parathyroid hormone (PTH), perhaps arising from phosphate retention and reduced generation of calcitriol. The elegant studies of Slatopolsky, Bricker and colleagues have shown that restriction of dietary phosphate in proportion to the magnitude of fall in glomerular filtration rate (GFR) can largely prevent the development of 2° hyperparathyroidism in dogs with experimental renal failure (3,4). It was postulated that serum P transiently increases as GFR falls early in the course of renal failure; increments in serum P would lower blood Ca and thereby increase PTH secretion; PTH would decrease tubular reabsorption of PO_4 and cause phosphaturia. Serum P and Ca levels would return to normal, but only at the expense of a higher PTH level. This process would repeat itself as renal failure progressed until the limit of inhibition of tubular PO_4 reabsorption is reached, i.e. GFR below 25-30 ml/min; then persistent hyperphosphatemia would occur. There is a problem with this theory as originally proposed in that serum P levels are normal or even low in patients with modest renal insufficiency. When marked hyperphosphatemia occurs in advanced renal failure, there is no question that hypocalcemia and increments in serum immunoactive PTH (iPTH) levels can be directly related to serum P levels (5).

Other data suggest that altered vitamin D metabolism contributes to altered Ca and P homeostasis in uremia; reduced generation of calcitriol could also play a role in causing 2o hyperparathyroidism, with a reduction in intestinal Ca absorption contributing to hypocalcemia and increased PTH secretion. Some studies have shown that serum calcitriol levels are normal in patients with modest renal failure (GFR above 40 ml/min) (6); however, children with moderate renal failure have subnormal $1,25(OH)_2D$ levels (7). Moreover, even "normal" levels are lower than would be expected in a situation with elevated iPTH levels. PO_4 metabolism has an important effect to regulate the generation of 1,25(OH)2D3 (8); thus, in renal failure, PO4 retention could reduce the synthesis of $1,25(OH)_2D$; through an effector mechanism that is not yet apparent, increased PTH secretion and 2o hyperparathyroidism could occur. Thus, it is not possible to separate "PO_4 retention" from alterations in "vitamin D metabolism" in a consideration of the pathogenesis of the 2o hyperparathyroidism of renal failure (Figure 1).

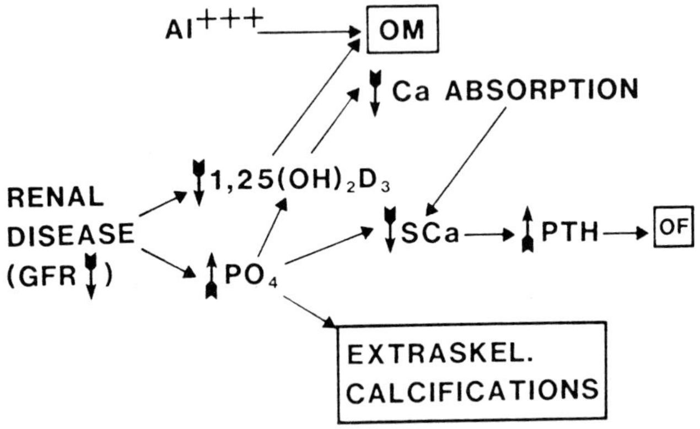

FIGURE 1. Scheme showing the proposed pathogenesis of 2° hyperparathyroidism and osteomalacia in renal failure. ABBREVIATIONS: GFR, glomerular filtration rate; OM, osteomalacia, OF, osteitis fibrosa; and SCa, serum calcium.

As reported by Brown and et al (9), abnormalities of parathyroid cell function have been identified in uremic patients with 2o hyperparathyroidism. Both hyperplasia, with increased cell number, and alterations of cell function exist; the latter is identified by a right-ward shift of the "set point", or the ambient Ca level in the incubation media causing a half maximal suppression of PTH release by the isolated the parathyroid cells. Such an abnormality has been found in cells from 70-80% of parathyroid glands taken from patients with ESRD (9). The factors responsible for this shift in "set point" are unknown. Clinical observations in dialysis patients that elevated serum iPTH levels are often not reduced until the serum Ca exceeds normal are consistent with a right-ward shift of the "set point," in vivo (10).

Since serum iPTH levels are often used to evaluate the status of patients with ESRD, it is important to emphasize a major effect that renal failure has on the results of such assays; which often employ antisera which recognize the mid- or carboxyl-terminus of the PTH molecule. Normally, filtration at the renal glomerulus plays a major role in clearing these PTH fragments from plasma, and they can exhibit substantial accumulation in the plasma of uremic patients (11). Sad to say, data are not available for most immunoassays to indicate what is "normal" level of iPTH in renal failure. The practice of immunoassay laboratories to include results from all dialysis patients as having secondary hyperparathyroidism in an figure showing the relation between serum iPTH and serum Ca is to be deplored. Such a designation is of little value in the differentation of a dialysis a patient with overt secondary hyperparathyroidism from one without. Data showing the relation between serum iPTH levels and a target organ response, such as histo-morphometric findings on bone biopsy, are needed before serum iPTH assays can be used intelligently and ideally for the management patients with renal failure.

PATHOGENESIS OF OSTEOMALACIA IN END-STAGE RENAL FAILURE

Osteomalacia can develop in patients with renal failure for several reasons: These include marked PO_4 depletion and hypophophatemia, coexistent nutritional deficiency of vitamin D, and the use of anticonvulsant drugs. Moreover, the calcitriol deficiency that is present in renal failure may make uremic patients more prone to develop osteomalacia. However, the most common factor associated with vitamin D-refractory osteomalacia in renal patients is aluminum accumulation in bone. The data supporting aluminum as an pathogenic factor are overwhelming: 1) Aluminum, from both dialysate and that absorbed from the intestine, is retained in the absence of kidney function; 2) there is a stong association between the aluminum content in water used to prepare dialysate and the incidence of osteomalacia in dialysis patients. 3) Aluminum accumulates along the calcification front of bone; moreover, little or no tetracycline uptake occurs at sites where there is aluminum accumulation; 4) aluminum injections can cause osteomalacia in animals; 5) inadvertent infusions of aluminum in solutions for parenteral nutrition solutions can cause osteomalcia in man; and 6), treatment with the chelating agent, desferrioxamine, which can remove aluminum, cause improvement of anecdotal cases of dialysis osteomalacia. The magnitude of the problem of bone disease associated with aluminum accumulation is unknown. It is possible that some other retained substance could also cause low-turnover osteomalacia in patients with uremia and a loss of excretory capacity. Whether renal patients with refractory osteomalacia will be identified without aluminum accumulation will be of great interest.

MANAGEMENT OF CALCIUM METABOLISM IN RENAL FAILURE

SECONDARY HYPERPARATHYROIDISM: With recognition of the importance of both preventing hyperphosphatemia and maintaining serum Ca levels within an acceptable range, there are certain well defined goals in clinical practices (Table I). The first is prevention of hyperphosphatemia; this is achieved both by reducing dietary PO_4 and by using PO_4-binding antacids. Control of hyperphosphatemia can prevent or reverse the extraskeletal calcifications that were common during the early years of dialysis; also, PO_4 restriction can aid in controlling 2° hyperparathyroidism. Once serum P is controlled, attention should be directed toward raising the serum Ca to normal. The

TABLE 1. Management of Mineral Metabolism in ESRD: Principles

I. Control Serum P (4.0-5.5 mg/dl) -Restrict diet PO_4 (<1 g/d) -PO_4-binding gels II. Adequate Ca Intake (#I 1st) -Dialysate Ca (3.0-3.5 mEq/L) III. Vitamin D sterols (#I 1st) -Rx of 2° hyperparathyroidism -Hypocalcemia -Prevent bone disease (*) -Children with ESRD Forms: Sterol with 1α-OH group is preferred.	IV. Miscellaneous -Water purification: to remove Al, F; control Mg, Ca. -Normalize blood pH -Normalize serum Mg -Avoid anticonvulsants -Chelate Al (*) V. Parathyroidectomy -Overt 2° hyper-parathyroidism -Failure of # I, II and III. -Calciphylaxis

* Place in management not established.

methods employed to raise serum Ca to normal include the use of dialysate Ca levels adjusted so there is no net Ca loss from the patient, i.e., 3.3-3.7 mEq/L, and Ca supplements in the diet. In addition, the active vitamin D sterols (calcitriol, dihydrotachysterol, 1-alpha-(OH)-vitamin D_3, and calcifediol (25-OH-D_3)) may be used. Their use varies from place to place, with marked differences in the standard of practice. Other papers in this session will focus on clinical effects of the active vitamin D sterols. Finally, parathyroidectomy is the treatment of choice in certain patients with overt 2o hyperparathyroidism. Space constraints preclude inclusion of indications for surgical intervention. However, careful evaluation to exclude the presence of vitamin D-refractory osteomalacia, which is often accompanied by hypercalcemia (12), is very important; this syndrome either fails to improve and may worsens after parathyroidectomy (12,13).

PREVENTION OF OSTEOMALACIA: As Ackrill et al note, appropriate water treatment must be used for patients undergoing hemodialysis. However, the occasional development of this syndrome in uremic patients who have never undergone dialysis indicate that ingestion of aluminum-containing compounds may be the source of aluminum. When one encounters aluminum-associated osteomalacia, rigid dietary phosphate restriction and reduction in the dose of PO4-binders is indicated. The use of Ca-carbonate to reduce PO4 absorption has been employed, as indicated by the abstract of Moriniere et al; the use of desferrioxamine is discussed by Ackrill et al.

Other management procedures are carried out in clinical practice but with no absolute proof of their efficacy. These include correction of acidosis, prevention of hypermagnesemia, and avoidance of fluoride in dialysate. The loss of vitamin D sterols either into urine of patients with the nephrotic syndrome or into peritoneal dialysate during treatment with continuous ambulatory peritoneal dialysis (CAPD) may add to vitamin D requirements; however, there are no data on the efficacy of replacement treatment under these conditions.

UNANSWERED QUESTIONS AND PROBLEMS IN RENAL FAILURE: A patient list of unanswered questions, related to mineral metabolism in uremia is given in Table 2. A number of critical questions must wait for answers. Some have been chosen for this symposium, while others must await further study and more time for their consideration.

TABLE 2. Some unanswered questions concerning renal osteodystrophy

I. Pathogenesis: -How does PO_4-retention act? -What is mechanism for the "set point" shift? -How important is PTH as a "uremic toxin?" -What is role of acidosis? II. Types of bone diseases: -What is significance of these? III. Prevention: -When to restrict diet PO_4? -When to add calcitriol?	IV. In managing establised ESRD, -Use of D sterols: When to use? Which to use? Do their effects differ? How do they act? -When to add Ca supplements? -When to do parathyroidectomy? V. With "Dialysis Osteomalacia," -Are there causes other than aluminum? -How can Al be removed? -How is Al absorbed? -Does Al removal help? -Do high PTH levels help? -What are safe and effective PO_4-binders lacking Al?

REFERENCES:

1. Coburn. J.W. and Slatopolsky, E. (1981): In: The Kidney, 2nd Edition, p. 2213. Editors: B.M. Brenner & F.C. Rector. Saunders, Philadelphia, PA.
2. Coburn, J.W. (1980): Kidney Internat. 17, 677.
3. Slatopolsky, E., Caglar, S,. Pennell, J.P. et al (1972): Kidney Internat. 2, 147.
4. Rutherford, W.E., Bordier, P., Marie, P., et al (1977): J. Clin. Invest. 60, 332.
5. Fornier, A.E., Arnaud, C.D., Johnson, W.J. et al (1971): J. Clin. Invest 50, 599.
6. Slatolpolsky, E., Gray, R., Adams, N.D. (1979): In: Vitamin D; Basic Research and its Clinical Application, p. 1209. Editors: A.W. Norman et al. W. de Gruyter, Berlin.
7. Portale, A.A., Booth, B.E., Tsai, H.C et al (1982): Kidney Internat. 21, 627.
8. Hughes, M.R., Haussler, M.R., Wergedal J. et al (1975): Science 190, 578.
9. Brown, E.M. (1981): In: Hormonal Control of Calcium Metabolism, p. 35. Editors D.V. Cohn et al, Exerpta Medica, Amsterdam.
10. Coburn, J.W., DiDomenico, N.C., Bryce, G.F. et al (1982): Clin. Res., 30, 539A.
11. Hruska, K.A. Martin, K., Mennes, P., et al (1977): J. Clin. Invest. 60, 501.
12. Hodsman, A.B., Sherrard, D.J., Wong, E.G.C., et al (1981): Ann. Int. Med. 94, 629.
13. Felsenfeld, A.J., Harrelson, J.M., Gutman, R.A. (1982): Ann. Int. Med. 96, 34.

UREMIC OSTEODYSTROPHY: CLASSIFICATION, CAUSE AND TREATMENT

D. Sherrard, S. Ott, N. Maloney, D. Andress, J. Coburn

University of Washington, Seattle, WA, and UCLA, Los Angeles, CA, U.S.A.

I. BACKGROUND

The connection between kidney disease and bone disease has been known since the nineteenth century. Early reports commented not only on the disorder but also on its response to cod liver oil long before cod liver oil was known to be a rich source of the then unknown Vitamin D (1).

Parathyroid: Subsequent studies reviewed the bone histology and clinical picture describing a variety of bone lesions (1,2) which were variously ascribed to Vitamin D abnormalities and hyperparathyroidism. In the 1960's and 1970's several investigators developed assays for parathyroid hormone (PTH). It quickly became known that most patients with renal failure had extremely high levels of this hormone, providing support for those who favored hyperparathyroidism as the cause of renal osteodystrophy. Bricker developed the hypothesis that with renal failure hyperparathyroidism was the physiologic "trade-off" for control of phosphate (3). Considerable experimental data provided support for this thesis and it was thought that this was the pathophysiology of renal osteodystrophy.

Vitamin D: But research in Vitamin D metabolism was equally creative in this era. A liver produced metabolite, 25 hydroxy vitamin D, was characterized and, like the dinosaur, achieved transient pre-eminence. The renally derived metabolite, 1,25 dihydroxy vitamin D (calcitriol), was soon shown to be crucial. While numerous other vitamin D metabolites have been identified and many analogs synthesized, calcitriol is the most potent and continues to be regarded as the major, if not only, physiologically active form of the vitamin. Actually this work has called into question its status as a vitamin; its physiology leads most investigators to regard it as a hormone (1)

The studies into both PTH and vitamin D have converged as investigators have tried to understand renal osteodystrophy. Certainly both of these hormonal systems are greatly disturbed when the kidneys fail and their abnormalities are connected. PTH is the trophic hormone for calcitriol, inducing its production by the kidney in response to a decrease in calcium level. As the kidneys degenerate, rising PTH levels encourage greater production of calcitriol per cell from the diminishing renal mass. For a time this maintains adequate circulating levels of calcitriol. Eventually inadequate renal mass can no longer maintain these normal levels and then hypocalcemia occurs. This hypocalcemia has at least 2 causes: 1) failure of gut absorption due to lack of calcitriol; 2) failure of bone resorption which requires both calcitriol and PTH. The hypocalcemia further worsens the hyperparathyroidism. The low calcitriol levels may also aggravate hyperparathyroidism (recent unpublished studies by Slatopolsky support the idea that calcitriol participates in feedback inhibition of PTH).

Other Factors: While abnormalities of vitamin D and PTH predominate in the pathophysiology leading to renal osteodystrophy other factors may play a role. The concentrations of calcium and phosphate, by themselves, can affect bone. Low levels of either one will inhibit mineralization of osteoid in patients with normal renal function. Acidosis impairs osteoid mineralization in normal subjects. In addition, magnesium abnormalities may interfere with tissue response to PTH while uremia itself (perhaps due to accumulation of toxic waste products) inhibits many cellular processes (2).

Dialysis Effects: The treatment of end-stage renal disease may also contribute. Dialysis patients are subjectd to large infusions of heparin with each treatment. This agent induces osteopenia when given continuously; it is unknown whether intermittent use is harmful. The alkali, acetate, is also given to these patients in large quantities as a substitute for bicarbonate. Whether this might interfere with normal apatite production is unknown (2).

Transplantation, too, confers potential problems. Adrenal steroids needed to prevent rejection certainly cause serious bone disease. With steroids superimposed on whatever bone problems have occurred prior to receiving a renal transplant, transplant patients have inordinate morbidity from bone disease, particularly aseptic necrosis of the hip (2).

II. BONE HISTOLOGY AND PATHOPHYSIOLOGY

Bone Histology: Initial studies of bone histology in renal patients revealed excess osteoid and infiltration of the marrow with fibrosis. Sometimes one of these lesions predominated, sometimes the other and sometimes they were combined. There seemed to be a geographic distribution of the various lesions. In sunnier climates the fibrotic lesion was more common while in more temperate areas osteomalacia was more frequent.

Using tetracycline labels bone formation could be determined. This information permitted the recognition of high and low bone formation lesions. Either of these lesions could be associated with excess osteoid, though in only the former was fibrosis seen while in the latter osteoid excess was more severe. Tetracycline labeling allowed us to demonstrate that in some cases the excess osteoid was mineralizing rapidly (high bone formation). The usually mild osteoid excess results from a slight disparity between its production and subsequent mineralization. The osteoid excess, associated with low bone formation, is a result of a similar disparity in the opposite direction. Both osteoid production and mineralization are impaired, the latter to a greater extent.

Later, a third severe lesion was described. Mixed uremic osteodystrophy included both marked osteoid excess (not the modest increase usually seen with renal osteitis fibrosa) and dense marrow fibrosis. This lesion was associated with a marked PTH elevation and a low bone formation rate.

All of these 3 lesions were seen in patients who had suffered from uremia and/or been on dialysis for many years. Patients with a shorter duration of disease generally had a mild lesion characterized only by a slight increase in osteoid and little or no fibrosis. Subsequently tetracycline labeling permitted the identification of 2 lesions in this group. In one (mild) bone formation is normal to elevated. In the other (aplastic) bone formation is suppressed. The histologic differences between these 5 groups are summarized in Table I.

TABLE I. Histologic Features of Renal Osteodystrophy

Group	Fibrosis Area (1)	% Mineralization (2)	Bone Formation (3)
Mild	< 0.5%	> 85%	> 30%
Aplastic	< 0.5%	> 85%	< 30%
Malacic	< 0.5%	< 85%	< 30%
Mixed	> 0.5%	< 85%	< 50%
Fibrotic	> 0.5%	> 85%	> 100%

1) As a percent of tissue area
2) As mineralized bone area/total bone area
3) As a percent of normal

Pathophysiology: To explain why these lesions occurred, concomitant developments in parathyroid and vitamin D metabolism were helpful. Quite early it became apparent that the normal and high bone formation pictures (mild and fibrotic lesions) were related and associated with increased PTH levels. These lesions appeared to be on a continuum. As parathyroid dysfunction worsened patients progressed from the mild to fibrotic picture. Successful therapy of the hyperparathyroidism resulted in a reversal.

The mixed lesion was initially enigmatic, but as data accumulated an explanation presented. These patients had PTH levels similar to those in the fibrotic group, presumably accounting for the similar degree of fibrosis. The calcium times phosphate product was significantly lower than in patients with other lesions. This reduction in available mineral presumably interferes with mineralization (Table 2).

The low bone formation lesions remained a mystery. In general PTH levels were low, but neither the reason for this nor the low bone formation was apparent. A co-existence of aluminum excess with fracturing osteomalacia was reported from other centers (5), but our own unit was proven to be free of aluminum contamination in the water (dialysate water was shown to be the source of aluminum in these reports). Nonetheless, when we were able to determine the aluminum content of the large number of biopsies we have collected, it became apparent that aluminum levels were much higher in the low bone formation lesions (ref. 4, 5; Table 2). In some instances, patients with mild lesions progressed to aplastic or osteomalacic as aluminum accumulated over a series of several biopsies. In other cases, control of hyperparathyroidism, together with increasing bone aluminum, resulted in osteomalacia.

Finally, while most of the patients with the aplastic lesion had high bone aluminum levels, in a few aluminum was undetectable. This mystery may be explained by recent observations in a dialysis unit heavily contaminated with aluminum. In this unit (cf. Ricanati, et al, reported elsewhere in this symposium) a much higher proportion of osteomalacia and aplastic bone disease was found than is usually seen. Several of the aplastic patients had low levels of bone aluminum both by histochemical stain and atomic absorption. Serum levels in these patients were strikingly high - in the range often seen in patients with high bone levels. Thus, it seems likely that cellular function is affected by the level in body fluids. These patients' osteoblasts may be inhibited by the ambient aluminum levels. Presumably with continued exposure bone levels would reflect this.

Table 2. Biochemical Features and Bone Aluminum Levels in Renal Osteodystrophy

Group	PTH(1)	Ca x P(2)	Bone Al(3)
Mild	2-3x	52	+
Aplastic	<1	53	++
Malacic	<1	52	+++
Mixed	4-6x	44	+
Fibrotic	4-6x	53	+

1) As multiples of normal, intact or N-terminal assays
2) Calcium and Phosphate in mg/dl
3) Relative amounts (see references 4 and 5 for actual levels)

Certainly data from parathyroid studies support this. In tissue culture studies of parathyroid cells, PTH release is markedly inhibited when aluminum is added to the culture medium (6). Such data may not only explain the low PTH levels seen in these patients, it also supports our hypothesis that circulating aluminum levels may have an effect on bone cells before bone levels themselves are particularly elevated.

Thus, the etiology of the major bone lesions seen in renal patients appears to be explained (Tables 1, 2). While other factors may play a contributory role, PTH, aluminum exposure, and levels of calcium and phosphate are the primary determinants of the bone pathology.

III. TREATMENT

First of all, prevention of hyperparathyroidism is important. Control of phosphate and maintenance of calcium level using high dialysate calcium, supplemental oral calcium, and vitamin D all appear useful (1,2). These measures will often control the hyperparathyroid bone lesions. Extensive fibrosis may resolve and, when a low calcium x phosphate product is corrected, mineralization of osteoid occurs quickly. .

Unfortunately, despite ideal management hyperparathyroidism may develop and progress. We must conclude that there are yet other factors besides calcium, phosphate and vitamin D which are involved in PTH suppression. In such patients we still must resort to parathyroidectomy. Our present practice is to do a subtotal excision, since total removal (with resultant hypoparathyroidism) potentiates the development of osteomalacia. In addition, we generally transplant the remnant to the arm where further excision is less hazardous if hyperparathyroidism recurs (5 of 40 operated patients have had recurrence over the last 7 years).

In addition, there is another problem with the therapy. Phosphate control is achieved by dietary selection and by the use of aluminum compounds taken orally. The aluminum forms a precipitate with phosphate in the bowel preventing its absorption. Unfortunately, a small, but significant amount of aluminum is absorbed and is a source of aluminum in some patients who develop aluminum toxicity.

Aluminum Toxicity: Prevention is the first measure to take. Water used to prepare dialysate fluid must be free of aluminum (levels must be less than 15 µg/L in the dialysate). It is imperative to maintain such water quality and to document regularly that the aluminum levels are low.

Aluminum gels for phosphate control are an important additional risk. Such therapy must be minimized with attention paid to keeping the phosphate level no lower than necessary. Calcium and magnesium compounds may partially replace aluminum compounds as "phosphate binders," but usually will not provide sufficient control by themselves.

Treatment of aluminum excess with the chelator, desferrioxamine (as discussed elsewhere in this symposium) is usually effective and apparently safe. Therapy is, however, prolonged, time-consuming and expensive. Nonetheless, such treatment not only provides strong confirmation of the toxicity of aluminum, it is also the only reliable approach to managing what had been an almost universally fatal disorder.

Summary and Recommendations: From these comments, it is clear that we have made remarkable progress both in the understanding and treatment of renal osteodystrophy in the last 15 years. It is also clear that several problems remain. These include the clarification of parathyroid suppression. We do not yet understand the physiology of this process well enough to reliably prevent hyperparathyroidism. Perhaps other measures (e.g., involving the autonomic nervous system, other activators or suppressors, membrane transport regulators, etc.) will be necessary to achieve our goal.

Phosphate control using aluminum is hazardous in some patients. Until renal failure is preventable, phosphate control will be essential. It is important to develop other means to control phosphate.

Finally, tangential to renal osteodystrophy is the problem of metastatic calcification. Usually (but not always) associated with a high calcium x phosphate product, patients with chronic uremia frequently develop soft-tissue calcifications. Serious consequences may occur if such deposits occur in the heart, lungs or blood vessels. Functional impairment can result from large peri-articular deposits.

Thus, as progress continues, we look forward to information that will help us with the resolution of these serious, continuing problems in our patient population.

REFERENCES

1. Ott, S.M. and Sherrard, D.J. (1983): In: Renal Bone Disease. Editors: G. Catto and J.W. Coburn. Martinus Nijhoff, Amsterdam. (In press).
2. Sherrard, D.J., Rattazzi, T. and Ott, S.M. (1982): In: Current Nephrology, p. 57. Editor: H.C. Gonick. John Wiley and Sons, New York, NY.
3. Bricker, N.S., Slatopolsky, E., Reiss, E., et al. (1969): Arch. Inter. Med., 123, 543.
4. Maloney, N.A., Ott, S.M. and Sherrard, D.J. (1982): Renal osteodystrophy revisited. Presented at the American Society of Bone Mineral Research. San Francisco, CA.
5. Ott, S.M., Maloney, N.A., Coburn, J.W., et al. (1982): N. Engl J. Med. 307, 709.
6. Morrissey, J., Rothstein, M., Mayer, G. and Slatopolsky, E. (1982) Kidney Int. 21, 138A.

Discussion of paper on Renal Osteodystrophy by D.S. Sherrard

M. PARFITT: You implied that if serum calcium is maintained, uremic patients develop osteitis fibrosa, whereas osteomalacia ensues if the serum calcium falls. Could you elaborate on this?

D. SHERRARD: I am reporting the association we observed rather than explaining the pathophysiology. Patients with "mixed" uremic osteodystrophy have a lower serum calcium phosphate-product, a mean of 42, compared to the other groups. You will recognize that this product is actually above normal; thus dialysis patients may require higher concentrations of these ions for bone mineralization. The other renal failure groups with bone disease had a higher product. Occasionally we have seen patients with a mixed lesion with a very low value; such low values are rare in patients with typical fibrotic lesions. Thus, this has been an attempt to characterize our observations.

C. NORDIN: You imply that the stimulus to the parathyroid gland to cause osteitis fibrosa is not a low serum calcium and that osteomalacia rises from either low calcium or from another factor such as aluminum.

D. SHERRARD: With the hyperosteoidosis seen in the mixed lesion, I believe that a reduced calcium or low calcium-phosphate product is a major feature. Also, factors other than a low serum calcium are involved in hyperparathyroidism; thus, we have followed dialysis patients for several years who have normal or even a slightly elevated serum calcium level, yet serum PTH levels have steadily increased with time.

M. PARFITT: We have seen patients with intestinal malabsorption who are similar to your "aplastic" group, but we do not know whether they have aluminum accumulation. The term, "aplastic" is a nice way to describe this lesion. Can osteomalacia, as we now define it, occur during the evolution of chronic renal failure before patients began on dialysis? We have seen patients with excess osteoid, wide osteoid seams, and high osteoid volume, who have supranormal mineralization rates on double tetracycline labeling. Thus, they have high bone formation rates and do not have osteomalacia.

D. SHERRARD: I think that moderate hyperosteoidosis may be a phase in the evolution of renal bone disease. If there are high serum PTH levels, the patients usually exhibit some fibrosis. On the other hand, if there is increased osteoid and absolutely no peritrabecular fibrosis, the patients usually have reduced bone formation and do not fare well. The patients that we call "osteomalacic" do not resemble nutritional vitamin-D deficiency osteomalacia, when some evidence of secondary hyperparathyroidism usually coexists. The dialysis patients with low turnover have an isolated osteoid increase and little or no evidence of hyperparathyroid changes.

C. NORDIN: Is all the osteomalacia in renal failure related to aluminum accumulation?

D. SHERRARD: In dialysis patients, this certainly seems so. I have shown only the data from our aluminum stain, but results with the measurement of aluminum in bone using atomic absorption spectroscopy have confirmed these findings. Certainly, other factors can cause osteomalacia, but we have not seen these, particularly in the patients referred to us for evaluation of bone disease; those with osteomalacia all have large amounts of aluminum.

C. NORDIN: Apart from the uptake of aluminum via dialysis and from phosphate binders, do you think it is possible that plasma aluminum can increase due to the fall of GFR and may not be related to increased intake?

D. SHERRARD: There is normally a small amount of urinary aluminum excretion in individuals with normal renal function, and so retention may contribute. However, I believe one must also have increased entry of aluminum into the body.

USE OF $1,25(OH)_2D_3$ IN THE TREATMENT OF RENAL OSTEODYSTROPHY IN PATIENTS WITH MODERATE RENAL FAILURE

Shaul G. Massry, Helen Gruber, Arif S. Rizvi, David Sherman, David A. Goldstein and Joseph M. Letteri

Division of Nephrology and Departments of Medicine, University of Southern California School of Medicine, Los Angeles, CA, U.S.A. and Nassau County Medical Center, East Meadow, NY, U.S.A.

Data reported from our laboratory suggested that phosphate retention in patients with moderate renal failure may interfere with the ability of these patients to augment the production of $1,25(OH)_2D$ to meet their increased need (1). A state of relative vitamin D deficiency develops leading to defective mineralization (2, 3), skeletal resistance to the calcemic action of parathyroid hormone (PTH) (4), and defective intestinal calcium absorption (3, 5). These abnormalities produce hypocalcemia and secondary hyperparathyroidism, which in turn will enhance bone resorption. Indeed, dietary phosphate restriction in proportion to the fall in glomerular filtration rate (GFR) in patients with moderate renal failure is adequate to reverse and correct the abnormalities in divalent ions in these patients (1, 3).

However, achieving the proper and adequate dietary phosphate restriction and successful patient compliance with the dietary regimen may prove difficult to attain. Since available data suggest that dietary phosphate restriction exerts its effect through increased production of $1,25(OH)_2D$ (1), it is obvious that an alternative therapeutic approach would be supplementation of $1,25(OH)_2D_3$. Indeed, preliminary studies demonstrated that the oral administration of 0.5 μg/day of $1,25(OH)_2D_3$ for six months to patients with moderate renal failure corrected the abnormalities in divalent ions and bone metabolism (6).

The present study reports the results of therapy with $1,25(OH)_2D_3$ in a larger population of patients with moderate renal failure. Patients with GFR between 15 and 55 ml/min and without significant proteinuria were asked to participate and only those who signed an informed consent entered the study. The duration of the study was one year. The patients were assigned in a double blind fashion to a placebo group and a treatment ($1,25(OH)_2D_3$) group. At the time of this report, 36 patients have been enrolled in the study with 14 having a GFR between 35 and 55 ml/min and 22 with a GFR between 15 and 35 ml/min. Twenty-three patients have already completed one year of study with 12 in the placebo group and 11 in the treatment group. The dose of $1,25(OH)_2D_3$ ranged between 0.5-1.0 (0.8±0.06) μg/day.

The blood levels of PTH were elevated in all but two patients with a mean value of 37±4 μleq/ml (normal: <10), and there was a significant inverse relationship between blood levels of PTH and GFR. The blood levels of 25OHD were normal while those of $1,25(OH)_2D$ were normal in patients with GFR greater than 35 ml/min. In those with GFR less than 35 ml/min, the blood levels of $1,25(OH)_2D$ were low but low normal values were encountered in six of the 22 patients.

The majority of patients showed evidence of bone disease secondary to hyperparathyroidism and/or defective mineralization. The abnormalities due to bone disease were more frequent and severe in patients with GFR below 35 ml/min. The bone histology showed the following abnormalities: a) an increase in the number of osteoclasts (osteoclast index) and in the surface density of bone osteoclast interface; there were significant correlations between these parameters and the blood levels of PTH, b) variable degrees of endosteal fibrosis, c) increased number of osteoblasts (osteoblast index), d) increased osteoid area, and e) prolonged mineralization lag time.

After a year of placebo treatment, there were no significant changes in the blood levels of calcium, inorganic phosphorus and alkaline phosphatase. The blood levels of PTH remained elevated. There was a decline in GFR in all but two patients with a mean fall of 16±3.8%, $p<0.01$; this reflected the natural spontaneous progression of renal insufficiency that occurs in patients with renal diseases. The abnormalities in bone histology either worsened or remained unchanged.

Treatment with $1,25(OH)_2D_3$ for one year produced a significant rise in the blood levels of calcium. All patients but one had at least one episode of mild hypercalcemia and three patients had two hypercalcemic episodes. Cessation of therapy for a few days or reduction of the dose of vitamin D metabolite was adequate to reverse the hypercalcemia. The blood levels of inorganic phosphorus fell initially and remained low for several months; they rose again to base line values by the 10th-12th months of therapy. There was a gradual decline in the blood levels of alkaline phosphatase. The blood levels of PTH fell in all but two patients and the mean decline was 38±9%, $p<0.01$; there was significant inverse correlation between the fall in the blood levels of PTH and the rise in the blood concentrations of calcium.

All but two of the treated patients displayed a rise in GFR with a mean increase of 12±3.2%, $p<0.01$. This is in contrast to the significant and spontaneous decline in GFR in the placebo group. This finding is interesting and important. It demonstrates that treatment with $1,25(OH)_2D_3$ may provide a therapeutic approach for the prevention of the natural progression of renal insufficiency.

Treatment with $1,25(OH)_2D_3$ resulted in either complete healing or marked improvement of all the abnormalities of bone histology including the manifestations of enhanced bone resorption and those of defective mineralization.

Our data demonstrate that treatment of patients with moderate renal failure with small doses of $1,25(OH)_2D_3$ is an effective therapy for the healing and the prevention of the progression of all the derangements in divalent ion metabolism. Such management may also provide a therapeutic tool for the prevention of the natural progression of renal insufficiency in patients with renal diseases.

REFERENCES

1. Massry, S.G. (1979): Pathogenesis of Secondary Hyperparathyroidism in Early Renal Failure: A Multifactorial System Including Phosphate Retention Skeletal Resistance to PTH, and Altered Vitamin D Metabolism: In: Vitamin D, Basic Research and its Clinical Application, p. 1203. Editors: A.W. Norman, K. Schaefer, D.V. Herrath, H-G. Grigoleit, J.W. Coburn, H.F. DeLuca, E.B. Mawer and T. Suda. W. de Gruyter, Berlin-New York.
2. Malluche, H.H., Ritz, E., Lange, H.P., Kutschera, J., Hodgson, M., Seiffert, U. and Schoeppe, W. (1976): Bone Histology in Incepient and Advanced Renal Failure. Kidney Internat. 9, 355.
3. Llach, F., Massry, S.G., Koffler, A., Malluche, H.H., Singer, F.R., Brickman, A.S. and Kurokawa, K. (1977): Secondary Hyperparathyroidism (2oHPTISM) in Early Renal Failure (ERN): Role of Phosphate (P) Retention. Clin. Res. 25, 507A.
4. Llach, F., Massry, S.G., Singer, F.R., Kurokawa, K., Kaye, J.H. and Coburn, J.W. (1975): Skeletal Resistance to Endogenous Parathyroid Hormone in Patients with Early Renal Failure: A Possible Cause for Secondary Hyperparathyroidism. J. Clin. Endocrinol. Metab. 41, 339.
5. Malluche, H.H., Werner, E. and Ritz, E. (1978): Intestinal Absorption of Calcium and Whole-Body Calcium Retention in Incipient and Advanced Renal Failure. Miner. Elect. Metab. 1, 263.

6. Healy, M., Malluche, H.H., Goldstein, D.A., Singer, F.R. and Massry, S.G. (1980): Effects of Long-Term Therapy with 1,25$(OH)_2D_3$ in Patients with Moderate Renal Failure. Arch. Intern. Med. 140, 1030.

USE OF ACTIVE VITAMIN D STEROLS IN END-STAGE RENAL FAILURE

J.W. Coburn, D.J. Sherrard, S.A. Ott, N.C. DiDomenico, G.F. Bryce, A.S. Brickman, L.W. Bassett, E.G.C. Wong, R.B. Miller, C.M. Bennett, R.H. Gold, O.N. Miller, S.A. Shupien, and P.C. Chang

Medical and Research Services, V.A. Wadsworth Medical Center and Dept. of Med., U.C.L.A. Sch. Med., Los Angeles, CA; V.A. Med. Ctr. & Univ. Wash, Seattle, WA; Roche Resch. Ctr., Nutley, N.J., and particpating institutions, U.S.A.

In patients with end-stage renal disease (ESRD), the generation of the renal hormone, 1,25-dihydroxy-vitamin D_3 (calcitriol), is reduced and its serum levels are undetectable or very low. Several physiologic derangements of mineral metabolism present in uremia could arise as a consequence of this deficiency of calcitriol; these include 1) impaired intestinal absorption of Ca, 2) impaired mineralization of bone, 3) the reduced calcemic response of bone to PTH, and 4), abnormal feedback suppression of PTH secretion by serum Ca. Thus, there are several theoretical reasons why highly active vitamin D sterols, such as calcitriol, should be used in the management of ESRD (1). This paper will focus on results with the use of calcitriol rather than other active vitamin D sterols for several reasons: 1) 1α-hydroxy-vitamin3_D has not had wide use in the U.S.; 2) dihydrotachysterol, which is used clinically, has not been extensively studied regarding its effects on bone and we have little experience with this sterol; 3) calcifediol (25-(OH)-vitamin D_3) seems to have substantial disadvantages because of its long half life, and experience with its use is limited in uremic patients.

OPEN TRIALS WITH CALCITRIOL IN SYMPTOMATIC OSTEODYSTROPHY

Several open trials with the use of calcitriol are reviewed in detail (2). In most, calcitriol was given to patients with symptomatic and often severe skeletal disease. Some of the effects of calcitriol observed in those with renal insufficiency are outlined in Table I. Treatment with calcitriol increases intestinal Ca absorption to normal or above; serum Ca concentration is increased secondary to increased Ca absorption, the increased skeletal response to the calcemic action of parathyroid hormone (PTH), or both.

Table I. ACTIONS OF $1,25(OH)_2D_3$ IN RENAL FAILURE

1. Increased intestinal Ca absorption.
2. Enhanced calcemic action of PTH on bone.
3. Increased serum Ca
   (arising from numbers 1 & 2 above)
4. Improved mineralization of bone (not if arising
   from aluminum accumulation).
5. Suppression of 2° hyperparathyroidism: From
   1) incr. serum Ca. & 2) ? direct parathyroid action.
6. Increased intestinal PO_4 absorption.
7. Other effects: improved myopathy; mucosal hypertrophy;
   growth simulation in children (mech. uncertain).

Suppression of 2° hyperparathyroidism can occur because of the rise in serum Ca and perhaps also from a direct effect of $1,25(OH)_2D_3$ on the parathyroid glands. The biochemical changes observed are often associated with improvement in both radiographic and histological features of 2° hyperparathyroidism (3). Substantial improvement of proximal myopathy has been noted during such therapy (4); this is surprising since receptors for calcitriol have not been found in muscle. Improved mineralization of osteoid has also occurred; however, this has been observed in patients with histologic evidence of both osteomalcia and osteitis fibrosa (the "mixed" disorder of Sherrard et al, above). A common "side effect" of therapy with the active vitamin D sterols is the appearance of hypercalcemia. Hypercalcemia has usually occurred: 1) when there has been substantial healing of the osteitis fibrosa, with reversal of the "hungry bone" syndrome, 2) when there is marked and overt hyperparathyroidism and there may be the need for surgical reduction of the mass of parathyroid tissue, and 3) in patients with vitamin D-refractory osteomalacia (5,6). Fortunately, the hypercalcemia usually reverses within a few days after withdrawal of treatment. Rare instances of persistent hypercalcemia remain unexplained as the plasma turnover of calcitriol is quite rapid. Another effect of calcitriol is to increase in absorption of PO4, and larger doses of PO4-binding antacids may be needed. In children with advanced renal failure, calcitriol or another active sterol is almost always required; otherwise, overt and symptomatic bone disease is almost universal in children with advanced renal failure.

With the application of the active vitamin D sterols to ESRD patients with symptomatic bone disease, it soon became apparent that some patients failed to respond, while others showed dramatic improvement. Peculiarly, patients with "pure" osteomalacia, a process that would be expected to respond to vitamin D, failed to improve (7). Such patients were subsequently identified as those with aluminum-associated, low-turnover osteomalacia (8); indeed, a retrospective analysis of the patients treated with calcitriol has indicated that aluminum accumulation in bone was the major factor associated with a poor response to therapy (9).

CONTROLLED STUDIES WITH CALCITRIOL IN DIALYSIS PATIENTS

Following the rather wide-spread introduction of these sterols into use, there have been several controlled trials, particularly in patients lacking the marked disease encountered in the early reports. Questions asked were whether these sterols could prevent the development of bone disease and what were the ill effects of such therapy. In a double-blind controlled study of 98 asymptomatic dialysis patients with normal bone X-rays, we (10) compared calcitriol with placebo given for a 30 month treatment period, the dosage was increased every 2 months from 1 to 4 capsules/day (1 cap = 0.25 ug or placebo). All patients received oral $CaCO_3$ providing 1 g Ca/day, vitamin D_3, 400 IU/day, and $Al(OH)_3$-gel to maintain serum P between 3.5 and 5.5 mg/dl. The dosage of sterol was not increased if serum Ca was 11.2-11.8 mg/dl but it was stopped to be re-initiated at a lower dose if serum Ca exceeded 11.8 mg/dl. Follow-up evaluation included serial radiographs and bone mineral content (BMC) of the mid- and distal radius, measured every 4 months. Serum iPTH (Ch 9 antiserum) was measured monthly and serum Ca and P, twice monthly.

During the treatment period, serum Ca rose from 9.4 ± 0.6 to 10.2 ± 0.5 mg/dl (mean±SD) in those receiving calcitriol; corresponding serum P levels were 4.7 ± 0.9 and 5.1 ± 0.7 mg/dl, respectively. In the placebo-treated group, comparable levels of serum Ca were 9.5 ± 0.6 and 9.7 ± 0.6 mg/dl, while serum P levels were 4.7 ± 0.9 and 4.9 ± 0.7 mg/dl, respectively. Serum levels of $1,25(OH)_2D$ increased from 7.7 ± 7.0 to 16.5 ± 5.9 pg/ml in the former group but were unchanged in the placebo-treated patients. In comparison to placebo, calcitriol suppressed iPTH in more patients than did placebo (60% vs. 27% of the placebo patients), and fewer calcitriol-treated patients exhibited a increase in serum iPTH (11% vs. 39% in the placebo group). Among the 25% of the study group who entered with lower serum iPTH levels (<130ulEq/ml), none showed worsened X-rays and far fewer exhibited significant decreases in BMC during the follow-up period. However, patients entering the study with serum iPTH levels above 130ulEq/ml, and in particular those with rising iPTH levels during follow-up, were more likely to develop erosions on X-ray and/or have a significantly decreasing BMC. Conversely, those with decreasing serum iPTH levels did not develop erosions nor exhibit significant decreases in BMC. Serum iPTH was generally not suppressed unless serum Ca exceeded 10.0-10.5 mg/dl, observations compatable with a right-ward shift in the "set-point" in many patients. The sub-group of placebo-treated patients showing a decrease in serum iPTH had an increase in Ca from 8.99 ± 0.25 to 9.39 ± 0.39 mg/dl (mean+SE) with $CaCO_3$ treatment (11); thus, this sub-group exhibited suppression of serum iPTH at an expected serum Ca. The only side effect of calcitriol treatment was asymptomatic hypercalcemia which rapidly reversed on stopping therapy. Radiographic evidence of soft-tissue calcifications was no more common in either treatment group (12).

The results of this study indicate the risk of developing 2° hyperparathyroidism, as indicated by overt radiographic findings, can be significantly lowered by treatment with calcitriol. Also, fewer patients showed a progressive reduction in bone mineral content, measured in cortical bone of the appendicular skeleton. These benefits were more apparent in patients at higher "risk," as evaluated by the serum iPTH levels at the time of entry into the study. These observations also point to the heterogeniety of 2° hyperparathyroidism in patients with end-stage renal failure. They also point to a risk of progression of 2° hyperparathyroidism in certain patients despite "ideal" conservative management. The development of hypercalcemia during calcitriol therapy in the face of serum $1,25(OH)_2D$ levels that remain subnormal suggest the existence of significant alterations of Ca homeostasis in such conditions with absent renal function.

In another controlled study which admitted symptomatic dialysis patients and those with with abnormal radiographs, Memmos et al (13) noted significant reversal in 2° hyperparathyroidism, as indicated by serum iPTH levels and hand radiographs, in those receiving calcitriol compared to placebo. Also, Berl et al (14), who studied patients with more severe skeletal disease, showed a significant improvement in histologic changes of 2° hyperparathyroidism in the patients receiving active sterol. Thus, the data available from controlled studies indicate that the features of 2° hyperparathyroidism can be significantly improved by treatment with calcitriol; hypercalcemia, which is usually asymptomatic and rapidly reversible, is more probably frequent than in those with normal renal function.

EFFECTS OF 24,25-DIHYDROXY-VITAMIN D_3 IN RENAL FAILURE

24,25-dihydroxy-vitamin D_3, a naturally occurring vitamin D sterol of uncertain function, is largely generated in the kidney, and its plasma levels are reduced in patients with advanced renal failure. Over the past several years, we have accumulated preliminary experience with the use of this sterol. We have treated two groups of ESRD patients with this sterol: 1) those with vitamin D-refractory osteomalacia and 2) those with overt and symptomatic 2° hyperparathyroidism; the latter were chosen because they were poor risks for surgery, had recurrence after initial parathyroidectomy or were those whose parathyroid glands could not be found at surgery. Thus, they were chosen because of failure of other therapeutic modalities. The patients with "dialysis osteomalacia" were those subsequently identified as having marked aluminum accumulation (8). With the administration of $24,25(OH)_2D_3$, in doses of 5 to 20 ug/day, nearly half of patients with "dialysis osteomalacia" have shown improvement of symptoms; moreover their bone biopsies showed a significant improvment in mineralization. The patients who improved also had a reduction in serum Ca and often an increase in serum alkaline phosphatase activity, In most patients, the dosage of calcitriol was increased when serum Ca fell (9). In the patients who showed no clinical response, there were no changes in serum biochemical parameters nor in bone biopsy results. The reason for the improvement in some of these patients, who exhibited the characteristic aluminum accumulation, remains unexplained.

In the uremic patients with osteitis fibrosa and markedly elevated serum iPTH levels who were treated with $24,25(OH)_2D_3$, we noted no clinical improvement, no change in serum iPTH levels nor in the abnormalities noted on bone biopsy. Such observations do not indicate that this sterol, when given to patients with significant 2° hyperparathyroidism, can cause significant suppression of parathyroid activity (16).

ACKNOWLEDGEMENT: Supported in part by USPHS Grants AM 72204, AM 14750, and research funds from the Veterans Administration.

REFERENCES:

1. Coburn, J.W. & Slatopolsky, E.(1981): In: The Kidney. 2nd Ed. p. 2213. Editors, B.M. Brenner & F.C. Rector, W.B. Saunders Co., Philadelphia.
2. Massry, S.G., Goldstein, D.A., & Malluche, H.H. (1980): Kidney Internat. 18, 409.
3. Coburn, J.W. (1980): Kidney Internat. 17, 677.
4. Henderson, R.G., Russell, R.G.G., Ledingham, J.G.G et al (1974): Lancet 1, 379.
5. Hodsman, A.W., Wong, E.G.C., Sherrard, D.J. (1981): Ann. Int. Med. 94, 629.
6. Boyce, B.F., Fell, G.S., Elder, H.Y. et al (1982): Lancet 2, 1009.
7. Coburn, J.W., A.S. Brickman, D.J. Sherrard et al (1977): In: Endocrinology of Calcium Metabolism. p.27. Excerpta Medica, Amsterdam.
8. Hodsman, A.W., Sherrard, D.J., Alfrey, A.C. (1982): J. Clin. Endocrinol. 54, 539.
9. Ott, S.M., Maloney, N.A., Coburn, J.W. (1982): New Engl. J. Med. 307, 709.
10. Coburn, J.W., DiDomenico, N.C. & Bryce, G.F. et al (1982): In: Vitamin D: Chemical, Biochemical and Clinical Endocrinology of Calcium Metabolism, p.833. Editors A.W. Norman et al. Walter de Gruyter, Berlin.
11. Coburn, J.W., DiDomenico, N.C., Bryce, G.F. et al (1982): Clin. Res., 30, 539A.
12. DiDomenico, N.C., Bassett, L.W., Gold, R.H. et al (1982): In: Vitamin D: Chemical, Biochemical, and Clinical Endocrinology of Calcium Metabolism, p. 877. Editors; A.W. Norman et al. W. deGruyter, Berlin.
13. Memmos, D.E., Eastwood, J.B. & Talner, L.B. et al (1981): British. Med. J. 282, 1919.
14. Berl, T., Berns, A.S. & Huffer, W.E. et al (1978): Ann. Int. Med. 88, 774.
15. Hodsman, A.W., Wong, E.G.C., Sherrard, D.J., et al (1983): Amer. J. Med. 74, 407.
16. Ott, S.M., Recker, R.R., Coburn, J.W., et al (1983): Kidney Internat. 23, 107.

SUPPRESSION OF SECONDARY HYPERPARATHYROIDISM BY $1,25(OH)_2D_3$

Eduardo Slatopolsky, Carol Weerts, Benjamin Thielan, Tilde Galceran and Kevin Martin

Renal Division, Department of Medicine, Washington University School of Medicine, St. Louis, MO, U.S.A.

The kidney plays a key role in the metabolism of parathyroid hormone and vitamin D, the two main hormonal systems responsible for the regulation of calcium and phosphate balance. In patients with chronic renal disease, these intricate and complex feedback mechanisms are disrupted. Thus, alterations in bone and mineral metabolism become apparent. Bone biopsies performed in patients with advanced renal failure have demonstrated the presence of osteitis fibrosa, osteomalacia, or a combination of these two pathological processes in the majority of patients.

Secondary hyperparathyroidism is frequently observed in patients with chronic renal disease. Chief cell hyperplasia of the parathyroid glands and high levels of radioimmunoassayable parathyroid hormone (i-PTH) are among the earliest findings affecting mineral metabolism in patients with chronic renal failure. Mild elevations in i-PTH in serum have been reported in patients with only slightly abnormal renal function (GFR 60 to 80 ml/min) (1,2). Although many factors are responsible for the regulation and secretion of parathyroid hormone, it seems that in patients with renal insufficiency the most important cause for the development of secondary hyperparathyroidism is a reduced serum ionized calcium.

Recent interest in a possible direct effect of vitamin D metabolites in the regulation of parathyroid hormone secretion was stimulated by demonstration of receptors for 1,25-dihydroxy D_3 in the parathyroid cells (3) and by the isolation of a calcium-binding protein (4). Since PTH appears to influence the metabolism of vitamin D, stimulating the synthesis of 1,25-dihydroxy D_3 (5,6), one could speculate that a negative feedback system could operate directly or indirectly as a control mechanism for PTH secretion. Thus, in the case of severe renal insufficiency the question is whether the inability to suppress the secretion of PTH is due in part to a decrease in 1,25-dihydroxy D_3 levels per se or exclusively to hypocalcemia. Many attempts have been made to demonstrate a direct effect of vitamin D or its metabolites on parathyroid hormone secretion. Divergent results have been published. Specifically, it has been reported that 1,25-dihydroxy D_3 inhibits (7,8,9), stimulates (10,11) or has no effect (12,13) on PTH secretion. We performed studies in vitro (14) using normal bovine parathyroid gland slices and isolated parathyroid cells. Both carboxy terminal and amino terminal radioimmunoassays for PTH were employed. No effect of 1,25-dihydroxyD_3 on PTH secretion was found during the four hour incubation of parathyroid slices in variable external calcium concentrations. The results from dual RIA measurements also show no effect of 1,25-dihydroxy D_3 on PTH secretion by isolated parathyroid cells during 90-150 minutes incubation with variable calcium concentrations. In addition, extensive analysis by polyacrylamide gel electrophoresis show no effect of 1,25-dihydroxy D_3 on the secretion of PTH fragments. The vitamin D metabolite also did not affect cyclic AMP generation. Since our studies were performed in tissues obtained from normal bovine parathyroid glands, in animals which are not deficient in 1,25-dihydroxy D_3, and furthermore the studies were performed during short periods of incubations in vitro, we decided to study the effects of 1,25-dihydroxy D_3 on PTH release in uremic patients. We entertained the possibility that the chronic administration of this metabolite of vitamin D may still have a direct effect on PTH release. Moreover, since 1,25-dihydroxy D_3 for intravenous use became available to us, we decided to study its potential effect on dialysis patients.

METHODOLOGY

We selected 20 patients with hypocalcemia maintained on chronic hemodialysis. In the control part of the studies blood was obtained before dialysis three times a week for a period of three weeks. In the treatment period 1,25-dihydroxy D_3 was given intravenously at the end of each dialysis for a period of 8 weeks. The starting dose was 0.5 µg and gradually was increased to a maximum of 4 µg per treatment. Finally, a second control post-treatment period was continued for an additional three weeks. Blood samples were obtained for total and ionized calcium, magnesium and phosphorus. PTH was measured with our chicken antibody CH9. This antibody recognizes the C terminal, middle region, and the intact PTH molecule.

RESULTS

The mean serum calcium increased from 8.5 mg/100 ml to 9.4 and with a peak response of 10.9 mg/100 ml during 1,25-dihydroxy D_3 administration. In the post-treatment period serum calcium decreased to a mean of 9.0 mg/100 ml. In general, there was a tendency for serum phosphorus to increase during 1,25-dihydroxy D_3 administration. Magnesium, on the other hand, remained fairly constant during the entire study in all patients. <u>Every single patient had a substantial decrease in the levels of PTH during 1,25-dihydroxy D_3 treatment and the mean decrement was 70%.</u> After 1,25-dihydroxy D_3 was discontinued, PTH increased in every single patient (Fig. 1). After three weeks of treatment, there was gradual rise in the levels of ionized calcium. Concomitantly, there was a significant decrease in the levels of i-PTH. However, it would seem that early during the administration of 1,25-dihydroxy D_3 before there was any significant increase in ionized calcium, already there was a decrease in the levels of i-PTH. Table 1 illustrates the results in a representative patient in which the levels of ionized calcium and i-PTH are compared during the control part of the studies and early course of administration of 1,25-dihydroxy D_3 before substantial changes in calcium can be observed. As is depicted in Table 1, there was no change in the levels of ionized calcium; however, the levels of parathyroid hormone decreased from control values of 764 $\pm$ 46 µlEq to 329 $\pm$ 59 µlEq.

CONCLUSIONS

Thus, the present studies demonstrate that $1,25(OH)_2D_3$ has remarkable suppressive effect on the release of PTH. Likely, the effects are mainly due to elevation in serum calcium to the upper limits of normal. However, it would seem that in addition to the calcemic effect, 1,25-dihydroxy D_3 per se modified the secretion of PTH. It is known that parathyroid glands obtained from uremic patients have a shift in the set point for calcium, requiring a higher concentration of ionized calcium than normal parathyroid glands for the suppression of PTH release. These studies raise the possibility that 1,25-dihydroxy D_3 may affect the regulation of PTH secretion by making the parathyroid gland more sensitive to calcium. Obviously, further studies are necessary to clarify this point.

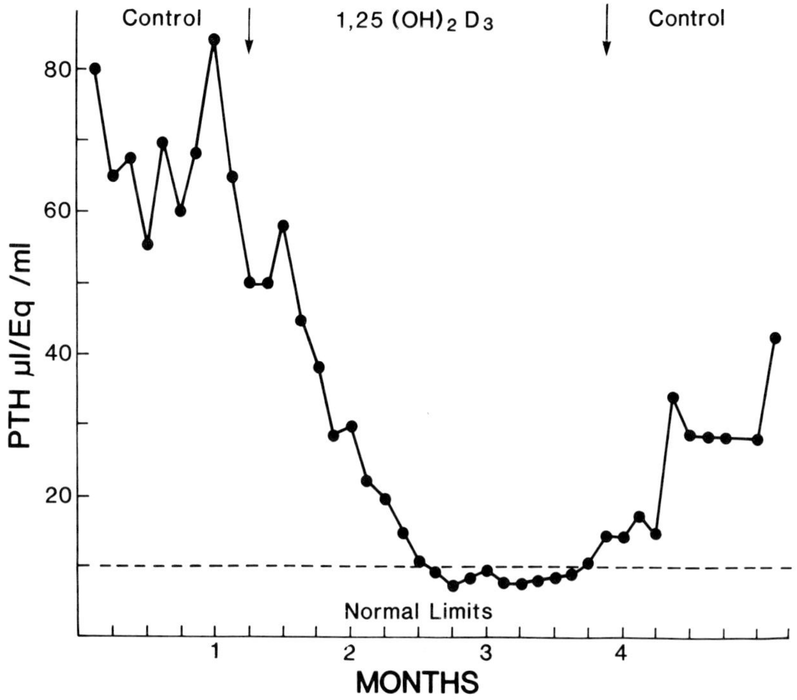

Figure 1. The effects of $1,25(OH)_2D_3$ on i-PTH in a uremic patient. During control studies i-PTH was increased 6-8 fold above baseline. During the administration of intravenous $1,25(OH)_2D_3$, the levels of serum i-PTH returned to normal. After $1,25(OH)_2D_3$ was discontinued i-PTH again increased 3-4 times above normal.

TABLE 1. Relationship between ionized calcium and i-PTH in a uremic patient before and after the intravenous administration of $1,25(OH)_2D_3$

	Control		$1,25(OH)_2D_3$	
	Ca^{++} mg/dl	PTH µEq/ml	Ca^{++} mg/dl	PTH µEq/ml
	4.86	752	4.72	229
	4.52	857	4.86	457
	4.82	768	4.60	343
	4.62	784	4.18	332
	4.76	691	4.74	276
	4.64	744	4.48	336
	4.68	715	4.98	345
	4.56	794	4.86	342
	4.58	748	4.68	330
	4.68	790	4.62	296
M	4.67	764	4.67	329
SD	±0.11	± 46	±0.23	± 59

REFERENCES

1. Reiss, E., Canterbury, J.M., and Bilinsky, R.T. (1968): Trans. Assn. Amer. Phys., 81, 104.
2. Arnaud, C.D. (1973): Kidney Internat., 4, 89.
3. Brumbaugh, P.F., Hughes, M.R., and Haussler, M.R. (1975): Proc. Natl. Acad. Sci. U.S.A., 72, 4871.
4. Oldham, S.B., Fischer, J.A., Shen, L., and Arnaud, C.D. (1974): Biochemistry, 13, 4790.
5. Rasmussen, H., Wong, M., Bikle, D., and Goodman, D.B.P. (1972): J. Clin. Invest., 51, 2502.
6. Garabedian, M., Holick, M.F., DeLuca, H.F., and Boyle, I.T. (1972): Proc. Natl. Acad. Sci. U.S.A., 69, 1673.
7. Chertow, B.S., Baylink, D.J., Wergedal, J.E., Su, M.H.H., and Norman, A.W. (1975): J. Clin. Invest., 56, 668.
8. Henry, H.L., Taylor, A.N., and Norman, A.W. (1977): J. Nutr., 107, 1918.
9. Madsen, S., Olgaard, K., and Ladefoged, J. (1981): J. Clin. Endocrinol. Metab., 53, 823.
10. Canterbury, J.M., Lerman, S., Claflin, A.J., Henry, H., Norman, A., and Reiss, E. (1978): J. Clin. Invest., 61, 1375.
11. Oldham, S.B., Smith, R., Hartenbower, D.L., and Henry, H.L. (1978): Adv. Exp. Med. Biol., 103, 509.
12. Llach, F., Coburn, J.W., Brickman, A.S., Kurokawa, K., Norman, A.W., Canterbury, J.M., and Reiss, E. (1977): J. Clin. Endocrinol. Metab., 44, 1054.
13. Tanaka, Y., DeLuca, H.F., Ghazarian, J.G., Hargis, G.K., and Williams, G.A. (1979): Min. Electr. Metab., 2, 20.
14. Golden, P., Greenwalt, A., Martin, K., Bellorin-Font, E., Mazey, R., Klahr, S., and Slatopolsky, E. (1980): Endocrinology, 107, 602.

Discussion of papers by Massry, Coburn and Slatopolsky

O. MILLER: Dr. Slatopolsky, what was the calcium intake in your patients? Were you giving calcium supplements?

E. SLATOPOLSKY: We gave supplements with the calcium intake between 0.55 and 1.3 g per day.

O. MILLER: Concerning the calcium intake that is recommended with calcitriol therapy, we carried out trials with calitriol in Japan, where calcium supplements were not given; the incidence of hypercalcemia was only 5% in a large study. This compares to our experience with hypercalcemia in about 30% of patients when we used calcium supplements. In retrospect, I believe we should not have used calcium supplements in such cases; I think this has a lot to do with how much calcitriol can be tolerated, whether given IV or oral.

M. DREZNER: Whether by design or not, an implicit assumption from several of these discussions is that $1,25(OH)_2D$ has a unique effect in this disease. Would you comment of the use of other vitamin D sterols and whether they are equally as successful as $1,25(OH)_2D$?

J. COBURN: This was not by design; $1,25(OH)_2D$ has been used in most studies carried out to date. I am not aware of any controlled comparisons of vitamin D sterols. Large doses of vitamin D, itself, can produce the beneficial effects, but it is much slower to act and much more hazardous to use because of its long half life. Dihydrotachysterol may also have effects similar to $1,25(OH)_2D$, with the exception that hypercalcemia can persist for a longer period following drug withdrawal. $1\alpha(OH)$ vitamin D has effects similar to $1,25(OH)_2D$, but this is not available in the United States.

E. SLATOPOLSKY: Most of us would agree that $1,25(OH)_2D$ is the drug of choice for suppression of secondary hyperparathyroidism. There may be disagreement regarding the treatment of other manifestations of renal osteodystrophy. Thus, I personally favor 25-hydroxyvitamin D in patients with osteomalacia that is not induced by aluminum; this problem usually improves with 25-hydroxyvitamin D.

Finally, in experimental studies in dogs with reduced renal function, we were not able to suppress secondary hyperparathyroidism with $24,25(OH)_2D$; after one year of uremia, they had very high levels of PTH despite treatment with $24,25(OH)_2D$.

D. SHERWOOD: Dr. Slatopolsky, I am puzzled by the implication that one has to give $1,25(OH)_2D$ parenterally to get the effect on PTH. The obvious difference between oral and intravenous $1,25(OH)_2D$ is that the sterol might have direct access to the intestinal receptors when taken orally. Certainly one could avoid this problem with oral 1-α(OH)D or dihydrotachysterol. Is there any special effect of giving $1,25(OH)_2D$ intraveneously?

E. SLATOPOLSKY: I was very surprised to see the dramatic changes occurring after such a short period of therapy, particularly since we measured iPTH with a C-terminal assay. I don't have an explanation for the differences.

J. COBURN: One difference between the oral administration compared to intravenous may be the slight increase in the plasma levels of $1,25(OH)_2D$ with oral treatment; thus the values were often subnoraml in patients given oral treatment despite the development of hypercalcemia. The intravenous administration would cause a transient high plasma levels of $1,25(OH)_2D$, which might have different effects on vitamin D receptors in the parathyroid glands. I would caution that suppression might not occur in every case; thus we have given intravenous calcitriol to selected patients who are candidates for parathyroid surgery for overt and severe secondary hyperparathyroidism. In the first two patients so treated, we were not able to suppress serum iPTH.

L. SHERWOOD: Dr. Slatopolsky, an extension of your argument about this effect of $1,25(OH)_2D$ would depend on the study of parathyroid glands from uremic patients or animals to see whether $1,25(OH)_2D$ has a direct effect. Have you done this?

E. SLATOPOLSKY: We are doing this at present. We believe that $1,25(OH)_2D$ may shift the "set point" back toward normal, not by affecting PTH secretion per se but by making the glands more sensitive to calcium. We are conducting these studies in uremic patients who are undergoing parathyroid surgery and also in an uremic dog model.

L. SHERWOOD: What is the etiology of the hypercalcemia in patients with aluminum overload? Is it due to the failure of calcium to enter bone?

J. COBURN: I believe that aluminum inhibits the entry of calcium into bone, although the mechanism for this is unknown.

S. MASSRY: Dr. Slatopolsky, you have shown that PTH is reduced by 60-70% at the end of the study. Is there a justification to inject the $1,25(OH)_2D$? This seems cumbersome; is it not simpler to give it by mouth?

E. SLATOPOLSKY: We simply inject the $1,25(OH)_2D$ three times weekly at the end of dialysis via the existing intravenous line. Thus, we do not ask the patient to take any added medications. They are happy not to take another medication since many already take twenty and forty pills per day.

H. MALLUCHE: Dr. Massry, I did not understand the classification of the bone disease in your patients. Did they all have osteitis fibrosa? I ask this to understand the discrepancy between the unequivocal beneficial effects of $1,25(OH)_2D$ in your patients compared to Dr. Coburn, who found a subgroup of patients with progression of parathyroid overactivity. Also, what were the serum phosphate levels in your patients?

S. MASSRY: Before therapy, these patients had increased bone resorption and defective mineralization, findings similar to those you reported several years ago in a general population of patients with moderate renal failure.

The serum phosphorus levels were not elevated and remained normal until the end of therapy; then the mean value increased to about 4.5 mg/dl.

There has been discussion of osteomalacia that is not responsive to $1,25(OH)_2D$; I think we should clearly make a distinction from a group of patients with "pure" osteomalacia. Many renal failure patients have a component of osteomalacia or hyperosteoidosis in their bone biopsy; this type of osteomalacia, as a component of overall bone disease, usually responds to $1,25(OH)_2D$. Dr. Malluche, when he was in Southern California, reported that twelve dialysis patients with substantial osteomalacia responded well after six months of therapy with $1,25(OH)_2D$. Three years later, in unpublished data, the bone is almost completely healed. Thus, our renal failure patients with hyperosteoidosis responded well to $1,25(OH)_2D$. I believe that the "unresponsive osteomalacia" applies to a small group of patients, perhaps 10%-20% of dialysis patients.

Moreover, we can't give $1,25(OH)_2D$ to them because hypercalcemia develops; if we could give $1,25(OH)_2D$ without causing hypercalcemia, they might respond.

J. COBURN: Dr. Massry, did you give aluminum hydroxide to your patients with moderate renal failure? If so, did you find aluminum in the bone biopsies? I am concerned whether treatment with calcitriol may affect the aluminum level in bone because of a need for more aluminum hydroxide.

S. MASSRY: Most of our patients had a GFR of about 20 ml/min; they did not have hyperphosphatemia, and they were not treated with phosphate binders. Among the 40 patients, there was only one with a bone biopsy showing a positive aluminum stain.

R. LANG: I have seen patients with non-suppressible hyperparathyroidism who were give $1,25(OH)_2D$; they then showed a decrease in bone mass. It is known that $1,25(OH)_2D$ can increase bone resorption. Did Dr. Massry or Dr. Coburn look at the bone volumes in their patients, particularly those with severe hyperparathyroidism?

J. COBURN: Trabecular bone volume was examined in those with bone biopsies, and there were no changes. Moreover, bone mineral content measured with photon absorptiometry in the mid and distal radius decreased in fewer patients given $1,25(OH)_2D$ compared to the placebo-treated group. Although $1,25(OH)_2D$ can produce bone loss in vitro, I do not believe that this occurs in vivo. In uremic patients classified as having a "mixed disorder" with both osteomalacia and osteitis fibrosa, there has been improved mineralization during calcitriol therapy. Thus, bone resorption did not occur with the low doses of $1,25(OH)_2D_3$ we used.

S. MASSRY: We have not seen it either.

THE MANAGEMENT OF ALUMINIUM RELATED OSTEOMALACIA IN RENAL FAILURE

Peter Ackrill, John Ball and J. Philip Day

Withington Hospital, Manchester, and The Departments of Rheumatology and Chemistry, Manchester University, U.K.

Since Alfrey first described the syndrome of dialysis dementia in 1972 there has been increasing evidence that aluminium accumulation in chronic dialysis patients may lead to a variety of toxic clinical manifestations. Included among these is a particular form of osteomalacic bone disease previously known as fracturing dialysis osteodystrophy. More recently it has become known as aluminium related or aluminium associated osteomalacia and, as the title implies, the mechanism of the aluminium involvement remains to be elucidated.

The condition appears to occur exclusively in patients with chronic renal failure usually appearing after many months on chronic haemodialysis but it is now being recognised in patients not previously dialysed and also in patients on C.A.P.D. The typical features are bone pain, particularly in the feet, heels and knees, less commonly the hips and shoulders, multiple non-healing fractures especially of the ribs and pelvis, and proximal myopathy. Serum alkaline phosphatase and immunoreactive PTH levels tend to be normal or only slightly raised. Characteristically, small doses of Vitamin D produce hypercalcaemia without bone healing. Histologically the picture is that of osteomalacia with increased osteoid volume, little osteoblastic activity and a markedly reduced mineralisation front. Aluminium can easily be demonstrated histochemically particularly at the junction of mineralised bone and osteoid.

In our experience whenever the case history of such a patient is examined a source of aluminium exposure will invariably be found. The source is either the dialysate or medication. Thus the aluminium content of the dialysate water supply may be naturally and consistently high (up to 100 ug/l) when obtained from certain sources or may be intermittently and unpredictably high (up to 1500 ug/l) when the process of alum flocculation is used by the water authorities to remove organic colouring matter. Contamination of the dialysate concentrate may occur both from the ingredients themselves or during manufacture. Pierides and others have described leaching of aluminium from the Redy cartridges used for regenerating dialysis fluid, and contamination of the replacement fluids used during haemofiltration and plasmaphoresis has been recognised.

Controversy continues regarding what is a safe dialysate aluminium concentration and we have shown that in order to achieve a negative aluminium balance during haemodialysis, the aluminium levels should at least be below 14 ug/l(less than 0.5 umol/l.). We feel this level is critical not only in preventing transfer into the patient but also to allow excretion of aluminium accumulated from other sources. Aluminium absorption from prescribed oral phosphate binders undoubtedly occurs and accounts for the demonstration of dialysis encephalopathy in previously undialysed patients. Although these cases are rare there is clearly a potential for aluminium accumulation whenever these agents are prescribed and similarly following ingestion of self-administered commercial antacids of which the physician may be unaware.

As already mentioned it is possible to remove small amounts of aluminium (approximately 100 ug/hour) by conventional dialysis alone. However in patients who have accumulated large quantities of aluminium the amounts removed compared with the total body burden is likely to be small.

Currently the only method available for removing substantial quantities of aluminium during dialysis is by chelation with Desferrioxamine (DFO), an agent used extensively for the treatment of iron overload. In-vitro experiments in our laboratory have shown that aluminium binds strongly to DFO ($K = 10^{22}$) in a 1:1 molar ratio and its dialysance is consistent with a molecular weight of approximately 600 Daltons. Administered intravenously during haemodialysis, DFO causes an acute rise in serum aluminium the level being maximal immediately prior to the following dialysis and the level falling successively with each subsequent dialysis. The absence of apparent toxicity associated with the very high serum aluminium levels which develop may be explained by the high degree of binding. The amount of aluminium removed during dialysis may be estimated by repeated analysis of the aluminium content of dialysate entering and leaving the dialyser. As might be expected, this amount is related to the prevailing serum aluminium level and is determined by the characteristics of the dialyser.

The technique of aluminium removal by chelation with DFO was first introduced for the treatment of dialysis encephalopathy but recently a number of authors have described their experience of its use in the treatment of aluminium related osteomalacia. Brown and his co-workers (2) reported dramatic clinical improvement in their 2 patients. Walking sticks were discarded and the patients returned to gardening. They emphasised the rapid response to treatment but contrary to subsequent reports they were unable to demonstrate reduction in bone aluminium content.

A similarly striking clinical response has been reported by Ihle and his colleagues (3) and also by ourselves (1). In both these studies aluminium removal from bone was clearly demonstrated both qualitatively using distinct histochemical techniques and quantitatively by analysis using flameless atomic absorption spectrophotometry.

A typical biochemical response to treatment is illustrated by one of our own cases in figure 1. This shows the serial changes in serum calcium and alkaline phosphatase in a patient exposed to a high dialysate aluminium level for many years. Repeated attempts to treat his bone disease with Vitamin D resulted on each occasion in unacceptable hypercalcaemia without clinical improvement. Prior to treatment he had gross proximal myopathy, little bone pain, but radiographically there were pseudo fractures in the pubic rami and multiple rib fractures. Bone biopsy showed osteomalacia. During the period of DFO therapy the serum calcium fell and serum alkaline phosphatase rose. He developed generalised bone pain and a further bone biopsy showed active osteitis fibrosa and disappearance of his osteomalacia. Subsequently following treatment with Vitamin D his serum alkaline phosphatase returned to normal without the development of hypercalcaemia, and he became pain free and fully ambulant.

In all three studies referred to there have been marked histological changes following DFO, with reduction or disappearance of osteomalacia and either the emergence of or the progression of pre-existant osteitis fibrosa. In many cases it appears that Vitamin D therapy has subsequently been required. In his comprehensive study Ihle compared his DFO treated group with a similar group treated by transplantation alone. The transplanted patients likewise showed clinical and biochemical improvement with a marked reduction in bone aluminium content but it also appeared that this particular group showed a greater return towards normal of their bone histology. It was speculated that the presumed normal physiological levels of Vitamin D in these patients might be an important factor.

Prior to the introduction of DFO, treatment of aluminium associated toxicity was confined to reduction of aluminium exposure. Nevertheless following the application of reverse osmosis or de-ionisation to the dialysate water supply and by reduction of aluminium ingestion, not only has there been a marked reduction in the number of new cases presenting with symptoms but also considerable improvement in some of the affected patients (4,5). It should be emphasised that such measures are equally important during and after a period of DFO therapy.

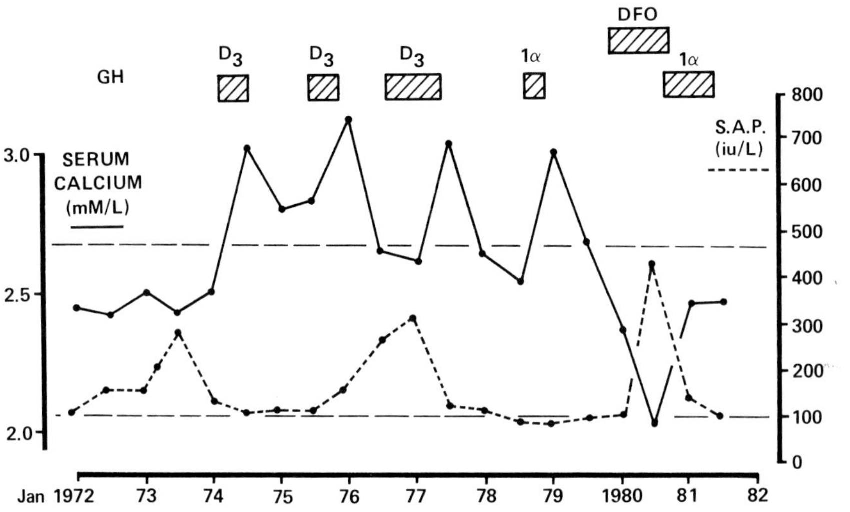

Figure 1. Serial changes in serum calcium and serum alkaline phosphatase (S.A.P.) in a patient with aluminium related osteomalacia during intermittent treatment with Vitamin D (D_3, 1 Alpha) and Desferrioxamine (DFO).

The place of DFO in the overall strategy of the treatment of aluminium osteomalacia has yet to be determined. The side effects reported during its use for iron chelation include allergic reactions, abdominal pain, posterior cataracts and retinal changes similar to those seen in retinitis pigmentosa. Such side effects have not been reported during aluminium chelation probably due to the low doses used but this could be relevant in the treatment of children. We have seen exacerbation of bone pain following DFO administration and increased seizure frequency during treatment of severe dialysis encephalopathy. Nevertheless it would appear that DFO is safe and can be dramatically effective in the treatment of severe symptomatic bone disease. The apparent ability of DFO to improve mineralisation may ultimately enable the mechanism of aluminium involvement in these cases to be understood.

Renal transplantation appears to be a useful if not a better alternative but in our experience there is a definite risk of precipitation of dialysis encephalopathy in patients with a heavy body burden of aluminium and in such cases it may be preferable to reduce this with DFO prior to admission to transplant waiting list.

Prevention must nevertheless be the mainstay of treatment and in this respect the most needed substance is a non-toxic non-aluminium containing phosphate binder.

ACKNOWLEDGMENTS

We would like to acknowledge the following from our own laboratories whose work has been freely reported without due recognition in this review text:

Z. Benzo, J. Denton, F.M. Garstang, K.C. Hodge, P.J. Metcalfe, and R.A. Romero-Martinez.

We wish to thank the Medical Research Council and the Withington Hospital Kidney Unit Endowment Fund for financial support to some of these projects. We also wish to thank Mrs.G.M.Williams who kindly typed the manuscript.

REFERENCES

1. Ackrill, P., Day, J.P., Garstang F.M., Hodge, K.C., Metcalfe, P.J., Benzo, Z., Hill, K., Ralston, A.J., Ball, J. and Denton, J. (1982): Proc. EDTA, 19, 203.
2. Brown, D.J., Dawborn, J.K., Ham, K.N. and Xipell, J.M. (1982): Lancet, 2, 343.
3. Ihle, B.U., Buchanan, M.R.C., Stevens, B., Becker, G.J. and Kincaid-Smith, P. (1982): Proc. EDTA, 19, 195.
4. Leather, H.M., Lewin, I.G., Calder, E., Braybrooke, J. and Cox, R.R. (1981): Nephron, 29, 80.
5. Pierides, A.M., Edwards, W.G., Cullum, U.X., McCall, J.T. and Ellis, H.A. (1980): Kidney International, 18, 115.

Discussion following paper by P. Ackrill

J. COBURN: I would like to comment on the experience of Dr. Alfrey and ourselves regarding the dialysis of aluminum. We were totally unable to remove aluminum during standard hemodialysis. The plasma concentrations of aluminum going into and coming from the dialyzer were almost identical because of the very high plasma protein binding of aluminum. Thus, our data contrasts to what you reported and to data reported from Vienna.

A. HODSMAN: Continuous ambulatory peritoneal dialysis (CAPD) is an effective way of removing desferoxamine (DFO) that is complexed to aluminum. We saw a five-fold greater removal of aluminum each day compared to a single hemodialysis with a cuprophane membrane; moreover CAPD has the advantage of being done 6 or 7 days a week. We noted significant increases in hemoglobin during a 3-6 month treatment with DFO. Have you observed the same phenomenon?

P. ACKRILL: Of the 8 patients we followed, nearly half showed an increased hemoglobin. One patient, whose hemoglobin was 5g/dl with monthly transfusions had a hemoglobin of 11g/dl without any transfusions after eight months of DFO therapy. The original report from Glasgow indicated that the anemia associated with aluminum overload was invariably associated with a low MCV. This has not been our experience. The hemoglobin rose even in patients with a normal mean corpuscular volume.

M. KLEEREKOPER: Dr. Slatopolsky has shown that aluminum inhibits PTH release by the glands; I wonder whether DFO might have its beneficial effect simply by "turning on" the parathyroid glands rather than be removing aluminum from bone.

E. SLATOPOLSKY: Certainly, an effect of DFO to remove aluminum from these patients has been demonstrated. Dr. Morrissey, in our laboratory, studied parathyroid cells in vitro and found that aluminum inhibited the release of PTH; he then washed them to remove aluminum and incubated them in a low calcium medium. The parathyroid cells then responded with a normal PTH release. Thus, there was no apparent persistent effect of aluminum. We don't understand the mechanism of this aluminum effect.

M. FRIEDLANDER: Dr. Massry, what happened to urinary calcium excretion in your patients with moderate renal insufficiency who received calcitriol?

S. MASSRY: The mean daily calcium excretion increased from 18 mg to 150 mg/day.

J. COBURN: I suspect that patients with residual function are tolerant to larger doses of 1,25$(OH)_2$D than are patients with end-stage renal failure, where there is no outlet for an increased calcium load.

J. O'RIORDAN: Dr. Coburn, the results of your prophylactic study are similar to those we conducted over a 3-4 year period. I am not really convinced that we produced any significant improvement in our patients, even though we lowered the serum iPTH levels. Do you feel that you improved your patients?

J. COBURN: That is an important question. The patients in our study were asymptomatic prior to entry into the study and they generally remained that way. The major change we saw was the lack of appearance of erosions on bone x-ray. There were three patients in the study who were judged by their physicians as "treatment failures"; parathyroidectomy was done in two, both having received placebo. A third patient, who was receiving 1,25$(OH)_2$D, was found to have aluminum-associated osteomalacia. Thus, among 100 pateints, there were 2 or 3 who worsened despite good conventional treatment of their end-stage renal failure.

In 25% of the patients receiving placebo with the lowest iPTH levels, there were no problems, and the iPTH levels in many could be reduced further with oral calcium carbonate. It is uncertain, however, how you can predict who these patients might be.

J. POTTS: For those interested in how to establish a diagnosis of aluminum accumulation, would it be possible to use the desferoxamine-induced increase in blood aluminum level as an alternative to bone biopsy to establish whether a patient has aluminum retention?

P. ACKRILL: We haven't studied this, but there was a presentation from Drs. Milliner and Coburn last evening, which showed a close association between the increment in plasma aluminum after DFO and bone aluminum content. In one patient treated with DFO for a long time, the magnitude of rise in serum aluminum following the same dose of DFO decreased with time. During the last few months of treatment, the pre-test plasma levels fell, this suggests that the freely available aluminum had been removed.

M. PARFITT: Dr. Ackrill, in some of your patients, osteitis fibrosa got worse as you gave DFO. Was this due to increased PTH secretion or due to increased responsiveness of the bone to PTH?

P. ACKRILL: The serum PTH levels rose during this period and then fell when we gave vitamin D.

A. MUDDE: We obtained good results utilizing DFO for patients with osteomalacia; however, as Dr. Ackrill noted, we observed a rise in serum aluminum after each dialysis. Also, we noted clinical deterioration with more convulsions in two patients with dialysis encephalapathy; and these two patients ultimately died; this occurred as the plasma aluminum levels rose.Is it possible that the infusion of DFO mobilized aluminum with further aluminum accumulation in the brain?

P.ACKRILL: This was a worry when we first used DFO; initially we restricted its use to those with encephalopathy. In these patients, there can be an increase in seizure activity during the first few weeks of therapy. We controlled this by giving diazapam prophylactically during dialysis and by reducing the dialysis hours. Ultimately, the patients all improved. Because of the very high binding affinity of DFO for aluminum, it would seem unlikely that there is a risk of transferring aluminum to other organs in the body.

What is uncertain is whether it would be better to give repeated small doses of DFO rather than giving it once a week, as we have done in the past; this question is under study at present.

O. MEHLS: Is there any information on whether the aluminum bound to DFO is lost in the feces? When we gave DFO for iron overload in children on dialysis, we found that most of the iron bound to DFO was lost in the feces.

P. ACKRILL: There are no data available on stool losses of aluminum after DFO administration. A very small amount of aluminum is lost during conventional dialysis, i.e., 100-200 micrograms per dialysis. However, when we followed patients with regular dialysis for several years, we demonstrated the loss of aluminum from bone with a change in bone histology. Thus, it is possible that considerable aluminum is lost in the stools.

Regarding the method for DFO administration, we have developed a method for measuring free DFO as opposed to bound DFO, which can only be measured as "plasma aluminum." When one infuses DFO into the arterial line, some is lost into dialysate as unbound DFO. If, however, one gives DFO into the intravenous line, the DFO becomes bound, and free DFO does not appear in the circulation. Similarly, when you give DFO to the patient, it all becomes bound to something, iron, aluminum or perhaps another metal.

Whether the DFO should be given before or after dialysis is still worthy of study I don't believe available data which indicate that you remove more aluminum if you give the DFO after dialysis.

C. NORDIN: Regarding the cause of the low $1,25(OH)_2D$ levels in renal failure, raised by Dr. Coburn, I applied multiple regression analysis to this problem, and I evaluated the regression between serum $1,25(OH)_2D$ levels with a group of variables in patients with chronic renal failure. The degree of renal failure was not a determinant of the serum $1,25(OH)_2D$ level. The most important determinant was plasma phosphorus level; the second most important variable was plasma bicarbonate, and the third most important was the level of 25-hydroxyvitamin D. Thus the degree of renal failure itself, does not seem to be a determinant except as it affects these three variables.

Dr. Coburn, you said that you produced only small increments in plasma $1,25(OH)_2D$ levels when you treated with calcitriol. What do you mean by that? Treatment with $1,25(OH)_2D$ produces a peak blood level about two hours after taking the dose; then there is a rapid decay with a 12 hour half-life. Thus, there is no measurable increase in blood level 24 hours after a given dose. When were your blood levels drawn?

J. COBURN: The blood levels of $1,25(OH)_2D$ were measured four to eight hours after the last dose; the average serum level increased from 8 pg/ml to 17 pg/ml. Some patients had values above 20 pg/ml, but most were below this level.

There are prospective data in individual renal failure patients by Portale, et.al.; they found that dietary phosphate restriction produced a rise in plasma $1,25(OH)_2D$ levels to normal or above in children with moderate renal insufficiency. Others have found that unless the GFR is below 40 or 50 ml/min., the serum $1,25(OH)_2D$ levels in adults are not decreased. Thus, several factors can affect serum $1,25(OH)_2D$ levels in these patients.

XI NON-PARATHYROID HYPERCALCEMIA

NON-PARATHYROID HYPERCALCEMIA

Moderator, John T. Potts, Jr.

Department of Medicine, Harvard Medical School and Massachusetts General Hospital, Boston, MA, U.S.A.

INTRODUCTION: HYPERCALCEMIA IN MALIGNANCY

J. POTTS: There has been increasing clinical interest in the hypercalcemia of malignancy in the last decade. Clearly the disease entity is important from the point of view of differential diagnosis. It is important to know whether a given patient who presents with hypercalcemia has malignancy as the cause -- or has a more benign disorder, such as hyperparathyroidism or sarcoidosis. Hypercalcemia can be life-threatening and must often be treated by general measures even before the diagnosis is known; more definitive therapy requires a firm diagnosis.

Clinically, of course, malignancy is often evident due to a variety of systemic symptoms and obvious signs and manifestations of the tumor. Clinicians concerned with differential diagnoses of hypercalcemia, however, appreciate that occasionally the presence of the malignancy is not obvious. There may be an occult tumor with a slow clinical course, such as hypernephroma. Alternatively, for example, in an individual with chronic obstructive pulmonary disease, radiological detection of a lung tumor may be difficult and the symptoms of chronic disease difficult to distinguish from the presence of malignancy.

In such cases, we turn to our differential biochemical criteria. How good are they as aids in the differential diagnosis of hypercalcemia and how can they be applied definitely and efficiently in deciding that malignancy is the cause of the hypercalcemia? Here, I believe, we still find a considerable amount of disappointing confusion and uncertainty, although recently some progress and considerable clarification are evident. There appears to be general agreement that in many cases of hypercalcemia and malignancy, the biologically responsible agent is not parathyroid hormone. There is great fundamental interest in the chemical and biological nature of the tumor-derived factors which are responsible for the hypercalcemic syndrome(s). Such knowledge may provide clues to the physiological roles of the substances (assuming overproduction of naturally occuring factors) and may even contribute to the knowledge of basic mechanisms of oncogenic transformation. Current theories of oncogenesis suggest that overproduction of substances normally produced in cells occurs as a "down-stream" effect of excessive action of promotors or enhancers. In this regard, the association, preferentially, of only certain types of tumor with hypercalcemia may reveal interesting features of genetic translocation in tumor cells responsible for hypercalcemia.

There is a lengthy and sometimes confusing history of clinical observations with the problem of tumor hypercalcemia. Albright called attention to the peculiar "parathyroid like" features of tumor hypercalcemia in 1941. Dr. Lafferty made a very important clinical contribution, the definition of the syndrome of pseudohyperparathyroidism, in his excellent review in 1966. Dr. Arnaud and his colleagues reported finding around 1972 detectable or slightly elevated immunoreactive PTH in most malignancies. But then, just a year or two later, Dr. Powell and his colleagues in our group, found that immunoreactive PTH was not detectable in blood or tumor extracts in most patients with malignancy and hypercalcemia. It rapidly became apparent that we were involved with a very confusing situation, which is still unresolved today. There is frequent detection of parathyroid hormone in the circulation of these patients by many, but not all, laboratories, despite the growing evidence that whatever the responsible tumor-derived agents are, they are not biologically identical to active parathyroid hormone in the blood. (Hence, parathyroid hormone levels might have been expected to be undetectable.)

If one observes the long period of time (2-4 decades) between initial clinical interest in this problem and the only recent clarification concerning results with certain clinical tests ($1,25(OH)_2D$, fasting urinary calcium and bone biopsies) applied to these patients, it is evident that there has been a long, frustrating period of uncertainty concerning the etiology of the hypercalcemia of malignancy. Dr. Sherwood, in studies that were performed with Dr. Aurbach, Dr. O'Riordan, and myself at NIH 20 years ago, had evidence that some of the tumors contained parathyroid hormone. Drs. Tashjian and Munson had similar findings. Dr. Singer today reviews evidence concerning the frequency with which immunoreactive PTH can be detected in tumor extracts. Despite this evidence, many clinical and laboratory features noted in hypercalcemic patients with cancer suggest parathyroid hormone is not the responsible mediator of the hypercalcemia. Hence, attention has begun to focus on identification and isolation of tumor-derived agents that act as bone resorbing factors and are distinct from parathyroid hormone.

Clinically, Drs. Stewart and Broadus and their colleagues, as well as other groups, as reviewed by Dr. Broadus today, have made useful advances by simultaneous application in differential diagnosis of hormonal assays and related biochemical techniques. These studies are aimed at improving clinical diagnostic efforts with existing techniques while awaiting the results of fundamental studies of tumor-derived hypercalcemic factors. Such efforts have revealed useful distinctions in findings between patients with the hypercalcemia of malignancy versus those with hypercalcemia due to hyperparathyroidism. There are disagreements among groups regarding certain results that must reflect variations in patient population or differences in techniques. Separation between groups is not absolute, but multidiscriminant analysis is useful, many now feel.

One can say with greater confidence in 1983 concerning tumor hypercalcemia that parathyroid hormone is not biologically responsible, at least in most cases. The increased or normal circulating immunoreactive PTH detected by many, but not all, laboratories may mean that inactive or incomplete PTH is being secreted as a type of tumor marker. Alternatively, low levels of hormone may still be secreted by suppressed glands at concentrations detectable by some assays. Finally, the abnormalities in blood proteins associated with malignancy may be affecting immunoassay results in a totally non-specific fashion. Goltzman and colleagues illustrate that this confusion with regard to the nature of circulating "PTH-like" material in patients with malignancy is evident even in the cytochemical bioassay (see Session I).

There is still not a clear consensus regarding the practical usefulness of applying a series of special assays, other than the parathyroid hormone radioimmunoassay, because of continuing disagreement, reflected in the presentations and comments of the panelists and audience, concerning some of the results seen by different groups. Cost effectiveness of the approach is not clear. The best direction for the future seems likely to derive from present efforts to isolate and chemically characterize the non-parathyroid tumor substances responsible. Specific assays for these tumor factors should be useful.

Several different lines of evidence seem to point to multiple factors, distinct from one tumor to another. Tumor-derived growth factors, peptides of molecular weight several times larger than parathyroid hormone, and peptides also distinct from parathyroid hormone but similar to it in molecular size, have been identified by different groups. Only when these agents have been fully characterized will it be clear whether there is indeed a multiplicity of responsible factors. Certain evidence points to action of the factor through the parathyroid hormone receptor with stimulation of cyclic AMP as central to the mechanism of action of the tumor-derived hypercalcemic factors. Others, however, as summarized by Bringhurst and colleagues, find bone resorbing activity in the absence of increased cyclic AMP production at the levels of the substance required to resorb bone in _in vitro_ assays. Hence, even in the basic studies of the nature of tumor factors, there is not a single direction evident in present research efforts.

HUMORAL HYPERCALCEMIA OF MALIGNANCY

Arthur E. Broadus and Andrew F. Stewart

Departments of Internal Medicine, Yale University and West Haven Veterans Hospital, New Haven and West Haven, CT, U.S.A.

There is reasonable agreement that malignancy-associated hypercalcemia (MAHC) results from two general mechanisms: 1) local osteolytic hypercalcemia--hypercalcemia which is based on bone resorption mediated by tumor cells metastatic to (e.g., breast carcinoma) or occurring primarily in (e.g., multiple myeloma) the skeleton and 2) humoral hypercalcemia of malignancy--hypercalcemia which results from the systemic effects of a factor(s) produced by tumor cells remote from bone. As used in this review, the terms local osteolytic hypercalcemia (LOH) and humoral hypercalcemia of malignancy (HHM) represent a biochemical rather than a clinical classification scheme, even though they have rather clear-cut clinical correlates (1). That is, patients either do or do not display biochemical evidence of a circulating calcemic factor and are so classified.

Our original clinical series included 50 patients with MAHC, 15 patients with primary hyperparathyroidism (1° HPT) and hypercalcemia of comparable severity, and 15 non-hypercalcemic patients with similar malignancies as a "control" group (1). The most surprising single finding of this series was the apparent frequency of HHM, this mechanism being identified in 82% of the patients studied. The features of this syndrome included: 1) an increase in nephrogenous cyclic AMP (NcAMP), 2) a reduction in TmP/GFR, 3) a marked mean increase in fractional calcium excretion, 4) a marked reduction in circulating 1,25-$(OH)_2D$, and 5) normal or undetectable serum iPTH in each of four region-specific assays. The features in the patients with LOH were: 1) markedly reduced NcAMP, 2) variable results for TmP/GFR, and 3) mean values for fractional calcium excretion, plasma 1,25-$(OH)_2D$, and serum iPTH which were essentially identical to those observed in the patients with HHM. Each of the patients in the local osteolytic group had a massive skeletal tumor burden, whereas bone metastases were either absent or confined to a few small lesions in the patients in the humoral group.

Given the importance of the results for NcAMP in this classification scheme, several points merit emphasis. One doesn't usually anticipate truly bimodal data when dealing with biological syndromes of this complexity, yet bimodal results were seen. The reason for this lies in the nature of the determination, in that a value for NcAMP of zero is as reproducible technically as one which is several-fold elevated. Because of stress and/or a degree of azotemia, the plasma concentration of cAMP is frequently moderately elevated in patients with MAHC, and in such patients results for cAMP excretion are less easily interpreted than those for NcAMP.

In the course of subsequent work, we have studied a total of 125 patients with MAHC. Results for NcAMP were elevated in 100 patients and depressed in 25 patients, with the other findings in these two populations being as described above. In addition, the size of the "control" group of patients with a malignancy has been enlarged to a total of 50 patients, with an aggregate biochemical data base which is quite normal. In related studies, several patients were restudied after either anti-hypercalcemic therapy or following successful anti-neoplastic therapy (2). As one would anticipate, successful anti-neoplastic therapy resulted in a normalization of the biochemical indices of the humoral syndrome, whereas anti-hypercalcemic therapy did not.

In collaboration with David Goltzman in Montreal, we attempted to corroborate our biochemical classification scheme by assaying plasma for activity in the cytochemical bioassay (CBA) for PTH (3). The CBA results were ten-fold higher on the mean in the patients with elevations in NcAMP than in the patients with suppressed values for NcAMP. The results, however, were not bimodal; whether the explanation for this overlap is technical or biological is unknown. On gel filtration, CBA activity in the plasma from patients with HHM ran ahead of the bioactivity in plasma from patients with 1° HPT. In addition, this bioactivity was only slightly inhibited by preincubation with an antiserum to PTH, whereas the activity in comparable samples from patients with 1°HPT was entirely eliminated (3).

The implications of the data presented above with respect to the tissue source of the calcium in patients with HHM were confirmed by bone histomorphometry (4). These specimens revealed striking osteoclastic bone resorption, together with indices of bone formation and mineralization which were markedly reduced. This pattern of almost complete "uncoupling" differed dramatically from the changes observed in biopsies obtained from patients with 1°HPT. Whether this uncoupling should be viewed as entirely a consequence of the biological actions of the calcemic factor in question or is multi-factorial in nature remains unclear.

Taken together, these various findings provide a rather clear picture of the pathophysiological mechanisms responsible for the hypercalcemia in both the local osteolytic and humoral categories of MAHC. Both syndromes represent basically "resorptive" forms of hypercalcemia, the principal differences being the nature and site of production of the bone-resorbing factors. In both syndromes, the PTH-1,25-$(OH)_2D$ axis is appropriately suppressed and fractional calcium excretion is increased. The circulating material in patients with HHM shares with native PTH the ability to stimulate adenylate cyclase activity and phosphaturia in the proximal nephron as well as osteoclastic bone resorption, but it differs from PTH in its immunochemical and chromatographic behavior, in its relative inability to stimulate 1-hydroxylase activity and calcium reabsorption in the distal nephron, and in its aggregate influence on the skeleton.

The data from the patients with HHM studied in vivo provide a general strategy for study and isolation of the responsible factor(s) in vitro. Our own investigations in this area are broadly-based, but the discussion here will be confined to human tumors as studied in three detection systems: 1) a canine renal cortical adenylate cyclase assay, 2) the CBA for PTH, and 3) a conventional bone-resorbing assay.

Extracts from tumors obtained from patients defined as having HHM _in vivo_ contain potent adenylate cyclase-stimulating activity _in vitro_ (Fig. 1), this having been observed in 14 of 15 tumors examined to date. Tumors obtained from patients with LOH contain no such activity, and "control" tumors also contain little or no activity (5). The tumors with adenylate cyclase-stimulating activity also have activity in the cytochemical assay, and both activities are completely inhibited by the competitive inhibitor, [Nle,^{8},^{18},Tyr^{34}]bPTH-(3-34) amide (Fig. 2). Preincubation of tumor extracts with a panel of five different anti-PTH antisera, including four with amino-terminal reactive determinants, resulted in no loss of adenylate cyclase-stimulating activity. More purified material contains potent bone-resorbing activity (unpublished observations). Physical studies indicate that the material is a protein with a molecular weight several times larger than native PTH. Present preparations are approximately 5000-fold purified.

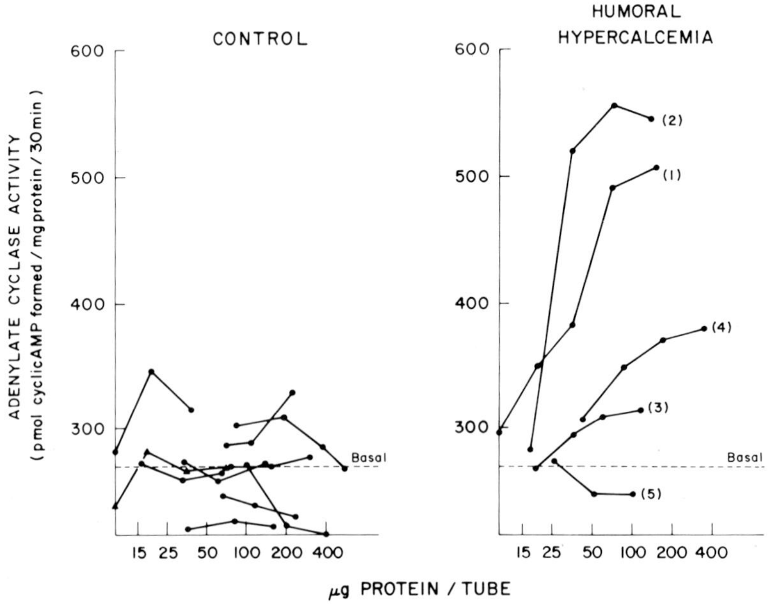

Figure 1. Adenylate cyclase-stimulating activity in extracts from control tumors (left panel) and from tumors obtained from patients with HHM (right panel) (6).

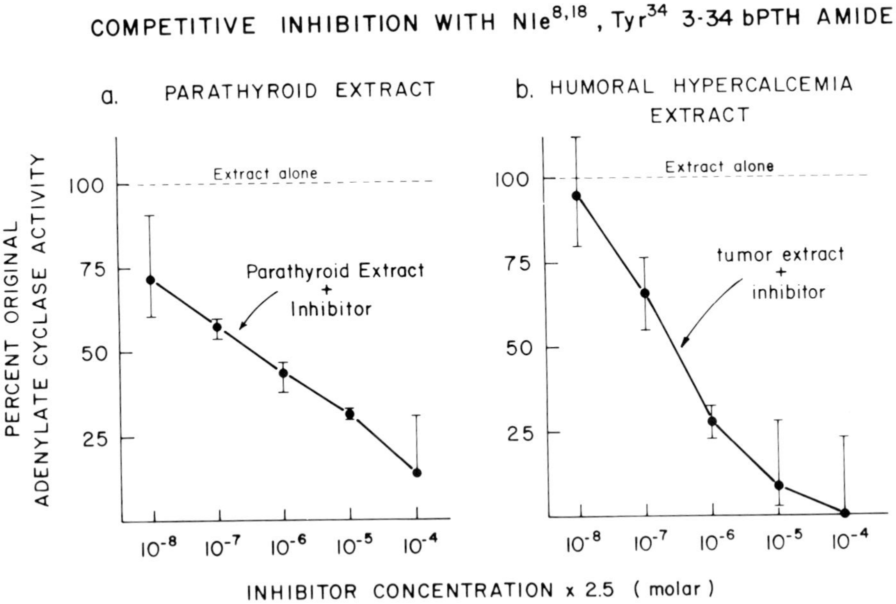

Figure 2. Competitive inhibition of a parathyroid adenoma extract (left panel) and a tumor extract (right panel) with [Nle,8,18,Tyr34]bPTH-(3-34) amide (6).

REFERENCES

1. Stewart, A.F. Horst, R., Deftos, L.J., Cadman, E.C., Lang, R. and Broadus, A.E. (1980): New Engl. J. Med., 303, 1377.
2. Stewart, A.F., Romero, R., Schwartz, P.E., Kohorn, E.I. and Broadus, A.E. (1982): Cancer, 49, 2389.
3. Goltzman, D., Stewart, A.F. and Broadus, A.E. (1981): J. Clin. Endocrinol. Metab., 53, 899.
4. Stewart, A.F., Vignery, A., Silvergate, A., Ravin, N.D., LiVolsi, V., Broadus, A.E. and Baron, R. (1982): J. Clin. Endocrinol. Metab., 55, 219.
5. Stewart, A.F., Insogna, K.L., Goltzman, D., and Broadus, A.E. (1983): Proc. Natl. Acad. Sci. USA, 80, 1454.

HUMORAL HYPERCALCEMIA OF MALIGNANCY: ROLE OF PARATHYROID HORMONE AND PROSTAGLANDIN E_2

Frederick R. Singer, Charles F. Sharp, Jr., Elizabeth Ryzen, and Robert K. Rude

Orthopaedic Hospital/University of Southern California Bone and Connective Tissue Laboratory and University of Southern California School of Medicine, Los Angeles, CA, U.S.A.

Fuller Albright first proposed that ectopic production and secretion of parathyroid hormone by nonparathyroid tumors could account for hypercalcemia in patients with minimal or no skeletal metastases. Beginning in the mid 1960's reports of extractable parathyroid hormone in nonparathyroid tumors began to appear, an apparent confirmation of Albright's hypothesis [1]. In a few patients simultaneous sampling of the arterial and venous supply of the tumor revealed somewhat higher levels of immunoreactive parathyroid hormone in the venous drainage, further support for the concept of ectopic parathyroid hormone secretion.

Refinement of and increased availability of radioimmunoassays for parathyroid hormone have surprisingly resulted in conflicting views on the concept of "ectopic hyperparathyroidism." Utilizing mid region or carboxyl-terminal radioimmunoassays serum immunoreactive parathyroid hormone levels are usually within the normal range or low [2]. The normal levels could be interpreted to be consistent with inappropriate secretion of the hormone and to be responsible for the hypercalcemic state. However, amino-terminal assays usually find low or undetectable hormone levels in hypercalcemic cancer patients [3]. These paradoxical results could be explained by the observation that hypercalcemia induced by calcium infusion in the bovine species suppresses secretion of intact parathyroid hormone while allowing release of carboxyl-terminal fragments. Thus, sensitive mid region or carboxyl-terminal assays could detect biologically inactive circulating hormonal fragments secreted by the suppressed normal glands of hypercalcemic cancer patients. It should be emphasized that a frankly elevated parathyroid hormone level in a hypercalcemic cancer patient strongly suggests the presence of a second disorder, primary hyperparathyroidism [3].

Patients with primary hyperparathyroidism often have a constellation of abnormalities in addition to elevation of serum immunoreactive parathyroid hormone concentrations. These include elevation of nephrogenous cycle AMP, a lowered renal tubular maximum for phosphorus reabsorption, hyperchloremic acidosis, elevated serum $1,25(OH)_2D$ concentrations, increased osteoclastic bone resorption and increased bone formation on bone biopsy. Studies of these parameters in patients with humoral hypercalcemia of malignancy have recently revealed that patients with this syndrome exhibit striking differences from those with classical primary hyperparathyroidism. Although the cancer patients may present with elevated nephrogenous cyclic AMP [3, 4] and lowered renal tubular maximum for phosphorus reabsorption [4], these abnormalities are not specific for the state of hyperparathyroidism. Elevated nephrogenous cyclic AMP almost always is found in the absence of elevated serum parathyroid hormone concentrations and is also present in some normocalcemic cancer patients with normal parathyroid hormone levels [3, 5]. Renal phosphorus wasting is a feature of all forms of true hypercalcemia since elevation of the ionized calcium concentration directly inhibits renal tubular conservation of phosphorus. Strong evidence against the hypothesis of "ectopic hyperparathyroidism" as a common cause of humoral hypercalcemia of malignancy is provided by the common findings of metabolic alkalosis [1], low serum $1,25(OH)_2D$ concentration [4] and increased osteoclastic bone resorption without compensatory increased osteoblastic activity in most patients [6]. Taken with the parathyroid hormone radioimmunoassay data, these important parameters of parathyroid hormone activity provide strong evidence against a frequent role for parathyroid hormone in the pathogenesis of humoral hypercalcemia of malignancy. What still needs to be fully explained is the relatively common finding of immunoreactive parathyroid hormone in tumor extracts of both hypercalcemic and normocalcemic cancer patients [7]. It is likely that in most cases synthesis but not secretion of parathyroid hormone accounts for these findings.

Attention turned to the possible role of prostaglandin E_2 (PGE_2) in humoral hypercalcemia of malignancy in 1972 after discovery of the first animal model of hypercalcemia, fibrosarcoma in the mouse [8]. Injection of fibrosarcoma cells into host animals produced hypercalcemia and elevated serum PGE_2 levels, both of which were reversed by drugs which inhibited prostaglandin synthesis. Subsequently several studies implicated PGE_2 in patients with humoral hypercalcemia of malignancy [8]. Patients with hypercalcemia, elevated plasma PGE_2 or urinary PGE_2 metabolite, and few or no skeletal metastases were also found to respond to prostaglandin synthesis inhibitors. Patients with skeletal metastases were unresponsive to therapy despite demonstration of lowered urinary PGE_2 metabolite in one study.

It is unclear how often PGE_2 secretion by tumors accounts for hypercalcemia in cancer patients. Patients with PGE_2-mediated hypercalcemia apparently do not have elevated nephrogenous cyclic AMP levels and may therefore not represent a frequent form of humoral hypercalcemia of malignancy. However, we have recently treated 10 hypercalcemic patients with few or no skeletal metastases with a five day course of ibuprofen and observed resolution of hypercalcemia in 5 patients (unpublished observations). Since a single passage of PGE_2 through the pulmonary circulation results in clearance of more than 90% of PGE_2, the tumors thought to produce hypercalcemia by a PGE_2-mediated mechanism must secrete enormous amounts of PGE_2. An alternate explanation is that tumors may produce a hypercalcemic factor whose mechanism of action is to stimulate endogenous bone prostaglandin synthesis and, in consequence, hypercalcemia. We have previously reported that several tumor extracts from hypercalcemic patients produced bone resorption in bone organ cultures which was inhibited by indomethacin [9]. Possible candidates for the tumor factor include epidermal growth factor and platelet-derived growth factor, both of which cause prostaglandin dependent bone resorption in vitro.

REFERENCES

1. Skrabanek, P., McPartlin, J. and Powell, D. (1980): Medicine, 59, 262.
2. Riggs, B.L., Arnaud, C.D., Reynolds, J.C. and Smith, L.H. (1971): J. Clin. Invest., 50, 2079.

3. Rude, R.K., Sharp, C.F., Jr., Fredericks, R.S., Oldham, S.B., Elbaum, N., Link, J., Irwin, L. and Singer, F.R. (1981): J. Clin. Endocrinol. Metab., 52, 765.
4. Stewart, A.F., Horst, R., Deftos, L.J., Cadman, E.C., Lang, R. and Broadus, A.E. (1980): N. Engl. J. Med., 303, 1377.
5. Kukreja, S.C., Shemerdiak, W.P., Lad, T.E. and Johnson, P.A. (1980): J. Clin. Endocrinol. Metab., 51, 167.
6. Sharp, C.F., Jr., Rude, R.K., Terry, R. and Singer, F.R. (1982): Cancer, 49, 1449.
7. Sharp, C.F., Jr., Rude, R.K. and Singer, F.R. (1982): Program of the Sixty-fourth Annual Meeting of The Endocrine Society, p. 428.
8. Metz, S.A., McRae, J.R. and Robertson, R.P. (1981): Metabolism, 30, 299.
9. Minkin, C., Fredericks, R.S., Pokress, S., Rude, R.K., Sharp, C.F., Jr., Tong, M. and Singer, F.R. (1981): J. Clin. Endocrinol. Metab., 53, 941.

RECOMBINANT DNA TECHNOLOGY AND THE HUMORAL HYPERCALCEMIA OF MALIGNANCY

Henry M. Kronenberg

Department of Medicine, Massachusetts General Hospital and Harvard Medical School, Boston, MA, USA

The factor(s) that cause most cases of the humoral hypercalcemia of malignancy have not yet been purified. Several groups have made rapid progress in characterizing the factor(s) by developing sensitive *in vitro* assays that allow detection of small amounts of biologically active material. Traditional techniques of protein chemistry are being used with some success to purify and characterize the biologically active molecules. While these efforts are likely to succeed, they have been slowed somewhat, because human tumor tissue is only sporadically available, and the amounts of tissue are limited. Animal models provide large amounts of tissue, but may or may not correspond to human disease. Cultured cells and tumors grown in nude mice promise to provide large amounts of human tissue, but the stability of the production of the hypercalcemia-inducing factor(s) in these systems is problematic. Further, because the tumors may not make large amounts of the factor(s), the purification may prove difficult. For these reasons, the use of recombinant DNA technology may usefully complement traditional approaches to the study of the humoral hypercalcemia of maligancy.

What can we hope to accomplish with recombinant DNA technology? First, the purification and sequence analysis of the relevant gene may prove easier than the purification and sequence analysis of the protein. Second, we should be able to produce the protein in micro-organisms and cultured cells. This should provide us with large amounts of the human proteins that might otherwise not be available. Finally, we should be able to put the gene into tumors that do not cause hypercalcemia and then create animal models of human humoral hypercalcemia.

The methods for cloning DNA copies of messenger RNA are now straightforward. A mixture of mRNA molecules is isolated from a tissue, and the mRNA sequence is copied into a double-stranded DNA sequence in a series of enzymatic steps. This DNA is then inserted a vector--a bacterial plasmid, for example--and then introduced into *E. coli*. Each resultant bacterial colony or clone contains copies of one paticular plasmid. Each colony therefore carries copies of one particular DNA sequence representing a part of the initial mixed population of mRNAs. By simply isolating individual bacterial colonies on petri dishes, the DNAs representing each particular mRNA in the initial population from the tissue are physically separated and thereby purified. The problem of isolating the DNA sequences representing the factor(s) causing humoral hypercalcemia then reduces to that of telling which DNA sequences encode that protein.

Table I lists the assays that can be used to decide which DNA sequence encodes a particular protein. If the protein of interest has already been purified, several sensitive and specific assays can be used. From the protein's amino acid sequence, using the genetic code, several possible DNA sequences encoding the protein can be deduced. Portions of these sequences can then be synthesized chemically, and these short oligonucleotides can then be made radioactive and used to bind to the particular bacterial colonies encoding the protein of interest. Alternatively, the bacteria may be synthesizing small amounts of the protein of interest, if appropriate plasmid construction strategies were used. Antiserum that recognize the protein can be used then to bind to the particular bacterial colonies that synthesize the desired protein.

The methods described so far require that the protein of interest has already been purified. Since the protein causing malignant hypercalcemia has not yet been purified, these methods will only be helpful in the future. In contrast, we may already be able to take advantage of assays that use cloned DNA to bind specifically to particular complementary mRNAs from cell extracts, thereby allowing purification of the mRNAs. These purified mRNAs are then translated into proteins that can be recognized as those causing humoral hypercalcemia. These assays use the information transfers associated with nucleic acid hybridization (cloned DNA to mRNA) and protein synthesis (mRNA to protein) to change the problem of assaying particular DNA sequences back to the original problem of assaying particular protein sequences. Cloning DNA thereby trades one problem for another: Cloning DNA solves the problem of purifying individual proteins, but makes great demands on the sensitivity and specificity of assays for detecting factors causing humoral hypercalcemia.

Are the assays currently available for detecting the factors causing humoral hypercalcemia sufficiently sensitive and specific? Obviously the most specific assay would involve the

TABLE I. Assays to determine which cloned DNA encodes a factor causing humoral hypercalcemia

---

*1. Hybridization to radioactive synthetic oligonucleotide encoding a portion of the factor.

*2. Immunological detection of the factor synthesized in bacteria

3. Hybridization to mRNA which is subsequently translated into protein <u>in vitro</u> with detection of the protein by
   - *a. antibody precipitation
   - *b. physico-chemical characteristics--size, iso-electric point, etc.
   - c. biochemical assays--stimulation of renal or bone cell adenylate cyclase (with inhibition by PTH 3-34), specific binding to bone or renal membranes, stimulation of PTH-like activity in guinea pig kidney, binding to growth factor receptors

* indicates a requirement for at least partial purification of the protein.

---

production of hypercalcemia by infusion into animals or people of the putative factor.

The factor would have to be active at doses of factor that yield blood levels of the factor actually found in patients. (Since humoral factors work through the bloodstream rather than locally, this stringent criterion is needed.) While this assay must ultimately be used before any factor can be declared the cause of humoral hypercalcemia of malignancy, the assay is both too insensitive and cumbersome to be used for the initial purification of the factor. Instead, a number of in vitro assays are being used. Bone resorption assays have the important advantage of measuring an activity clearly related to the hypercalcemia exhibited in patients, but these assays are also relatively insensitive and cumbersome. More sensitive assays include stimulation of adenylate cyclase from renal membranes or bone cells, stimulation of glucose-6-phosphate dehydrogenase in guinea pig kidney slices, binding to PTH receptors on bone or renal cell membranes, and binding to growth-factor receptors on cellular membranes. Other participants in this symposium discuss the merits of each of these assays. The assays all reflect activities measured in patients with humoral hypercalcemia of malignancy. Several of the assays seem to be measuring PTH-like activity, since the activity can be blocked by the presence of PTH(3-34), an antagonist of PTH action. The use of each assay reflects the assumption that one protein causes both hypercalcemia and the activity measured in vitro. Only when the proteins are purified can this assumption be validated.

Which assays should be used to detect activity among the products of mRNA-directed protein synthesis? The ideal assay would be easy to perform, very sensitive, and certainly specific for the protein causing humoral hypercalcemia. None of the assays fulfills all of these criteria, so it is not surprising that a consensus in the field has not yet been reached.

How much protein can we hope to synthesize using mRNA from tumors? This question cannot be answered with precision, but data from analogous studies is helpful. Colman and Morser (1) showed that *Xenopus* oocytes injected with unpurified interferon mRNA secrete 2.5 pg interferon/oocyte/hr. Since oocytes stably synthesize mRNA products for 24 hours, and the injection of 50 oocytes is straightforward, 3 ng of specific protein can be synthesized using this approach. It is reasonable to hope that several of the assays already discussed are sufficiently sensitive to detect nanogram amounts of biologically active hypercalcemia-inducing factor.

Obviously, the more that is known about the protein of interest, the easier it is to characterize mRNA translation products. Even if the protein is not pure, characteristic migration on gels or columns, or monoclonal antibody can be used to identify proteins synthesized in vitro without demanding biological activity.

The major limitation of the use of recombinant DNA technology, of course, is the requirement that the factor of interest be a protein. The work of several investigators presented at this symposium certainly suggests that this assumption is valid. More problematic is the ability of cell-free systems to synthesize the protein in a way that results in bioactivity. For example, if the protein has two non-identical subunits encoded by two different genes, no one gene product will yield bioactivity. Further, some kinds of cruical post-translational modifications--

phosphorylation, glycosylation, peptide cleavage--may not be carried out by available *in vitro* systems. These constraints are less important if amino acid sequence data or antibodies are available.

It seems certain that at some point the powerful techniques of the molecular biologist will contribute to the characterization of the factor(s) causing humoral hypercalcemia. Whether this contribution will come before or after the protein has been purified will be determined by experiments now in progress in a number of laboratories.

REFERENCES

1. Colman, A., and Morser, J. (1979): Cell, 17, 517.

BONE-RESORBING ACTIVITY RELEASED *IN VITRO* BY TUMORS CAUSING HYPERCALCEMIA OF MALIGNANCY

F. Richard Bringhurst, Barbara E. Bierer and Gino V. Segre

Endocrine Unit and Department of Medicine, Massachusetts General Hospital, Boston, MA, U.S.A.

The cause of the accelerated bone resorption and hypercalcemia frequently observed in patients with malignancy remains obscure. Metastases to bone, although common, frequently occur without accompanying hypercalcemia (1). Release by tumor tissue of circulating factors responsible for increased bone resorption seems clearly established for those cases without skeletal metastases where the hypercalcemia responds to extirpation of the tumor. The postulated involvement of circulating prostaglandins, ectopic parathyroid hormone (PTH) or osteoclast activating factor in the humoral hypercalcemia of malignancy (HHM) has not been strongly supported by clinical studies of patients with this syndrome, however, and the mechanism of the hypercalcemia in most cases of HHM is unexplained.

Many patients with HHM display features consistent with PTH excess (2,3), and involvement of the PTH receptor-adenylate cyclase complex in the HHM syndrome has been suggested by recent reports that tumor-cell conditioned medium and extracts of tumor tissue from patients with HHM activate adenylate cyclase in isolated renal membranes (4,5). Inhibition of this activity by a synthetic inhibitor of PTH receptor binding has been offered as further evidence for the involvement of the PTH receptor in HHM. On the other hand, radioimmunoassays directed against the biologically active region of the PTH molecule do not detect PTH-specific sequences in these preparations. Moreover, elevated urinary cyclic AMP excretion has been reported in many cancer patients without hypercalcemia (6), and other clinical features of HHM, including elevated fractional excretion of calcium, suppression of 1,25-(OH)2-D, and a marked discordance between osteoblastic and osteoclastic activity on bone biopsy (2), are not consonant with present understanding of PTH action. These considerations suggest that humoral agents which do not interact with the PTH receptor may be important in the pathogenesis of HHM.

Our general approach to the problem of HHM has been to identify and characterize bone-resorbing factors released directly *in vitro* by cultured tumor tissue obtained at surgery from patients with cancer-associated hypercalcemia. By establishing stable cell lines from such tumors, we hope to facilitate the further purification, characterization and structural identification of tumor-cell products which cause bone resorption *in vitro* and, presumably, hypercalcemia *in vivo* .

Bone resorption is quantitated by the release of radioactive calcium from neonatal mouse calvarial bones during 72 hours *in vitro*. Effects on cyclic AMP production are evaluated in the same system, after short-term (10-20 min) incubations, by cyclic AMP radioimmunoassay of calvarial extracts. In this system, bone resorption and cyclic AMP production are stimulated coordinately by bPTH at concentrations between 10^{-9}M and 10^{-7}M.

We have detected substantial bone-resorbing activity in conditioned medium from primary cultures of tumor tissue from 6 of 7 patients with hypercalcemia of malignancy (Table 1). In 4 of these 6, tumor-cell secretion of nondialyzable resorbing activity has persisted beyond the first month of continuous culture. The only tumor tissue which has so far failed to release bone-resorbing activity was obtained from a patient with advanced non-Hodgkin's lymphoma.

TABLE 1. Effects of tumor-conditioned media on mouse calvarial bone resorption and cyclic AMP production

TUMORS	DILUTION	^{45}CA RELEASE	C-AMP
Malignant Melanoma	1:10	3.6	0.9
Transitional Cell Bladder	1:20	3.1	0.9
Oat Cell Lung	1:20	1.8	1.1
Squamous Cell Skin	1:20	1.7	0.8
Giant Cell Bone	1:20	1.6	?
T-Cell Leukemia	1:5	1.6	1.0
Non-Hodgkin's Lymphoma	1:10	1.1	?
Bovine PTH(1-34), 100 nM		3.2	9.0

(Results expressed as treated/control ratios.)

In the case of the melanoma, sufficient tumor was obtained to permit extensive characterization of the bone-resorbing activity in the primary culture medium. This material caused a dose-related stimulation of calvarial bone resorption which was maximal at a dilution of 1:20 in the bioassay. The resorbing activity was shown to be non-dialyzable, acid-precipitable, protease-sensitive and resistant to extraction by organic solvents. It was heat-stable and survived freezing, lyophilization, and prolonged incubation in buffers ranging in pH from 2 to 9. The resorption induced by this factor was completely inhibited by calcitonin (1 ug/ml) and by use of bones killed by repetitive freeze-thawing. The activity was unaffected by cortisol (1 uM) or indomethacin (2 mM) in the assay medium. Gel-filtration chromatography suggested a molecular weight of approximately 12,500 daltons. No PTH was detectable in the crude medium by either of two PTH immunoassays or by a sensitive cytochemical bioassay. At concentrations maximally effective in stimulating bone resorption, the melanoma medium caused no activation of cyclic AMP production by the calvarial bones or by ROS 17/2 clonal rat osteosarcoma cells. Melanoma medium also failed to activate adenylate cyclase in isolated canine renal membranes.

We have studied the effect on calvarial cyclic AMP production of culture medium from 5 of the tumors which release resorbing activity *in vitro*. In no case was a cyclic AMP response detectable at concentrations of medium which clearly caused resorption of these bones (Table 1).

We believe that tumors associated with hypercalcemia frequently release soluble macromolecular factors which lead directly to accelerated bone resorption and that these factors are thus responsible for the appearance of hypercalcemia *in vivo*. Our observations suggest that, unlike PTH, these factors stimulate bone resorption without an accompanying increase in bone-cell cyclic AMP. It is possible that the substances released by these tumors might exhibit activity in more sensitive renal-membrane adenylate cyclase assays. Nevertheless, the bone resorption which they induce in calvaria in vitro appears to be mediated independently of the classical PTH receptor/adenylate cyclase complex.

REFERENCES

1. Ralston, S., Gardner, M.D., Fogelman, I. and Boyle, I.T. (1982): Lancet, 2, 903.
2. Stewart, A.F., Horst, R., Deftos, L.J., et al. (1980): New Engl J Med, 303, 1377.
3. Goltzman, D., Stewart, A.F. and Broadus, A.E. (1981): J Clin Endocrinol Metab., 53, 899.
4. Stewart, A.F., Insogna, K.L., Goltzman, D. and Broadus, A.E. (1983): Proc. Natl. Acad. Sci. USA, 80, 1454.
5. Strewler, G.J., Williams, R.D. and Nissenson, R.A., (1983): J Clin Invest., 71, 769.
6. Rude, R.K., Sharp, C.F., Fredericks, R.S., et al., (1981): J Clin Endocrinol Metab., 52, 765.

DISCUSSION: NON-PARATHYROID HYPERCALCEMIA

Moderator: John T. Potts, Jr

Department of Medicine, harvard medical School and Massachusetts General Hospital, Boston, MA, U.S.A.

J. POTTS: I would like to turn to the clinical issues and ask about certain confusing issues raised in the presentations by Drs. Broadus and Singer. I might start by asking them if they would return to the dilemma of unexplained differences in findings among groups regarding a bimodal distribution of nephrogeneous cyclic AMP in patients with hypercalcemia and malignancy and the related issue, levels of nephrogenous cyclic AMP in normocalcemic patients with cancer.

A. BROADUS: We used a biochemical classification. Yet, as I also indicated, there are clinical correlates. We do not regard a solitary or a few bone metastases as necessarily indicating a local osteolytic mechanism. The patients that we classify biochemically as having local osteolytic disease on bone scan, radiological survey, or on autopsy findings, always have a massive tumor burden in bone. The patients in the humoral group never have that presentation in our experience. Roughly half of them will have a few isolated lesions on bone scan, but that is all.

F. SINGER: We do see some normocalcemic patients who have high nephrogenous cyclic AMP. We also see some patients that we classify as humoral hypercalcemia, who have a low nephrogenous cyclic AMP. I have no explanation for the difference.

R. JOSSE: In a large number of patients that we have looked at, approximately 55 hypercalcemic cancer patients with an appropriate number of control subjects, we have been unable to see a bimodal distribution. We find a spectrum of changes whether we look at patients with or without metastases. I find it quite surprising that there is such a bimodal distribution in your data, yet it appears quite convincing.

I would like to make a point about the bone histology that one sees in a group of hypercalcemic cancer patients. Again we have noticed a spectrum of findings. If one looks at patients with multiple myeloma there is clearly massive bone resorption with very little evidence of bone formation. However, if one studies patients with solid tumors, there is a spectrum of histologic changes in which one sees generally increased bone resorption, but also occasionally increased bone formation. With tumor metastatic to bone, in most cases, one finds primarily localized osteolysis and increased bone resorption without evidence of increased bone formation.

A. BROADUS: We did not show any material from patients with metastatic cells in bone. We see precisely the same findings you mentioned. The data which I showed were specifically from patients with humoral mechanisms for hypercalcemia. We excluded patients with tumor cells in bone.

G. SEGRE: Dr. Singer, you seemed to confirm some of the data that we published previously regarding control of hypercalcemia. Prostaglandin synthetase inhibitors seem to play a role in the control of hypercalcemia in patients who have solid tumors without bony metastases.

The question I have for Dr. Singer concerns the discrepancies in results achieved using radioimmunoassays versus mass spectrographic analysis for estimation of prostaglandin production. Do you have any comments about why there are these discrepan- cies between the two methodologies?

F. SINGER: One of the problems with prostaglandin assays has been the deterioration of tracer during the incubation period. Another problem we have found is that if you attempt to use either silica or LH-20, you will find artifacts that appear to arise from these materials. Certainly the mass spectrographic method is the most advanced technique, but the assay is difficult and not easily applicable. Unfortunately, no investigators are measuring urine for prostaglandin metabolites at the current time. I can't really answer your question, except to say that anyone who attempts to measure prostaglandin E or its metabolites in the blood or urine has a difficult task.

L. RIGGS: The observation that you have found that the parathyroid hormone antagonist, PTH(3-34), blocks the adenylate cyclase response to your tumor factors suggests that the substance is binding with PTH receptors, yet Dr. Kronenberg has told us that the cDNA probe studies are negative.

How much of a structural difference in homology between the putative hypercalcemic factor(s) and mature PTH would still allow binding of the former to the PTH receptor, yet not give a positive result with the cDNA probes?

H. KRONENBERG: I don't think anyone really knows the structural variation in peptide sequence that is tolerated for binding to the receptor. Hybridization assays should be compared with radioimmunoassays. Nucleic acid hybridization is something that we think we understand. While in controlled circumstances hybridization assays may be more specific than radioimmunoassays, what is clear with regard to nucleic acid hybridization involving long stretches of DNA is that there is a tremendous sensitivity to the presence or absence of short stretches of perfect homology. If a stretch of 50 base pairs in a sequence of 500 nucleotides is perfectly homologous to 50 pairs of a probe, binding will be easily detectable. If the 50 homologous base pairs are scattered along a 500 base pair stretch, no binding will occur. There are, therefore, stringent limits as to what we can conclude about the negative nucleic acid hybridization studies.

Loosely speaking, that means that the sequences of PTH and the factor causing humoral hypercalcemia probably differ by at least 30% or so at the nucleic acid level, as a minimum. Such an estimate is only approximate, particularly when you realize that the genetic code is degenerate (several codons for the same amino acid). Two proteins actually could be more similar than predicted from hybridization studies. If, for example, there are ten amino acids that really represent considerable peptide homology, we could have missed them entirely.

J. POTTS: On this important point that Dr. Riggs raises, we can say that the material that might be related to PTH is not detected by immunoassays for PTH nor detected by hybridization assays. Nonetheless, the factor(s) has this interesting property that cyclic AMP generation by the factor in vitro in renal membranes is blocked by the 3-34 PTH peptide. What these findings mean, in terms of binding by the factor to the PTH receptor, is of great interest since the overall findings concerning similarity of the tumor factor(s) and PTH do not point in the same direction.

S. POSEN: I would like to ask Dr. Broadus if he is surprised by the clear bimodal distribution between the humoral and non-humoral hypercalcemia patients? Given the natural history of cancer, would we not expect humoral factors responsible for the hypercalcemia of malignancy to persist even if the patient subsequently develops metastases?

A. BROADUS: I'm not surprised at all by our bimodal data, and we continue to see it. We have now done studies in 125 patients which nears our limit of exhaustion, and we see the same data. I cannot explain why other workers do not see it. It does not exclude the presence of other hidden mechanisms or a few individual patients with different factors that would be misclassified by our scheme, which is basically biochemical in nature. However, it would be less than a few percent. You asked whether the presence or absence of bone metastases in any way alters our definition. In my view, no. Take a patient with a serum calcium of 14 mg who has a localized renal cell carcinoma. Six months later with the same tumor and the same calcium value, the patient now has bone metastases. Perhaps an added mechanism based on local stimulation in bone is in effect, but I don't think the fundamental mechanism has changed.

J. COBURN: Prostaglandins have certain effects which should be recalled; thus prostaglandins clearly play a role in maintaining normal renal blood flow and function in a number of pathological states. Thus the use of prostaglandin inhibitors can cause a marked decrease in renal function, particularly in conditions with volume depletion and/or in hypercalcemia. There is a good study showing that renal function in hypercalcemic animals becomes markedly depressed when prostaglandin inhibitors are superimposed upon the hypercalcemia. So, even if prostaglandins play a role in causing hypercalcemia, prostaglandin inhibitors may not be appropriate therapy for many patients.

A. KORKOR: Dr. Broadus, the humoral factor that you find seems to mimic the effects of PTH on kidney in terms of cyclic AMP generation, but it does not stimulate $1,25(OH)_2D$ synthesis. The mechanism by which the hormone stimulates the 1α-hydroxylation is thought to be linked to cyclic AMP production. Do your observations imply that such a linked relation is not present or do you have any other explanation for the apparent discrepancy?

A. BROADUS: The answer to that is not known. Based on the *in vivo* data, the tumor factor(s) is like PTH, in some respects, *in that* it stimulates renal cyclic AMP generation and phosphaturia. However, it does not stimulate the 1α-hydroxylation of 25(OH)D. Neither does it stimulate distal tubular reabsorption of calcium, and its aggregate effects on bone are quite different from those of PTH. My interpretation at this time is that there may be a definite humoral factor-receptor interaction, but we have to have pure material in hand to test this possibility rigorously and definitively.

XII ECTOPIC CALCITRIOL PRODUCTION INCLUDING SARCOIDOSIS

ECTOPIC CALCITRIOL PRODUCTION INCLUDING SARCOIDOSIS

Moderator: John T. Potts, Jr

Department of Medicine, Harvard Medical School and Massachusetts General Hospital, Boston, MA, U.S.A.

INTRODUCTION

J. POTTS: The questions that our speakers will address are the following: Does extra-renal production of $1,25(OH)_2D$ occur, and if so, is it of physiologic significance, particularly the placental production of $1,25(OH)_2D$? To what extent is there consensus that excessive production of $1,25(OH)_2D$ is responsible for the hypercalcemia of sarcoidosis?

HYPERCALCEMIA AND BONE DISEASE ASSOCIATED WITH SARCOIDOSIS

Michael F. Holick

Vitamin D Laboratory, Endocrine Unit, Massachusetts General Hospital, Harvard Medical School, Boston, MA and Department of Nutrition and Food Science, Massachusetts Institute of Technology, Cambridge, MA

INTRODUCTION

Sarcoidosis is a multisystem granulomatous disorder of unknown etiology that most commonly affects young adults, although it can occur in young children and in elderly adults (1). There is no particular sex predilection, and it usually presents itself as erythema nodosum or acute uveitis or hilar adenopathy that is discovered on a routine roentgenogram of the chest (2). The diagnosis is established by histologic evidence of widespread noncaseating epitheloid-cell granulomas and is supported by clinical and radiologic evidence of a multisystem disease and a positive Kveim--Siltzbach skin test (1,2).

HYPERCALCEMIA

Various biochemical abnormalities are often associated with sarcoidosis. Harrel and Fisher in 1939 were the first to report an association between sarcoidosis and hypercalcemia (3). Depending on the series, hypercalcemia with a serum calcium concentration above 11 mg/dl has been reported in as little as 2 percent and as high as 35 percent of patients with sarcoidosis (1,2,4,5). The cause of the hypercalcemia was an enigma until Anderson and his colleagues (6) showed that three patients with sarcoidosis and hypercalcemia were absorbing more calcium from the gastrointestinal tract than would healthy controls. Furthermore, they noted the serum calcium of one patient increased from 12.6 mg/dl to 16.3 mg/dl after receiving 9000 IU of vitamin D_2 daily for ten days, suggesting to them that the gastrointestinal tract of this patient was hypersensitive to vitamin D. The serum calcium of this and of three other hypercalcemic sarcoid patients was decreased when corticosterone was administered.

Although this observation was confirmed and expanded upon (7,8), little new information about the cause of the hypersensitivity of the intestine to small doses of vitamin D until the 1970s when it was appreciated that vitamin D was biologically inert until it was metabolized in the liver to 25-hydroxyvitamin D and then in the kidney to 1,25-dihydroxyvitamin D (9). The development of assays for these metabolites prompted several investigators to determine whether the "hypersensitivity to vitamin D" was indirectly due to an acquired defect in vitamin D-metabolism. Several reports appeared, suggesting that the circulating concentrations of 25-OH-D were normal, but the concentrations of 1,25-$(OH)_2$-D were abnormally elevated (10,11). It was well known that sarcoid patients were more prone to the development of hypercalcemia in the summer and fall. In 1979 Papapoulous et al. (12) reported the case of a patient with sarcoidosis who developed hypercalcemia during the summer months at a time when the 25-OH-D increased in the normal range, whereas the circulating concentrations of 1,25-$(OH)_2$-D increased markedly in to the supranormal range and was coincident with the occurrance of hypercalcemia. An increase in corticosterone therapy caused the serum calcium and 1,25-$(OH)_2$-D to return to the normal range. Hence, it appeared that the hypersensitivity to vitamin D was due to an abnormality in 25-OH-D metabolism. Inappropriately elevated 1,25-$(OH)_2$-D concentrations in the circulation maintained a high efficiency in the intestinal absorption of calcium even in the presence of hypercalcemia. Until recently, it was unknown whether the elevated circulating concentrations of 1,25-$(OH)_2$-D was, due to a defect in the regulation of the renal metabolism of 25-OH-D to 1,25-$(OH)_2$-D or an ectopic site capable of metabolizing 25-OH-D to 1,25-$(OH)_2$-D. Evidence to support the latter hypothesis was provided by Barbour and colleagues (13) when they reported that during an episode of hypercalcemia an anephric patient with sarcoidosis had an elevated serum 1,25-$(OH)_2$-D concentration. Steroid therapy (40 mg of prednisone a day) decreased the circulating concentration of 1,25-$(OH)_2$-D, and, in turn, the serum calcium concentration returned to normal. Thus, this patient was able to metabolize 25-OH-D to 1,25-$(OH)_2$-D strongly supporting the hypothesis that the etiology of the hypercalcemia associated with sarcoidosis is due to an unregulated ectopic synthesis of 1,25-$(OH)_2$-D. Although not yet proven it is most likely that the ectopic site is the sarcoid granulomas.

BONE INVOLVEMENT

Sarcoidosis of the bone is usually seen in patients who have chronic, persisent, irreversible, multisystem disease. Radiologic evidence of bone involvement with sarcoidosis occurs in about 5 percent of the patients (1,2,4,14,16). Most commonly, a generalized osteopenia is observed of the small bones of the hands, and to a lesser extent, those of the feet and wrists. However, sarcoidosis of the bone can present as punched-out lytic lesions or less frequently as osteosclerotic lesions (14-20).

CONCLUSION

Sarcoidosis is a multisystem disease that can potentially affect every organ system in the body. Because the symptoms and biochemical abnormalities associated with this disease are so nondescript the diagnosis is often missed. This is especially true for patients presenting with hypercalcemia and lytic or sclerotic bone lesions. Usually an extensive tumor workup is initiated before a diagnosis of sarcoidosis is entertained especially when the chest reontgenogram is found to be normal which is seen in about 3 to 5 percent of patients with disseminated sarcoidosis (1). To date, this is the only acquired disease that can potentially cause an ectopic unregulated synthesis of 1,25-$(OH)_2$-D. An understanding of the biochemistry and molecular biology of the derepression and activity of this extrarenal 25-OH-D-1-hydroxylase may provide a unique insight into the physiology of this important enzyme.

REFERENCES

1. Mayock, R.L., Bertrand, P., Morrison, C.E. and Scott, J.H. (1963) : Am. J. Med., 35, 67.
2. Siltzbach, L.E., James, D.G., Neville, E., Turiaf, Battesti, P., Sharma, P. and Hosoda, T. (1974) : Am. J. Med., 57, 847.
3. Harrell, G.T. and Fisher, S. (1939) : J. Clin. Invest., 18, 687.
4. Holick, M.F. (1982) : N. Engl. J. Med., 20, 1257.
5. Goldstein, R.A., Israel, H.L., Becker, K. and Moore, C. (1971) : J. Am. Med. Assoc., 51, 21.
6. Anderson, J., Dent, C.E., Harper, C. and Philpot G.R. (1954) : Lancet, 2, 720.
7. Henneman, P.H., Dempsey, E.F., Carroll, E.L. and Albright, F. (1956) : J. Clin. Invest., 35, 1229.
8. Bell, N.H. and Bartter, F.C. (1967) : Acta Endocrinologica, 54, 173.

9. Holick, M.F., Potts, J.T. Jr. (1983) : In: Harrison's Principles of Internal Medicine, 10th edition, p. 1944. Editors: K.J. Isselbacher, R.D. Adams, E. Braunwald, R.G. Petersdorf and J.D. Wilson. McGraw-Hill, New York, New York.
10. Bell, N.H., Stern, P.H., Pantzer, E., Sinha, T. and DeLuca, H.F. (1979) : J. Clin. Invest., 64, 218.
11. Chesney, R.W., Hamstra, A.J., DeLuca, H.F., Horowitz, S., Gilbert, E.F., Hong, R. and Borcherding, W. (1981) : J. Pediatr., 98, 919.
12. Papapoulos, S.E., Clemens, T.L., Fraher, L.J., Lewin, I.G., Sandler, L.M. and O'Riordan, J.L.H. (1979) : Lancet, 1, 627.
13. Barbour, G.L., Coburn, J.W., Slatopolsky, E., Norman, A.W. and Horst R.L. (1981) : N. Engl. J. Med., 305, 440.
14. Rohatgi, P.K. and Archutowska-Kempka, M. (1981) : Arch. Neurol., 38, 261.
15. Bodie, B.F., Kheir, S.M. and Omura, E.F., (1980) : J. Am. Acad. Dermatol., 3, 401.
16. Silver, H.M., Shirkhoda, A. and Simon D.B. (1978) : Chest., 72, 238.
17. Teirstein, A.S., Wolf, B.S. and Siltzbach, L.E. (1961) : N. Engl. J. Med., 265, 65.
18. Turner, O.A. and Weiss, S.R. (1969) : Am. J. Roentgenol Radium Ther. Nucl. Med., 105, 322.
19. Bonakdarpour, A., Levy, W. and Aegerter, E.E. (1971) : Am. J. Roentgenol Radium Ther. Nucl. Med., 113, 646.
20. Young, D.A. and Laman, M.L. (1972) : Am. J. Roentgenol Radium Ther. Nucl. Med., 114, 553.

VITAMIN D METABOLISM IN SARCOIDOSIS

J.L.H. O'RIORDAN

Department of Medicine, Middlesex Hospital, London, England

Since our original opportunity to follow a patient who developed hypercalcemia spontaneously, following prolonged exposure to sunlight, we have had the opportunity to study other patients with hypercalcemia and sarcoidosis along with Roger Smith in Oxford and Lawrence Sandler and Larry Fraher at the Middlesex Hospital.

The features of these patients at the time that they are hypercalcemic is that the concentration of 25-OH-D is strictly within the normal range, while the measured concentration of $1,25(OH)_2D$ is elevated.

Treatment with steroids in one form or another makes the patient quite quickly normocalcemic; this is associated with a decrease in the concentration of $1,25(OH)_2D$. I might say that clearly it is necessary to characterize the material believed to be $1,25(OH)_2D$ most carefully. We have used an immunoassay that is particularly selective for one hydroxylated compound.

The pattern of change in one patient revealed a striking response to small doses of hydrocortisone (60 milligrams a day). Calcium fell to normal as did $1,25(OH)_2D$. No change whatsoever occurred in the concentration of 25-OH-D. Steroid therapy was stopped and the concentration of calcium and $1,25(OH)_2D$ rose to abnormally high levels again.

In normal subjects, there is no relationship between the concentration of 25-OH-D and $1,25(OH)_2D$. By contrast, in the patients with hypercalcemia and sarcoidosis, there is a correlation between the concentration of $1,25(OH)_2D$; there is an abnormal substrate/product relationship in these patients at the time that they are hypercalcemic. This relation does not exist when normocalcemia has been achieved by treatment with steroids. Now, steroids have, I think, a number of actions in reducing the concentration of $1,25(OH)_2D$ in sarcoidosis. At a time when the patients are hypercalcemic, the concentration of $1,25(OH)_2D$ rises quickly after administration of an oral dose of several micrograms of calcitriol metabolite and does not fall to normal within 48 hours.

When these same patients are challenged in the same way, with several micrograms of calcitriol when they are normocalcemic on steroids, the rate of rise of $1,25(OH)_2D$ is normal and it clears much more rapidly from the circulation. So, it is possible that steroids are affecting the metabolism of calcitriol (or endogenous $1,25(OH)_2D$).

The original patient that we studied became hypercalcemic when exposed to sunlight. It has been know for years that patients with sarcoidosis are hypersensitive to sunlight. If we mimic sunlight in another patient by giving 3,000 units of vitamin D daily, there is a rise in the concentration of serum calcium, which follows a rise in the concentration of $1,25(OH)_2D$. If one stops the vitamin D, the calcium returns to normal as the concentration of $1,25(OH)_2D$ falls. So, the change in serum calcium is vitamin D-dependent.

We had an opportunity to look at another patient with sarcoidosis at the time when he was hypercalcemic and the initial concentration of $1,25(OH)_2D$ was already elevated. When vitamin

VD was given, the concentration of 25-OH-D rose progressively. The concentration of $1,25(OH)_2D$ also rose futher, as you would expect from the previous patient. When steroids were added and the vitamin D challenge continued, there was a precipitous fall in the concentration of $1,25(OH)_2D$, followed by a fall in the concentration of calcium to normal.

Time doesn't permit me to consider the source of the putative $1,25(OH)_2D$. We have looked at the changes in D metabolites in patients who are anephric (these are not patients with sarcoidosis). We have evidence that when the subjects were given 1 mg vitamin D_3 daily for one month, there were not only increases in the concentration of 24,25 and 25,26 dihydroxy metabolites, but also evidence in two of three patients that $1,25(OH)_2D$ became detectable. I agree that it is important to verify that the metabolite that reacts in the assays as $1,25(OH)_2D$ is indeed the authentic metabolite. The material detected in high concentration in patients with sarcoidosis comigrates with authentic $1,25(OH)_2D$, for example, on variety of chromatographic systems, including reverse phase hplc. I look forward to the views of others concerning these issues.

ECTOPIC PRODUCTION OF 1,25-DIHYDROXYVITAMIN D

T. Kenney Gray, William Mentz, Juliette Wait and Galen Barbour. University of North Carolina School of Medicine, Departments of Medicine & Pharmacology, Chapel Hill, NC 27514; and Medical Services, V.A. Medical Center, Hampton, VA. and Department of Medicine, Eastern Virginia School of Medicine, Norfold, VA.

The ectopic production of 1,25-dihydroxyvitamin D (1,25$(OH)_2$D is synonymous with the extra-renal synthesis of this metabolite of vitamin D. The extra-renal synthesis of 1,25$(OH)_2$D was first postulated to occur in the fetoplacental unit. Soon after this postulate was described, the synthesis of 1,25$(OH)_2$D was described in placental tissues of human and rat origin. Later cells isolated from chick calvariae and human bone were reported to synthesize 1,25$(OH)_2$D in vitro. The cells used in these experiments were heterogeneous in nature. Furthermore, it is unknown if cells in bone have this capacity in vivo. Persistance of 1,25$(OH)_2$D in the circulation of a nephrectomized animal would be compelling evidence for the extra-renal synthesis of 1,25$(OH)_2$D if one could be certain of the specificity of the techniques used to isolate and assay putative 1,25$(OH)_2$D. Recent reports from two laboratories failed to show the formation of 1,25$(OH)_2$D when 25(OH)D was administered to acutely nephrectomized laboratory rats. In a related study employing the model of a nephrectomized, dialyzed pig a compound that reacted in a 1,25$(OH)_2$D assay was present in the circulation. Paradoxically in the same model (^{3}H-26,27)-25(OH) D_3 was not metabolized to (^{3}H-26,27)-1,25$(OH)_2D_3$, suggesting that the assayed compound was not authentic 1,25$(OH)_2$D. Some investigators have reported that 1,25$(OH)_2$D can be detected in the circulation of patients with chronic renal failure or of nephrectomized patients. Many others report undetectable levels of 1,25$(OH)_2$D in such patients. This controversy will not be settled until the specificity and sensitivity of the various assays used by these investigators are delineated and standardized.

The extra-renal synthesis of 1,25$(OH)_2$D in a bilaterally nephrectomized patient with sarcoidosis was postulated two years ago. The basis for this postulate was persistant 1,25$(OH)_2$D in the circulation of this patient despite nephrectomy. This postulate prompted us to study the in vitro metabolism of 25(OH)D by macrophages obtained by brochoalveolar lavage from patients with sarcoidosis and normal volunteers. Freshly isolated macrophages incubated with (^{3}H-26,27)-25$(OH)D_3$ for 60 min. converted the substrate to a radioactive peak which comigrated with authentic 1,25$(OH)_2$D on HPLC system employing hexane:n-propanolol (9:1,v/v). When the radioactivity comigrating with 1,25$(OH)_2$D was collected and rechromatographed on a HPLC system using different solvents, it did not comigrate with authentic 1,25$(OH)_2$D. This unidentified metabolite was formed by cells obtained from normocalcemic patients with sarcoidosis and normal volunteers. We did not have the opportunity to obtain pulmonary macrophages from patients with sarcoidosis and hypercalcemia. These unexpected findings led us to consider the possibility that the novel metabolite of 25(OH) D_3 formed by the pulmonary macrophages might occur in vivo and be mistakenly identified as 1,25$(OH)_2$D. To test this possibility we incubated aliquots of the novel metabolite in a radioimmunoassay for 1,25$(OH)_2$D. Displacement of the radioligand in a fashion paralleling the standard curve was associated with quantities of novel metabolite calculated to range from 5 to 60 picograms. This result and our previous findings showed that the novel metabolite of 25$(OH)D_3$ was not separated from 1,25$(OH)_2$D by the commonly used HPLC system employing hexane:n-propanolol (9:1,v/v) and that the novel metabolite cross-reacted in an assay for $1,25(OH)_2D$. These findings support the contention that one or more metabolites of vitamin D may be present in the circulation of nephrectomized patients and might be mis-identified as $1,25(OH)_2D$. New metabolites whose chemical structure has been defined are known to cross-react with $1,25(OH)_2D$ in the competitive protein binding assay that employs the chick mucosal receptor protein. Given the description of metabolites that interfere in assays previously believed to be specific for $1,25(OH)_2D$, it is clear that the question of the extra-renal synthesis of $1,25(OH)_2D$ will not be resolved until techniques capable of separating native $1,25(OH)_2D$ from other metabolites present in the circulation and assays with established specificity are employed. Until then, the question of the ectopic or extra-renal production of $1,25(OH)_2D$ remains an interesting and perplexing issue.

DISCUSSION: ECTOPIC CALCITROL PRODUCTION INCLUDING SARCOIDOSIS

A. NORMAN: As of now, by my count, there are at least 23 chemically characterized metabolites of vitamin D. We reported two new ones several weeks ago at the Federation Meetings. These are both metabolites of $1,25(OH)_2D$ which are made in the intestine. These are the first two metabolites of $1,25(OH)_2D$, in my opinion, that show significant interaction with intestinal receptors. $1,25(OH)_2$-24-oxo-D_3 binds, as well as 1,24R,-$25(OH)_3$-D_3; the other metabolite, $1,23,25(OH)_3$-24- -D_3 binds less well. Both metabolites are able to stimulate intestinal calcium absorption in the chicken and to mobilize bone calcium. While there is a hypothesis that abnormal metabolism of vitamin D in sarcoidosis causes hypercalcemia due to increased levels of $1,25(OH)_2D$, as Dr. Gray summarized, we need to be careful to clearly ascertain whether the substance that mediates the hypercalcemia is truly $1,25(OH)_2D$. Thus, I agree with Dr. Holick that mass spectrometry of any putative metabolite indeed needs to be done. I think Dr. Gray, in light of his studies with macrophages from patients with sarcoid, would agree with that conclusion.

J. O'RIORDAN: I would accept that the total identification of the hypercalcemic factor has not yet been achieved, and we would be delighted to have some of Dr. Norman's new sterols to study. All I can say is that so far we have not been able to separate the abnormally produced vitamin D metabolite from $1,25(OH)_2D$, but we are continuing to try. Like Dr. Gray, I have been confused by the published literature. I can say though that our own data looks much clearer.

M. PARFITT: Some old clinical observations may help individuals in deciding where to pursue this work on sarcoidosis further. In tropical Queensland there is an interesting situation which is unique with respect to sarcoidosis. First, it is the only part of the world where predominantly light skinned people spend many hours of the day working in the tropical sunlight. Second, a compulsory annual chest x-ray was required for the entire population. A large number of patients with subclinical sarcoidosis were detected who had only hilar adenopathy. In this subclinical group of patients, the incidence of hypercalcemia was 40% and the incidence of hypercalciuria was 80%. I think the observations of Dr. O'Riordan enable me, retrospectively, to interpret those data. I suggest that anyone who wants to pursue this matter further should arrange to do a sabbatical leave in Queensland, Australia.

J. COBURN: Hypercalciuria is a much more sensitive indicator of the effects of $1,25(OH)_2D$ than hypercalcemia. Hypercalcemia is more likely to develop during exogenous administration of $1,25(OH)_2D$ when renal function is reduced.

K. GRAY: If the material responsible for hypercalcemia in sarcoidosis is $1,25(OH)_2D$, Dr. Coburn's remarks are appropriate. If it is not 1,25$(OH)_2D$, the material isolated may not produce hypercalcemia.

F. SINGER: Dr. John Adams recently reported studies in 5 patients with sarcoidosis. A 1,25$(OH)_2D$-like substance was found in the macrophages of patients with sarcoidosis. From all the information available this material looks like 1,25$(OH)_2D$.

XIII OSTEOPOROSIS – PATHOGENESIS, PREVENTION AND TREATMENT

OSTEOPOROSIS: AN OVERVIEW

C. Conrad Johnston, Jr., M.D.

Pathogenesis

Osteoporosis is the most common of the metabolic bone diseases. A number of papers were presented indicating the progress made in this field, relating both to the pathogenesis of the disease and to its prevention and treatment.

Dr. Nordin reported additional data to support his model that bone volume is determined by an independent variable--bone formation rate--and volume-dependent variable--fractional bone resorption. In this case, mean-seam width was used as an index of formation in biopsies from a group of premenopausal women in a state of equilibrium, when formation and resorption are balanced. Again, previously reported correlations were found. Dr. Nordin feels that age-related bone loss is associated with an increase in resorption, and that this increase is more marked in that subset of the population who develop osteoporosis. The principal disagreement here is with the methods used to estimate rates of resorption and bone formation--measurement of resorption and formation surfaces. Many investigators feel that rates cannot be derived from static surface measurements. Nordin emphasizes the importance of the model, formation as an independent variable, and believes that substitution of other measures of rates (i.e., calcification rate derived from tetracycline labeling), would only shift the curve, and would not alter the fundamental concept. Clearly, additional data using multiple methods to correlate change over time will be needed to finally resolve this dilemma.

Dr. Parfitt addressed from a new perspective the important problem of age-related loss of trabecular bone. Is this loss of trabecular bone due to a decrease in the number (density) of trabeculae, or to decrease in the thickness of individual trabeculae? His studies indicate that both mechanisms are, in part, responsible; but, loss of trabeculae is the predominant mechanism, both for age-related loss and for the more marked deficit found among osteoporotics. A reduction in the mean-wall thickness of individual structural units can explain the thinness of individual trabeculae, but not total loss of the structure. He suggests that during the accelerated phase of bone loss shortly after menopause, osteoclasts perforate trabeculae; thus, there is no remaining structure upon which new bone can be rebuilt. A similar mechanism may be responsible for endosteal bone loss.

Studies utilizing tetracycline labeling as a measure of bone apposition indicate that osteoblast function declines with age in normals, and, to a more marked degree, in osteoporotics. At menopause, there is an increase in bone remodeling which persists for some time. Among some who will develop osteoporosis, the rapid remodeling ceases, for unknown reasons; and, this cessation may be a factor important in fracture pathogenesis. He suggests that some osteoporotics start with low bone mass at maturity, and have a prolonged phase of accelerated bone loss, with a consequence of low bone mass and fracture. These individuals would have high remodeling on biopsies taken at the time of fracture. Another population has rapid loss, but is unable to compensate, and decreased remodeling is found on biopsy; thus, the heterogeneity of morphometric variables in osteoporosis can be explained.

Dr. Parfitt presents a new hypothesis which places great emphasis on loss of structural elements due to increased osteoclast activity. This phenomenon occurs years before fracture; thus, prevention and treatment must focus on the years associated with rapid bone loss, shortly after the menopause. Dr. Nordin stresses increased resorption as the primary event responsible for bone loss in osteoporosis. Measured variables are derived from static measurement of bone surfaces at the time of fracture. Parfitt emphasizes that most of the bone loss is due to removal of structural elements during the rapid phase of bone loss after the menopause, and this loss is due to osteoclast penetration of existing trabeculae. Could the increased resorption surfaces seen by Nordin reflect the previous activity postulated by Parfitt? Clearly, additional studies are necessary, but the focus of research should shift from the patient with the disease--fracture--to the individual losing bone at a rapid rate some years before the morbid event.

Low bone mass is one of the principal determinants of osteoporotic fractures, and Robert Heaney reviewed the complex mechanisms responsible for determination of bone mass in the aging individual. Four elements are important: 1) peak bone mass achieved; 2) remodeling balance; 3) remodeling rate, and 4) time. Many factors may affect the first three of these variables to produce the bone mass found at any point in time.

Mechanical loading, perhaps acting through a direct or an indirect stimulation of osteoblasts (thereby producing a positive remodeling balance), may be important, both in attainment of peak adult bone mass, and in subsequent rates of loss. With age, there is a reduction of peak strains induced, rate of strain, and also, diversity of activity performed. These factors may lead to a negative remodeling balance and bone loss.

Remodeling rates may be determined primarily by parathyroid hormone secretion. In the presence of a negative remodeling balance, such as is found with aging individuals, an increase in remodeling rate would lead to a more rapid loss of bone. Increased effective calcium intake will suppress parathyroid hormone (PTH), and thus, remodeling. It is not entirely clear whether calcium intake within the usually expected range affects bone loss, but inadequate intake certainly could accelerate loss caused by other factors. Other nutrients may negatively affect calcium balance, as well, especially excessive intakes of protein and alcohol.

Estrogen deficiency is associated with accelerated bone loss, although the mechanisms are not clear. Remodeling rates are increased by estrogen withdrawal, and in the presence of a negative remodeling balance, more rapid loss would ensue. Estrogen also appears to affect calcium homeostatic mechanisms leading to more effective absorption from gut, renal calcium conservation, and a blunted PTH effect on bone.

Calcitonin may play a role in age-related bone loss, but this role remains to be clearly delineated; also, accumulation of structural errors, such as perforation of trabeculae by excessive osteoclastic resorption (as suggested by Parfitt), may be important.

Clearly, many factors are important in the determination of bone mass, and it is only through a better understanding of these mechanisms that a rational approach to prevention of bone loss can be derived.

It has generally been assumed that osteoporotic fractures of the vertebrae, distal radius, and hip are of similar pathogenesis. Riggs, however, suggests that there are several osteoporotic syndromes. Type 1 osteoporosis is associated with excessive trabecular bone loss leading to vertebral collapse fractures and to Colles fractures, especially among women aged 50 to 65 years of age. It is postulated that estrogen deficiency leads to an increased sensitivity of bone to the action of PTH, and that this activity causes loss of bone. The calcium mobilized with bone loss reduces PTH secretion, but not sufficiently to prevent excessive bone loss; however, since serum PTH concentration is reduced, less $1,25(OH)_2D_3$ is synthesized by the kidney, and calcium malabsorption ensues. Since all women are estrogen-deficient after menopause, and no measured difference in sex hormone concentrations has been found between the majority who do not develop osteoporosis and the small group who do, Riggs postulates that there is some undefined intrinsic abnormality of bone which predisposes to excessive loss with estrogen deficiency. Nordin has suggested that the osteoporotics have more marked calcium malabsorption, but this should lead to increased secretion of PTH, and Riggs has found PTH concentrations to be low in this group, compared to controls; thus, the predisposing factors remain to be determined.

Type 2 osteoporosis is associated with loss of both trabecular and cortical bone, and eventuates in both hip and vertebral fractures. It occurs primarily in individuals over age 75, and although more common in women, also affects men. It is postulated that there is a primary defect in $1,25(OH)_2D_3$ synthesis, leading to calcium malabsorption and secondary hyperparathyroidism with increased bone turnover. Since there is a negative remodeling balance at individual sites, bone loss occurs.

There is accumulating evidence from Riggs, his associates and others that the different fracture syndromes generally associated with osteoporosis may be due to different mechanisms of bone loss. This concept is important in designing effective programs for prophylaxis and treatment. Clearly, we would not wish to introduce a therapeutic program to prevent one fracture type which would lead to an enhanced chance of developing another fracture syndrome.

The important clinical problem of steroid-induced osteoporosis was reviewed by Avioli. Glucocorticoids seem to produce, primarily, loss of trabecular bone and thus, vertebral fractures. The effect is dose- and time-dependent, but can occur with as little as 7 mg of Prednisone a day, or its equivalent. Those particularly at risk are growing children, postmenopausal women, and those receiving other drugs which may affect the skeleton, such as anti-convulsants. Glucocorticoids have multiple effects which are responsible for bone loss, including impaired calcium absorption, increased calcium excretion by the kidney, and impaired osteoblast function.

No effective means is currently available to prevent these complications, other then reduction in dose and time of administration, when possible. A new glucocorticoid under development, Deflazacort, shows promise of being less deleterious to mineral homeostasis than currently available drugs.

Prevention and Treatment

The treatment of osteoporosis must be considered both from the standpoint of prevention of bone loss and therapy of the patient after fracture has occurred. Lindsay reviewed the evidence that administration of estrogen can prevent loss of bone in postmenopausal women. This effect has been demonstrated, using a number of techniques which measure both cortical and trabecular bone. On therapy, bone loss can be prevented up to eight years, when slow loss may begin. When estrogen is withdrawn, loss ensues, but is no greater than the loss occurring after natural menopause. Administration of estrogen is also associated with less loss of height and fewer vertebral deformities than occur in placebo-treated controls. Christiansen has also noted that a combination of estrogen and progesterone prevents cortical bone loss. The principal problem of prophylaxis with estrogen is the determination of who should receive the drug, since it is not without toxicity. Christiansen has found that there is a population of rapid bone losers that, he predicts, will develop osteoporosis. These women have lower estrogen concentrations, higher serum alkaline phosphatase, and higher urinary hydroxyproline/creatinine ratios than those losing more slowly. This problem requires additional study, but these data provide promising leads to the development of a simple screening procedure for the selection of women for prophylactic estrogen therapy shortly after the onset of menopause.

Chesnut and associates have demonstrated that administration of calcitonin to patients with osteoporotic fractures leads to an increase in total body calcium, measured by neutron activation. This increase persisted for 18 months, but by 26 months, the rate of gain was not sustained. There was no change in regional bone mass measured by photon absorptiometry. The calcitonin was well tolerated by the patients, with few adverse reactions. This group has also demonstrated that administration of Stanozolol to a similar population of postmenopausal osteoporotic patients is associated with a significant increase in total body calcium at 26 months on therapy. The magnitude of the increase in calcium retention seemed to persist throughout the study. Analysis of biochemical and histologic data suggested that the effect of the drug was to stimulate bone formation. There were transient elevations in SGOT in a number of patients, as well as some evidence of increased facial hair, ankle edema, and hoarseness. In neither of the studies were there sufficient numbers of patients to determine whether there was a reduction in fracture incidence.

Meunier presented data on 57 osteoporotic patients treated for two years with a combination of sodium fluoride, calcium, and vitamin D. No control group was included. Fifty-six percent of the patients experienced relief from back pain after two years on therapy. The incidence of vertebral fracture was lower in the second year of treatment than in the first, and the mean annual increase in the radiological vertebral index was also reduced during the second year. There were no significant changes in the biochemical parameters measured. Bone biopsies were performed before and after treatment in 11 patients classified as good responders. These biopsies showed that there was a marked increase in the osteoid surfaces and osteoblastic surfaces, without an increase in the resorption surfaces. There was a marked increase in trabecular bone volume in these biopsies. The newly-formed bone was lamellar in character. No microradiographs were performed, but there is some evidence in the literature to suggest that the newly-formed bone is not as well calcified as is normal bone. Side effects consisted of mild GI irritation in 22% of the patients and transient periarticular pain in 33% of the patients, but only 7% of the patients discontinued therapy because of adverse reaction. Some of the patients treated with fluoride did not appear to respond to the therapy. Dr. Meunier found that some of these showed no response on formation surfaces, while others had increased formation surfaces, but did not gain bone. The mechanisms for these changes remain to be elucidated.

Initial studies have been undertaken to evaluate the effect of $1,25(OH)_2D_3$ in the treatment of osteoporosis and these were reviewed by Dr. Gallagher. Some evidence suggests that postmenopausal osteoporotics have a low concentration of $1,25(OH)_2D_3$. When this drug was given in a preliminary study, there was a significant increase in bone volume at 24 months, measured on iliac crest biopsies. The calcium balance improved, so that it became positive after six months; but subsequently, a less positive balance was found. There appeared to be a significant decrease in vertebral fractures in the treated group. Additional studies will be necessary to evaluate this therapeutic agent in the treatment of osteoporosis.

A new approach to the treatment of osteoporosis has been developed, and is currently under evaluation. The "ADFR" method was reviewed by Dr. Frost. An agent known to activate bone remodeling is administered in pulsatile fashion, in order to simultaneously activate a number of the bone remodeling units; then, a medication which will depress osteoclastic activity during the resorptive phase is administered, thus reducing the amount of bone removed. Subsequently, a free period is allowed, so that the osteoblasts will replace their programmed quantum of bone. Since the osteoclasts have removed less bone, bone balance will be positive. The entire sequence can then be repeated. This method was developed based on the current understanding of bone function as an organ. Preliminary data from animal studies appears to indicate that the sequence will produce its desired effect.

Clearly, progress has been made over the past decade in our understanding of osteoporosis. Use of the bone biopsy has led to a better understanding of the pathogenesis of age-related bone loss, although controversy still remains. It is apparent that efforts should be focused on that period of rapid bone loss which occurs shortly after menopause, to clarify our understanding of this phenomenon. Many factors may be important in the development of maximum adult bone mass and its subsequent rate of loss, including mechanical loading, hormonal influences, and nutrition factors. These all provide fertile areas for additional research during the next few years. The fracture syndromes generally associated with osteoporosis may be due to different pathogenic mechanisms; thus, an approach to prevention and treatment may require awareness of this heterogeneity. Therapeutic modalities for the patient with osteoporosis are growing, with evidence accumulating that fracture rates can be reduced. The application of the ADFR theory may allow even further advances. Progress is being made to identify patients who will subsequently be at risk of fracture; thus, a rational prophylaxis can be designed. Clearly, the next decade should provide exciting, new insights into the pathogenesis and treatment of osteoporosis.

THE DETERMINANTS OF BONE VOLUME IN YOUNG ADULTS

J. Aaron, K. Sagreiya, D. Carter and B.E.C. Nordin

M.R.C. Mineral Metabolism Unit, Leeds
and Department of Endocrinology, Royal Adelaide Hospital, Adelaide

INTRODUCTION

In previous publications (1,2,3) we have suggested that trabecular bone volume at equilibrium is determined by the relationship between bone formation rate on the one hand and fractional bone resorption on the other. In these previous papers, we relied on the total forming surface as the measure of bone formation rate. We now present a further analysis of the samples from 40 young normal adults in which we have been able to use seam width as a measure of appositional rate. The results serve to strengthen our original hypothesis.

CLINICAL MATERIALS AND METHODS

The analysis is based on iliac crest samples taken with a 7 mm internal diameter trephine from 21 females below the age of 49 and 19 males below the age of 55 who died after a short illness not known to affect bone metabolism. The samples were fixed in 10% buffered formalin, embedded in methyl methacrylate and cut into 48 sections with a Jung heavy duty microtome. Four fields of each of 16 sections were examined with a Zeiss integrating eyepiece. Trabecular bone volume was determined by point-counting (magnification x 50); forming (osteoid-covered) and resorption (crenated) surfaces by intercept-counting (x 80); and mean seam width by direct measurement (x 400).

Trabecular bone volume (V) is expressed in mm^3/mm^3 of total volume; total surface (TS), forming surface (FS) and resorption surface (RS) in mm^2/mm^3 of total volume; and the latter also as a percentage of total surface (%RS); and mean seam width in microns.

In a separate clinical study on 86 cases with a variety of metabolic disorders other than osteomalacia, double tetracycline labelling was employed and the appositional rate determined from the mean space between the labelled bands.

RESULTS

Simple Regression Analysis

The relationship between mean seam width and appositional rate in the 86 clinical cases is shown in Fig. 1. The correlation is highly significant ($r = .693$: $P < .001$), as previously noted by Parfitt (4). We conclude that it is possible to use mean seam width as a measure of appositional rate in the absence of osteomalacia. The mean values of the measured variables in the 40 cases are shown below. None of the differences between the males and females is significant, and the data from the two sexes have therefore been pooled.

	AGE(yrs)	V(mm^3)	FS(mm^2)	SW(u)	RS(mm^2)	TS(mm^2)	%RS
Mean	41.4	.22	.21	9.1	.15	2.9	5.7
S.E.	9.3	.01	.15	2.0	.07	0.10	0.45

The significant correlations are those between total resorption surface and formation surface ($r=.689:P<.001$); between resorption surface and total surface ($r=.493:P<.002$); and between volume and total surface ($r=.382:P<.02$). None of the correlations with age is significant. Seam width is inversely but not significantly related to total volume.

The relation between total forming and total resorption surface in the 40 cases is shown in Fig. 2. As indicated above, the correlation is highly significant, as would be expected if these were real measures of bone formation and resorption in subjects in bone equilibrium. The mean value of FS is about 1.5 times the mean value of RS, which suggests that the resorption front advances about 50% faster than the formation front if the bone is in equilibrium.

Multiple Regression Analysis

Our model postulates that bone volume at equilibrium is determined by the relation between bone formation rate and fractional bone resorption. The regression of volume on forming surface and total resorption surface is given by the equation

$$V = 16.5\ FS^* - 18.5\ RS + .22 \quad (R = .368^*)$$

The correlation with RS is negative but not significant. This is what would be expected; the ratio of FS to RS determines whether a subject is losing or gaining bone but does not determine the equilibrium volume. However, regression of volume on forming surface and percent surface resorption yields are more significant result:

$$V = 23.3\ FS^{**} - 1.2\ \%RS^{**} + .23 \quad (R = .502^{**})$$

When total surface is regressed in this way on forming surface, seam width and resorption surface (absolute or fractional), the only significant correlation to emerge is the positive one between total surface and resorption surface already described.

It is also possible to calculate bone lifespan from our model; at equilibrium, the lifespan in days is the volume in mm^3 divided by the daily bone formation rate in the same units. FS is the forming surface and SW is a measure of appositional rate so FS x SW is a measure of the bone formation rate. Since the mean value of FS is .21 mm^2 and the mean seam width is 9.1 μ, the mean product is about 1.9 x 10-3 mm^3 which represents the formation rate per twenty days, if a calcification lag time of twenty days is assumed, or 0.95 x 10-4 mm^3/day. Since the mean bone volume is .21 mm^2, the mean lifespan is about 2,000 days (.21/.95x10-4). The lifespan is inversely related to percent surface resorption, as would be expected from the model, but because the product of lifespan and fractional resorption rate should be constant we have plotted log lifespan against log %RS as shown in Fig. 3. This yields a correlation coefficient of

-.504 ($P < .001$). A higher r value is obtained (-.637) by applying the Spearman correlation coefficient to the original data. A high fractional resorption is bound to shorten lifespan. (The same is true of red cell survival; a haemolytic anaemia may be due to a fault in the red cells or in the environment).

Fractional surface resorption is not of course synonymous with fractional volume resorption but might be expected to be related to it. In young normal adults at bone equilibrium, the bone formation and resorption rates must be equal, and BFR divided by volume in this group therefore represents fractional volume. When this is plotted against surface resorption, it transpires that %RS is numerically very close to % volume resorption per 100 days (Fig. 4).

DISCUSSION

It is clear that the data are compatible with the proposed model, i.e. that bone volume is determined by the relationship between an independent variable - bone formation rate - on the one hand and a volume-dependent variable - fractional bone resorption - on the other. At high percentage calcification fronts, the bone formation rate must be the product of the forming surface and the appositional rate, and we have used mean seam width as a measure of the latter. This yields a mean bone formation rate of about 10-4 mm^3 per day per mm of whole biopsy volume and a mean lifespan of about six years.

As far as resorption is concerned, the positive correlation between formation and resorption surface is what would be expected in cases at bone equilibrium (which is what we assume these young adults to be) and suggest that these two variables are appropriate measures of the bone formation and resorption rates. There is no method at present of actually measuring the advance of the resorption front and therefore no way of expressing resorption rate as a fraction of volumes. It is clearly appropriate, however, to express resorption surface as a fraction of total surface because these two variables are closely related, and it is highly likely that fractional volume resorption rate is a function of fractional surface resorption. This presumably explains why (as would be expected from the model) fractional surface resorption yields higher inverse correlations with bone volume (on multiple regression analysis) than does total resorption surface.

REFERENCES

1. Nordin, B.E.C., Aaron, J., Speed, R. and Crilly, R.G. Bone formation and resorption as the determinants of trabecular bone volume in postmenopausal osteoporosis. Lancet 2, 277-279, 1981.
2. Nordin, B.E.C., Aaron, J. A New Model for Osteoporosis. In: Vitamin D. Chemical, Biochemical and Clinical Endocrinology of Calcium Metabolism. Walter de Gruyter & Co. Berlin, 1982, pp. 921-923.
3. Nordin, B.E.C., Aaron, J., and Speed, R. A New Model for Osteoporosis. In: Osteoporosis. Eds. J. Menczel et al. Wiley, New York, 1982, pp. 21-25.

4. Parfitt, A.M., Mathews, C., Rao, D., Frame, B., Koleerekoper,M. and Villanuva, A.R.
Impaired osteoblast function in metabolic bone disease.
In: Osteoporosis: Recent advances in pathogenesis and treatment. Eds. H.F. DeLuca et al, University Path Press, Baltimore, 1981, pp. 321-330.

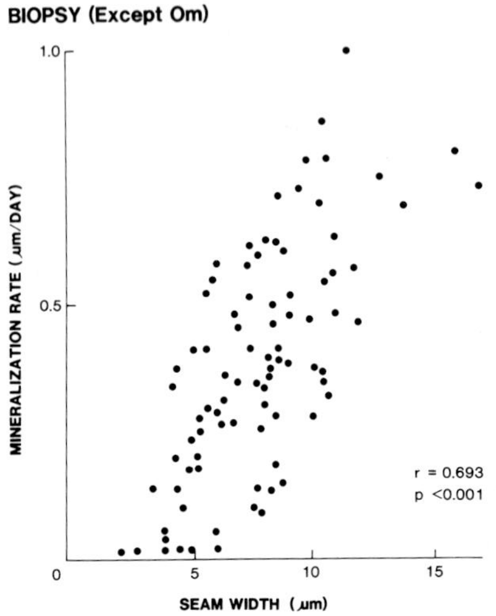

Fig. 1: The relation between seam width and appositional rate in 86 cases of metabolic bone disorder other than osteomalacia.

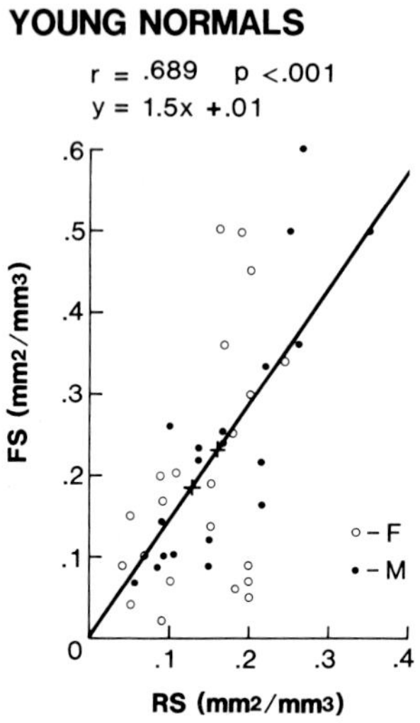

Fig. 2: The relation between total resorption surface and total forming surface in 40 young normal adults.

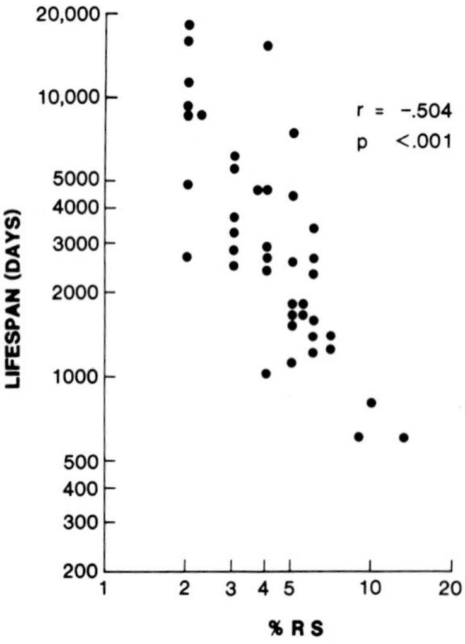

Fig. 3: The relation between percent resorption surface and lifespan in 40 young normal adults.

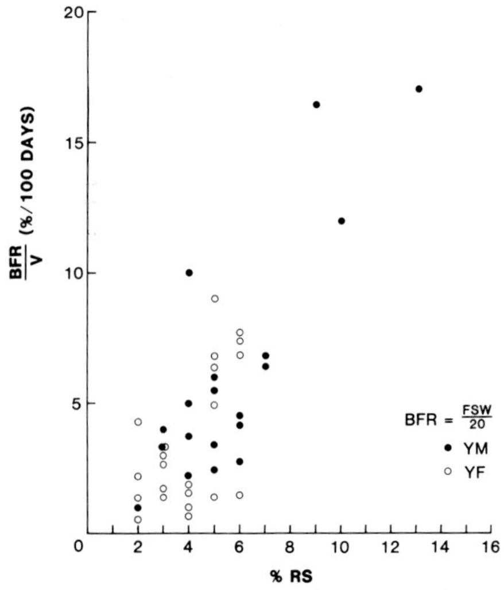

Fig. 4: The relation between percent resorption surface and percent of bone volume being formed per 100 days in 40 young normal adults.

Discussion after C. Nordin presentation:

P. MEUNIER: What do you designate as formation surfaces - osteoblast surfaces with mineralization fronts, or total osteoid surfaces?

C. NORDIN: For this analysis, I have used the total osteoid-covered surface. It would give slightly different values, but wouldn't affect the principle if I used forming surfaces with mineralization fronts. I am going to reanalyze the data on that basis, but it won't make any major difference in substance.

H. FROST: Kinetic studies using double labeling have repeatedly shown that the rates of formation do not reliably relate to the fraction of the surface covered by osteoid in osteoporotic patients with no mineralization defect.

S. OTT: We have looked at bone biopsies from 23 osteoporotic women who have normal mineralization. The apposition rate is normal, but the percent of the osteoid-covered surface that takes up tetracycline labels varies from 3 to 90%. A significant number of the biopsies have less than half of the osteoid-covered surface taking up tetracycline labels.

C. NORDIN: The principle of the model is that bone formation is an independent variable. I applied the principle in the simplest possible way by using percent resorbing surfaces and total forming surfaces. I am prepared to believe that it could be applied by taking only the surfaces with mineralization fronts; or again, only the surfaces that take up the tetracycline labels. It would shift all my points slightly to the left or slightly to the right, but it is unlikely that it would make any difference to the concept of the model. Dr. Parfitt showed me yesterday how he uses tetracycline-labeled surfaces, and I am quite prepared to accept that as an improvement, but a lot of my material is obtained post-mortem.

J. IVY: If you are looking at crenated bone surfaces, the length of time after resorption has occurred until new formation starts may vary tremendously. If you are looking at patients with osteoporosis, the resorption may have occurred 5 to 10 years previously.

C. NORDIN: The fact remains that crenated surface, which I take to be resorption surface or a measure of resorption, is twice as high relative to total formation surface in postmenopausal women that it is in premenopausal women, and the bone volume is reduced by almost half in the postmenopausal, as compared to the premenopausal subjects. This is an extraordinary coincidence if what you say is correct.

MICROSTRUCTURAL AND CELLULAR BASIS OF AGE RELATED BONE LOSS AND OSTEOPOROSIS

A.M. Parfitt, C.H.E. Mathews, A.R. Villanueva, D.S. Rao, M. Rogers, M. Kleerekoper, B. Frame

Henry Ford Hospital, Detroit, MI U.S.A.

It is obvious that for bone loss to occur the rate of total body bone resorption must exceed the rate of total body bone formation. In terms of the quantum concept, this imbalance must be focal and must apply to the average remodeling cycle on any surface that is losing bone (1). The relative contributions of increased number and/or activity of osteoclasts and decreased number and/or activity of osteoblasts to focal imbalance remains controversial. We have approached this problem in two ways - first, by defining more accurately the structural changes that occur in trabecular bone with age and in osteoporosis and second, by relating abnormalities of bone cell function demonstrated and inferred, to the observed structural changes.

We partition trabecular bone volume (TBV) into two components, an index of the thickness of structural elements (mean trabecular plate thickness - MTPT) and an index of the number of structural elements (mean trabecular plate density - MTPD). MTPT is obtained indirectly by standard stereologic calculations applied to perimeter and area measurements in the two-dimensional section. MTPD is obtained by dividing volume by thickness according to the equation MTPD(/mm) = TBV%/MTPT (μm)x10. MTPD is numerically equal to one-half the surface density (bone surface area/unit volume of tissue), but expresses a different concept in different units. MTPD is an index of the frequency with which a scanning line will intersect the two dimensional profiles of structural elements and is the reciprocal of the mean distance between structural elements in a single direction of scanning. In 78 normal subjects there was a significant linear fall in TBV with age in both sexes and this was due mainly to a fall in MTPD with a much smaller change in MTPT. The further reduction in TBV in 70 female patients with osteoporosis and compression fractures, was due mainly to a further reduction in MTPD. This indicates that the loss of trabecular bone with age and the further loss in patients with osteoporosis is due mainly to complete removal of some structural elements, those remaining being only slightly reduced in thickness but more widely separated. Reduction in thickness made a more significant contribution to the bone loss in 30 male patients with vertebral compression fractures and in 50 patients of both sexes with hip fracture. In some normal subjects, mean trabecular thickness appears to increase with age, presumably as a compensatory mechanism in response to a reduction in plate density. Failure of this process may contribute to the structural changes in osteoporosis.

The reduction in mean wall thickness with age is a likely explanation for the reduction in mean trabecular thickness, but it is unlikely that this mechanism can be responsible for complete removal of structural elements. First, significant reduction in MTPD occurs before there has been any significant fall in MTPT. Second, the frequency distribution of directly measured thickness showed no accumulation with age of thinner than normal structural elements (2). Third, mean interstitial bone thickness increases with age (3), but a decrease is necessary for complete removal. Fourth, the range of values for mean wall thickness, the frequency of remodeling activation and the duration of the remodeling cycle indicate that complete loss of a structural element as the end result of progressive thinning would take far too long to account for the observed rate of fall in MTPD. Consequently, the most plausible disorder of bone cell function to explain removal of entire structural elements is increased depth of osteoclastic resorption cavities leading to focal perforation of trabecular plates, as previously suggested by Arnold (4). This process could account for the stepwise reduction in trabecular bone mineral density observed by computed tomography (4) and probably occurs during the first 3-5 years after menopause when there is both kinetic and biochemical evidence of increased bone resorption, and when bone loss is most rapid. A similar mechanism probably underlies loss of cortical bone. Mean net bone loss at the cortical endosteal surface in the metacarpal is 50 μm/yr (6), but the maximum loss explainable by reduced mean wall thickness is less than 10 m/yr. The role of greatly enlarged subendosteal resorption cavities in cortical bone loss is well established (4,7).

We also made kinetic measurements after double tetracycline labeling in 46 patients with postmenopausal osteoporosis and vertebral compression fracture and 42 healthy white females. Thirty-five patients were completely untreated and 11 were receiving a calcium supplement of 0.5-2.0 g/d; there was no significant difference in any measurement between the two groups so that the results were pooled. In the normal subjects there was a significant fall with age in the mineral apposition rate, the fraction of osteoid labeled, and the product of these two measurements, referred to as corrected apposition rate, which in the absence of osteomalacia is an index of the mean rate of matrix synthesis by individual teams of osteoblasts. For all three measurements the mean values in the osteoporotic patients were significantly below age-predicted values based on the regressions on age in the normal subjects. This indicates that osteoblast function declines with age, and has declined more in patients with osteoporosis. This decline is partly the result of fewer osteoblast precursors because of the age-related shift from hematopoietic to fatty marrow, and possibly also reflects a defect in the transmission or detection of a coupling signal, whether biochemical or biophysical (6,8). Whatever the reason, defective osteoblast function is the likely explanation for the lower mean wall thickness in patients with osteoporosis than in normal subjects of the same age (9).

In the normal subjects there was a modest increase in bone formation rate after menopause, whether expressed per unit of bone surface, per unit of bone volume, or per unit of tissue volume, but a relatively greater increase in osteoclast covered surface and in resorption rate calculated indirectly, assuming the rate of bone loss indicated by the regression of TBV on age. In the patients with osteoporosis, the bone formation rate expressed in the same three ways was significantly lower than expected for age, even though osteoid surface was not reduced. The results were similar in patients with and without a calcium supplement. Indirectly calculated bone resorption rate, based on several different models and assumptions was significantly lower than in normal subjects of similar age. There was a similar difference in direction and magnitude between osteoporotics and control subjects in osteoclast covered surface, but not in total crenated surface. The variance in the patients with osteoporosis was significantly greater than in normal subjects, and in a few patients bone formation rate and indirectly calculated resorption rate were significantly increased. In addition to defining the remodeling state in patients with osteoporosis, these data indicate that osteoid surface is not a valid index of formation rate and crenated surface is not a valid index of resorption rate in these patients (10).

CONCLUSIONS

1. After menopause total body bone resorption increases, as evidenced by kinetic, biochemical and histologic indices but total body bone formation increases less than in other high turnover states such as hyperthyroidism.
2. Increased depth of osteoclastic resorption cavities leads to perforation

of trabecular plates, which initiates removal of entire structural elements, leaving those that remain more widely separated. As a result there is less surface available for bone formation, and bone loss occurring by this mechanism is largely irreversible, emphasizing the need for prevention.

3. Rapid bone loss precipitated by estrogen deficiency and occurring by this mechanism is a necessary, but not a sufficient, condition for the occurrence of clinical osteoporosis and fractures.

4. Osteoblast function declines with age, with a reduction in both the rate and the amount of matrix synthesis by each osteoblast team, so that both mean wall thickness and the thickness of residual structural elements slowly decline with age.

5. In patients with osteoporosis and compression fractures, the structural changes in trabecular bone are qualitatively similar but more severe.

6. In osteoporosis matrix synthesis by each osteoblast team is further reduced in rate and amount, a magnification of the age-related trend, but remodeling activation and bone formation rate are also substantially reduced, a reversal of the age-related trend.

7. The transition from the postmenopausal increase in bone remodeling to the osteoporotic decrease in bone remodeling is unexplained, but it is likely to be one of the factors that selects patients who fracture from among the totality of women who lose bone.

8. Some patients with vertebral osteoporosis had too little bone to start with and have normal bone remodeling by the time of fracture, some had prolonged accelerated bone loss and have increased remodeling by the time of fracture, and some are unable to repair or compensate for accelerated bone loss and have decreased remodeling by the time of fracture. In this manner the histologic heterogeneity of osteoporosis can be reconciled with a unified concept of histopathogenesis.

9. It is impossible to construct a single mathematical model that expresses bone remodeling and bone mass as functions of time which applies to patients with osteoporosis as well as to normal subjects.

10. In most patients with osteoporosis mechanical weakness and fracture mainly reflect structural damage sustained many years earlier. The remodeling state at the time of biopsy may not be related to the reasons why the patient lost bone, but may be important in determining the response to treatment.

REFERENCES

1. Parfitt, A.M. (1979): Editorial, Calc. Tiss. Int. 28, 1.
2. Wakamatsu, E. and H.A. Sissons (1969): Calc. Tiss. Res. 4, 147.
3. Courpron, P. (1981): Orthop. Clin. North Am. 12, 513.
4. Arnold, J.S. (1970): In: Osteoporosis, p.80. Editor: U.S. Barzel. Grune and Stratton, N.Y.
5. Ruegsegger P. and M. Dambacher. This volume.
6. Parfitt, A.M. (1980). Henry Ford Hospital Medical Journal 28, 95.
7. Wu, K., and H.M. Frost (1967): J. Lab. Clin. Med. 69, 810.
8. Parfitt, A.M. (1982): Metabolic Bone Disease and Related Research 4, 1.
9. Darby, A.J. and P.J. Meunier (1981): Calc. Tiss. Int. 33, 199.
10. Nordin, B.E.C., Aaron, J., Speed R., and Crilly, R.G. (1981). Lancet ii, 277.

Discussion after M. Parfitt's presentation:

C. JOHNSTON: Dr. Parfitt, I think the most important information that you have presented is that there is an irreversible loss of trabecular bone due to osteoclastic resorption which occurs years before we see the patient.

M. PARFITT: I agree that the importance of distinguishing between the number of structural elements and the thickness of the elements is that once they have gone, they cannot be replaced. There is no surface available on which the osteoblast can build, whereas, if the bone trabeculae are just thin, at least the potential exists for reexpanding them to a normal size.

C. JOHNSTON: Could the resorption surface that Dr. Nordin sees be a marker for this process?

M. PARFITT: Yes, I suspect that total resorption or crenated surfaces are remnants of increased resorption that was completed at some time in the past.

C. NORDIN: For the record, I will define very briefly the area of disagreement. The changes at the menopause, which we define as beginning at age 50, are similar in our two analyses. We diverge when we come to the osteoporotic fracture cases, but only in one respect. I agree that, taking the group as a whole, there is reduced formation in the crush fracture cases. Where we differ is that Dr. Parfitt considers there is no increase in resorption, however you express it, compared to the normal menopausal woman. Our data show very clearly that there is a further increase of resorption in osteoporosis. It comes down to a fundamental difference in how we calculate resorption. I don't believe it is possible to measure resorption rates, unless individuals are in equilibrium. Then you can measure formation rates and deduce resorption rates. I have made no attempt to calculate resorption rate in any but young patients in equilibrium. I have said to Dr. Parfitt in the past, and will say it again now, that I cannot accept the way he is calculating resorption rates. The increase in resorption we find, compared to normal postmenopausal women, is highly compatible with our hydroxyproline data, which show very clearly that there is increased resorption in the osteoporotic patient.

M. PARFITT: In contrast to Dr. Nordin, I solved the differential equation resulting from his model, and the rates of resorption were calculated according to his model, with the assumption that the osteoporotics are losing 20% faster than the rate you would expect from the regression of trabecular bone volume on age.

P. MEUNIER: Postmenopausal osteoporosis is a heterogeneous disorder. We have found about 30% with high-remodelling disease (with increased resorption surfaces and increased appositional surfaces), about 20% with osteoblastic depression, and about 50% with no detectable abnormality. So, I think if we mixed all these patients in a single population, it would be difficult to interpret the physiology. Separating the three types also may be helpful in choosing proper treatment.

M. PARFITT: I agree about the heterogeneity. The variance of all the measurements in osteoporosis is increased. Although I didn't comment on it, I hope this was apparent from the standard deviations on my slides. The increased variance may not only be due to increased variation between subjects, but also to greater anatomical variation between one site and another. Also, the variance is no greater in the patients with osteoporosis than in patients who have a presumed single cause for this disease, such as primary hyperparathyroidism. I agree that the state of remodelling at the time of the biopsy may be helpful in deciding what treatment the patient should have. Finally, using the formation rate measured by tetracycline labeling, only about 5% have increased remodelling.

J. COMPSTON: All previous studies in normal subjects have shown no change in mineral apposition rate with age. Could your different results relate to the way your subjects were selected?

M. PARFITT: Yes, that is entirely possible. One cannot select individuals for biopsy by a random process. However, a fall in apposition rate with age was previously observed by Frost in the rib.

J. COMPSTON: Do your figures for bone formation rate agree numerically with Dr. Nordin's calculations from his model?

M PARFITT: I have not made that calculation.

J. REEVE: Could increased scatter about the mean value for trabecular plate thickness account for plate loss?

M. PARFITT: In 1969 Wakamatsu and Sissons measured the thickness of structural elements directly in autopsy material from normal subjects and found, just as we did, that there was very little reduction in thickness but a substantial increase in separation. They found no increase in very thin elements, less than 5% were thinner than 50 µm at all ages. If the mechanism for complete loss is an exaggeration of thinning, there should be an increase in the number of very thin structures with age.

DETERMINANTS OF AGE-RELATED BONE LOSS

Robert P. Heaney, Creighton University, Omaha, NE, U.S.A.

Human bone mass usually reaches its peak value sometime between ages 30 and 40, and thereafter declines with advancing age. This decline is particularly rapid in women in the 5-15 years following menopause. Reduction in bone mass comes about through bone remodeling, a process which is quantized in discrete packets throughout the skeleton. For bone mass to decrease significantly, these remodeling packets must, on average, resorb more bone than they replace by formation; and the overall rate of remodeling must be of sufficient magnitude to allow the imbalance at each remodeling locus to sum to appreciable changes in total skeletal mass.

Peak adult mass is the best available predictor of subsequent bone mass during aging. The principal factor known to influence peak achieved bone mass is genetic endowment. Probably mechanical loading and adequacy of nutrition are important in permitting full realization of genetic potential, but, within the usual range for adult activity and diet, direct evidence for their role is not yet available.

Thus bone mass at any age after the fourth decade can be expressed as the resultant of four elements: 1) peak bone mass achieved, 2) average remodeling balance, 3) remodeling rate, and 4) time. All other factors which influence age-related bone loss do so by affecting one or more of the first three. Principal among the factors affecting bone loss after the adult peak has been achieved are 5) mechanical loading; 6) nutritional status, especially effective calcium intake; 7) hormonal status, especially estrogen withdrawal at menopause; and 8) accumulated structural errors produced in successive waves of remodeling.

Mechanical loading acts principally to stimulate osteoblasts so that the formative phase of remodeling exceeds prior resorption. The exercise which often accompanies mechanical loading may also enhance release of somatotrophin, which both increases remodeling rate and stimulates osteoblasts in its own right. In any event, it is clear that bone mass declines with disuse, on one the hand, and increases with heavy loading on the other, and both changes seem to be substantially reversible in normal adult humans. Muscle mass decreases proportionately with bone during normal aging, and it seems likely that decreased physical activity with advancing age is a major cause of both changes. In any event, decreased mechanical loading presents the perimenopausal female with a bone remodeling status in which average balance at each remodeling locus is negative, and in which the aggregate rate of bone loss thus depends upon the remodeling rate.

Because the time constant for remodeling in adult bone is on the order of 0.5-1.5 years, there is a phase lag between actual skeletal mass and that mass directly needed for current mechanical loads. During the declining years of life this phase lag results in a buffer of excess bone, relative to current needs. This buffer constitutes the major protection against the unusual loads of falls and injuries; it is itself inversely related to remodeling rate.

Other things being equal the principal determinant of remodeling rate is parathyroid hormone (PTH). High effective calcium intakes, by suppressing endogenous PTH release, also suppress bone remodeling rate. It is less clear whether variations in calcium intake within the usual range of dietary variation have an appreciable effect on age-related bone loss. Nevertheless it is reasonably certain that inadequate intake exaggerates the rate of bone loss caused by other factors. Calcium intake is known to fall with age, and there is some evidence that absorption efficiency also falls, with the result being that effective intake falls even more than actual intake.

In this connection it is now recognized that other nutrients and many drugs interfere with calcium retention, and thus effectively increase the calcium intake requirement. Principal among these are diets high in protein and fiber, as well as excesses of alcohol, caffeine, and aluminum-containing antacids. High phosphorus intakes, contrary to some speculation, do not appear to affect calcium balance or to alter calcium intake requirement. Finally, calcium intake is important because it may limit achievement of the maximum genetic potential for peak bone mass.

Estrogen, by mechanisms not well understood, also suppresses overall remodeling rate, and hence prior to menopause minimizes the negative bone balance associated with decreased mechanical loading and maximizes the buffer of excess bond associated with the remodeling phase lag. But at menopause estrogen withdrawal leads to an increase in bone remodeling, and hence - with the average remodeling locus in negative balance - to an accelerated rate of bone loss. Further, estrogen acts on the calcium homeostatic mechanisms to enhance both calcium absorption from the diet and renal calcium conservation, as well as to blunt PTH-mediated calcium release from bone. Hence at menopause external calcium metabolism deteriorates and, unless calcium intake is quite high, bone comes to play a larger role in meeting the calcium needs of the extracellular fluid.

Somatotrophin, as already noted, both stimulates osteoblasts and increases overall remodeling rate. In excess, as in acromegaly, it leads to increased bone mass. Somatotrophin production declines with age, and while the precise role of this decrease in age-related bone loss remains unknown, these two age-related changes are at least concordant.

The role of calcitonin (CT) remains unclear. It had previously been reported that immunoreactive CT production falls with age, but recent studies using techniques which measure principally the intact circulating hormone, have not confirmed this finding. Similarly, estrogen has been shown to enhance CT release in response to hypercalcemia, and it has been speculated that the estrogen effect on bone remodeling is mediated through such CT release, but this suggestion remains unconfirmed and it seems unlikely, on other grounds, to be a full and satisfactory explanation for the estrogen effect in bone.

A further factor in age-related bone loss, analogous to aging effects in other tissues, is the accumulation, through successive cycles of bone remodeling, of what can perhaps be called "structural errors". Principal among these would be perforation of trabecular plates in cancellous bone and the excavation of overlarge resorption cavities during Haversian remodeling in compact bone. Both changes appear to be at least partly irreversible.

In normal remodeling, osteoblastic new bone formation is confined to surfaces previously eroded by osteoclastic resorption. When trabecular plates are perforated, the rim remaining around the perforation presents less surface for subsequent osteoblastic work than would have been the case if only a shallow excavation had been made in the trabecular plate. Thus aging in trabecular bone seems to consist in part of a one-way conversion of plates to spicules. In Haversian remodeling, wall thickness of newly deposited bone is limited by the need to nourish the ring of osteocytes most distant from the central canal, and when the diameter of the resorbed cavity is large, the resulting central canal at completion of the remodeling cycle is large also. Thus Haversian remodeling during aging results in increased microscopic porosity in cortical bone. Neither the trabecular nor the cortical process needs be considered abnormal per se: each may represent simply one tail of a distribution of remodeling events. Their significance lies in their effective irreversibility and hence in their tendency to accumulate over time.

The interplay of these several factors, as outlined in the foregoing, is depicted schematically in the following figure.

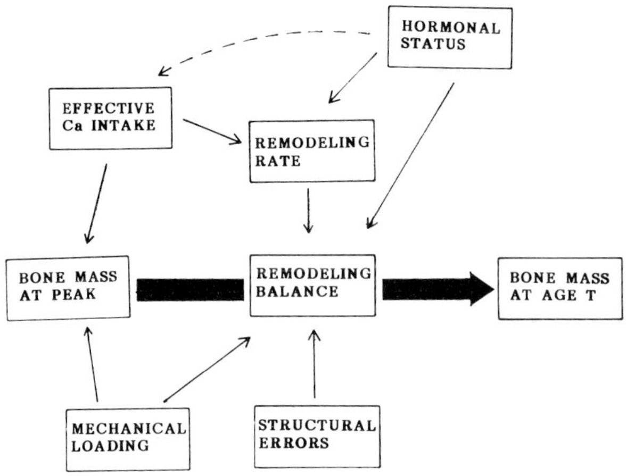

Discussion after R. Heaney's presentation:

C. JOHNSTON: Are you suggesting that mechanical loading decreases in the population, and if that were prevented, then age-related bone loss would be prevented?

R. HEANEY: I am suggesting that mechanical loading does decrease in the general population with aging. I submit to you that this is a fact of every-day experience. If that were reversed, I would predict that age-related bone loss would be much reduced, except for the impact of such things as the irreversible structural errors which occur with remodelling as Dr. Parfitt has stated.

R. LINDSAY: What is the relative importance of total bone mass at maturity in comparison to subsequent rate of loss?

R. HEANEY: I will refer that question to Dr. Johnston.

C. JOHNSTON: The genetic component, which as we previously reported, may include prenatal environmental influences, is large but I can't give a percent figure. It requires further longitudinal studies.

L. LANYON: There are at least three components of an individual's activity rating that could contribute to age-related bone loss. One is the peak strain induced. Most elderly people are less active and develop lower peak strains. The second is the rate of strain, and old people are generally less vigorous than young people. And the third is the diversity of activity, and although some old people do some very diverse things, the general trend is to greater uniformity. Another point is that perhaps we are getting a pessimistic view by looking at iliac bone biopsies. In bone with greater load bearing maybe it is possible for cancellous bone to reestablish continuity.

R. HEANEY: Your first comment represented in greater detail the data of everyday experience to which I referred earlier. Concerning your second point, I think one needs to postulate only effective irreveresbility, not an intrinsic irreversibility for the structural changes.

E. MEEMA: We measured the muscle mass of the forearm and the bone mass of the radius in women, both in relation to aging and to menopause. In both cases, bone mass was lost one decade before muscle mass was lost, which does not support the importance of mechanical factors.

R. HEANEY: That may have been the wrong muscle mass to measure, inasmuch as the forearm muscles, if I recall my anatomy, are working more on the hand and wrist than they are on the forearm bones, so that perhaps it should have been the upper arm muscles that would have related best with the forearm bones.

R. NORDIN: My only point of disagreement is that I don't find any fall in calcium absorption among normal women at menopause. A quick question: how do you explain the very striking rise in fracture rates with age, if the loss of bone is proportional to the loss in soft tissue?

R. HEANEY: It takes a large number of studies, correcting for calcium intake, to see this effect since there is such a large spread of data. I cannot explain the temporal discontinuity in fracture rates. It is unlikely that muscle mass changes as precipitously as the Colles fracture rate.

HETEROGENEITY OF INVOLUTIONAL OSTEOPOROSIS: EVIDENCE FOR TWO DISTINCT OSTEOPOROSIS SYNDROMES

B. Lawrence Riggs, L. J. Melton III, and H. W. Wahner

Endocrinology Research Unit, Division of Endocrinology and Metabolism and Internal Medicine, Department of Medical Statistics and Epidemiology, Section of Diagnostic Nuclear Medicine, Mayo Clinic and Mayo Foundation, Rochester, MN, U.S.A.

Bone responds to adverse stimuli in a limited number of ways. Thus, osteoporosis may be the final common response of bone loss from various types of abnormalities in bone and calcium metabolism. In this communication, we summarize evidence which suggests involutional osteoporosis can be divided into two distinct syndromes. Type I osteoporosis occurs in a relatively small subset of postmenopausal women who are 51 to 65 years of age. Less frequently, a similar syndrome occurs in men of comparable age. Type II osteoporosis occurs in a large proportion of women or men who are older than 75 years of age. Osteoporosis occurring in the decade from 66 to 75 years may represent a combination of both types. We prefer the terms Type I osteoporosis and Type II osteoporosis to the more familiar terms of postmenopausal osteoporosis and senile osteoporosis which we feel are semantically inadequate.

TYPE I OSTEOPOROSIS

This classic form of the disease was described in 1940 by Dr. Fuller Albright and his associates and characteristically occurs in women within 10 to 15 years of menopause. Less commonly, men are affected with a form of osteoporosis that is otherwise indistinguishable from that occurring in postmenopausal women. Vertebral fracture is the main clinical manifestation of this type of osteoporosis but Colles' fracture of the distal radius occurs frequently. Both of these fracture sites contain large amounts of trabecular bone.

We (1) have recently evaluated bone mineral density (BMD) in the appendicular and axial skeleton in 105 normal women and in 27 women, ages 51 to 65 years, with vertebral fractures due to the osteoporosis using single and dual photon absorptiometry (Table 1). At a site in the radius which contains predominantly cortical bone, mean BMD was only slightly lower than normal and only 4 of the osteoporotic women were below the age-adjusted normal range. Discrimination was much better, however, for the lumbar spine, which consists primarily of trabecular bone and 20 of the 27 women had values below the normal range. These findings strongly suggest that patients with Type I osteoporosis have lost disproportionately large amounts of trabecular bone from the axial skeleton. Thus, this syndrome may be equivalent to that which Nordin has called accelerated osteoporosis (1).

Table 1. Mean Z-scores in women with osteoporotic fractures. The Z-score is the deviation in standard deviations from the age-regression for normal women.

	N	Radius	Lumbar spine	Femoral neck
Ages 51-65 years				
Only vertebral fractures	27	-0.75†	-1.92¶	--
Ages >75 years				
Hip ± vertebral fractures	22	+0.41	+0.24	0.31*
Only vertebral fractures	19	-0.30	-0.50	--

For difference from predicted normal: $^*P \leq 0.05$, $^\dagger P \leq 0.01$, ¶$P \leq 0.001$

For Type I osteoporosis, the predilection for women and the temporal proximity of the menopause implicate estrogen deficiency as an etiologic agent. Longitudinal studies of appendicular, mainly cortical, bone loss after oophorectomy have shown accelerated bone loss (total of about 8% over predicted) for about 7 years (3). The extent of axial, mainly trabecular, bone loss due to estrogen deficiency is controversial but may be quantitatively similar to appendicular bone loss (4). The negative calcium balance induced by menopause is associated with an increase in bone turnover, with bone resorption increasing more than bone formation (5). The mechanism by which menopause accelerates bone loss is now better understood than formerly. Heaney's and Nordin's groups have theorized that estrogen deficiency might increase responsiveness of bone to circulating endogenous PTH. Direct evidence supporting this mechanism was provided by our demonstration (6) that estrogen treatment of women with Type I osteoporosis decreased bone resorption (assessed by microradiography of biopsy specimens) but increased serum iPTH. It has been suggested that the menopause decreases calcitonin secretion (7); if so, this would be an additional factor which exacerbates bone loss.

We have found that parathyroid function is normal or decreased in most patients with Type I osteoporosis (8). This does not preclude a permissive or sustaining role for PTH in maintaining bone resorption, however, because when estrogen is deficient, bone resorption is enhanced. Indeed, hypoparathyroid women have denser vertebrae at any age than do normal women (9). A consistent feature of Type I osteoporosis is subnormal calcium absorption. In untreated patients with postmenopausal osteoporosis, we found that circulating levels of 25-hydroxyvitamin D (25-OH-D) were normal but that levels of serum 1,25-dihydroxyvitamin D ($1,25(OH)_2D$) were significantly reduced (10). In addition, reduction in calcium absorption correlated positively with reduction of serum $1,25(OH)_2D$ and administration of a small and probably physiologic dose of $1,25(OH)_2D$ normalized calcium absortion. These data suggest that impaired metabolism of 25-OH-D to $1,25(OH)_2D$ is mainly responsible for the observed decrease in calcium absorption. Decreased production of $1,25(OH)_2D$ in osteoporosis does not appear to be a primary (intrinsic) defect of renal 25-OH-D 1α-hydroxylase activity, however, as we have found that following administration of parathyroid extract, the increase in serum $1,25(OH)_2D$ was similar in both control and Type I osteoporotic subjects (11). Although all of these findings have not been confirmed uniformly, they are sufficiently consistent to suggest the model shown below for Type I osteoporosis. The resultant changes in calcium metabolism, therefore, are the secondary consequences of increased bone loss.

TYPE I OSTEOPOROSIS
("Postmenopausal" Osteoporosis)

Estrogen deficiency → Incr. bone loss ← Other factors

Incr. bone loss
↓
Decr. PTH secretion
↓
Decr. $1,25(OH)_2D$ production
↓
Decr. calcium absorption

Because all postmenopausal women are relatively estrogen deficient but only some develop osteoporosis, factor(s) in addition to menopause must determine individual susceptibility. In a matched group of postmenopausal women with and without vertebral compression fractures, we were unable to find any significant difference in serum concentations of a battery of 12 different hormones, including free estradiol, free estrone, free testosterone, and androstenedione (12). Nor could we confirm the suggestion that such differences were present only below the age of 65 years. Thus, we still favor our original theory (13) that subjects who develop postmenopausal osteoporosis have an intrinsic abnormality that predisposes to accelerated bone loss in the absence of estrogen.

TYPE II OSTEOPOROSIS

The type of osteoporosis occurring in persons 75 years of age or older differs clinically from the type previously described. Hip fracture, which is uncommon in Type I osteoporosis, assumes great clinical importance in Type II osteoporosis. The female:male ratio of affected persons decreases to 2:1 and the disorder is much more prevalent. Among the very elderly, about 50% in women and 25% in men (14) have fractures of the vertebrae or hip.

As assessed by dual photon absorptiometry, the overall decrease in BMD during life is 42% in the lumbar spine (mainly trabecular bone) and 58% in the femoral neck (mixed cortical and trabecular bone). By age 75 years, virtually the entire population of aging women had BMD values at both sites which were below the theoretical fracture threshold. For 26 elderly women with hip fractures, BMD of the femoral neck was only slightly decreased (Table 1) and all individual values were within the age-adjusted normal range. In these same subjects, BMD values at the midradius, distal radius, and lumbar spine did not differ significantly from those for age-comparable normal subjects. From these data, we conclude that patterns of trabecular and cortical bone loss differ between the two osteoporotic syndromes. In contrast to Type I osteoporosis, which is characterized by accelerated and disproportionate loss of trabecular bone, Type II osteoporosis is characterized by a proportionate loss of both cortical and trabecular bone and a rate of loss similar to that of the general population. Thus, Type II osteoporosis corresponds well to Newton-John and Morgan's (15) model: as age-related bone loss progresses, an increasing number of the aging population have BMD values below the fracture threshold; and those elderly men and women with BMD in the lower part of the normal distribution will have a greater risk for fracture.

For Type II osteoporosis, there appear to be two major causes--impaired bone formation and secondary hyperparathyroidism. First, from the fourth decade of life onward, less bone is formed than is resorbed at individual remodeling foci, and this imbalance increases with aging (16). Second, serum iPTH increases in both men and women with aging (8,17). This is not a consequence of decreased renal function because partial correlation coefficients showed that serum iPTH did not correlate with glomerular filtration rate at a fixed value for age (8). Rather it seems more likely that it is due to the well documented age-related decrease in calcium absorption (see Gallagher et al. (10) for review). We (10) have found that serum $1,25(OH)_2D$ also decreases in elderly persons and that intestinal adaptation to lower intakes of dietary calcium (a process mediated by changes in serum $1,25(OH)_2D$) is impaired. The defect of calcium absorption in aging rats has been shown to be due to decreased $1,25(OH)_2D$ production resulting from a primary defect in 25-OH-D 1α-hydroxylase activity (18,19). Our recent finding of a subnormal rise in serum $1,25(OH)_2D$ after PTH infusion in elderly women which was even less in elderly women with hip fracture (20) suggests that patients with Type II osteoporosis also have a primary, age-related defect in metabolism of 25-OH-D to $1,25(OH)_2D$. Our observation that serum bone Gla-protein and other biochemical markers increase with aging (20), suggests that secondary hyperparathyroidism may increase bone turnover. Because bone formation remains decreased at level of individual remodeling foci, increased bone turnover would result in increased bone loss.

TYPE II OSTEOPOROSIS
("Senile" Osteoporosis)

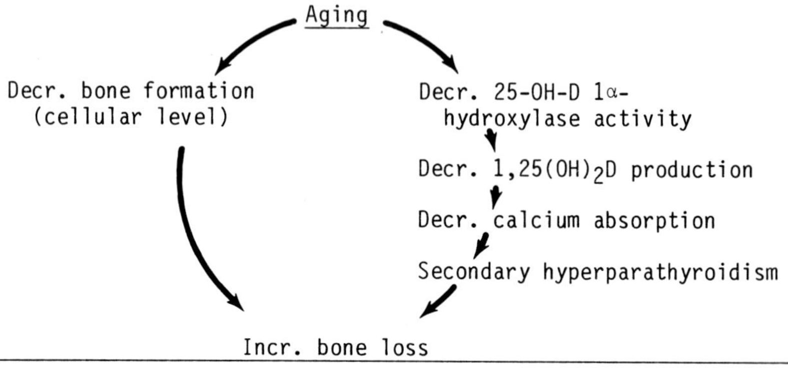

CONCLUSIONS

Osteoporosis occurring in women within the first 15-20 years after menopause and that occurring in men and women older than 75 years differs with respect to epidemiology, patterns of cortical and trabecular bone loss, parathyroid function, and cause. These differences (summarized in Table 2) are sufficiently large as to warrant separate classification as distinct syndromes.

Table 2. Summary of differences between Type I osteoporosis and Type II osteoporosis.

	Type I	Type II
Age	51 to 65 yrs*	> 75 yrs*
Sex ratio	F 6:1 M	F 2:1 M
Bone loss: type	Mainly trabecular	Trabecular and cortical
rate	Accelerated	Not accelerated
Fracture type	Mainly vertebral	Both vertebral and hip
Parathyroid function	Decreased	Increased
Calcium absorption	Decreased	Decreased
Metabolism of 25-OH-D to $1,25(OH)_2D$	Secondary decrease	Primary decrease
Major etiologic factors	Menopause	Decreased bone formation Secondary hyperparathyroidism

*Both types occur in decade from 66 to 75 years

REFERENCES

1. Riggs, B.L., Wahner, H.W., Seeman, E., Offord, K.P., Dunn, W.L., Mazess, R.B., Johnson, K.A. and Melton, L.J. III (1982): J. Clin. Invest., 70, 716.
2. Nordin, B.E.C. (1971): Br. Med. J., 1, 571.
3. Lindsay, R., Hart, D.M., Forrest, C. and Baird, C. (1980): Lancet, 2, 1151.
4. Mazess, R.B. (1982): Clin Orthop., 165, 239.
5. Heaney, R.P., Recker, R.R. and Saville, P.D. (1978): J. Lab. Clin. Med., 92, 964.
6. Riggs, B.L., Jowsey, J., Goldsmith, R.S., Kelly, P.J., Hoffman, D.L. and Arnaud, C.D. (1972): J. Clin. Invest., 51, 1659.
7. Hillyard, C.J., Stevenson, J.C. and MacIntyre, I. (1978): Lancet 1, 961.
8. Gallagher, J.C., Riggs, B.L., Jerpbak, C.M. and Arnaud, C.D. (1980): J. Lab. Clin. Med., 95, 373.
9. Seeman, E., Wahner, H.W., Offord, K.P., Kumar, R., Johnson, W.J. and Riggs, B.L. (1982): J. Clin. Invest., 69:1302.
10. Gallagher, J.C., Riggs, B.L., Eisman, J., Hamstra, A., Arnaud, S.B. and DeLuca, H.F. (1979): J. Clin. Invest., 64, 729.
11. Riggs, B.L., Hamstra, A. and DeLuca, H.F. (1981): J. Clin. Endocrinol. Metab., 53, 833.
12. Davidson, B.J., Riggs, B.L., Wahner, H.W. and Judd, H.L. (1983): Obstet. Gynecol., 61, 275.
13. Riggs, B.L., Jowsey, J., Kelly, P.J., Hoffman, D.L. and Arnaud, C.D. (1973): Clin. Endocrinol. Metab., 2:317.
14. Melton, L.J. III and Riggs, B.L. (in press): The Osteoporotic Syndrome: Detection and Prevention. Editor: L.V. Avioli, Grune & Stratton, Inc., New York.
15. Newton-John, H.F. and Morgan, D.B. (1968): Lancet, 1, 232.
16. Lips, P., Courpron, P. and Meunier, P. (1978): Calcif. Tissue Res., 26, 13.
17. Wiske, P.S., Epstein, S., Bell, N.H., Queener, S.F., Edmondson, J. and Johnson, C.C., (1979): N. Engl. J. Med., 300, 1419.
18. Horst, R.W., DeLuca, H.F. and Jorgenson, N. (1978): Metab. Bone Dis. Rel. Res., 1, 29.
19. Armbrecht, H.J., Zenser, T.V. and Davis, B.B. (1980): J. Clin. Invest., 66, 1118
20. Tsai, K.S., Kumar, R. and Riggs, B.L. Unpublished data.
21. Delmas, P.D., Stenner, D., Wahner, H.W., Mann, K.G. and Riggs, B.L. (in press): J. Clin. Invest.

Discussion after L. Riggs' presentation:

C. JOHNSTON: In Type 1 osteoporosis the estrogen deficiency may have been more severe than in the controls immediately after menopause, but the difference may not persist after the bone had been lost.

L. RIGGS: Yes, we have to explain why there is a 2 to 1 predominance of females over males, and I suggest that this is a reflection of the rapid bone loss that occurred in all women at the time of the menopause or several years thereafter.

R. HEANEY: You stated that the Type 2 patients are part of the normal population and that their parathyroid hormone levels are higher. Are you suggesting that these levels are simply the high end of a normal distribution?

L. RIGGS: That's right. They are not significantly higher, but there is a trend to higher values that are proportional to the somewhat lower values for bone density.

C. NORDIN: I agree with most of what you say, but you have left out a very important factor. You and I , and many others, have reported that calcium absorption is significantly lower in osteoporotics than in controls. I showed that in Leeds over many years and have exactly the same results in Adelaide. That is the main missing factor that accounts for the accelerated bone loss in crush fracture osteoporosis.

L. RIGGS: Our data suggest the decrease in calcium absorption is a consequence of an increase in bone resorption, and is not a primary defect.

O. SCHAADT: We found in normal women a highly significant decrease in the lumbar spine BMC after the age of 50, but in the femoral shaft, with predominantly cortical bone, the bone mineral loss was not significant until the age of 65 or 70. I think this is in agreement with your findings. Also, patients with fracture of the femoral neck demonstrate a significant decrease in BMC of the femoral shaft, but not of the lumbar spine.

L. RIGGS: As a group, our patients with hip fracture have a significantly decreased mean value for bone mineral; but in contrast to Type 1 osteoporosis, they are all individually within the normal distribution.

R. LINDSAY: Does Type 1 osteoporosis predispose to Type 2 osteoporosis?

L. RIGGS: Yes, I think so.

STEROID-INDUCED OSTEOPOROSIS

Louis V. Avioli

Division of Bone and Mineral Metabolism, The Jewish Hospital of St. Louis at Washington University, School of Medicine, St. Louis, Missouri, U.S.A.

Since compound E (cortisone) was administered to the first patient with rheumatoid arthritis on September 21, 1948, the anti-inflammatory and immunosuppressive effects of glucocorticoid medications have proven both therapeutic, and in many instances, life-saving. An analysis of the results obtained after 34 years of experience with pharmaceutical preparations of glucocorticoid drugs reveals beneficial responses in a variety of connective tissues and immunoproliferative disorders such as rheumatoid arthritis, systemic lupus erythematosis, necrotizing vasculitis, glomerulonephritis and other syndromes characterized by polyarthritis and polymyalgia rheumatica. In each instance, the primary art of therapy has been to control the disease, alleviate the symptoms, and reduce the morbidity. Indications for the use of glucocorticoid medications should be conditioned primarily by the extent of the clinical problem. The physician should be constantly aware that treatment with synthetic glucocorticoid analogues, although advantageous for controlling the inflammatory and/or immunoproliferative manifestations of the disease in question, is not designed to eliminate the actual cause of the disease. Thus, glucocorticoid therapy will prove of maximal benefit primarily in clinical disorders (with either local or systemic inflammatory manifestations) which are self-limited, or when used with other forms of medications which also possess the capacity of inducing a remission of the underlying disease process.

The anti-inflammatory activity of cortisone is the result of its conversion to hydrocortisone in the body. Hydrocortisone, or cortisol, is the primary glucocorticoid product secreted by the adrenal cortex. Because of the undesirable side-effects of cortisol which result from sodium retention, a variety of synthetic derivatives of cortisol have been produced. The major synthetic analogues of cortisol which have become available for clinical use are prednisone, prednisolone, methyprednisolone, triamcinolone, dexamethasone, paramethasone and betamethazone. These compounds have varying anti-inflammatory potencies which can be correlated with their plasma half-lifes. The duration of action of cortisone and cortisol is short with biologic half-lives of 8-12 hours; prednisone, prednisolone and methylprednisolone are intermediate in action with biologic half-lives of 12-36 hours; dexamethazone, betamethazone and paramethasone are longer acting compounds with biologic half-lives of 36-72 hours. Despite the decreased capacity for sodium retention which characterizes the synthetic glucocorticoid analogues, it should be stressed that the other undesirable side effects of these compounds are proportional to their anti-inflammatory effects which conditions the overall clinical response. The adverse effects of glucocorticoid therapy include a variety of metabolic, gastrointestinal, cardiovascular, ocular, cutaneous, musculoskeletal, endocrine, central nervous system and infectious disorders (1). Although anyone of these side-effects may prove disadvantageous for the patient who is subjected to long-term steroid therapy, the most potentially disabling adverse effect is the development of osteopenia (reduced bone mass) with a consequent increased propensity to bone fractures (2-5). This complication occurs with doses as low as 7 mg of prednisolone per day (2). This glucocorticoid effect is due primarily to an impairment in calcium absorption, increases in urinary calcium excretion and a direct anti-anabolic and catabolic effect of glucocorticoids on the skeletal tissue (6-10). The bone loss produced by all the synthetic glucocorticoid analogues has a characteristic distribution: it is more severe in those regions of the skeleton having a higher content of trabecular bone (e.g. the vertebrae and ribs) and is less striking in the long bones which are composed predominantly of less metabolically active cortical bone (3,6). As a result, rib fractures and compression deformities of the vertebrae are quite common in patients subjected to long-term treatment regimens with the synthetic glucocorticoid analogues. The incidence of symptomatic bone disease in patients treated with currently available synthetic glucocorticoids is dose-related, and time dependent. It is also highest in growing children during periods of increased bone turnover and rapid longitutional growth, post-menopausal women, who normally have moderate degrees of osteoporosis because of increased age and estrogen deficiency, and in patients taking medications such as anticonvulsants which also affect bone adversely (11). These skeletal deformities and the morbidity and pain associated with recurrent fractures are often more incapacitating than the underlying disease process which necessitated glucocorticoid therapy.

There is no question that the glucocorticoids have played a prominent if not dominant role in the therapy of a variety of clinical disorders since a patient with rheumatoid arthritis was treated with cortisone in 1948. Physicians must respect that, despite the continued appearance of "newer and more potent" synthetic analogues of the cortisol molecule with less salt retaining effects, the subtle skeletal effects of these potent drugs still confront the unsuspecting patient. A detailed understanding of the clinical pharmacology and the nature and extent of the potential complications that occur with each of the synthetic analogues is essential before any therapeutic regimen is either initiated or continued for prolonged periods. In this regard we should begin to recognize the potential attributes of a new glucocorticoid analogue, deflazacort. Deflazacort, a drug which resulted from the structural modification of the prednisolone compound (12), now appears to offer the physician the unique opportunity of prescribing glucocorticoid treatment with the anticipation of a good therapeutic response and mineral alterations in bone metabolism. Recent studies in patients requiring glucocorticoid treatment reveal that deflazacort is less injurious to calcium absorption and bone metabolism than prednisone or betamethazone in equipotent dosages (13-18). Until diseases such as rheumatoid arthritis, lupus erythematosus, and chronic asthma are considered preventable, we must rely on glucocorticoid compounds to retard the progression of disease activity and minimize patient symptomatology. In any case, the glucocorticoid which serves both of these purposes with the least effect on bone and calcium absorption should be the ultimate drug of choice.

REFERENCES

1. Axelrod, L. (1976): Med. 55, 39.
2. Reid, D.M., Kennedy, N.S.J., Smith, M.A., Tothill, P., Nuki, G. (1982): Brit. J. Med., 285, 330.
3. Howland, W.J., Pugh, D.G., Sprague, R.G. (1958): Radiology, 71, 69.
4. Curtiss, P.H., Clark, W.S., Herndon, C.H. (1954): J.A.M.A., 156, 467.
5. Saville, P.D., Kharmosh, O. (1967): Arth. Rheum., 10, 423.
6. Hahn, T.J., Boisseau, V.C., and Avioli, L.V. (1974): J. Clin. Endo. Metab., 39, 274.
7. Jowsey, J., Riggs, B.L. (1970): Acta. Endocrin., 63, 21.
8. Laake, H. (1960): Acta. Endocrin., 34, 60.
9. Wajchenberg, B.L., Periera, V.A., Kieffer, J. (1969): Acta Endocrin., 61, 173.
10. Hahn, T.J., Halstead, L.R., and Haddad, J.G. (1977): J. Lab. Clin. Med., 90, 399.
11. Hahn, T.J. and Hahn, B.H. (1976): Seminars in Arthritis and Rheumatism, 6, 1965.
12. Alessandro, A., Antonio, P., Giuseppe, B. and Valeria, P. (1980): European Journal of Drug Metabolism and Pharmacokinetics, 5, 207.
13. Hahn, T.J., Halstead, L.R., Strates, B., Imbimbo, B., and Baran, D.T. (1980): Calcif. Tissue Intl., 31, 109.
14. Caniaggia, A., Marchetti, M., Gennari, C., Vattimo, A. and Nicolic, F.B. (1977): Int. J. Clin. Pharmacol., 15, 126.
15. Bernini, M., Nardi, P., Fusi, L., Imbimbo, B., Montagnani, M., and Gennari, C. (1982): Calcif. Tissue Intl., 34, 586.
15. Vattimo, A., Lore, F. and Nuti, R. (1982): Calcif. Tissue Intl., 34, 585.
17. Lo Cascio., V., Bonnuci, E., Imbimbo, B., Adami, S., Bullanti, P., Galvanini, G., and Scuro, L.A. (1982): Calcif. Tissue Intl., 34, 582.
18. Russell, J.E. and Avioli, L.V. (1982): Calcif. Tissue Intl., 34, 580.

Discussion after L. Avioli's presentation:

O. MEHSL: You referred to calcitriol treatment of patients with glucocorticoid osteoporosis. Dr. Ritz and I treated renal transplant patients with calcitriol and found no increase in bone mass in comparison to untreated patients.

CAN ESTROGEN THERAPY PREVENT BONE LOSS

R. Lindsay

Regional Bone Center, Helen Hayes Hospital, W.Haverstraw, NY, College of Physicians and Surgeons, Columbia University, NY, NY, U.S.A.

Since Albright's classical description of postmenopausal osteoporosis, the role of sex hormones in prevention of bone loss and fracture has been hotly debated. Poor designs and inadequate technical methods were but two of the factors which contributed to the continuing controversy surrounding the subject. Only in the past 10 years have studies appeared in the literature of sufficient merit to allow us to define the role of ovarian failure and sex hormone replacement in pathogenesis and prevention of osteoporosis respectively.

Cross sectional studies in which bone mineral content in the female population is compared to age usually have indicated that maximal bone mass occurs around 30 years with a linear or curvilinear decline thereafter. When the data is presented in this fashion, little if any acceleration of bone loss is observed in the 45-55 year age range, the expected average age of the menopause. When the data is presented differently, however, with premenopausal and postmenopausal women presented separately, and bone mass in the postmenopausal group presented as a function of years since menopause, a definite significant acceleration of bone loss is often observed. Recent prospective data of patients undergoing oophorectomy has shown a significant rise in bone turnover during the year following the operation. In addition, serum alkaline phosphatase, including calcium and hydroxyproline all increase in postmenopausal or oophorectomized women confirming the more active state of the skeleton in these women.

In the 1970's, several prospective double-blind studies demonstrated using single beam photon absorptiometry, radiogrammetry and radiological densitometric techniques, that provision of estrogen therapy prevents bone loss in young post-menopausal or oophorectomized women (Table 1). These initial studies, mostly of 2 to 5 years duration have proved to be reproducible in other laboratories, and every prospective study in young women has demonstrated using these non-invasive techniques to estimate bone mass, that estrogens, at best in this relatively short term, inhibit bone loss. Our recent data, using a non-invasive technique to measure bone turnover has confirmed the original suggestion by Riggs that bone resorption is quickly and effectively reduced by estrogen followed by a slower fall in bone formation. Serum alkaline phosphatase, including calicum and hydroxyproline are also, as would be expected, lowered by estrogen treatments.

In one long-term prospective study the biochemical effects of estrogen have been shown to continue for at least 5 years, and after a mean of 9 years, estrogen therapy prevented the height loss, which was evident in a placebo treated group (Table 2). This reduction in height was associated with evidence of structural changes in the spine measured in lateral radiographs. Two investigations into the dose-response relationship of estrogen on bone loss have indicated that 0.625mg conjugated equine estrogens or its equivalent is

TABLE 1.

AUTHOR	YEAR	TYPE OF STUDY	DURATION	ESTROGEN EFFICACY
Aitken	1973	Prospective Double Blind	1 year	Yes
Lindsay	1976	Prospective Double Blind	5 years	Yes
Recker	1977	Prospective Double Blind	2 years	Yes
Horsman	1977	Prospective Double Blind	2 years	Yes
Lindsay	1980	Prospective Double Blind	9 years (mean)	Yes
Christiansen	1980	Prospective Double Blind	2 years	Yes

Selective recent studies to determine the efficacy of estrogen in preventing bone loss in postmenopausal or oophorectomized women.

TABLE 2. The effect of long-term estrogen treatment on height, weight and vertebral morphometry of lumbar Vertebra 2.

		TREATMENT		
		Estrogen (n = 58)	Placebo (n = 42)	Significance
Height (cm)	Original	160.8 ± 1.1	161.0 ± 1.3	ns
	Final	160.7 ± 1.2	160.1 ± 1.4*	ns
Weight (kg)	Original	62.4 ± 2.2	64.4 ± 0.7	ns
	Final	61.7 ± 1.9	67.6 ± 2.5	$p<0.02$
Bone Mineral Content (Radius) mg/mm		78.9 ± 2.1	80.4 ± 1.9	
		77.2 ± 1.9	72.8 ± 1.6*	$p<0.01$
Anterior Vert Height⁺(mm)		36.4 ± 1.4	34.1 ± 1.2	$p<0.1$
h/H^+		0.87 ± 0.02	0.80 ± 0.02	$p<0.06$
Wedge Angle $(^o)^+$		2.96 ± 0.64	4.62 ± 0.71	$p<0.05$

* $p<0.01$ from initial value

$^+$ Final measurements only

h/H is ratio of central vertebral height to posterior height sufficient to retard bone loss in the majority of individuals. While all estrogens appear to be effective in reducing bone loss, if given in appropriate doses, the effect does not appear to be estrogen specific. Certain progestogens and androgens may also reduce the rate at which bone is lost.

When estrogen therapy is terminated bone loss begins again. In one study the rate of bone loss following removal of estrogen was at least equivalent to that occurring immediately following the menopause. However, one other study designed more specifically to investigate the effect of estrogen withdrawal, demonstrated a recurrence of bone loss at a rate equivalent only to that of the placebo treated group without evidence of an acceleration. As far as is known, estrogens continue to impede bone loss for as long as they are given, however, in the longest study to date some evidence was presented suggesting that after 8 years therapy in young women a slow loss of bone supervened despite continuation of estrogen therapy. The importance of this finding is as yet unclear, but it may represent the onset of an age dependent, sex-hormone independent phenomenon.

The mechanism by which estrogens act on bone is as yet unclear. Undoubtedly bone turnover is reduced, but estrogens do not appear to act directly on bone, since as yet true estrogen receptors have not been identified in bone. It is possible that estrogens modify the secretion of effects of the hormonal triad which control calcium homeostasis, parathyroid hormone, calcitonin and the vitamin D system. Subtle changes in circulating levels of the hormones have been identified in special circumstances. In patients calcitonin levels have been shown to increase during pregnancy and after estrogen treatment. In therapy at least such an increment in calcitonin secretion and the likely subsequent effects on PTH and 1,25 dihydroxyvitamin D could account for most if not all of the effects of estrogen on bone. However, it is also possible that estrogen could modify bone turnover by modulating activity or secretion of the local messengers within bone such as prostaglandins or peptides although direct evidence of such an effect is lacking.

Undoubtedly good evidence exists that in postmenopausal or oophorectomized women estrogens reduce the rate of bone loss and may protect against individual failure in the vertebral bodies. The evidence that such long-term therapy will prevent fractures, is less good relying mostly on case control and retrospective studies. However, if the assumption that the bone loss occurring with aging is mainly responsible for the rise in fracture incidence with age, then it seems reasonable that when bone loss is retarded, i.e., using estrogens, then the increase in fracture incidence should be prevented.

REFERENCES

1. Aitken, J.M., Hart, D.M., Lindsay, R. (1973): British Medical Journal, 515-518.
2. Lindsay, R., Hart, D.M., Aitken, J.M., MacDonald, E.B., Anderson, J.B., Clarke, A.C. (1976): Lancet i, 1038-1041.
3. Recker, R.R., Saville, P.D., Heaney, R.P. (1977): Annals of Internal Medicine, 87, 649-655.
4. Horsman, A., Gallagher, J.C., Simpson, M., Nordin, B.E.C. (1977): British Medical Journal ii, 789-792.
5. Lindsay, R., Hart, D.M., Forrest, C., Baird, C. (1980): Lancet, 1151-1154.
6. Christiansen, C., Christensen, M., McNair, P., Hagen, C., Stocklund, K., Transbol, I. (1980): European Journal Clin. Investigation 10,000-000.

A MODEL FOR ESTABLISHING OPTIMAL PROPHYLAXIS AND TREATMENT IN POSTMENOPAUSAL OSTEOPOROSIS

Claus Christiansen, Paul Rødbro* and Lone Tjellesen

Department of Clinical Chemistry, Glostrup Hospital, University of Copenhagen, and *Department of Clinical Physiology, Aalborg Hospital, Denmark

Bone metabolism in postmenopausal osteoporosis is characterized by a negative calcium balance where bone resorption is greater than bone formation (1): i.e. a negative calcium balance at a quicker rate of bone turnover (1,2). The increased bone formation is reflected by an increase in alkaline phosphatase owing to heightened osteoblastic activity (2,3).

Oestrogen treatment can reverse bone loss in women with postmenopausal osteoporosis. This has been shown in recent studies where the bone loss was estimated on the bone mineral content of the forearm (4). The few available reports on serum alkaline phosphatase in postmenopausal osteoporosis suggest that the positive calcium balance at the start of oestrogen treatment results from a rapid fall in bone resorption and a more protracted fall in bone formation (3). To investigate these differing rate changes, we studied the serum alkaline phosphatase concentration as a function of time in early postmenopausal women receiving oestrogens. In addition we studied the relationship between bone mineral content, urinary hydroxyproline, and serum alkaline phosphatase in order to see whether it was possible to propose a model for development of optimal prophylaxis and treatment in postmenopausal osteoporosis.

PARTICIPANTS AND METHODS

All participants in the study were informed verbally and in writing about the trial and all gave their written consent. The participants were divided into 5 groups:

Group 1 consisted of five normally menstruating women, aged 23-29 years, from the laboratory staff. They were studied throughout one menstrual cycle (range 26-35 days). Fasting blood samples were taken each day for one menstrual cycle.

Group 2 consisted of 82 normal premenopausal women, aged 23-45 years (mean age 32.5 years). None of these women received oral contraceptives.

Group 3 consisted of 114 healthy female volunteers. They had passed a natural menopause six months to three years before. For the first study (study I) the 114 women were allocated to receive cyclical female hormones (high dose, see footnote) or placebo. After two years' of treatment the participants continued in a second study (study II) for one year. The women in both groups were randomised into four subgroups: continued hormone treatment or placebo, and continued placebo or hormone treatment. All participants received 0.5 g calcium (Sandoz) daily during both studies (4).

Group 4 comprised 92 healthy volunteers in their early menopause. They had passed a natural menopause 2.5 to 5 years previously, and had not received hormonal treatment since their menopause (3).

The participants were allocated by random sampling numbers into four treatment groups with groups 1 to 3 receiving sequential female hormones (see footnote), and the fourth identical-looking placebo tablets. In addition all participants received 0.5 g calcium (Sandoz) daily. The treatment was given for 12 months. All participants in groups 3 and 4 were examined at the start of treatment and at 3-month intervals between the 16th and 22nd day of the tablet cycles throughout the year of treatment. Group 5 comprised 54 women all aged 70 years (5). Serum alkaline phosphatase was measured by an enzymatic method (Merckotest R, 3344). Serum E_2 was determined by radioimmunoassay.

RESULTS

The results for serum E_2 and alkaline phosphatase in relation to ovulation in group 1 are shown in Fig. 1 A, which demonstrates the well known oestradiol peak leading up to ovulation time. The figure also shows that alkaline phosphatase in these young women is constant and independent of serum oestradiol. On a larger time scale (Fig. 1 B) serum alkaline phosphatase is constant in premenopausal women (group 2). Fig. 1 C demonstrates that untreated postmenopausal women have higher than normal mean values of serum alkaline phosphatase and that these high mean values become normal during hormone treatment. The fall in mean alkaline phosphatase is protracted and when hormone treatment is stopped the mean serum alkaline phosphatase rises slowly above normal. The data in Fig. 1 D show that the decrease in mean serum alkaline phosphatase during hormone treatment is independent of the hormone dose within the range used.

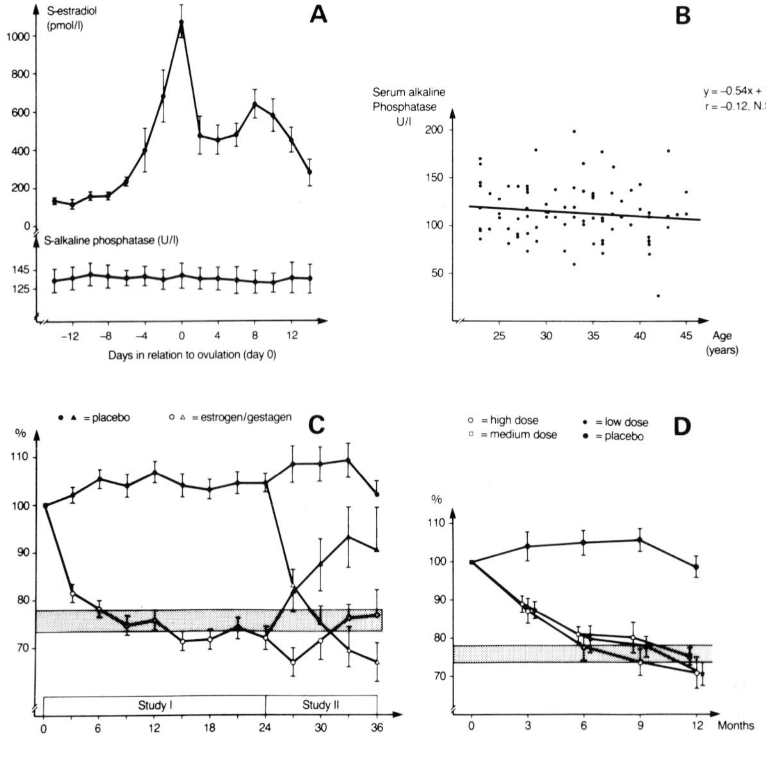

DISCUSSION

On the basis of published data including that from our departments and the present study it is possible to propose a model for establishing optimal prophylaxis and treatment of postmenopausal osteoporosis. Longitudinal and cross-sectional studies have shown that in premenopausal women BMC remains constant, whereas after the menopause it falls exponentially.

Furthermore, both urinary hydroxyproline/creatinine (index of bone resorption) and alkaline phosphatase (index of bone formation) increase after the menopause, the former relatively more than the latter (leading to a negative calcium balance). Finally, we know that urinary hydroxyproline/creatinine is constant in the postmenopausal years, whereas serum alkaline phosphatase increases significantly (6). This may tentatively be interpreted as a decrease in negative calcium balance with age (when calcium balance is expressed in absolute figures). These combined data could constitute the first part of the model (Fig. 2 A): The hatched area symbolises total bone loss estimated from the difference in bone formation and bone resorption. The slope of the BMC curve at any one time (i.e. rate of bone loss) is reflected as the distance between formation and resorption.

Moreover, we have data showing that serum alkaline phosphatase slowly decreases to normal levels during oestrogen treatment (Fig. 2 B), and oestrogens increase BMC (3). After long-term treatment fasting urinary hydroxyproline/creatinine becomes normal (3). The increase in BMC can thus be explained by a more rapid fall in urinary hydroxyproline/creatinine than in serum alkaline phosphatase, i.e. bone resorption is greater than bone formation. This part of the

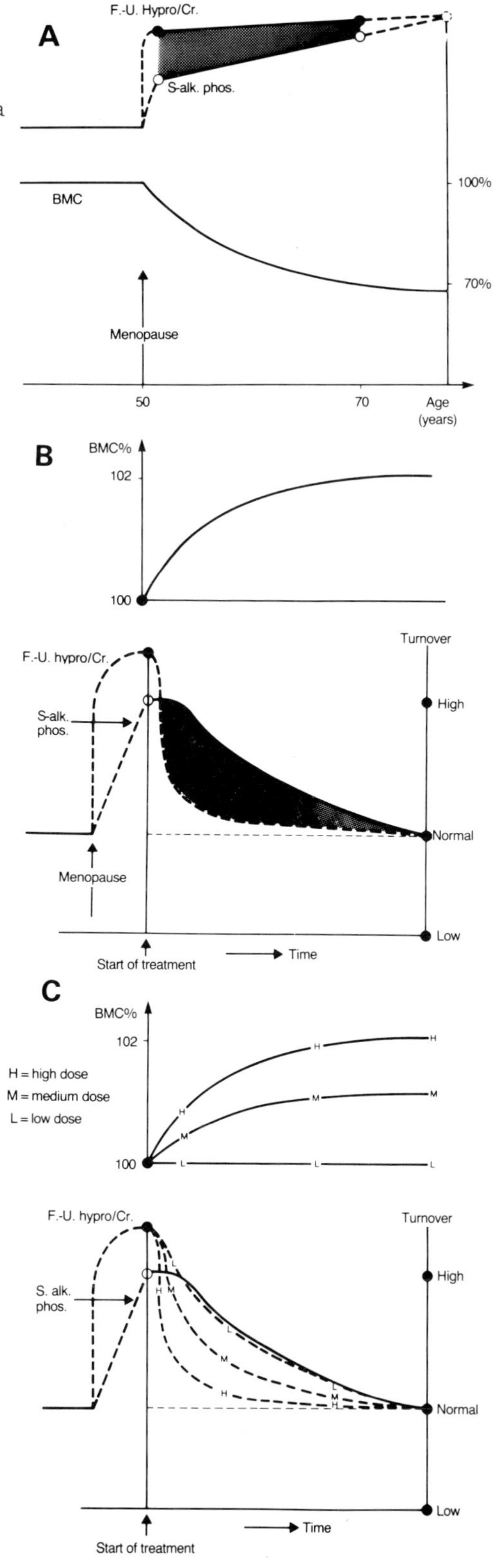

model is illustrated in Fig. 2 B (around the menopause time axis). The hatched area between the urinary hydroxyproline/creatinine and the serum alkaline phosphatase curves reflect the positive calcium balance mirrored in the BMC curve. The slope of the BMC curve at any one time in the figure reflects the distance between urinary hydroxyproline/creatinine and serum alkaline phosphatase. Furthermore, the model can be supported by our recent data on dose response on BMC during oestrogen treatment (7). We showed (Fig. 2 C) that a low dose, L, (1 mg E_2) stops the bone loss but does not increase BMC, whereas moderate, M, (2 mg E_2), and high, H, (4 mg E_2) doses both increase BMC, the higher dose most markedly. Since our present data show that there is no dose response on serum alkaline phosphatase, the combined data leave only one possible explanation: that there must be a dose response on urinary hydroxyproline/creatinine during E_2 treatment, i.e. a dose response on bone resorption. This part of the model is demonstrated in Fig. 2 C, where the curves for urinary hydroxyproline/creatinine are postulated. This model indicates that oestrogen treatment of postmenopausal bone loss must be initiated early on if the aim is to maintain BMC at premenopausal levels.

REFERENCES

1. Heaney, R.H., Recker, R.R. and Saville, P.D. (1978): J. Lab. Clin. Med. 92, 964.
2. Crilly, R.G., Jones, M.M., Horsman, A. and Nordin, B.E.C. (1980): Clin. Sci. 58, 341.
3. Christiansen, C., Christensen, M.S., Larsen, N.-E. and Transbøl, I. (1982): J. Clin. Endocrinol. Metab. 55, 1124.
4. Christiansen, C., Christensen, M.S. and Transbøl, I. (1981): Lancet i, 456.
5. Jensen, G.F., Christiansen, C. and Transbøl, I. (1982): Clin. Endocrinol. 16, 515.
6. Christiansen, C., Rødbro, P. and Tjellesen, L. (1983): Clin. Sci. (Submitted).
7. Christensen, M.S., Hagen, C., Christiansen, C. and Transbøl, I. (1982): Am. J. Obstet. Gynecol. 144, 873.

Footnote: days 1-12: 4 mg, 2 mg, or 1 mg 17β-oestradiol + 2 mg, 1 mg, or 0.5 mg oestriol for high dose, medium dose or low dose, respectively; days 13-22: 1 mg norethisterone acetate in all doses; days 23-28: 1 mg 17β-oestradiol in high dose and medium dose + 0.5 mg oestriol in these doses. No hormones in low dose days 23-28.

Discussion following Drs. Lindsay's and Christiansen's presentations:

C. JOHNSTON: Dr. Christiansen has presented a promising method for identifying those in the population with rapid bone loss, but it would be difficult to apply all the measurements to the general population. If you had to select three determinations which are available and inexpensive, which would you choose?

C. CHRISTIANSEN: I would choose fat mass calculated from height and weight first, then urinary hydroxyproline, and last serum alkaline phosphatase.

C. NORDIN: Dr. Christiansen, there is an extraordinary discrepancy between the total body calcium and total body potassium data in men and women shown by you and Dr. Heaney. Dr. Heaney showed no fall in the calcium/potassium ratio with age in women, and you showed a marked fall in women with age. Can you resolve this difference?

C. CHRISTIANSEN: The validity of the measurements of total body potassium can be looked at in another way. If the GFR and the serum creatinine do not change with age, the serum creatinine can be used an an estimation of lean body mass, or muscle mass. Our data for lean body mass and GFR data from the literature gives exactly the same slopes, so I think that our data are correct.

C. NORDIN: Dr. Lindsay, with all the evidence that has been gathered by yourself, Dr. Christiansen, and ourselves, and now by Dr. Genant and Ettinger that estrogens do that same thing to the spine as to the peripheral bones, it would be extraordinary if you couldn't use peripheral bone measurements to assess the rate of bone loss in the skeleton as a whole, including the trabecular bone in the spine. Of course, the rates won't be the same, but I know of no study showing that a person losing rapidly in the peripheral bone is not also losing rapidly in the spine, or that if you stop the bone loss in the periphery, you will not stop bone loss in the spine.

R. LINDSAY: In cohort studies, you can use almost any measurement that you want; but our recent data using dual energy photon absorptiometry in the spine and single energy photon absorptiometry in the periphery shows that in an individual although the changes are in the same direction, they aren't necessarily positive or negative at both sites. But, if you slow the loss in the periphery in a group of subjects, you will also slow the loss in the center in the group.

H. GENANT: In Dr. Lindsay's last slide, although there was a strong correlation between the two measurements sites for the group, the dispersion about the regression line was so great that the predictive errors was about .7 or .6, so that one cannot predict the rate of spinal loss in the individual patient based upon the peripheral measurement except with highly precise CT as Dr. Hangartner has shown.

M. PARFITT: Dr. Christiansen, what dose of flouride showed no prophylactic effect?

C. CHRISTIANSEN: We use 20 mg. per day of sodium flouride.

L. RIGGS: The failure of flouride to prevent bone loss is related to the site of measurement. Flouride has its main effect on trabecular bone in the vertebrae, and this is an example, Dr. Nordin, of a treatment regimen where there is a discrepancy between the two scanning sites. Over a 5-year period, bone mineral density will decrease after flouride therapy at the distal radius; but, will increase in the spine.

J. KANIS: There are many biological precedents for disparities in trabecular and cortical bone mass changes. Flouride is one, but other examples are parathyroid hormone, and the combination of phosphate and calcitonin. So, changes at one site do not mean that equal changes occur in the same direction at other sites.

J. BUCHANAN: Dr. Lindsay, I was a bit discouraged to see the escape from estrogen prophylaxis after 8 to 10 years. Was that related changes in life style, such as dietary calcium intake or exercise?

R. LINDSAY: The life style of the treated and placebo groups are changing in the same way. I believe we are seeing age-dependent bone loss.

F. LAFFERTY: Dr. Lindsay, the 19-nor-progestational agent that prevents bone loss has potential androgen effects and I am concerned about adverse long-term effects on the cardiovascular system. Have you studied Provera (medroxyprogesterone) instead?

R. LINDSAY: Yes. We looked at Provera, and were disappointed with its effect, although other groups have shown that Provera is effective.

O. SCHAADT: In normal women, we found a high correlation between BMC in the forearm, the lumbar spine, and the femoral neck. In osteoporotic women, however, the correlation between the peripheral skeleton and the axial skeleton disappears, but the correlation between different sites in the peripheral skeleton is still significant.

ANABOLIC STEROIDS, AND CALCITONIN, IN THE TREATMENT OF POSTMENOPAUSAL OSTEOPOROSIS

Charles H. Chesnut III, David J. Baylink, Helen E. Gruber, Joel Ivey, Meredith Matthews, Wil B. Nelp, Karen Sisom

Division of Nuclear Medicine, Departments of Medicine and Radiology, University of Washington, Seattle, WA, U.S.A., and Mineral Metabolism Laboratory, American Lake Medical Center, Tacoma, WA, U.S.A.

INTRODUCTION

For a therapeutic modality to achieve efficacy in the treatment of postmenopausal osteoporosis, it should ideally satisfy a number of conditions. Such a modality should slow bone resorption and/or stimulate bone formation with a subsequent increase in bone mass and decrease in fractures, should be associated with relatively few side effects, and should be easily administered, at a reasonable expense. Also, the mechanism of action of the therapeutic program should be reasonably well understood. Based upon previous studies (1, 2) from our laboratories synthetic salmon calcitonin, and the anabolic steroid stanozolol, satisfy a number, but not all, of these criteria.

STUDY DESIGN

In previous clinical trials 50, and 44, Caucasian females with clinical postmenopausal osteoporosis and spinal compression fractures were randomized into calcitonin, or stanozolol, treated or control groups. The anabolic steroid study was double blind; multiple parameters were utilized in each study to assess both efficacy and mechanism of action. Subjects were studied for 25-29 months.

RESULTS

In terms of defining calcitonin's efficacy, total body calcium (TBC) by neutron activation analysis (a measurement of total bone mass) increased significantly ($p<.01$) from baseline through 18 months of study participation in the treated group (figure 1). Significant losses in TBC were noted in the control group through 18 months; by 26 months, however, the rate of increase in TBC noted in the treated group through 18 months was not sustained. Regional bone mass measurements by single photon absorptiometry techniques revealed no significant changes through 26 months in either treated or control groups. Analysis of spine radiographs revealed new vertebral compression fractures in 3 treated patients, and no new compression fractures in the control group, during the first year of study. In the second year 3 new compression fractures occurred in the treated group, and 2 new fractures were noted in the control patients in the same time period. This observed distribution of fractures in treated and control groups was not statistically significant ($.05>p<.07$, Fisher's exact test), but it must be recognised that both the number of subjects and observation periods were too small to validly assess fracture frequency.

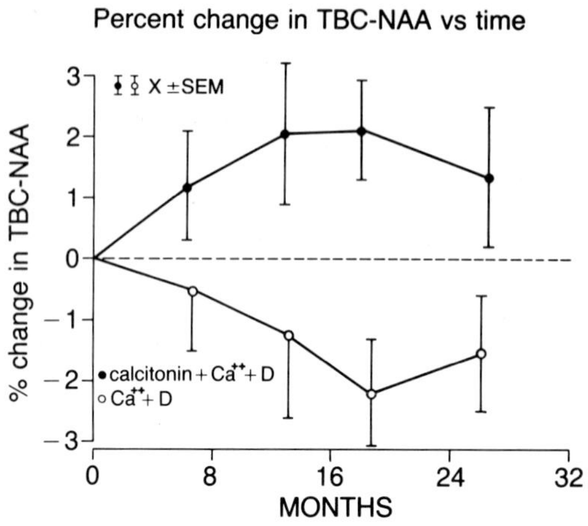

Figure 1. Percent change in total body calcium (grams) as a function of treatment time in treated and control patients. (1)

In terms of defining stanozolol's efficacy, TBC increased from baseline through study completion in the treated group by a mean 4.4%; a mean .01% increase was noted in the control group for the same period (figure 2). Such changes were significant in the treated ($p<.01$), but not the control, group; changes from baseline in TBC between the 2 groups were significantly different ($p=.03$). Also, analysis of the mean differences between treated and control groups in percent TBC change from baseline revealed the magnitude of the mean difference to increase throughout the study; drug effect therefore appeared to persist throughout the entire study. As in the calcitonin trial, no significant changes in regional bone mass measurements were noted; a significant correlation ($r=.5$, $p<.05$) was however observed between slope changes in regional bone mass and in TBC (total bone mass). In addition, no new spinal compression fractures were noted in the treated group throughout the period of study participation; 3 new spinal fractures occurred in the control group over a similar time. However, as with the calcitonin trial such a distribution of fractures was not statistically significant ($p=.07$, Fisher's exact test), but again only a limited number of patients were studied.

Analysis of urine, serum, and bone histology data, in combination with the previous TBC and radiographic findings, provides a number of postulated mechanisms of action for the 2 therapeutic entities. For calcitonin: increased calcitonin (exogenously administered) results in decreased bone resorption (as confirmed on bone biopsy), leading to the observed transient increase in TBC. In greater detail the decrease in bone resorption results in an observed decrease in serum calcium and a subsequent documented increase in iPTH levels. Further, a secondary decrease in serum phosphorus, a postulated increase in 1,25-$(OH)_2$ cholecalciferol (possibly due to increased iPTH levels), an increase in calcium absorption, and a subsequent increase in urinary calcium were documented in the study.

For stanozolol the following mechanism of action can be hypothesised: stanozolol increases total urinary cyclic AMP (observed in the study) possibly resulting in a decrease in urinary calcium excretion (observed). Serum calcium subsequently rises (documented) leading to an observed decrease in iPTH levels. A decrease in bone resorption would consequently be expected, although such a decrease was not documented on bone biopsy (the biopsies were however obtained 26-29 months after the onset of therapy, and a transient decrease in bone resorption within 3-6 months of therapy onset can not be ruled out). Stanozolol does appear to directly increase bone formation, as suggested in the treated group (p=.06) by an increase in the rate of bone formation on iliac crest bone biopsies at study conclusion, and by a significant increase in non-dialyzable hydroxyproline (a marker for bone formation) at 17 months of study participation. The net effect of stanozolol's actions on these remodeling parameters would be to increase total bone mass (as documented by the increase in TBC), and theoretically to stabilize the spine's structural integrity and prevent further fractures.

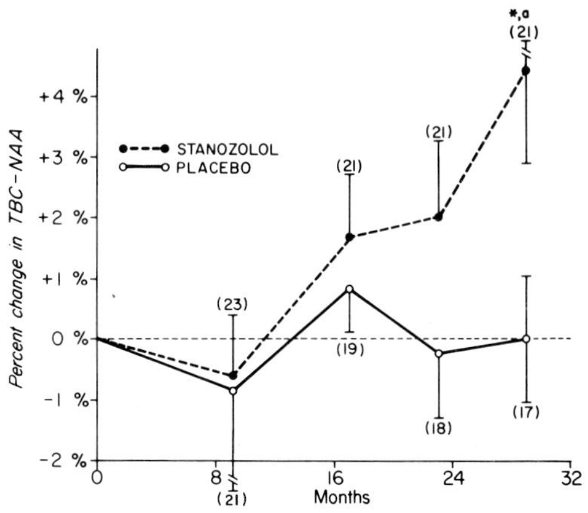

Figure 2. Percent change in total body calcium as a function of treatment time in treated and control patients, mean ±SEM. (2)
():n
*: significantly different from baseline, p<.01
a: change from baseline between treated and control groups significantly different, p=.03

ADVERSE REACTIONS

A number of mild adverse reactions occurred in the calcitonin study in response to calcitonin injections, primarily facial flushing and local inflammatory reactions at the injection site. In the stanozolol study significant but transient elevations of SGOT, and a number of clinically adverse reactions (increase in facial hair, ankle edema, hoarseness, and/or acne), occurred (interestingly, 30% of the placebo group developed similar clinical findings during the study). In neither the calcitonin nor the stanozolol study were these reactions sufficiently severe to cause total termination of therapy.

ADDITIONAL STUDIES

Recently available data (3) suggest an additional relationship of calcitonin, and possible calcitonin deficiency, to postmenopausal osteoporosis: while basal calcitonin levels appear similar in osteoporotic and age-matched normal females, a possible deficiency in calcitonin reserve (response of calcitonin to calcium infusion) in osteoporotic females has been noted. This latter finding supports the hypothesis of calcitonin deficiency as an etiologic factor in osteoporosis, and would reinforce the potential usefulness of calcitonin in this disease.

Additional studies (4, 5) further documenting stanozolol's stimulation of bone formation have appeared, both from our laboratory and from other laboratories. In addition, a recent study (6) notes a reduction in high density lipoproteins, and elevation of low density lipoproteins, following stanozolol therapy, with such changes reversible following therapy discontinuation.

CONCLUSIONS

Currently, the positive attributes of synthetic salmon calcitonin in the treatment of postmenopausal osteoporosis include its overall safety and lack of significant side effects, and its slowing of bone mass loss (at least transiently) through 12-16 months. Such attributes would be of definite benefit for the usage of calcitonin as prophylaxis in postmenopausal osteoporosis (i.e., to prevent the loss of bone in individuals with relatively normal bone mass, who have not as yet developed fractures). Calcitonin's negative attributes include its expense, its questionable ability to diminish fractures (although no significant data in this regard were available from the current study, it is unclear whether an agent such as calcitonin which only slows bone mass loss can be expected to prevent further fractures in individuals with substantially reduced bone mass), and its apparent association with a "resistance" to its effectiveness after a finite period of time. This apparent resistance is particularly worrisome, and was documented in the recent calcitonin study by two general data trends: first, the significant urine and serum changes (except for serum iPTH) occurred early in the study (4-6 months) and the affected parameters were no longer changing by the end of the study; and second, TBC tended to decrease in treated patients at the end of the study. The possibility of marked physiologic change(s) occurring between 12 months and the end of the study must be considered; possibilities which might account for the cessation of response to calcitonin include resistance to calcitonin action due to the development of antibodies, a loss of receptor sites for calcitonin (possibly due to excessive dosage and/or duration of calcitonin administration), and/or normal bone remodeling sequences (i.e., decreasing bone resorption may have eventually led to decreasing bone formation).

In conclusion, at the present time synthetic salmon calcitonin appears to possess rather limited usefulness for the long term treatment of postmenopausal osteoporosis, and indeed there would be concern as to whether such an agent should be used as primary therapy in individuals with reduced bone mass and previous fractures. It should however be noted that calcitonin's relative safety is a definite advantage, and justifies further work addressing the problems of expense, route of administration, and drug resistance. Such work should be particularly directed at identifying the cause of the apparent resistance (is it due to a lack of available receptors?) and whether it may be possible to overcome this resistance with reduced dosage, and cyclical therapy, regimens. Previous data from our laboratories with clodronate, another agent whose primary mechanism of action is a decrease in bone resorption, does suggest that an intermittent, "pulsing" dosage regimen may be more efficacious, as compared to continuous therapy.

The positive attributes of stanozolol in postmenopausal osteoporosis therapy include a significant and persistant increase in total bone mass as assessed by TBC (probably by an increase in bone formation and a decrease in urinary calcium excretion), an acceptable cost, and oral administration.

While no significant fracture data was available from the previous stanozolol study, the absence of new spinal fractures in the treated group is encouraging. Whether other anabolic steroids other than stanozolol show similar effects in postmenopausal osteoporosis is unclear, but presumably some benefit would accrue from their usage in this disease.

The negative attributes of stanozolol are primarily related to its side effects. It should be noted however that the previous trial's adverse reactions were in general relatively mild, and were not unacceptable to patients primarily concerned with the morbidity of osteoporosis. The significance of a transiently elevated SGOT is unclear; no other abnormal liver function tests were noted. The observed lipid changes are of concern regarding possible atherogenic potential, although the relationship of such lipoprotein changes to acceleration of atherogenesis is at present purely theoretical (6). It may not be wise to institute stanozolol for the long term prophylactic therapy of osteoporosis (for example, in the perimenopausal or immediately post-menopausal female); in the person with established postmenopausal osteoporosis with reduced bone mass and fractures (in whom restoration of previously lost bone mass is necessary to prevent further fractures) the risk of the drug in terms of its lipid effect, compared to the morbidity of the osteoporosis process, may well justify its usage. Overall, the risk-benefit ratio of stanozolol in the postmenopausal osteoporosis female appears acceptably low.

REFERENCES

1. Chesnut, C.H., Baylink, D.J., et al (1981): In: Calcitonin 1980, p. 247. Editors: A. Pecile, Excerpta Medica.
2. Chesnut, C.H., Ivey, J.L., Gruber, H.E., et al (1983): In Press, Metab.
3. Taggart, H.M., Chesnut, C.H., Ivey, J.L., et al (1982): Lancet, 8270, 475.
4. Farley, J.R., Chesnut, C.H., Baylink, D.J., (1982): Clin. Chem., 27, 2002.
5. Beresford, J.N., Gallagher, J.A., Poser, J., et al (1983): In: XVII European Symposium on Calcified Tissues, Abstracts, 97.
6. Taggart, H.M., Applebaum-Bowden, D., Haffner, S., et al (1982): Metab. 31, 1147.

TREATMENT OF IDIOPATHIC OSTEOPOROSIS WITH SODIUM FLUORIDE

P.J. Meunier, K. Galus, D. Briançon, C. Edouard, S.A. Charhon

INSERM Unit 234, Faculty Alexis Carrel and Department of Rheumatology. Edouard Herriot Hospital. LYON. France

The ideal therapeutic approach to osteoporosis (OP) responsible for vertebral fractures (VF) is the use of an agent which not merely slows the rate of bone loss but rather increases trabecular bone mass to an extent that the VF rate decreases. Although many therapeutic agents have been investigated in OP, very few are known to substantially increase trabecular bone mass. Fluoride appears to be one of them, as evidenced by the massive increase in bone density which characterizes bone fluorosis.

Fluoride was introduced for the treatment of OP 22 years ago (1), but the efficacy and safety of long-term fluoride treatment in OP is still a matter of debate. Most published studies have been conducted on relatively small numbers of patients, for variable times (1 to 120 months), using doses of sodium fluoride (NaF) ranging from 10 to 100 mg daily, with or without supplements of calcium and/or vitamin D given in varying doses. For these reasons, no clear guidelines have as yet emerged on the potential benefit of NaF therapy in OP. In addition, the drug is cheap to manufacture, not protected by patents, and therefore commercially not an attractive proposition.

The present study was carried out in order to better analyze the magnitude and the mechanisms of the anabolic effects of NaF on the trabecular bone of the axial skeleton in idiopathic OP. We used an unvarying protocol, combining NaF, calcium and vitamin D, to treat a group of 57 osteoporotic patients for 2 years. The number of patients was large enough for valid statistical analysis of the data. The efficacy of the treatment was evaluated radiologically from the changes noted in the VF rate, and histologically by bone histomorphometry on transiliac biopsies after tetracycline double labelling. In addition, a more detailed histomorphometric analysis was carried out in 11 patients who were classed as good responders on the basis of a 33% increase in trabecular bone volume and the absence of further VR. This detailed analysis consisted of measurements of the mean wall thickness (MWT) of trabecular packets, osteoblastic surfaces, singly and doubly tetracycline labeled surfaces and lamellar thickness.

MATERIALS AND METHODS

48 female and 9 male patients, all having at least one collapsedvertebra due to idiopathic OP were treated for 2 years. Each received 50 mg of NaF per day (25 mg b.i.d., given one hour before meals in the form of a gastric acid-resistant capsule), 1 gm of elemental calcium (Ca) per day (given at least 3 hours before or after NaF) and 8000 IU of vitamin D2. All patients were seen every 3 months for clinical, radiological and biochemical follow up.

The effects on the VF rate were evaluated by using a radiological vertebral index (RVI) measured on lateral X-ray films of the thoracic and lumbar spine. RVI takes into account the number and seriousness of the vertebral deformities found on 15 vertebrae, from T3 to L5. The vertebral body is graded "1" when normal, "2" when biconcave, and "4" when crushed or having a fractured plate.

The biochemical effects were determined from measurements of serum Ca, phosphorus, alkaline phosphatase, creatinine, parathormone, fluoride (F) and of urinary Ca, F and hydroxyproline.

The histomorphometric analysis of trabecular bone was obtained on pre- and post-treatment transiliac biopsies, according to previously published methods (3). Were measured : trabecular bone volume (TBV), osteoid volume (TOV), osteoid surfaces (TOS), the thickness index of osteoid seams (TIOS), osteoclastic resorption surfaces (TORS), the calcification rate (CR), the MWT of trabecular packets, osteoblastic surfaces, i.e. per cent of total trabecular surfaces (TTS) covered by either plump osteoblasts (POBS) or flat osteoblasts (FOBS), per cent of TTS covered by single (SLS) or double tetracycline labels (DLS), and the mean thickness of a pair of lamellae (LT), i.e. one bright and one dark lamella seen under polarized light.

RESULTS.

. Clinical. All patients had back pain before treatment. 56 per cent had a complete relief of back ache after 2 years of therapy and 22 per cent had a reduction of pain.

. Changes in the vertebral fracture rate (Table 1). The incidence of VF was lower in the second year of treatment than in the first and the mean annual increase in the RVI was also reduced during the second year of therapy.

TABLE 1. Changes in the vertebral fracture rate evaluated by the incidence of new vertebral fractures (VF) and the mean annual increase of the RVI in 57 osteoporotic patients treated for 2 years with NaF-Ca-vitamin D.

	N	Number (%) of patients with new VF		Mean annual increase of RVI	
		1st year	2nd year	1st year	2nd year
Female	48	16 (33)	5 (10)	1.5 ± 2.3	.8 ± 2.8
male	9	3 (33)	1 (11)	1.3 ± 2.2	.7 ± 1.7

. Biochemical effects. No significant changes were noted in any of the parameters listed above except for serum and urine fluoride levels. After 3 months therapy serum F levels attained a plateau at about 0.20 mg/l. Urinary F increased slowly but steadily during the 24 months of therapy, reaching a mean value of about 7 mg/24 hrs.

. Effects on bone histology (Tables 2 and 3). The most striking change was a marked increase in the osteoid surfaces (TOS) and osteoblastic surfaces (POBS and FOBS). In contrast resorption surfaces (TORS) did not increase significantly and the result of this uncoupling in bone remodeling was a marked increase in TBV. The newly formed bone was lamellar and the augmentation of TBV was caused by a significant increase in both the mean wall thickness of trabecular packets and mean thickness of matrix lamellae. The calcification rate did not change significantly while the osteoid seam thickness index increased moderately. When expressed in percent of total trabecular surfaces POBS and FOBS increased markedly, but when expressed in per cent of osteoid covered surfaces these osteoblastic surfaces decreased. This suggests an increased birthrate of osteoblasts at the tissue-level, but a possible toxic effect of long-term fluoride therapy on the osteoblasts, at the cell-level.

TABLE 2. Changes in mean values for histological variables after 2 years of combined therapy NaF-Ca-vit. D (females with idiopathic osteoporosis).

	TBV (%)	TOS (%)	TIOS	TORS (%)	CR (μm/day)
Pre-treatment	9.9±3.8	20.7±9.9	14.5±7	5.3±2.7	.59±.19
Post-treatment	15.9±8.6	50.7±20.6	19.2±7.9	5.8±3.2	.52±.22
n° cases	29	37	37	34	40
$p <$	.001	.001	.02	ns	ns

TABLE 3. Changes in mean values for histological variables after 2 years of combined therapy in 11 responders.

	TBV (%)	MWT (μm)	POBS (%)	FOBS (%)	SLS (%)	DLS (%)	LT (μm)
Pre-treatment	8.7±2.3	35.1±8.6	.6±.6	2.6±1.3	2.9±1.6	1.8±1.5	6.50±.45
Post-treatment	17.0±7.9	40.8±9.4	1.4±1.5	10.1±6.1	4.6±5.2	2.7±2.9	6.94±.42
$p <$	.01	.01	.05	.01	ns	ns	.001

. Side effects. These consisted of mild gastrointestinal irritation (22 per cent patients) and transitory periarticular pains (33 per cent). Treatment had to be discontinued because of adverse side effects in 7 per cent of patients. One patient, a 78 year old patient with mild renal failure (serum creatinine 142 μmol/l) developed bilateral non traumatic femoral neck fractures. She had stopped calcium and vitamin D supplementation after 15 months of combined therapy. The first fracture occurred 5 months and the second 6 months later. At this time the second bone biopsy revealed morphological and dynamic evidence of osteomalacia, with mottled periosteocytic lacunae on the microradiographs.

DISCUSSION

Our results are in agreement with the main studies in the literature which described a decrease in the rate of new vertebral fractures (4, 5, 6), and there is no doubt that NaF is a pharmaco logically active drug with particular effects on axial bone mass. In contrast, fluoride has been shown to have little effect on the cortical bone of the appendicular skeleton, and in a previously published study we did not find any change in bone density measured on the distal radius by photon absorptiometry in 26 osteoporotic patients treated for 2 years with the combined therapy NaF-calcium-vitamin D (2). Another controversial question about fluoride therapy concerns the possible existence of a mineralization defect of bone in treated osteoporotic patients. A retardation of osteoid mineralization has been demonstrated in few patients treated with doses of NaF greater than 40 mg daily and this can be minimised by the concurrent administration of calcium supplements and vitamin D. From our histological results this mineralization defect could be due to a direct toxic effect of NaF at the individual cell level on an increased osteoblast population. It is well-known that osteoblasts are directly involved in osteoid mineralization. Finally, the two main contraindications of NaF therapy for osteoporosis are osteomalacia and renal failure, because of the risk of a too high level of fluoride retention.

Other major questions remain concerning the optimal daily dose of NaF, the optimal duration of treatment, the necessity of the combination with Ca and/or vitamin D, the intermittent or continuous use of NaF and the identification of potential responders and non-responders. Studies are presently conducted to address these questions.

Despite these uncertainties, and after 10 years of experience, we feel that the benefits of the combined therapy of NaF-calcium-vitamin D outweighs its adverse effects in the management of trabecular osteoporosis responsible for vertebral fractures.

ACKNOWLEDGEMENTS

The authors extend their appreciation to Dr J.A. Kanis, Dr Z.F.G. Jaworski, and Dr C. Schnitzler for their helpful suggestions. They thank Laboratoires UPSA for kindly providing sodium fluoride.

REFERENCES

1. Rich, C. and Ensink F. (1961) : Nature (Lond.), 191, 184.
2. Briançon, D. and Meunier P.J. (1981) : Orth. Clinics N. America, 12, 629.
3. Meunier, P.J. (1983) : In : Annual Advances in Bone and Mineral Research p 191. Editor : W. Peck. Excerpta Medica, Amsterdam - Oxford - Princeton.
4. Riggs, B.L., Seeman, E., Hodgson, S.F., Taves D.R. and O'Fallon M.O. (1982) : New Engl. J. Med., 306, 446.
5. Reutter, F.W. and Olah, A.J. (1978) : In : Fluoride and Bone, p 249. Editors : B. Courvoisier and A. Donath. Hans Huber, Bern.
6. Jowsey, J. (1979) : In : Osteoporosis II, p 123. Editor : U.S. Barzel. Grune and Stratton, New York.

THE USE OF CALCITRIOL (1,25 DIHYDROXYVITAMIN D) IN OSTEOPOROSIS

J.C. GALLAGHER

Creighton University School of Medicine, Omaha, NE 68131 USA

INTRODUCTION

Two major studies have reported that a large proportion of patients with osteoporosis have impaired calcium absorption. In about one third of patients the absorption problem is so marked that the fecal calcium exceeds the calcium intake (1,2). This defect in absorption appears to be rather specific to calcium and suggests that the cause may lie in the regulatory process which controls absorption. Since 1,25 $(OH)_2D$ is the major hormone controlling calcium absorption, then it might be expected that serum 1,25 $(OH)_2D$ levels would be lower than normal in osteoporosis. On the other hand if the absorptive defect in the gut were the primary problem then serum 1,25 $(OH)_2D$ levels should be normal. A number of recent studies have now demonstrated abnormalities in vitamin D metabolism in osteoporosis. About 60-70% of osteoporotics have reduced serum levels of 1,25 $(OH)_2D$ but not 25-OH-D. Indirect attempts to stimulate 1,25 $(OH)_2D$ production by placing patients on a low calcium diet have shown that the response in osteoporotics is impaired when compared to normals (3). Direct stimulation of 1,25 $(OH)_2D$ production by the kidney using injections of parathyroid hormone did show an increase in one study, (4) but no response in another study(5). Although there is an overlap between the serum 1,25 $(OH)_2D$ levels of normals and osteoporotics various explanations may account for this finding. Some of the overlap can be attributed to individual variation in dietary calcium intake. We previously showed a significant correlation between calcium intake and serum 1,25 $(OH)_2D$ levels in normal subjects but not in osteoporotics (2). If serum 1,25 $(OH)_2D$ levels in normals are adjusted to a constant calcium intake, the normal range for serum 1,25 $(OH)_2D$ narrows from 20-53 pg/ml to 24-43 pg/ml. When osteoporotic values are compared to these adjusted normal range then a larger proportion of patients (13 out of 27) lie below the normal range than did previously (7 out of 27). Another confounding aspect is that normal subjects themselves may be developing osteoporosis, thus blurring the distinction between the two groups. There does appear to be a small group of osteoporotic patients who have low calcium absorption with normal serum 1,25 $(OH)_2D$ levels. There is no obvious explanation for this finding particularly since they appear to respond normally interms of calcium absorption to treatment with synthetic 1,25 $(OH)_2D_3$.

EFFECTS OF TREATMENT WITH SYNTHETIC 1,25 DIHYDROXYVITAMIN D_3 (ROCALTROL)

Because it is likely that decreased calcium absorption

contributes to the negative balance found in osteoporotic patients, we recently completed a study at the Mayo Clinic in which we examined the short and long term effects of synthetic 1,25 dihydroxyvitamin D_3 (Rocaltrol) in patients with osteoporosis, the dose used being 0.25 ug twice daily,(6). Calcium absorption and balance always improved on treatment. Calcium balance increased by 53 mg/day after six months and by 32 mg/day after 24 months of treatment, although in the long term study the final calcium balance was slightly negative. In addition there was a significant increase in bone volume at 24 months as measured by bone histomorphometry on bone biopsies from the iliac crest. We also found that significantly less vertebral fractures occurred in the treated group than in the placebo group. (6) These preliminary results demonstrate that treatment with 1,25 dihydroxyvitamin D_3 in small doses can be effective in osteoporotic patients. The dose of Rocaltrol used in this study showed no significant decrease in renal function. Hypercalcemia and hypercalcuria were infrequent events leading to minor adjustments in three out of twenty patients in the dose.

There is interest in the idea that adminstering larger doses of 1,25 $(OH)_2D_3$ might result in increasing the degree of activation of bone cells, either by increasing numbers of osteoblasts or by increasing osteoblast function. This could lead potentially to increases in bone volume.

In order to treat osteoporotics with larger doses of 1,25 dihydroxyvitamin D_3 some restriction of calcium intake is necessary in order to avoid hypercalcemia. To establish the relationship between urine calcium excretion and the dose of 1,25 dihydroxyvitamin D_3, further tests in normal subjects and patients with osteoporosis were performed at varying doses. Urine calcium expressed as a proportion of the calcium intake was used as a measure of the dose response to 1,25 dihydroxyvitamin D_3. Some preliminary data is shown in Tablel.

TABLE I. Dose response effect of 1,25 $(OH)_2D_3$ on Urine Calcium expressed as a fraction of the Dietary Calcium. (mean values given)

Dose of 1,25 $(OH)_2D_3$	Urine Calcium/Calcium Intake	(N)
0.20 ug/day	0.22	(20)
0.50 "	0.30	(25)
1.00 "	0.48	(12)
2.00 "	0.75	(10)

The results in Table I show that the mean urine calcium excretion expressed as a fraction of the calcium intake is approximately 0.30 on a dose of 0.50 ug daily, 0.5 on 1.0 ug daily and 0.75 on 2.0 ug daily. In order to use a dose of 1,25 $(OH)_2$ D_3

1 ug twice daily, it was estimated from the dose response that the calcium intake would need to be restricted to 400 mg daily and that the predicted urine calcium would be about 75 percent of the intake, namely 300 mg per day.

Six patients were given 1.0 ug twice daily of 1,25 dihydroxyvitamin D_3 in combination with a calcium intake of 400 mg. There was an increase in serum and urine calcium in all patients. Hypercalcemia occurred in one patient and hypercalcuria occurred in another patient. When the dose was reduced to 0.75 ug twice daily in those two patients serum and urine calcium returned to normal. Urine hydroxyproline was measured and showed no increase during the first six weeks but a small increase by the six months. Serum immunoreactive parathyroid hormone showed a decrease in all patients. The provisional results on bone histomorphometry in these patients showed that marked activation of bone occurred in three out of four patients. This was expressed in two cases by dramatic increases in the number of double tetracycline labels accompanied by large increases in osteoid forming surfaces. Although we saw a small increase in activation frequency after six weeks, it appeared to take another two to three months before the more marked effect was seen.

CONCLUSIONS

A review of the published results on serum 1,25 $(OH)_2D$ levels in osteoporotics shows an overlap between osteoporotics and normals. Most of the low values in normal subjects are due to their high calcium intake and represents the normal adaptation response (3). In osteoporotics, however, there is a failure in the adaptation mechanism and levels of serum 1,25 $(OH)_2D_3$ are low because of decrease production by the kidney (3). Thus, if the effect of calcium intake on serum 1,25 $(OH)_2D_3$ is taken into account in osteoporotics then the difference between them and the normal subjects becomes even greater. It is not clear yet why serum 1,25 $(OH)_2D$ levels are reduced in osteoporotics. It may be due to the lower parathyroid hormone levels found in this group, secondary to a slight hypercalcemia from increased bone resorption or there may be an age related decline in the ability of the kidney to produce 1,25 $(OH)_2D$. Now that measurements of serum 1,25 $(OH)_2D$ are readily available, future management of osteoporotics should probably concentrate on administering synthetic 1,25 dihydroxyvitamin D_3 to those patients in whom the serum levels are reduced (less than 35 pg/ml), since these are the patients with the lowest calcium absorption. Long term studies have shown that low doses of Rocaltrol (0.25 ug bid) can be used safely when combined with moderate dietary calcium restriction of around 800 mg per day. At this dose we found no significant changes in renal function after two years of treatment and a decrease in the occurrence of new vertebral fractures. The availability of the active metabolite 1,25 $(OH)_2D_3$ now makes this agent the treatment of choice in most conditions where vitamin D might be used. Although much more potent than vitamin D_2 or D_3, its short half life of a few hours means that side effects such as hypercalcemia can generally be controlled within 24 hours, in contrast to the effects of vitamin D_2 or D_3 where hypercalcemia has been known to last for days or weeks. However, because of its potency it is advisable when using 1,25 $(OH)_2D_3$ to monitor serum calcium and creatinine as well as 24 hour urine calcium every few weeks.

Acknowledgements: I would like to acknowledge Dr. Larry Riggs and Dr. Robert Recker with whom parts of these results are shared.

REFERENCES:

1. Gallagher, J.C., Aaron, J., Horsman, A., Marshall, D.H., Wilkinson, R. and Nordin, B.E.C. (1973) Clin. Endocinol. Metab. 2, 293.

2. Gallagher, J.C., Riggs, B.L., Eisman, J., Hamstra, A., Arnaud, S.B. and DeLuca, H.F. (1979) J. Clin. Ivest. 64,729.
3. Nordin, B.E.C., Peacock, M., Crilly, R.G., Francis, R.M., Speed, R. and Barkworth, S., (1981) In: Osteoporosis. Recent Advances in Pathogenesis and Treatment. ed. DeLuca, H.F. et al. University Park Press, Baltimore, p. 359.
4. Riggs, B.L., Hamstra, A. and DeLuca, H.F. (1981) J. Clin. Endocinol. Metab. 53, 833.
5. Slovik, D.M., Adams, J.S., Neer, R.M., Holick, M.F. and Potts, J.R. Jr. (1981) N. Engl. J. Med. 305, 372.
6. Gallagher, J.C., Jerpbak, C.M., Jee, W.S.S., Johnson, K.A., DeLuca, H.F. and Riggs, B.L. (1982) Proc. Natl. Acad. Sci. USA 79,3325.

OSTEOPENIA: THE ADFR TREATMENT

H. M. Frost, M.D.

Southern Colorado Clinic, 2002 Lake Ave., Pueblo, Colorado, U.S.A.

I. INTRODUCTION

The ADFR treatment of osteopenias (OPn), a particular form of a general concept named coherence treatment by the author, was conceived in 1977 by sigma bone group members at the University of Utah-sponsored bone workshop, Sun Valley, Idaho,[5] descriptions of it appeared in subsequent articles,[6-11] it has attracted some interest and animal and human studies of the concept are now underway in the United States and abroad. Because of that interest and some apparently encouraging early results, this symposium's program committee suggested a brief review of that treatment and its background.

IMPACT OF 19TH CENTURY ATOMISM ON THERAPEUTIC STRATEGY

The ADFR treatment described below embodies a general concept that can apply to many physiologic systems and problems, but its ADFR version can apply specifically to the osteopenias (OPn). As a morbid state characteristic of all osteoporoses (OPs), OPn (i.e., bone tissue volume deficits)[14] form a major problem in human medicine throughout the world and numerous efforts have been made to add bone to such skeletons in children as well as adults.

As for the strategy of those efforts, investigators in the previous century found that cells named osteoblasts form new bone tissue and cells named osteoclasts resorb already existing bone but, in the operational sense, they did not perceive any important biological organization superimposed on those facts. So, even in 1980, most people viewed bone tissue volume deficits as due <u>either</u> to excessive osteoclastic activity, <u>or</u> to defective osteoblastic activity.[10,11] That "either-or" idea contains a major hidden assumption: that all bone resorptive and formative activities occur independently of each other, so they are regulated independently of each other too. Given those assumptions, then attempting to restore bone to an OPn skeleton by seeking some continuous treatment that either retarded osteoclastic activity or stimulated osteoblastic activity seemed reasonable.

THE RESULTS OF TESTS OF ATOMISTIC STRATEGIES

Two sets of facts expose that atomistic viewpoint and strategy as flawed.

<u>First set</u>: Since about 1930 hundred of diverse continuous treatments of OPs patients have failed to add bone to their skeletons, excepting only treatments with fluoride.[1] Given their number, diversity and consistency, those failures leave little doubt that all had fundamental strategic flaws, yet the fact that the bone balance normally is positive on the periosteal envelope and negative on the trabecular envelope at the same time in the same bone and even in adults proves that real mechanisms do control the bone balance, so if we understood them we might be able to manipulate them for therapeutic purposes.[10]

<u>Second set</u>: This constitutes the complex intermediary organization (IO) of the skeleton, discovered by the author in the early 1960s. In the senses

of biological organization and physiologic importance, it fills the same essential roles in bone that the nephron does in kidney and its special mechanisms directly underlie the pathogenesis of all OPs.[2-11,14] However, due to some controversy the existence of that IO as an operational entity began to gain some general acceptance only after about 1980, and it still remains an enigma to most clinicians and investigators.

II. THE IO AND BONE BALANCE

The following features of that IO pertain to this text. In human adults most bone tissue turnover occurs in multi-cellular packets named BMU in which an initial Activating event makes a group of osteoclasts assemble and Resorb a packet of bone, followed by replacement by osteoblasts that Form a packet of new bone in the previous defect. Those A-R-F processes couple in such a way that the R and F always occur in the same place and in the sequence given, and on all skeletal envelopes in adults, and the amounts removed and formed in response to endocrine and other effects usually change in the same way, although often unequally.[11] In the normal human adult the positive bone balance on the periosteal envelope represents an excess of F over R per packet, while the negative balance on the cortical-endosteal and trabecular surfaces represents less F than R per packet.[3,4] That mechanism quantizes or makes both bone turnover and bone balance incremental rather than continuous processes. A special term, ΔB.BMU, signifies the size of any deficit or excess per completed BMU, and it specifically determines steady state bone balance on the adult's bone envelopes.[11] According to Parfitt, a normal adult skeleton has perhaps 10^5-10^6 such active remodeling units or BMU at any one moment.[12] Significantly, in the unchallenged skeleton these BMU are out of step with each other, i.e., temporally incoherent, as in the diagram below, left.

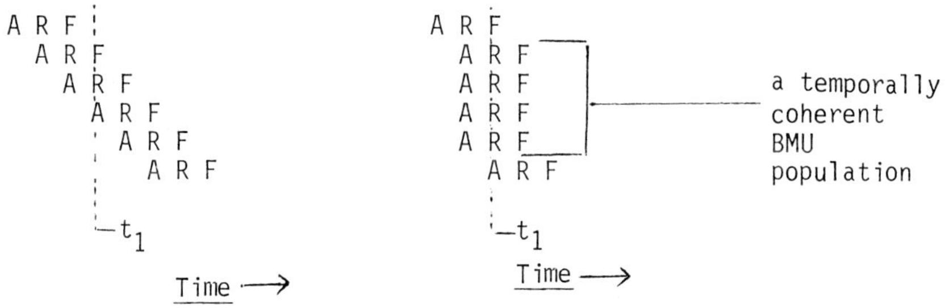

A drug given to such an incoherent skeleton will act on all 3 of the fundamental remodeling events at the same time, for at any moment it will affect activation, resorption and formation, although in different units depending on the stage they are in at that moment. Furthermore, under continuous treatment a drug will in time affect the A phase, then the R and finally the F phase of any and all individual BMU.

The MCN property. The first set of facts noted above means that whatever an agent (for example, calcitonin) may do to isolated 'clasts or 'blasts in tissue culture or related systems, in the intact living human it has little effect on bone balance so it affects both the R and F stages of intact, living BMU in the same way. Elsewhere the author calls this an MCN effect (multiple-chained-neutralizing), and it is a particular, ubiquitous and major property and function of the IO.[11] It, specifically, probably defeated the earlier mentioned past efforts to add bone to OPn skeletons by divers continuous treatments.

III. THE ADFR CONCEPT

The ADFR idea offers a simple stratagem to circumvent those MCN effects. Sharply pulsing the activation or "A" modality of the bone remodeling system makes a population of new BMU of nontrivial size begin throughout the skeleton at essentially the same time, so they progress in step or coherently in time through their subsequent R and F stages. Then a medication that Depresses osteoclast activity is given during the R phase of the BMU activity to make it resorb less bone than normal. At or before the switchover to formation the drug is then withdrawn to Free the F phase of the drug effect. That would make the ΔB.BMU parameter positive by allowing normal amounts of bone to deposit in smaller than normal holes, thereby creating permanent increments of extra bone. Repeating that manipulation adds further increments. Hence the ADFR treatment: activate-depress-free-repeat. The right side of the above diagram encodes the basic idea.

In theory of course, one could also use an agent that stimulates the BMU formation phase to construct an ADSR scheme of treatment (activate, depress, stimulate, repeat), and further variations of the idea can serve other purposes. Clearly too, the idea should generalize to any system for which the net output averaged over time sums the quantized effects of a series of sequential processes that occur in a fixed order over fixed time intervals. Hence the general concept of coherence treatment, already known by different terms to physicists, spectroscopists, oncologists and chemists. One apparently successful version has been tried in osteoporosis, although in retrospect the timings chosen in that study could be improved.[13]

To make the stratagem work requires drugs or other agents that can safely and effectively produce an activation pulse, that can depress the resorption phase without interfering with the basic ARF sequence, and knowing when and how long to give and when to withdraw the drugs. Such information can and has come from histomorphometric studies that follow one of the writer's histomorphometric algorithms,[2,11,14] but also the recent noninvasive, ultraprecise photon absorption and quantitative CAT scan methods of detecting changes in bone density could follow treatments of intact human volunteers over time, allowing us to study the pharmacologic and endocrinologic responses of the basic parameters, including the important ΔB.BMU parameter, that determine how the quantized bone remodeling and bone balance systems work *in vivo*. The need for such information offers a major and new challenge and opportunity for contemporary investigators, and with respect to methodology as well as to any data provided by it. When such information becomes available in quantity, the author suspects we will find that not all patients respond alike to a given treatment or drug, that some treatments that are safe in one group of patients can cause unacceptable risks in another, that the timings of the various ADFR steps must fit the age, sex, disease(s), drugs, and kind of OPn and OPs in question, and that current texts on skeletal regulation need drastic revision.

IV. CONCLUSION

Discovery of the skeletal IO and some of its novel properties have provided new and better insights into the pathogenesis and treatment of all skeletal disease, including but certainly not limited to the OPs and OPn. That both challenges and requires investigators of such problems to understand that IO, and to learn to think in terms of the newer and more holistic and productive skeletal physiology it has fathered. The use of sequential and intermittent treatment and investigative challenges, rather than continuous ones, could become one hallmark of that new holism.

REFERENCES

1. Briancon, D., Meunier, P.J.: Treatment of osteoporosis with fluoride, calcium and vitamin D. Orth. Clin. No. Amer. 12:629-648, 1981.
2. Frost, H.M.: Mathematical Elements of Bone Remodeling. Charles Thomas, Springfield, 1964.
3. Frost, H.M.: Bone Dynamics in Osteoporosis and Osteomalacia. Charles Thomas, Springfield, 1966.
4. Frost, H.M.: Bone Remodeling and its Relationship to Metabolic Bone Diseases. Charles Thomas, Springfield, 1973.
5. Frost, H.M.: Coherence treatment of osteoporoses. MS circulated to the sigma bone group in 1977.
6. Frost, H.M.: Treatment of osteoporoses by manipulation of coherent bone cell populations. Clin. Orth. Rel. Res. 143:228-244, 1979.
7. Frost, H.M.: Coherence treatment of osteoporoses by an ADFR Scheme. In: Osteoporosis, eds. H.F. DeLuca, H.M. Frost, W.S.S. Jee, C.C. Johnston, Jr. and A.M. Parfitt. University Park Press, Baltimore, 393-396, 1981.
8. Frost, H.M.: Coherence treatment of osteoporoses. Orth. Clin. N. Amer. 12:649-669, 1981.
9. Frost, H.M.: The osteoporoses in the 1980's: A field in flux. Int. Med. 3:65-93, 1982.
10. Frost, H.M.: Pharmacology and the osteoporoses. A field in flux. Meth. and Find. Exptl. Clin. Pharmacol. 5:5-16, 1983.
11. Frost, H.M.: The skeletal intermediary organization: A review. J. Met. Bone Dis. Rel. Res., in press.
12. Parfitt, A.M.: Stereologic basis of bone histomorphometry. In: Bone Histomorphometry: Techniques and Interpretation. Ed. R.R. Recker, C.R.C. Press, Boca Raton, 53-88, 1983.
13. Rasmussen, H.: Theoretical considerations in the treatment of osteoporosis. In: Osteoporosis, eds. H.F. DeLuca, H.M. Frost, W.S.S. Jee, C.C. Johnston, Jr. and A.M. Parfitt, Univ Park Press, Baltimore, 383-392, 1980.
14. Orthop. Clin. N. Amer. 12, 1981.

Discussion following Dr. Chesnut's, Meunier's, Gallagher's and Frost's presentations:

L. RIGGS: There are two developments on the immediate horizon that may make calcitonin therapy better than it now appears. The first is recombinant gene technology; at least one company has the gene for calcitonin, so we should soon have human calcitonin in large amounts, and hopefully resistance will be less. Second, Dr. Heath, from our group, by using better extraction techniques, has shown that the plasma level of calcitonin monomer is very low. A hundred units of calcitonin in a single injection, is a pharmacologic dose. Giving a more physiologic dose by continuous infusion, as insulin is sometimes administered in the treatment of diabetes, may be the way for the future.

Dr. Meunier, you are using relatively small doses of flouride, which is commendable; but with larger doses, up to 75 and 100 mg of sodium flouride a day, you will see a mineralization defect.

C. CHESNUT: Yes, I agree that 100 MRC units is probably excessive, and certainly daily administration may not be essential. Somewhere between 25 and 50 units may be the optimal dose, but this needs further study. I agree that human calcitonin may provide improved efficacy; however, it is our feeling that the resistance we see is not antibody-mediated, although we did not measure neutralizing antibodies.

J. BUCHANAN: Dr. Riggs presented earlier a concept of pathogenesis of osteoporosis starting with a primary increase in bone resorption, leading to systemic release of calcium and depression of PTH, calcitriol and GI absorption of calcium. If this is true, there would be some danger in administering calcitriol, which would reverse the compensatory response. Yet, Dr. Gallagher's results seem beneficial. Is there an explanation for this paradox?

C. GALLAGHER: Our results imply that calcitriol suppresses bone resorption primarily, and changes the flow of calcium from out of bone into bone. Incidentally, plasma calcitriol levels on treatment are typical in the range of 50 to 60 pg/ml on 0.5 μg/day; but there is considerable individual variation.

S. TOH: With regard to calcitonin resistance, using single photon absorptiometry we found that calcitonin treatment of Paget's disease slowed the loss of normal non-Pagetic bone over two years, but by the end of the third year of treatment, the effect was no longer apparent.

C. CHESNUT: That goes along with what we said - calcitonin can slow bone loss for a period of time, but the effect does not last indefinitely. Our single photon regional bone mass measurements did not change.

J. KANIS: Dr. Gallagher, you report that calcitriol appears to decrease fracture frequency. If I interpret your data correctly, you are converting patients to zero balance - preventing futher loss of bone, but not increasing bone mass.

C. GALLAGHER: Of all the measurements of calcium metabolism, the balance technique is probably the least sensitive. We did iliac bone biopsies and saw a significant increase in trabecular bone volume after two years.

C. JOHNSTON: Was this at the expense of the cortical bone?

C. GALLAGHER: We did not measure cortical bone loss, but Dr. Recker has some data showing that cortical bone loss is decreased on treatment with calcitriol.

H. FROST: Concerning bone pain and fractures in osteoporotic patients, an important point is consistently overlooked. Many assume that the propensity to bone fragility and fracture is due solely to loss of bone quantity, this is certainly important, but it is not everything. The other factor is skeletal micro-damage. The effect of decreased bone turnover and a prolonged value for sigma is an accumulation of micro-damage or micro-fractures, so with progressive weakening until a normal load finally causes a crush fracture. An activator, such as calcitriol, could reduce fractures by increasing bone turnover and repairing the micro-damage of bone, without necessarily increasing the quantity of bone.

A second problem of interpretation observed with fluoride treatment is that conventional histomorphometry ignores the degree of mineralization of the bone, which can have a significant effect on its mechanical properties and on its fragility. For that purpose, microradiography remains one of the best tools.

C. GALLAGHER: That would explain the much greater increase in bone volume with fluoride than with calcitriol; and yet, a comparable reduction in fracture rates with both treatments.

H. FROST: Also, it is part of the explanation why bone mineral content may not change when trabecular bone volume increases, aside from any difference between trabecular and cortical bone.

R. NEER: Dr. Meunier, are the effects of sodium fluoride on trabecular bone at the expense of cortical bone, or is there an increase in the total amount of bone? I understand that you saw no overall change in cortical bone density, but did the trabecular bone responders lose cortical bone?

P. MEUNIER: Cortical thickness showed no significant change in any group or sub-group, including responders. Cortical porosity, increased, but the error in the measurement is very large. Nevertheless, we do not recommend fluoride for patients with hip fracture.

J. REEVE: In our study with a synthetic fragment of parathyroid hormone 1-34, trabecular bone volume, measured by Dr. Meunier increased to a similar extent as with sodium fluoride, but the effect appeared about three times as fast. Similar results were found in normal greyhounds treated in a similar way with PTH injections, so the effect is not dependent on the treated subjects having osteoporosis. In neither of these studies did we see changes in peripheral cortical bone measured by photon absorptiometry. I have a serious concern about using serial fracture incidence in the same patient as a criterion of treatment success. Ruegsegger and Dambacher showed that loss of bone in osteoporosis was often episodic. If treatment is started at a time when bone is being lost quickly, it is predictable that the fracture incidence will fall, whether or not treatment modified the disease. That is why you need matched controls for this sort of study.

C. GALLAGHER: Half the patients in both the placebo and treatment groups were crossed over by randomization, but I agree that long-term comparison of placebo and treatment groups is the only way to be sure that a natural diminuation in fracture rate has not occurred. However, we're talking about a 75 to 80% reduction infracture rates, which is far outside spontaneous variation. Also, Riggs' historical control period was longer than one year. Finally, the episodic bone loss you mentioned was observed only in the extremities.

C. ANDERSON: The ADFR concept seems to work - in fact, it has worked so well for us that we were skeptical of our results; we saw an 80 to 120% increase in trabecular bone volume. But there needs to be considerable experimental work yet to find out the optimum timing of episodic therapy. If the ADFR is tailored to the actual value for sigma in the patient at the time of biopsy, sigma for both resorption and formation will decrease towards normal adult nonosteoporotic values.

H. FROST: The significance of sigma (the length of time it takes the average bone remodelling unit to progress from activation to completion) in the present context is that to get a steady-state effect from any treatment one has to maintain it for at least one sigma. In the symptomatic osteoporotic sigma is prolonged, so you have to treat for a minimum of two years. We saw earlier that the initial positive bone balance induced by calcitonin leveled off after two years - it was only a transient, not a persistent effect.

F. MELSEN: Dr. Meunier, we have treated 150 patients for five years with fluoride. Our results after two years are similar to yours. By study of microradiographs, we found that the newly formed bone was very loosely textured and contained very little mineral, but after five years of treatment, the abnormal bone had been replaced. Have you seen the same remodelling of the newly-created bone after treatment?

P. MEUNIER: Yes.

J. HARRISON: Was there any relationship between the bone histology before starting therapy and the response?

P. MEUNIER: We did not find any significant difference in the three groups. High-remodelling osteoporotics responded as well as normal or low-turnover patients. However, there are two types of non-responders. Some patients (about 10%) have no increase in formation surface, but 25% had a marked increase in formation surface, but despite this, did not gain bone. I think it's important to discuss response and non-response in terms of bone histology.

C. CHESNUT: We agree with Dr. Frost on ADFR. Our data suggests that intermittent pulse therapy has to be tested more thoroughly. We need to make better use of skeletal alkaline phosphatase as an index of bone formation and urinary hydroxyproline as an index of bone resorption to define the proper timing of the pulse. This is going to be a major area of research in the future.

XIV PAGET'S DISEASE

PAGET'S DISEASE

Moderator: Stephen M. Krane

Department of Medicine, Harvard Medical School and Massachusetts General Hospital, Boston, Massachusetts, U.S.A.

Paget's disease of bone has been studied extensively by many investigators interested in metabolic bone diseases. Yet it was pointed out by Albright and Reifenstein in 1948 that Paget's disease is not generalized and that normal bone can always be identified. The fact that Paget's disease is localized to some but not to all bones was offered as, "strong evidence against its being a metabolic or endocrine disorder" (1). Even if Paget's disease does strictly belong in the category of metabolic bone diseases, it has been possible to learn a great deal about bone turnover in this disorder and successfully use therapeutic agents to help patients clinically.

We assume that the initial event in Paget's disease is a focal resorption of existing normal bone (2). Histologically, this excessive resorption is shown by the increase in the scalloped resorption spaces (Howship's lacunae) filled with active osteoclasts that are larger and more multinucleated. Even in the earliest biopsies of pagetic lesions, however, there is evidence of increased osteoblastic activity with the deposition of lamellar or woven bone adjacent to areas of resorption, frequently on opposite surfaces. These events have been interpreted as indicating a marked increase in the "birth rate" of the so-called basic multicellular units of bone (3). Although bone resorption and formation are both increased, there is a greater relative increase in resorption as compared with normal bone. The "uninvolved" nonpagetic bone may not be entirely normal and show increased resorption and osteoid surfaces. The latter changes have been interpreted as due to secondary hyperparathyroidism (3).

If resorption is the initial event in Paget's disease and the increases in bone formation are coupled to the increases in resorption, then it would follow that if one decreases the resorption rate, the formation rate should also decrease. It has been possible, using three different types of agents (calcitonins, diphosphonates, and mithramycin), to decrease bone resorption in Paget's disease. Indices of bone formation decrease later than those of bone resorption. Although each of these drugs reduces osteoclast function and possibly the generation of new osteoclasts from precursor cells, the activity of the disease eventually returns to pretreatment levels following discontinuation of therapy. The pagetic lesion therefore is not cured. Recent evidence has suggested the possibility that Paget's disease is due to infection of osteoclasts or osteoclast precursors with a virus possibly related to measles or respiratory syncytial virus. F.R. Singer and B.G. Mills present the evidence for viral infection of pagetic cells and discuss the problems in identifying possible agents. If a virus is definitively identified, it will still be essential to prove that this agent is the <u>cause</u> of the disease and not simply a passenger. If the former is the case, <u>cure</u> of Paget's disease could be achieved only if the putative virus is eliminated or if the deleterious consequences of such infection (altered proliferation and function of bone cells) are reversed.

At the present time, it is necessary to deal with the clinical problems of Paget's disease. Although most patients are asymptomatic or the involvement is of relatively little consequence, others are candidates for therapy with either calcitonin, diphosphonates (bisphosphonates) or mithramycin, or possibly combinations of these drugs. Some of these clinical problems are listed in Table 1. Not all of these problems are responsive to drug therapy.

TABLE 1. Clinical problems in patients with Paget's disease of bone

1.	Pain over lesions
2.	Deformities
3.	Joint disease
4.	Neural compression
5.	Propensity to fracture
6.	Vascular effects (high bone flow, high cardiac output, "steal" syndromes)
7.	Disabling fatigue
8.	Hypercalcemia and hypercalciuria
9.	Hyperuricemia
10.	Tumors (reparative granulomas, malignant neoplasms)

For example, it is probable that joint disease such as pagetic coxopathy, once developed, will not be reversed by medical management but will eventually require and respond to total hip replacement. Other features are responsive, however, particularly pain over lesions demonstrable radiologically or by bone scan.

C. Nagant de Deuxchaisnes reviews certain aspects of the use of calcitonins, particularly with respect to their success in improving the focal lesion with apparent healing of the osteolytic disease and replacement with mineralized bone. O.L.M. Bijvoet discusses the use of the bisphosphonates and emphasize their extraordinary potency in inhibiting bone resorption. This has been demonstrated in numerous careful studies with etidronate disodium, and is reflected in the normalization of the abnormally high urinary hydroxyproline excretion. In Bijvoet's experience, use of etidronate disodium results in clinical improvement in most instances although some individuals have a temporary increase in bone pain. Fractures were not a problem in his series. There was an increase in osteolytic pagetic lesions in some individuals as stressed by Nagant de Deuxchaisnes. In contrast, APD (disodium [3-amino-1-hydroxypropylidene]-1, 1-bisphosphonate), the most potent of the available bisphosphonates appears to arrest osteolytic lesions and promotes filling in of defects. Unfortunately, APD has not been approved for use in most countries, including the U.S.A. Experience with mithramycin is reviewed by W.G. Ryan. This drug is effective in reducing abnormal chemical findings in Paget's disease and improves symptoms and abnormal bone scans. It is potentially the most toxic of available drugs and must be used with caution. The long term remissions that have occasionally been observed following a brief course of therapy have provided impetus for study of further potential uses of mithramycin alone or in combination with other agents.

REFERENCES

1. Albright, F. and Reifenstein, E.C., Jr. (1948): The Parathyroid Glands and Metabolic Bone Disease. Selected Studies. Williams & Wilkins, Baltimore.

2. Singer, F.R., Schiller, A.L., Pyle, E.B. and Krane, S.M. (1978): In: Metabolic Bone Disease, vol. 2, p. 489. Editors: L.V. Avioli and S.M. Krane. Academic Press, New York.

3. Meunier, P.J., Coindre, J.M., Edouard, C.M. and Arlot, M.E. (1980): Arthritis Rheum., 23, 1095.

WHAT IS THE ETIOLOGY OF PAGET'S DISEASE AND CAN WE CURE IT?

Frederick R. Singer and Barbara G. Mills

Orthopaedic Hospital/University of Southern California Bone and Connective Tissue Laboratory and University of Southern California Schools of Medicine and Dentistry, Los Angeles, CA, U.S.A.

THE ETIOLOGY OF PAGET'S DISEASE

Paget's disease of bone is a disorder whose underlying pathology appears to involve a localized activation of osteoprogenitor cells to differentiate into osteoclasts in one or more sites in the skeleton.

This results over a period of time in a radiologically apparent osteolytic lesion which advances slowly. After decades an entire bone may be involved with the disease process which has usually evolved into a dominantly osteosclerotic state. This occurs due to a local proliferation of osteoblasts which attempt to repair the result of the underlying osteolytic activity. For reasons which are unclear the exuberant bone formation of Paget's disease leads to an increase in bone mass. Because of the ensuing abnormal bone architecture, bones involved with Paget's disease are likely to become deformed and are susceptible to fracture. The nature of the signal for osteoblastic differentiation in Paget's disease is unknown but future studies will certainly focus on the possibility that the skeletal coupling factor recently described by Baylink and colleagues is involved.

Since the time of Paget a variety of hypotheses have been proposed to explain the etiology of the disease. These include disorders of inflammation, hormone secretion, vascular malformation, neoplasia and connective tissue metabolism. Until the present no significant evidence has been presented to support any of these theories. With the appreciation of the existence of slow virus infections of the nervous system, attention has been focused on whether Paget's disease is a similar entity (1). Slow virus infections of the nervous system such as subacute sclerosing panencephalitis, and Paget's disease share certain clinical and laboratory features which suggest a common type of pathogenesis. Both disorders have a prolonged clinical course, involvement of a single organ, familial predisposition, absence of an acute inflammatory process, giant cells in pathologic lesions and viral-like nuclear inclusions in affected cells. The latter observation has particularly stimulated studies searching for a viral etiology of Paget's disease.

Ultrastructural studies of the bone cells of almost 200 patients have revealed that the osteoclasts of each patient have characteristic nuclear and cytoplasmic inclusions which are not found in other bone cells, or in osteoclasts from a variety of metabolic bone diseases. These inclusions have a microtubular structure and most closely resemble viral nucleocapsids of the Paramyxoviridae family. The viruses of this family include measles, mumps, the parainfluenzas, and respiratory syncytial virus. A measles-like virus is responsible for subacute sclerosing panencephalitis so that there is precedent for a virus from this family to be involved in a human slow virus infection.

Morphological similarity of the nuclear inclusions of Paget's disease with viral nucleocapsids is not sufficient evidence for the presence of a virus in the Pagetic osteoclasts. For this reason more sophisticated methodology has been utilized to address the problem. Rebel and his colleagues utilized indirect immunofluorescence and immunoperoxidase staining techniques on decalcified bone sections to search for viral antigens (2). They found evidence of measles virus antigens in the osteoclasts of all patients studied with rabbit antisera to measles as well as serum from a patient with subacute sclerosing panencephalitis. In our own studies of bone biopsy specimens and cultured cells from surgical specimens we initially found negative results with measles antisera and positive results with several antisera to respiratory syncytial virus (3). Subsequently other measles antisera has given positive results in about 50% of specimens, and in some patients both measles and respiratory syncytial virus antigens were found in the same osteoclasts of serial sections. The finding of antigens of both viruses in some specimens is unexplained at this time since there is no known antigenic cross-reactivity between measles and respiratory syncytial virus. A mixed infection or viral recombination could account for the results, or the possibility exists that the putative viral agent is a previously unclassified virus of the Paramyxoviridae family.

Despite long-term culture of mononuclear cells obtained from surgical specimens, we have not been successful in isolating an infectious virus from Pagetic lesions. Nuclear inclusions are only occasionally found in cultured cells and budding off of complete virions from the cell membrane has never been observed despite the presence of antigens of respiratory syncytial virus in all but one cell culture. This suggests that the cultured cells we have studied are not sufficiently permissive for full expression of the viral genome. Unfortunately osteoclasts do not survive more than a few days in culture.

These early experiences with attempts to isolate an infectious virus from pathologic specimens of Paget's disease are reminiscent of the difficulty encountered in recovering an infectious virus from brain specimens of patients with subacute sclerosing panencephalitis. Only after repeated long-term cultivations of brain cells was it finally possible to isolate the measles-like virus from about 20% of specimens.

The problem in isolating an infectious virus is explained by the electron microscopic observations. The viruses of the Paramyxoviridae family are RNA viruses consisting of a central nucleic acid surrounded by a group of protein subunits termed the capsid. The combination of the central nucleic acid and associated capsid is the nucleocapsid. The final assembly of a complete infectious virus requires the addition of an outer envelope which is derived from cellular proteins. The electron microscopy of Paget's bone cells as well as brain cells of subacute sclerosing panencephalitis indicates only the nucleocapsid is present and it follows that isolation of an infectious virus would not occur until the outer envelope was present. We do have preliminary evidence for transmission of respiratory syncytial virus-antigens from cultured Pagetic cells to co-cultivated HEP-2 cells, a cell line used to rescue respiratory syncytial virus (4). However, electron microscopy has not demonstrated infectious virions in these cells.

Because of the encouraging results thus far obtained, studies to definitively demonstrate a viral presence in Paget's disease continue. These include utilization of monoclonal antibodies for more specific viral antigen identification, viral peptide and messenger RNA isolation and cDNA hybridization probes. In addition attempts to develop an animal model of Paget's disease by injecting bone cells into the skeleton of athymic nude mice is ongoing.

Should a virus be isolated and identified from Pagetic lesions many questions will remain. It will be necessary to demonstrate that the virus can induce the disease in animals. An evaluation of immunoregulatory function will be necessary to explain what accounts for an autosomal dominant inheritance of the disease in up to 50% of patients. Finally it will be important to determine which cells are the initial target of the virus, differentiated osteoclasts or precursors, and how does the virus produce a proliferation of osteoclasts? Such information would be useful in planning future studies of the treatment and prevention of this common bone disorder.

A CURE FOR PAGET'S DISEASE?

A variety of therapeutic agents, including the calcitonins, the diphosphonates and mithramycin, have been shown to produce clinical and biochemical remission in patients with Paget's disease (5). When available, histological evaluation indicates a variable reduction of the numbers of osteoclasts and osteoblasts in the lesions of treated patients. Despite the inhibitory effects of these agents on bone cells, the majority of studies indicate that the osteoclasts in treated patients still harbor the characteristic nuclear and cytoplasmic inclusions. Further evidence of a persisting viral presence is provided by the finding that viral antigens are still present in the osteoclasts as determined by immunohistologic techniques (2).

It is conceivable that complete eradication of osteoclasts from Pagetic lesions, if possible, would not allow persistence of a viral infection and thereby result in a "cure" of the disorder. At this time it is not possible to be certain whether this is a likely result since the initial target cell of the putative viral infection is not known. If osteoclast osteoprogenitor cells are the initial target cells a viral infection might persist in the absence of the differentiated cells. In addition it is not established that any form of therapy can completely and selectively eradicate all the osteoclasts from a Pagetic lesion. Complete suppression of bone cell activity might, in fact, be harmful since it would probably not permit resolution of the osteolytic lesions of Paget's disease. This is a well-documented effect of calcitonin therapy despite incomplete suppression of bone cell activity (5).

If Paget's disease can be shown to be a consequence of a viral infection of bone cells it seems reasonable to conclude that future therapy will revolve around anti-viral agents. Prevention of the disease may also be possible through specific immunization. It appears likely that we will continue to use a variety of suppressive drugs until the etiology of Paget's disease has been definitively established.

REFERENCES

1. Singer, F.R. (1980): Calcif. Tissue Int., 31, 185.
2. Rebel, A., Basle, M., Pouplard, A., Malkani, K., Filmon, R. and Lepatezour, A. (1980): Arthritis Rheum., 23, 1104.
3. Mills, B.G., Singer, F.R., Weiner, L.P. and Holst, P.A. (1981): Proc. Natl. Acad. Sci. (USA), 78, 1209.
4. Mills, B.G., Singer, F.R., Weiner, L.P. and Holst, P. (1981): In: Hormonal Control of Calcium Metabolism, p.410. Editors: D.V. Cohn, R.V. Talmage and J. L. Matthews. Excerpta Medica, Amsterdam.
5. Proceedings of the Kroc Foundation Conference on Paget's Disease of Bone (1980). Editors: R.D. Altman and F. Singer. Arthritis Rheum., 23, 1073.

Discussion following paper by F. Singer

S. KRANE: One of the problems, of course is that the finding of viruses or inclusions doesn't mean that this is the etiological agent, but could be a passenger as has been shown in other diseases.

J. SHAPIRO: In the cell cultures that you mentioned where you had positive fluorescence, what were the cells?

F. SINGER: They are probably related to osteoblast-like cells. Osteoclasts do not survive, which is one of the problems with long-term cell cultures. We believe the osteoclast is probably permissive for the full expression of the viral genome, but we culture mononuclear cells which contain alkaline phosphatase and also receptors for 1,25(OH)$_2$D, but we don't know their true nature. They are probably osteoprogentor cell osteoblasts, but we cannot prove it at this time.

J. SHAPIRO: I assume you don't see inclusions in these cells?

F. SINGER: All the cells exhibit positive immunofluorescence in all cultures that we have looked at, but it is difficult to find inclusions. We found them in four cultures from four different patients, but that is I think due to lack of permissiveness of the cells for the full expression of the viral genome.

J. SHAPIRO: How many specimens have you seen in which you cannot identify inclusions in osteoclasts?

F. SINGER: Occasionally Dr. Mills has to search for several weeks, but if she looks at enough osteoclasts all patients have them. I think investigators from other countries agree.

C. JACKSON: How do you explain the inheritance pattern that we see in Paget's on a virus hypothesis?

F. SINGER: I hesitate to speculate on that, although there are now two studies showing a linkage in some families with the HLA focus on, I believe, chromosome 6. If this is a viral disease, and I use the word "if" on purpose, there may be a mild immune abnormality; but that really remains to be seen after a viral etiology is proven.

DO CALCITONINS HELP PAGET'S DISEASE ?

Charles Nagant de Deuxchaisnes

Arthritis Unit, Department of Medicine, St-Luc University Hospital, Louvain University in Brussels, Belgium

Calcitonin (CT) remains at present the therapeutic agent of choice in Paget's disease, because it is the only medication available which is both effective and devoid of skeletal and systemic toxicity.

Its effectiveness is due to its antiosteoclastic effect. Receptors to CT have been described on the osteoclasts. In vitro, osteoclasts incubated on a glass or plastic substrate keep an intense ruffling activity. When CT is added, the osteoclasts come to quiescence : complete cessation of lamellipodial activity and pseudopod retraction is achieved within a few minutes and this in a reversible fashion (1). The osteoblasts remain unaffected and when they are added to the culture, the osteoclasts immediately regain their activity (2). In the rat, studies on the alveolar bone osteoclasts showed that CT first decreased the number of nuclei and then the number of osteoclasts, especially those attached to bone (3).

Focal bone resorption by giant multinucleated osteoclasts, containing the typical intranuclear inclusions, is the primum movens of Paget's disease. CT acts on the osteoclast number, size and function, as well as on the differentiation of the osteoprogenitor cells into osteoclasts. An action on osteoclast count and on their ultrastructure (retraction of the ruffled border) has been demonstrated already 30 min after CT injection in Paget's disease (4). Chronic administration of CT in pagetic patients also induced a significant decrease in the osteoclast count (5,6), osteoclast size (7), number of nuclei per osteoclast (6,7). Total resorption surface significantly diminished (6). There was less woven, and more lamellar bone (6).

This antiosteoclastic effect reflects itself by a decrease in the parameters of bone turnover (serum alkaline phosphatase and urinary output of total hydroxyproline) to circa 50 % of pretreatment values. They will fall into the normal range if they were not too elevated to start with, but will not do so if pretreatment levels were high. This is referred to as the *plateau phenomenon*, the exact mechanism of which is unknown. Secondary hyperparathyroidism and down-regulation of the receptors as possible causes have been ruled out. Perhaps the continued presence of unaffected osteoblasts prevents complete action of CT on the osteoclasts (cfr. experiments in vitro). The plateau phenomenon does in no way mean, however, that osteoclasts are not being inhibited. Indeed, during the plateau phenomenon, there is continued suppression of symptoms, progressive amelioration of the histological findings (8), and a continued progression from a focal negative to a focal positive bone balance on X-Rays (9). When CT therapy is withdrawn, the parameters of bone turnover return to pretreatment values after a period of about 6 mo. Very few cases do not respond to CT administration from the very beginning. They are referred to as *primary resistance* to CT. More cases lose some, and a few cases lose all of their initial response to CT. They are referred to as *secondary resistance*, or the *rebound phenomenon*, or also the *escape phenomenon*. Whether this reflects the presence of a more agressive group of oesteoclasts or whether CT loses its effect on the differentiation of the osteoprogenitor cells remains speculative. In vitro, escape ceases when cell proliferation in neonatal mouse calvaria is inhibited by γ-irradiation (10). This is consistent with the theory that escape is due to bone cell differentiation and recruitment of specific precursor cells, in response to stimulators of bone resorption, leading to the appearance of osteoclasts that are unresponsive to CT. When porcine (PCT) or salmin (SCT) calcitonins are used, secondary resistance should be distinguished from *antibody-based resis-*

tance. If anticalcitonin antibodies often appear during long-term administration of PCT or SCT, they seldom lead to clinical resistance, which manifests itself in circa 5 % of the cases, but in 22 % in one series (11), usually not before 2 years of therapy (12). The only valid proof that antibody-based resistance has occurred is a response to CT upon changing to an alternative calcitonin (13).

The first indication, and the most frequent one, for administering CT in Paget's disease is to relieve bone pain. That this can be accomplished successfully has been shown in a Multicenter double-blind trial (14), using 80 U/day of SCT 6 days/week for 3 mo. in 46 versus placebo in 36 patients matched for sex, age, duration of disease, prevalence of pain, decreased function, and increased local temperature. Improvement occurred in 60 % of the SCT group versus 15 % of the placebo group ($p<0.001$), improvement of function in 29 % of the SCT group versus 13 % of the placebo group ($p<0.01$), and decreased temperature in 45 % of the SCT group versus 11 % in the placebo group ($p<0.025$). Side-effects numbered 47 in the SCT group versus 7 in the placebo group. In open studies, relief of pain in 14 series of the literature which we have analyzed was observed on the average in 80 % (45-100 %) of the patients. Pain in the limbs was especially relieved, while low back pain and pain owing to osteoarthritis connected with Paget's disease were more resistant. Pain was usually relieved within a matter of weeks, and did not necessarily recur when therapy was interrupted. Early recurrence, within 6 mo. of CT withdrawal, was the exception rather than the rule, and in 50-77 % of the patients, pain had not recurred one year after cessation of CT therapy (15-17), pointing towards the possibility of discontinuous therapy for this indication. Spontaneous fractures do seldom occur during CT therapy. Yet this is the most frequent complication in Paget's disease (18), especially the dreaded femur fracture, whose prognosis may be grim, with an 18 % mortality and a 40 % non-union in the experience of Dove (19). Its exact incidence is unknown, but 31 such fractures in pagetic femurs (19 traumatic, 12 spontaneous) were observed in 737 patients treated with EHDP (20), an incidence of 4.2 %. We have only found one such fracture, a traumatic one (21), during CT therapy out of 497 patients, i.e. an incidence of 0.2 %. This is clearly an underestimation of the actual incidence of this fracture. It is probable, however, that CT does prevent the affected long bones from fracturing. CT is also especially useful in other complications of Paget's disease, such as immobilization hypercalcemia (22), high output cardiac failure (23), and symptoms due to or mimicking neurologic compression (24,25). It is unable to improve deafness, but prepares to orthopedic surgery by rapidly diminishing bone blood flow (26) and, more slowly, bone softness.

Side-effects are numerous, especially nausea and flushing, but mild, and they usually diminish with time. They at times are sufficiently unpleasant that about 10 % of the patients, especially women, will interrupt therapy. They are dose-dependent and more pronounced when CT is given intramuscularly than subcutaneously.

Paget's disease being a focal condition, it should also be approached focally to ascertain whether the diminution in bone turnover, as assessed biochemically, is *beneficial* to the pagetic lesions. Only through a careful radiographic documentation, collected prospectively, can this be accomplished, the bone scan being a blind method of evaluation. In doing so, reconstruction of those areas where bone resorption was apparent could be observed in 100 % of the cases within 4 mo. of the initiation of therapy (9,27,28). On high dosages, disease progression could be reversed. While the biochemical indices of bone turnover reached a plateau, the focal bone balance continued to improve radiologically. This effect was dose-dependent and highly reversible upon CT withdrawal. It could be reproduced in 100 % of the cases on retreatment with CT. It could not be reproduced neither with the diphosphonate EHDP (low dosages), nor with the combined therapy EHDP + CT (27,28). Only the second generation diphosphonate APD was able to induce positive focal bone balances (29). Using a particular scoring system explained elsewhere (27,28), a ratio between positive and negative signs (28) seen on X-Rays was determined, which was referred to as the "constructive index" (30). It was infinite for CT, 0.28 for EHDP (7.0 mg/kg/day), 0.96 for combined therapy CT + EHDP (7.4 mg/kg/day), and 12-20 for APD (600 mg/day). Whenever mineralization defects were produced by diphosphonates, the administration of CT healed them very rapidly, as if CT under those circumstances had mineralizing properties. Calcitriol in this situation did not achieve any radiologic improvement (28). A similar situation is seen in the rat where EHDP-induced lesions in the growth cartilage do not heal on calcitriol, but do so when CT is given (31). Our results with CT on X-Rays reinforce those obtained by Doyle et al. (32), and Woodhouse et al. (21). They have been confirmed by Murphy et al. (33), and Whyte et al. (34).

In summary, CT may improve Paget's disease clinically, biochemically, radiologically, and histologically. This effect is dose-dependent and reversible on withdrawal of therapy, although symptoms may not recur before long periods of time. Intermittent therapy is often sufficient, although continuous treatment may be indicated in some cases. Useful dosages are 50 U of SCT 3 times weekly to twice daily, or 0.5 mg (=50 U) of HCT 3 times weekly to twice daily. Any progress in the mode of administration of CT that would allow to avoid the parenteral route and that simultaneously would not produce any of the unpleasant side-effects, might make of CT not only an effective drug, devoid of skeletal and systemic toxicity, but also a popular one.

REFERENCES

1. Chambers, T.J. and Magnus, C.J. (1982) : J. Pathol., 136, 27.
2. Chambers, T.J. (1982) : J. Cell. Sci., 57, 247.
3. Baron, R. and Vignery, A. (1981) : Metab. Bone Dis. Rel. Res., 2, 339.
4. Singer, F.R., Melvin, K.E.W. and Mills, B.G. (1976) : Clin. Endocrinol., 5 (suppl.), 333s.
5. Singer,F.R., Rude, R.K. and Mills, B.G. (1977) : In : Human Calcitonin and Paget's Disease, p. 93. Editor : I. MacIntyre. Hans Huber Publishers, Bern.
6. Fornasier,V.L., Stapleton, K. and Williams, C.C. (1978) : Human Pathol., 9, 455.
7. Schulz, A., Delling, G., Kruse, H.P., Kuhlencordt, F. and Ziegler, R. (1977) : In : Molecular Endocrinology, p. 199. Editors : I. MacIntyre and M. Szelke. Elsevier/North-Holland Biomedical Press, Amsterdam.
8. Bordier, P., Figueroa, M. and Marie, P. (1974) : In : La Maladie de Paget. Symposium International, p. 155. Editor : D.J. Hioco. Armour Montagu, Paris.
9. Nagant de Deuxchaisnes, C., Rombouts-Lindemans, C., Huaux, J.P., Malghem, J. and Maldague, B. (1977) : In : Molecular Endocrinology, p. 213. Editors : I. MacIntyre and M. Szelke. Elsevier/North-Holland Biomedical Press, Amsterdam.
10. Krieger, N.S., Feldman, R.S. and Tashjian, A.H., Jr. (1982) : Calcif. Tissue Int., 34, 197.
11. Singer, F.R., Fredericks, R.S. and Minkin, C. (1980) : Arthritis Rheum., 23, 1148.
12. Hosking, D.J., Huddlestone, L.B., Clark, A.J., Johnson, S.K. and Martin, T.J. (1981) : Metab. Bone Dis. Rel. Res., 2, 315.
13. Martin, T.J. (1979) : Aust. N.Z.J. Med., 9, 36.

14. Bouvet, J.P. (1977) : Nouv. Presse Méd., 6, 1447.
15. Avramides, A., Flores, A., DeRose, J. and Wallach, S. (1976) : J. Clin. Endocrinol. Metab., 42, 459.
16. Martin, T.J., Jerums, C., Melick, R.A., Xipell, J.M. and Arnott, R. (1977) : Aust. N.Z.J. Med., 7, 36.
17. Evans, I.M.A., Banks, L., Doyle, F.H., Joplin, G.F., Pennock, J., Stevenson, J.C. and MacIntyre, I. (1980) : Metab. Bone Dis. Rel. Res., 2, 87.
18. Nagant de Deuxchaisnes, C. and Krane, S.M. (1964) : Medicine (Baltimore), 43, 233.
19. Dove, J. (1980) : J. Bone Jt Surg., 62-B, 12.
20. Johnston, C.C., Jr., Altman, R.D., Canfield, R.E., Finerman, G.A.M., Taulbee, J.D. and Ebert, M.L. (1983) : Clin. Orthop., 172, 186.
21. Woodhouse, N.J.Y., Chalmers, A.H., Wells, I.P., Dewbury, K.C. and Mohamedally, S.M. (1977) : Brit. J. Radiol., 50, 699.
22. Woodhouse, N.J.Y. (1972) : Clin. Endocrinol. Metab., 1, 125.
23. Henley, J.W., Croxson, R.S. and Ibbertson, H.K. (1979) : Aust. N.Z.J. Med., 9, 390.
24. Chen, J.R., Rhee, R.S.C., Wallach, S., Avramides, A. and Flores, A. (1979) : Neurology (Minneap.), 29, 448.
25. Douglas, D.L., Duckworth, T., Kanis, J.A., Jefferson, A.A., Martin, T.J. and Russell, R.G.G. (1981) ; J. Bone Jt Surg., 63-B, 495.
26. Wootton, R., Reeve, J., Spellacy, E. and Tellez-Yudilevich, M. (1978) : Clin. Sci. Mol. Med., 54, 69.
27. Nagant de Deuxchaisnes, C., Rombouts-Lindemans, C., Huaux, J.P., Devogelaer, J.P., Malghem, J. and Maldague, B. (1979) : In : Molecular Endocrinology, p. 405. Editors : I. MacIntyre and M. Szelke. Elsevier/ North-Holland Biomedical Press, Amsterdam.
28. Nagant de Deuxchaisnes, C., Maldague, B., Malghem, J., Devogelaer, J.P., Huaux, J.P. and Rombouts-Lindemans, C. (1980) : Arthritis Rheum., 23, 1215.
29. Nagant de Deuxchaisnes, C., Rombouts-Lindemans, C., Huaux, J.P., Esselinckx, W., Devogelaer, J.P., Withofs, H., Meersseman, F., Malghem, J. and Maldague, B. (1982) : In : Symposium CEMO IV "Diphosphonates and Bone", p. 303. Editors : A. Donath and B. Courvoisier. Editions Médecine et Hygiène, Genève.
30. Nagant de Deuxchaisnes, C., Rombouts-Lindemans, C., Huaux, J.P., Devogelaer, J.P., Malghem, J., Maldague, B., Withofs, H. and Meersseman, F. (1982) : Brit. Med. J., 284, 274.
31. Boris, A., Hurley, J.F., Trmal, T., Mallon, J.P. and Matuszewski, D.S. (1979) : Acta Endocrinol. (Kbh.), 91, 351.
32. Doyle, F.H., Pennock, J., Greenberg, P.B., Joplin, G.F. and MacIntyre, I. (1974) : Brit. J. Radiol., 47, 1.
33. Murphy, W.A., Whyte, M.P. and Haddad, J.G., Jr. (1980) : Radiology, 136, 1.
34. Whyte, M.P., Murphy, W.A., Haddad, J.G., Jr. and Avioli, L.V. (1981) : In : Calcitonin 1980. Chemistry, Physiology, Pharmacology and Clinical Aspects, p. 217. Editor : A. Pecile. Excerpta Medica, Amsterdam.

Discussion following paper of Charles Nagent de Deuxchaines

D. RAO: You mentioned that Paget's disease is localized, not generalized. We have presented data to indicate that the bone that is not involved radiologically or by bone scan is abnormal both by histomorphometry as well as by photon absorptiometry. Furthermore, we have evidence to suggest the presence of secondary hyperparathyroidism. Dr. Meunier has similar data so that the bone that is apparently normal seems to be involved from the effects of secondary hyperparathyroidism.

C. NAGENT DE DEUXCHAINES: What you say may be a consequence of Paget's disease, but when we treat Paget's disease we want to treat the focal disease. I am well aware of the data showing there is a secondary hyperparathyroidism in Paget's disease. Therefore, I am a little bit worried to give calcitonin which may enhance this effect by increasing parathyroid hormone secretion. However, as we know intermittent parathyroid hormone therapy may be beneficial in increasing trabecular bone volume.

C. JOHNSTON: What are the consequences of lytic lesions that you demonstrated? We have rarely seen them in our patients and they seem to have few consequences, but I think that question is still open. Your suggestion of intermittent calcitonin therapy is interesting. Could there be arguments made both for and against it? Do you have data at the present time that intermittent treatment is an effective way to treat the patient with calcitonin?

C. NAGENT DE DEUXCHAISNES: I think it may be effective. It may be effective for the symptoms. Maybe we should treat the patient for one year and wait until the symptoms recur. Maybe we won't have to give calcitonin again or we can defer for another year or eighteen months. Sometimes calcitonin has to be given again within a 3 to 6 month period. Many patients are well for a long time after treatment. On the other hand, if I treat for progression of the disease, then I tend to be more aggressive. I may repeat treatment again with higher doses than are necessary to keep the process under control. With regards the osteolytic lesions in patients on EHDP, the purpose of treating Paget's disease is to try to have a homogenous and healthy bone because fractures are certainly one of the main consequences of Paget's disease. I know of your study showing that a number of fractures have occurred during treatment with high doses of EHDP, but this does not reach statistical significance.

EHDP in the recommended doses does not enhance the fracture rate, but it may also be true that calcitonin prevents fractures. I think that there has been no formal study of that, but analyzing all the studies on calcitonin, it is very difficult to find one single femur fracture in pagetic bone during treatment with calcitonin.

P. MEUNIER: We have shown histologically that the mineralization defect induced by excessive doses of EHDP spontaneously and completely heals in three months. I am not sure if you can explain the healing of the observed mineralization defect to the effect of the calcitonin that you gave immediately after stopping the EHDP?

C. NAGENT DE DEUXCHAISNES: We had to give it immediately because the patient had severe pain and the patient did not want to wait until the fracture would spontaneously reverse.

When I show an x-ray after three months, it's to show how dramatic the changes are, but you can show a change after 15 days. When I read the published histologic data it doesn't disappear as quickly. It may be true that we are simply hastening the natural history of healing of the mineralization defect. After 15 days you can see that calcitonin heals the bone lesion. I don't think we have enough patients that have not experienced pain, and that have just had this fracture defect with giving calcitonin. The fracture doesn't reverse itself as quickly as when one gives calcitonin.

P. MEUNIER: Yes, except that we used tetracycline labeling and not x-rays. We have to decide what is the most sensitive method to evaluate a mineralization defect.

BISPHOSPHONATE TREATMENT FOR PAGET'S DISEASE OF BONE

Olav L.M. Bijvoet

Clinical Investigation Unit of the Department of Endocrinology, University Hospital, Leiden, the Netherlands

THE IMPORTANCE OF TREATMENT

Paget's disease of bone is a common affection in Anglosaxon countries. In Great Britain the prevalence is estimated to be more than 5% among hospital patients aged 55 years and over. In many other parts of the world it is considered rare and variations in the incidence have been reported within the same country. The fraction of patients with signs and symptoms relevant to the disease has been estimated at one twentieth (1).

The most frequent abnormalities are deformity - to be prevented by early treatment - and pain, over affected bones or resulting from complications. Involvement of the skull may lead to nerve deafness and headaches. Vertebral involvement may cause backpain, vertebral collapse and involvement of peripheral nerves. Long bones, when affected, may be painful, bow, fracture and stress adjacent joints. Treatment aims at prevention of deformity and complications, at improvement of bone structure, and at alleviation of pain.

Calcitonin was introduced for the treatment of Paget's disease in the mid-sixties (2). It will improve many of the clinical features of the disease and two of the most striking findings have been, that it often causes considerable pain relief and, that its use may be associated with some radiological improvement. Reasons to continue search for better treatment are initial or late resistance to calcitonin in a sizeable proportion of patients, the disadvantage of parenteral administration and - in a few patients - the occurrence of nausea as a side effect (8). The major problem is continued dependence on the drug, because arrest of treatment is inevitably associated with recurrence of the disease activity, loss of the structural improvement, and recurrence of pain (3,4). Moreover biochemically remissions are hardly ever complete unless disease activity was moderate to begin with (4).

THE BISPHOSPHONATES

The bisphosphonates may turn out to be the major pharmacological acquisition for modulation of bone metabolism and calcium homeostasis, after vitamin D. The name refers to a class of compounds with in common a core with the structure P-C-P, two phosphate groups directly linked to a single carbon. At present three of these have been studied in clinical practice. These are indicated as EHDP, APD and Cl_2MDP of these only EHDP (etidronate) has as yet reached the status of an official drug. This hangs together with the fact that EHDP is the longest known of this group.

EHDP Cl_2MDP APD

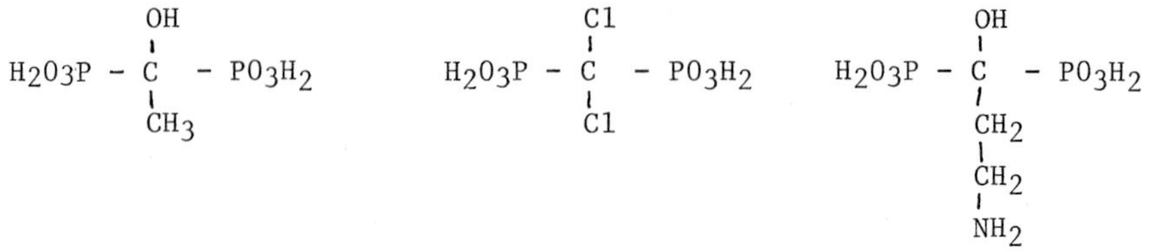

EHDP was originally synthesized in 1865 - 1887 (5,6). The compound has an unusually great ability to form bonds with free calcium and with bound calcium. Binding of bisphosphonates to crystal surfaces is responsible for an inhibitory effect on crystallization processes. Investigations of its effects in the mammalian species has led to discovery of biological effects (7,8) that, though perhaps relatable to the ability of bisphosphonates to form strong bonds with calcium, should not always be reduced to their ability to inhibit crystal growth and dissolution. The biological properties, most relevant in the present context are

a) Modulation of normal bone formation, resulting in the production of abnormal and insufficiently mineralized bone matrix (9). This is mainly characteristic of EHDP (10). It is interesting that concurrent administration of calcitonin may reduce expression of this effect in animals as well as in humans (11,12).

b) EHDP alone of the three bisphosphonates increases renal tubular reabsorption of phosphate, causing an increase of serum phosphate. The reason for this is unknown (13).

c) It was found that all three bisphosphonates possess the ability to inhibit bone resorption the order of potency being APD>Cl_2MDP>EHDP (10). In mammals the rates of bone formation and of bone resorption depend on each other - there are as yet ill understood local mechanisms of cell interaction that regulate the activity of the one in dependence of the activity of the other. This concept is used to explain why initial reduction of the rate of bone resorption after bisphosphonate administration is always followed by supposedly secondary reduction of the bone formation rate (10,14). The effect on osteoclastic bone resorption appears not to be due to inhibition of crystal dissolution, but the ability of the bisphosphonates to concentrate in bone due to affinity to bone mineral may be important (15). Some data suggest that in the case of Cl_2MDP, mineral bound Cl_2MDP may be cytotoxic to resorbing cells (15). EHDP and APD affect the ability of osteoclasts to resorb bone, even though formation rate of osteoclasts seems not to be reduced (10), except in Paget's disease where all bisphosphonates tend to reduce the abnormally increased number of bone cells (14,16,17).

d) As yet ill understood is the finding that APD and EHDP may possess anti-inflammatory effects. It has long been known that bisphosphonates may form large complexes with calcium in solution that, below a given concentration, remain soluble. It is thought that these complexes, rather than the ionized bisphosphonates, excert specific actions on macrophages or their precursors. Since it is now understood that macrophages share their precursors with osteoclast, the same mechanism of action may account for modulation of cellular immunity as well as modulation of bone resorption (15,18,19).

BISPHOSPHONATES IN PAGET'S DISEASE OF BONE

In Paget's disease a greatly accelerated rate of remodelling is combined with the development of structurally abnormal bone. The disease seems likely to be primarily a disorder of osteoclasts. The observation stands firm that the initial effect of administration of bisphosphonates in Paget's disease and the axis of their efficacy is a reduction of the rate of bone resorption. This is manifest in reduction or normalization of the abnormally increased urinary excretion rate of hydroxyproline (14). At the present stage of development EHDP or etidronate disodium is the only one of the three bisphosphonates available to the medical profession. We will therefore discuss the use of EHDP in Paget's disease. APD is, however, the most potent of the available bisphosphonates and its effects are more clearcut and less disturbed by secondary problems as these of EHDP. Since, in addition, our personal experience is closely associated with the development of APD, etidronate will be discussed in the light of, and after discussion of APD. Cl_2MDP is not discussed because clinical trials of this drug in Paget's disease were recently stopped for reasons not yet published.

APD

APD is disodium (3-amino-1-hydroxypropylidene)-1,1-bisphosphonate. It is administered orally at doses of 300 mg, twice daily (from 900-300 mg per day) (14). Our experience relates to 150 patients entered over the last 6 years. Detailed studies relating to about 15 per cent of these have been published (14). After starting APD a rapid fall of urinary hydroxyproline (OHP) occurs. The rate of fall is dose dependent. It is often possible to obtain normalisation of OHP within a fourtnight but in some patients, particularly the most severe ones, this may take anything up to three months. Serum alkaline phosphatase (AP) is considered to reflect osteoblast activity - and takes about three months to normalize when the reaction of OHP was rapid. When the decrease of OHP is slower, the fall of AP is retarded as well. The fall of AP probably reflects a biological adaptation of bone formation to reduced resorption rates and the delay may reflect the active period of normal osteoblasts. Initially we overtreated patients, continuing APD until after normalization of AP. More recent experience shows that treatment can be stopped as early as normal OHP is obtained and in the majority of patients subsequent biochemical and clinical remission will continue to complete itself automatically, without further drugs. The three months period during which bone formation is transiently in excess of resorption is characterized by transient reductions of serum and urine calcium, increase of parathyroid hormone levels in serum and of $1,25(OH)_2$-cholecalciferol and a positive calcium balance (14, 20). In bone biopsies osteoclast-counts and osteoblast-counts are reduced but do not always normalize; the thickness of osteoid always normalizes (14). Radiological changes in Pagetic bones are generally rewarding; particularly impressive may be reconstruction of cortical bone and re-definition of trabecular bone (18,21). On bone-scans uptake is generally reduced by 85% regardless of the initial intensity of uptake. Clinical improvement is characterized by normalization of increased temperature over affected areas often within a few weeks. Bone pains due to Paget's disease generally disappear within one to two months. Increase of pain is not observed. Improvement of neurological symptoms has been observed, but seldom improvement of hearing. With the exception of one patient (who previously had suffered fractures) and in whom an additional pathological fracture occurred after one month of treatment, healing normally despite continued treatment, we have never seen fractures in treated patients.

Remissions have continued despite arrest of treatment for varying periods, up to 6 years (which is the longest observation period). Recurrences have occurred at any time after arrest of treatment, from one month to 5 years, in two thirds. We have as yet been unable to find any criterium associated with a likelyhood of recurrence. However incomplete treatment entails a greater likelyhood of exacerbation. The rate at which biochemical or clinical changes occur, indicative of recurrence, is sufficiently slow to allow a 6 to 12 months delay between subsequent check-ups in the out patient department. Recurrences can be retreated with oral APD.

ETIDRONATE

Etidronate or EHDP is disodium (1-hydroxy ethylidene)-1,1-bisphosphonate. It has been administered orally at doses ranging from 1 to 20 mg per kg body weight (60-2000 mg per day)(22,23). With the highest doses OHP is progressively reduced until after 3 months normal values have been obtained in the majority. At the recommended dose, however, of 300 mg daily 50% fall of OHP is obtained, at 6 months with great variation between patients. Further prolongation of treatment will not improve results. A similar and proportional pattern of response is seen with measurements of serum alkaline phosphatase levels. A delay in the rate of reduction of serum alkaline phosphatase relative to OHP has also been noted. (22,23,24).

I have mentioned before that a particular property of EHDP, when given at doses effective on bone resorption is an adverse effect on the quality of new-formed bone resulting in the appearance of osteomalacia. This problem is particularly severe when EHDP is used at doses of 20 mg per kg body weight per day and can be considered responsible for a number of problems characteristic for Etidronate and which have been pertinently discussed in a recent critical evaluation (23).

a) There is a significant improvement in pain related to etidronate, but many patients do not respond and pain may develop over the site of Pagetic lesions within 4 to 6 weeks of initiating therapy, sometimes severe and disabling and persisting for months after the drug is withdrawn. The problem may be dose related, but since bisphosphonate absorption is low and may be very variable - monitoring effective dose is not too effective.

b) In our own group, encompassing around 300 to 400 patient-years of APD treatment we have only seen one case of pathological fracture. Apparently a number of patients have developed fractures while on treatment with etidronate (23,24). The problem may admittedly be dose related and there are authors who expressed reservations because they think there is insufficient information on the incidence of fractures in untreated patients.

c) Methods have been developed to insure maximum radiographic reproducibility (21,25). With such methods it has been found that treated with calcitonin or with APD show arrest of advancing osteolytic lesions and filling in of defects. With low doses of etidronate however more than half of patients developed increases of osteolytic lesions.

The manner in which I have summarized data shows evident reservation towards EHDP therapy. It is true that no comparative studies have been published and it is gratifying to know that a comparative study between EHDP, EHDP combined with calcitonin and APD is near completion in New-Zealand (26). Meanwhile it is good to recall what was mentioned earlier, that combination of calcitonin with low dose EHDP seems to reduce the severity of EHDP-induced osteomalacia (11,12). Our own data suggest that many patients using the combination treatment achieve normal or near normal bone turnover irrespective of the initial disease activity, with hydroxyproline excretion declining with a half time of about six weeks. Defective mineralisation has not been seen, and radiological results show a significant improvement over those with EHDP alone. One out of three patients from our own study reported in 1978 (12) have now remained in remission up to seven years, some of these with initially very active Paget's disease.

I would conclude that treatment with bisphosphonates is a great improvement relative to calcitonin in, that the oral treatment mode is easy, that results promise to be more complete and predictable, that relative short courses of treatment and at very long intervals are possible. In the future there might be no reason to withhold effective treatment in any patient

presenting with signs or symptoms of the disease. It is also evident that etidronate is not the final answer. As long as this is the only drug available, combination with calcitonin should be considered when patients present with osteolytic lesions or when EHDP treatment increases pain.
What we do not know is the consequence of the fact that these agents are likely to be retained in the skeleton for very long times.

REFERENCES

1. Hamdy RC: Paget's Disease of Bone. Praeger Sc. Eastbourne (1981) passim.
2. Bijvoet OLM, Jansen A: Lancet ii (1967) 472.
3. MacIntyre I, et al.: Arthritis and Rheumatism 23 (1980) 1139-1147.
4. Hosking DJ, Bijvoet OLM.: Therapeutic uses of calcitonin. In: Endocrinology of calcium metabolism, Edited by J. Parsons. Raven Press, New York,1982.
5. Menschutkin N: Ann.d.Chem.u.Pharm. 133 (1865) 317-320.
6. von Baeyer H, Hofman KA: Ber. Deutch. Chem. Ges. 30 (1897) 1973-1978.
7. Francis MD, Russell RGG, Fleisch H.: Science 165 (1969) 1264-1266.
8. Fleisch H.: Arthritis and Rheumatism 23 (1980) 1162-1171.
9. Flora L, et al: Metab. Bone Dis. Rel. Res 2S (1980) 389-407.
10. Reitsma PH, et al.: Calcif. Tiss. Int. 30(1980) 35-42.
11. Boris A, et al.: Acta Endocrinol. 91(1979) 351-361.
12. Bijvoet OLM, et al.:Metab. Bone Dis. Rel. Res 1 (1978) 251-261.
13. Recker RR, et al.: J. Lab. Clin. Med. 81 (1973) 258-266.
14. Frijlink WB, et al.: Lancet i (1979) 799-803.
15. Reitsma PH, et al.: J.Clin. Invest. 70 (1982) 927-933.
16. Meunier PJ, et al. Rev. Rhum. 42 (1975) 699-705.
17. Meunier PJ, Chapuy MC, Alexandre C.: Lancet ii (1979) 489-492.
18. Bijvoet OLM, et al.: Arthritis and Rheumatism 23 (1980) 1193-1204.
19. Bijvoet OLM, et al.: APD, Bisphosphonates, the bone resorbing and the mononuclear phagocyte system. In: Diphosphonates and bone. Edited by A.Donath and B. Courvoisier. Ed Médecine et Hygiène, Genève, 1982 pp. 328-333.
20. Adami S, et al.: Calcif. Tiss. Int. 34 (1982) 317-320.
21. Nagant de Deuxchaisnes C, et al.: Treatment of Paget's disease with the diphosphonate APD. A biological and radiological study. In: Diphosphonates and bone. Edited by A. Donath and B. Courvoisier. Ed. Médecine et Hygiène, Genève, 1982 pp. 303-327.
22. Hosking DJ: Brit. Med.J.. 283 (1982) 686-688.
23. Krane SM: Ann. int. Med. 96 (1982) 619-625.
24. Bijvoet OLM.: La pharmacologie humaine des bisphosphonates. In: Rapports du IVe congrès Latin de Rhumatologie. Eds. H. van Cauwenberge, P. Franchimont, L. Ruyters, G. Heynen. Masson et Cie, Paris, 1980, pp.167-196.
25. Nagant de Deuxchaisnes C, et al.: Arthritis and Rheumatism 23 (1980) 1215-1234.
26. Ibbertson HK, Fraser R. In preparation.

Discussion of paper following O. Bijvoet:

S. POSEN: Dr. Bijvoet, have you any audiometric data after treatment with your disphosphonate? I am asking this question because I am unimpressed with the effect of calcitonin on long-term hearing losses.

O. BIJVOET: That was a very appropriate question. I have never seen the hearing improve. We have very carefully measured audiograms. I think when a patient with Paget's disease already has hearing troubles it is not due to edema, but it must be due to compression of the nerve. I have the feeling that in most cases it is irreversible. I know of some instances of improved hearing troubles with calcitonin but I've never seen it with APD.

M. PARFITT: All of you have shown a significant reduction in the external diameter of the involved bone, like Dr. Doyle showed many years ago with human calcitonin. Now, how do you explain a local increase in bone resorption of that site produced by an agent whose main action is to decrease general bone resorption?

O. BIJOVOET: This is an important question. I showed you that it probably acts at not the level of bone mineral, not even at the level of the osteoclast, but at the level of differentiation of the preosteoclasts to the osteoclasts. In Paget's disease you see a reduction in the number of osteoclasts. On the other hand when you give APD to normals you do not see a significant reduction in bone resopriton.

MITHRAMYCIN TREATMENT OF PAGET'S DISEASE OF BONE
EXPLORATION OF COMBINED THERAPIES - PARTICULARLY SODIUM ETIDRONATE (EHDP)

Will G. Ryan

Section of Endocrinology and Metabolism, Department of Medicine, Rush-Presbyterian-St. Luke's Medical Center, Chicago, IL, U.S.A.

Since we introduced mithramycin for the treatment of Paget's disease in 1969 (1) we have treated approximately two hundred patients (some on multiple occasions) with it with generally salutary results. One patient who had been a porcine and salmon calcitonin treatment failure appears to have been cured of her Paget's disease (10 years in complete remission) as a result of a single ten day hospital course (1972) of mithramycin followed by twice weekly out-patient injections for about three months during which time her alkaline phosphatase (alk. phos.) became normal and has remained so up to the present. A bone scan was normal in 1979 (2). Unfortunately to our knowledge all other patients we have treated with mithramycin alone have relapsed - most within a year or two. However, none of these patients received the above regimen of intensive inpatient followed by prolonged outpatient therapy and this may provide at least the partial key to achieving prolonged remissions.

Faced with the prospect of treating patients with a very toxic agent every two or three years for the rest of their lives in order to achieve adequate control of their disease we have begun to explore combinations of this therapy with more benign agents - particularly sodium etidronate (EHDP) and this approach appears to be promising in that we are achieving more prolonged remissions. Our experience suggests that these two agents are at least additive and possibly synergistic in their effects on Paget's disease. We have explored outpatient therapy as well in order to be able to prolong courses of therapy as well as be able to reduce expenses. The most promising approach at present appears to be that of initially treating the patient with EHDP (400 mg/day initially but increasing to 800 mg/day if significant alk. phos. reduction is not achieved) for approximately six months in an effort to saturate the osteoclasts with the agent and make them as sick as possible. We then hospitalize the patient for an approximate ten day course of mithramycin ("the double whammy") (approximately one mg/day but raising or lowering this dose according to apparent tolerance or toxicity) with very careful daily monitoring of serum enzymes (GPT, GOT, LDH), creatinine, and platelets to judge toxicity. We currently administer the mithramycin as an eight hour infusion in the evening after the results of blood tests drawn that morning are assessed.

General guidelines for withholding the mithramycin are increases in serum enzymes to approximately ten times their upper limit of normal (the GPT seems to be the most sensitive in this regard), an increase of serum creatinine of 0.3 mg/dl, or an absolute value of 1.5 mg/dl or greater, a precipitous decrease in platelet count or an absolute level of 150,000/cmm, or any clinical sign (excessive nausea, fever etc.) which may indicate excessive toxicity.

It is usual to see significant increases in serum enzymes which are usually reversible within two to three days. Approximately five to ten percent of patients have an increase in serum creatinine which usually takes one to three weeks to revert to baseline values. Accordingly, we usually discharge the patient from the hospital as soon as we are reasonably sure the creatinine is not continuing to rise and will readmit for further therapy later if indicated. The only occasion in which we have observed a significant reduction in platelet

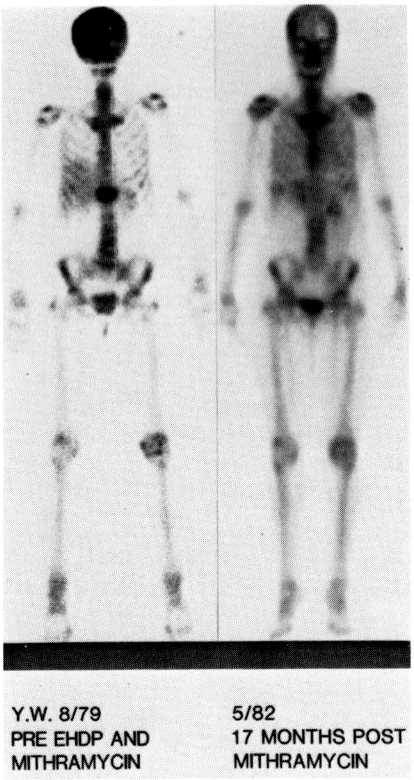

Figure 1. Bone scans taken prior to and at 17 months following hospital course of mithramycin after EHDP preloading. The obvious skull and vertebral disease activity are seen on the left. The scan on the right is read as normal. The patient is still in remission (May 1983) as judged by her normal serum alkaline phosphatase.

count was early in our experience when one patient received 50 mcg/kg/day of mithramycin for five days thru error and the platelet count decreased to 75,000/cmm. No bleeding occurred and recovery was uneventful. However, we recently have had mild to moderate urinary tract bleeding occur without a significant decrease in platelet count in two patients with underlying urinary tract disease. Thus a more careful assessment of platelet function may be indicated.

The other parameters followed during mithramycin therapy are serum calcium, phosphorous, and alk. phos. Hypocalcemia occurs less frequently in patients pretreated with EHDP but when significant is treated with oral or intravenous calcium as indicated. If serum phosphorous exceeds 5.0 mg/dl EHDP is discontinued during mithramycin therapy as we have the impression that this may be associated with enhanced nephrotoxicity. In two patients while the serum creatinine was rising the serum calcium and phosphorous also rose to abnormally high levels and then declined to normal concurrently with the serum creatinine.

Besides increasing the therapeutic effectiveness of mithramycin we have the impression that EHDP pretreatment may enhance toxic side effects and accordingly have reduced initial doses to one mg/day (or less if baseline serum creatinine exceeds 1.2) initially. We have had one bad experience resulting in death (a 78-year old man with limited spine disease but severe chronic pain unresponsive to EHDP alone) when mithramycin was given by the house staff without that mornings' parameters of toxicity having been drawn. Thus we have become even more cautious in administration of mithramycin in an effort to avoid more untoward experiences.

Approximately one third of patients (approximately 40) treated with this regimen have remained in remission to the present with two in apparent complete remission for over four years judged by normal alk. phos. and bone scans. (See Figure 1 on following page.)

In an effort to achieve higher remission rates we have begun to give follow up outpatient injections of mithramycin (approximately one mg. once or twice weekly) while continuing EHDP until the alk. phos. decreases to normal range for several weeks. Early experience with this appears promising but is too scanty at this point to state this with certainty. During this less intensive mithramycin therapy only serum creatinine and alk. phos. are monitored unless there are indications for other testing. We are also experimenting with the addition of other measures (methotrexate, radiation) in patients with extremely resistant disease.

These approaches to therapy are not recommended for patients who have disease which may be controlled adequately by more benign measures. They do however hold the promise of being effective for prolonged eradication of disease activity with resultant prevention of further bony deformity and disability in whom they are indicated.

REFERENCES

1. Ryan, W.G., Schwartz, T.B. and Perlia, C.P. (1969): Ann. Int. Med., 70:549.
2. Ryan, W.G. and Schwartz, T.B. (1980): Arth. & Rheum., 23:1155.

Discussion following paper of Dr. W. Ryan

G. RUSSELL: I think the evidence from both dichloromethylene - diphosphonate, APD, and certainly mithramycin support the contention that you may be able to have prolonged remission in the disease. I am concerned whether with sequential therapy you are actually accomplishing any more than if you allowed the full effect of the initial drug to be fully demonstrated. There is considerable evidence now that short exposures to either intravenous diphosphonates or oral diphosphonates will produce an effect on bone resorption with in a few days, but that a complete effect may take several months to achieve. If you administer your second drug in the latter phase of diphosphonate therapy you may not be achieving an additional affect by giving another agent.

W. RYAN: I think that's a possibility but, I do not know of many patients who have had prolonged responses to EHDP alone, and many of these patients had only a minimal response to the EHDP.

D. SHERRARD: Could you say something about the dose level of mithramycin you used?

W. RYAN: Mithramycin is definitely a very toxic drug that has to be used carefully. We have had one serious toxic reaction resulting in death, and so this is a therapy that should not be used lightly. I would say this therapy should be reserved for patients who have a disease which may be progressive and would result in extensive disability and deformity or who have failed both calcitonin and the EHDP therapy.

S. KRANE: Could you tell us how the patient with mithramycin toxicity died?

W. RYAN: He developed all the earmarks of mithramycin toxicity with low platelets and elevated liver enzymes.

XV IDIOPATHIC HYPERCALCIURIA

OVERVIEW:
IDIOPATHIC HYPERCALCIURA

Fredric L. Coe and Murray J. Favus

Idiopathic, normocalcemic hypercalciuria is certainly the commonest metabolic disorder observed in patients with calcium stone, and there is much evidence that hypercalciuria directly causes stones. The evidence relates high urine calcium levels to increased urine calcium oxalate supersaturation, and high supersaturation to genesis of calcium stones is widely accepted, and reviewed in the following three papers. There also seems to be a general consensus, drawn from many sources, that reduction of urine calcium level leads to a concomitant and impressive reduction of new stone production. At the moment, the principal uncertainties concern the mechanism by which urine calcium excretion is elevated and, in a related sense, the biochemical and clinical effects of measures that are taken to lower urine calcium in treatment of stone. Perhaps data that bear on the subject are presented by Dr. Lemann. He and his colleagues have shown clearly that administration of slight excesses of $1,25(OH)_2D_3$ to normal people causes fasting hypercalciuria and hypercalciuria on low calcium diet. On very low calcium diet, urine calcium level may exceed dietary intake. These data suggest that a modest disorder of vitamin D metabolism, that leads to a slight excess in the production of $1,25(OH)_2D_3$ could easily give rise not only to hypercalciuria but to an intolerance of low calcium diet. It could also give rise to fasting hypercalciuria, that could easily be confused with renal hypercalciuria.

Drs. Pak and Zerwekh, in describing their work, clearly indicate that on clinical study patients appear to divide themselves into those with predominant overabsorption of calcium and those who have fasting hypercalciuria and appear to have a defective renal tubule calcium reabsorption. Their clinical and laboratory observations clearly depict the heterogeneity of physiological response in the syndrome, and, interestingly, are quite compatible with the effects of $1,25(OH)_2D_3$ administration in normals. In noting response to treatment, Pak points out that patients with reduced renal calcium conservation seem to do very well with thiazide, and those who present principally with intestinal hyperabsorption probably can be treated with sodium cellulose phosphate.

Material from our own group is consistent with the Pak data and with the Lemann experiments in $1,25D_3$ administration. We observe and describe here a continuous spectrum of behavior in hypercalciuric subjects. At one end of the spectrum are patients who conserve very well when challenged with a low calcium diet and at the other end are patients who cannot conserve calcium well at all. Uniformly, hypercalciuric patients have low levels of serum PTH, and under conditions of low calcium diets the patients generally manifest a serum calcium level that is higher than that of normal subjects given the same diets. Despite the higher calcium level in the blood, and lower PTH, however, and equivalent levels of serum phosphorus, patients with hypercalciuria have the same levels of serum $1,25(OH)_2D_3$. The best explanation for the spectrum of behavior observed in hypercalciuria in response to low calcium diet is a subtle but persistent disorder of 1,25$(OH)_2D_3$ regulation.

If the following three papers are looked at as a group, and in the context of what is known about this disorder, the hypothesis emerges that a regulation disorder of 1,25$(OH)_2D_3$ may well be present, and may well explain the complex and variable behavior of patients. Probably, because of the wide range of behaviors, some can benefit from drugs that reduce calcium absorption and some benefit from thiazide. A final answer to treatment must await a definitive analysis of vitamin D metabolism, which still is not available.

IDIOPATHIC HYPERCALCIURIA

Fredric L. Coe

Nephrology Section, Department of Medicine, University of Chicago Pritzker School of Medicine, Chicago, IL, U.S.A.

Idiopathic hypercalciuria (IH) is defined by a daily urine excretion above 300 mg, men, 250 mg, women, or 4 mg/kg, either sex, normocalcemia, and the absence of an obvious systemic cause of hypercalciuria such as malignant tumor, sarcoid, vitamin D intoxication, immobilization, hyperthyroidism, Paget's disease, rapidly progressive osteoporosis, or drugs such as furosemide. Fifty percent of men and 75% of women with calcium oxalate renal stones have IH, compared to between 5-10% of otherwise normal people.

Idiopathic hypercalciuria is familial, and probably genetic. Favus and I have described sporadic hypercalciuria in rats, and Lau as well as ourselves has shown that selective in-breeding of hypercalciuric rats raises the frequency and severity of hypercalciuria in their offspring, in a pattern suggesting dominant inheritance.

Idiopathic hypercalciuria appears to cause stones by increasing urine calcium concentration and thereby raising urine supersaturation with respect to calcium oxalate, the main stone-forming crystal in the western world at this time. Higher supersaturation means a greater driving force for crystallization and therefore an increased risk of stones.

Urine calcium can be lowered by restricted calcium intake, by agents that interfere with calcium absorption such as sodium cellulose phosphate, or by thiazide diuretic agents. Thiazide appears to reduce urine calcium excretion, at least in part, by directly increasing renal tubule calcium reabsorption. Constanzo and her colleagues perfused segments of distal convoluted tubule, in situ, with a calcium Ringer's solution. Normally, the calcium concentration of collected fluid was 82% of that perfused. Chlorothiazide, intravenously or in the perfusate, lowered the ratio to about 50%.

One would expect that the chronic administration of thiazide to people with IH would reduce urine calcium losses, perhaps by raising tubule calcium reabsorption, and that reversal of hypercalciuria would lower calcium oxalate supersaturation, and this appears to be the case. By reducing urine supersaturation, thiazide lowers the thermodynamic driving force for crystallization and ought to reduce the risk of stone recurrence; this too has been confirmed, by clinical observation, in our own experience. Before treatment, new stones occurred at a rate of 68 stones/100 patient years at risk; during thiazide treatment, the rate fell to 7.0 stones/100 patient years at risk, a 10-fold reduction. The probability that chance alone would create so large a deviation of treatment stones from that predicted by the pretreatment rate and the number of patient years at risk during treatment is minute: x^2, 200; $p<.001$. Pak, Maschio and others have described similar results.

The link between stones and IH seems firmly established, by statistical association, mechanism, and response to treatment; but the very success of treatment has made the pathogenesis of hypercalciuria a very important issue for clinical investigators. As all of us begin to treat large numbers of patients who have IH and calcium oxalate stones, what will be the long-term systemic consequences Put more bluntly, where does the extra calcium go Thiazide lowers urine calcium by 100-300 mg/24 hr in patients with IH; does the intestinal tract decline to absorb the extra calcium, or is some of it retained in the body, in skeleton or soft tissues With a diet low in calcium, or when cellulose phosphate is used to reduce intestinal calcium absorption, what will the kidneys do Will they conserve calcium normally, or are endogenous calcium stores lost slowly into the urine Until recently, the conventional answer to these questions has been that IH has a dimorphic pathogenesis. Some patients have primary intestinal hyperabsorption and are best treated by restricted diet or cellulose phosphate; this has been termed 'absorptive' hypercalciuria. Others have defective renal tubule calcium reabsorption and require thiazide; this has been termed 'renal.' However, if all of the observations that have been made are viewed together, critically, the impression forces itself upon one's mind that hyperabsorption and defective renal tubule calcium conservation co-exist in virtually all patients, and that the basic pathogenesis of the disorder probably is more simple and more uniform than it has seemed to be.

There is little doubt that intestinal calcium hyperabsorption is a nearly universal characteristic of patients with IH. In balance studies, IH patients have increased net calcium absorption. Only one known hormone regulates intestinal calcium absorption, $1,25(OH)_2D_3$ ($1,25D_3$), so one might expect that $1,25D_3$ is elevated in IH, and that seems to be true.

Serum $1,25D_3$ levels of IH patients are higher than in normals, and higher $1,25D_3$ could account for their calcium overabsorption. Of course, it is always possible that there is some intrinsic intestinal disorder in IH that causes hyperabsorption, independent of $1,25D_3$, but given the generally elevated D_3 level, such a defect is difficult to prove.

To discriminate between these two mechanisms, a primary tubule defect or the effects of $1,25D_3$, we performed a low calcium diet experiment. Nine normal people and 27 patients with IH and calcium oxalate nephrolithiasis were fed a low calcium diet, LCD, 2 mg/kg/day of calcium. Blood and 24-hr urines were collected on the 7th, 8th and 9th days of the diet, as well as on a free choice diet for three days immediately prior to starting the LCD.

During days 7-9 of the LCD, normal people excreted less calcium than they ate, and the difference on each day between ingested calcium (I) and excreted calcium (E), I - E, was always above 0. Eating the same diet, the 27 patients excreted much more calcium, and values of I - E were, in most cases, near or below 0, indicating the loss of endogenous mineral in the urine. We reasoned that careful measurement of serum calcium on days 7-9 of LCD should permit distinction between reduced tubule calcium reabsorption due to non-$1,25D_3$ mediated reduction of parathyroid hormone (PTH) or an intrinsic defect, and the effects of inappropriate $1,25D_3$ elevation on bone. The former would exaggerate the normal fall in serum calcium provoked by LCD, as excessive urinary loss would be due to low PTH or a tubule defect and be superimposed upon inadequate intestinal absorption created by the LCD. If $1,25D_3$, however, were raising bone mineral efflux, it would thereby protect serum calcium from falling; at the same time, the high serum calcium would prevent a rise in PTH and thereby down-regulate fractional reabsorption of calcium (r(ca)). In other words, primary vitamin D excess would reduce PTH and r(ca) because bone calcium maintained serum calcium at an elevated level.

When normal people went from free choice diet (F) to LCD, serum calcium fell significantly, $p<.01$. The 27 patients, however, showed no fall in serum calcium so that during LCD the calcium level of patients exceeded that of normals significantly, $p<.001$. The only explanation for a higher serum calcium in patients despite urine calcium losses that exceeded their entire dietary intake is a stimulation of bone reabsorption, presumably by $1,25D_3$ in excess of PTH. Serum PTH of patients was below that of normals on both diets, $p<.001$, using a carboxy terminus assay of Louis Sherwood. On the free diet, serum $1,25D_3$ of patients was a bit above normal, as others have found, and during LCD patients had the same values as normals despite relative hypercalcemia and low PTH levels; in other words, $1,25D_3$ was in excess compared to PTH, as in our vitamin D-treated rats.

These data cannot exclude the simultaneous effects of inappropriately high $1,25D_3$ and a primary tubule defect that has reduced tubule calcium reabsorption. The PTH of our patients was clearly suppressed, so renal tubule calcium reabsorption would be physiologically down-regulated. Under such conditions, our intrinsic tubule transport disorder would merely be additive, and could not be separated from the effects of low PTH. What we can exclude is a sequence that begins with a tubule defect that provokes excessive calcium losses, hypocalcemia, subsequent $1,25D_3$ overproduction, and increased bone turnover, as serum calcium did not fall and therefore was supranormal and PTH was subnormal, at the very time that endogenous calcium was being lost in the urine.

Overall, in this study as in others, there was widespread evidence for inappropriately high $1,25D_3$, low PTH and defective calcium conservation during LCD. We also found subtle but significant evidence for tubule defects of phosphorus and magnesium reabsorption.

In IH, the main defect seems to be a disorder of renal cell $1,25D_3$ regulation, so the serum hormone level is inappropriate to calcium, phosphorus and PTH levels. Dietary calcium is over-absorbed; PTH is reduced; and when dietary supply of calcium is adequate simple $1,25D_3$-drive hyperabsorption is the main mechanism of hypercalciuria. However, if LCD is used to lower urine calcium, the $1,25D_3$ dysregulation is manifested; serum calcium does not fall normally because bone mineral maintains it, PTH is relatively suppressed, there is a failure of renal calcium conservation, and bone mineral can easily be lost.

Clinically, despite uncertainties about the nature of the vitamin D disorder and its relationship to the phosphate disorder, it seems clear that LCD and sodium cellulose phosphate must be used with great caution in the treatment of IH, and only in those patients who clearly can conserve calcium normally during LCD. Such patients seem to be a small minority, although this requires more study. Thiazide probably is a safer alternative.

SEPARATE PATHOGENETIC ORIGINS FOR ABSORPTIVE AND RENAL HYPERCALCIURIAS: DIFFERENT RESPONSES TO TREATMENT

Charles Y.C. Pak and Joseph E. Zerwekh

Section of Mineral Metabolism, Southwestern Medical School, The University of Texas Health Science Center at Dallas, 5323 Harry Hines Blvd., Dallas, TX, U.S.A.

There is continuing controversy concerning the pathogenesis of hypercalciuria associated with nephrolithiasis. It has been suggested that hypercalciuria is either renal or intestinal (absorptive) in origin, resulting from a "renal leak" or an enhanced intestinal absorption of Ca, respectively. A unifying scheme has attributed both renal and absorptive forms to a renal proximal tubular defect, characterized by varying degrees of Ca leak, phosphate leak and of accelerated 1,25-dihydroxyvitamin D (1,25-$(OH)_2D$) synthesis. The predominance of the defect in renal Ca handling would lead to renal hypercalciuria with secondary hyperparathyroidism. The prominence of renal phosphate leak or enhanced 1,25-$(OH)_2D$ synthesis may cause absorptive hypercalciuria, by stimulating intestinal Ca absorption, and by masking secondary hyperparathyroidism from the augmentation of intestinal absorption and skeletal mobilization of Ca.

We have favored separate etiologies for the hypercalciuria (Table 1).[1] For the two major forms, renal and absorptive hypercalciurias, we shall review data supporting separate pathogenetic origins. This separation has practical importance because of different responses to treatment.

Table 1. Classification of Hypercalciurias

Absorptive hypercalciuria Type I	27.8%
Absorptive hypercalciuria Type II	34.1
Absorptive hypercalciuria Type III (hypophosphatemia)	9.1
Renal hypercalciuria	9.1
Primary hyperparathyroidism	6.8
Fasting hypercalciuria with normal parathyroid function	13.1
Total	100.0

PATHOGENESIS OF RENAL HYPERCALCIURIA

The primary defect in renal hypercalciuria is presumed to be the impaired renal tubular reabsorption (renal leak) of Ca. The resulting decline in serum Ca, albeit occurring within the normal range, stimulates parathyroid function. The intestinal Ca absorption is usually increased consequent to PTH-dependent stimulation of 1,25-$(OH)_2D$ synthesis; this disturbance further contributes to the hypercalciuria. Thus, hypercalciuria is secondarily absorptive.

The following lines of evidence support the operation of this scheme:[2] (a) renal Ca leak, shown by fasting hypercalciuria in the setting of normocalcemia even following sodium deprivation, (b) an exaggerated natriuretic response to thiazide treatment, (c) secondary hyperparathyroidism, indicated by a high serum PTH and/or urinary cyclic AMP, correctable by thiazide treatment, (d) compensatory intestinal hyperabsorption of Ca from the PTH-dependent stimulation of 1,25-$(OH)_2D$ synthesis, demonstrated by the positive correlation between intestinal Ca absorption and serum 1,25-$(OH)_2D$ and restoration of normal serum 1,25-$(OH)_2D$ and intestinal Ca absorption by thiazide treatment, and (e) deleterious sequelae of PTH excess, indicated by reduced bone density and negative Ca balance encountered in some patients. That renal hypercalciuria does not coexist with renal phosphate leak and enhanced 1,25-$(OH)_2D$ synthesis is shown by the restoration of normal serum 1,25-$(OH)_2D$ from the correction of renal Ca leak with thiazide.

PATHOGENESIS OF ABSORPTIVE HYPERCALCIURIA TYPE I

The intestinal Ca absorption is presumed to be primarily increased in absorptive hypercalciuria Type I and Type II. Absorptive hypercalciuria Type I represents the classic presentation, where intestinal hyperabsorption and excessive renal excretion of Ca are encountered during a high as well as during a low Ca intake. This presentation excludes those with hypophosphatemia (Type III) or fasting hypercalciuria.

That this condition is intestinal and not renal in origin is suggested by:[2] (a) the high intestinal Ca absorption which exceeds urinary Ca, (b) normal/suppressed parathyroid function (serum PTH and urinary cyclic AMP), (c) lack of evidence for a disturbance in renal proximal tubular function, indicated by normal fasting urinary Ca, serum phosphorus and natriuretic response to thiazide, (d) selective intestinal hyperabsorption for calcium (not magnesium) and in jejunum (not ileum), patterns atypical for 1,25-$(OH)_2D$ action and hyperparathyroid states, (e) inappropriately low serum 1,25-$(OH)_2D$ for the level of intestinal Ca absorption and a lack of correlation between intestinal Ca absorption and serum 1,25-$(OH)_2D$, (f) inability of treatment by adrenocorticosteroids, thiazide, orthophosphate or potassium citrate to entirely correct the hyperabsorption of Ca, and (g) intact skeletal status, shown by normal serum alkaline phosphatase, gla- containing protein, urinary hydroxyproline, and bone density.

FASTING HYPERCALCIURIA WITH NORMAL PARATHYROID FUNCTION

In some patients with hypercalciuria, differentiation between absorptive and renal hypercalciurias may be difficult. Although fasting urinary Ca is high, indicative of renal Ca leak, parathyroid function is normal or suppressed, unlike in renal hypercalciuria. Whereas the lack of parathyroid function suggests increased Ca absorption, fasting urinary Ca is elevated unlike in absorptive hypercalciuria. There are several possibilities for this picture, including: (a) an incomplete clearance of absorbed Ca due to an inadequate dietary preparation prior to fasting urine collection, (b) relative insensitivity of the PTH assay used in detecting parathyroid stimulation, (c) altered "set point" for PTH release, and (d) excessive skeletal mobilization of Ca (e.g. hypophosphatemia and stimulated 1,25-$(OH)_2$D synthesis), and (e) secondary impairment of renal Ca reabsorption due to parathyroid suppression occurring from increased Ca absorption (e.g. from increased 1,25-$(OH)_2$D synthesis).

POSSIBLE COEXISTENCE OF PRIMARY INTESTINAL HYPERABSORPTION OF CA WITH RENAL PHOSPHATE LEAK AND HIGH 1,25-$(OH)_2$D SYNTHESIS

Serum 1,25-$(OH)_2$D has been reported to be high in one-third to one- half of patients with absorptive hypercalciuria. This disturbance was encountered in 28.9% of our patients with absorptive hypercalciuria Type I. Although renal phosphate leak could explain this rise, it has not been possible to consistently show that such a defect was present. However, the high serum 1,25-$(OH)_2$D may be corrected by orthophosphate therapy, suggesting an etiological role for renal phosphate leak.

Among hypercalciuric patients with normal serum Ca and parathyroid function, those with high serum 1,25-$(OH)_2$D had significantly higher fractional (intestinal) Ca absorption than those with normal serum 1,25-$(OH)_2$D (0.73 ± 0.08 vs. 0.68 ± 0.08, $p<0.05$), but equivalent fasting urinary Ca (0.08 ± 0.03 vs. 0.08 ± 0.04 mg/100 ml glomerular filtrate). Moreover, restoration of normal serum 1,25-$(OH)_2$D by orthophosphate decreased fractional Ca absorption in some patients (Fig. 1). The results suggested that high serum 1,25-$(OH)_2$D may have pathophysiological significance, and that it could contribute to the development of intestinal hyperabsorption of Ca in patients with absorptive hypercalciuria Type I. However, the intestinal Ca absorption remained high normal or elevated during orthophosphate therapy despite restoration of normal serum 1,25-$(OH)_2$D, supporting co-occurrence of primary hyperabsorption of Ca.

DIFFERENT RESPONSES TO TREATMENT

Thiazide.[2] In renal hypercalciuria, thiazide therapy "corrects" the renal Ca leak and restores normal parathyroid function, serum 1,25-$(OH)_2$D concentration, and fractional Ca

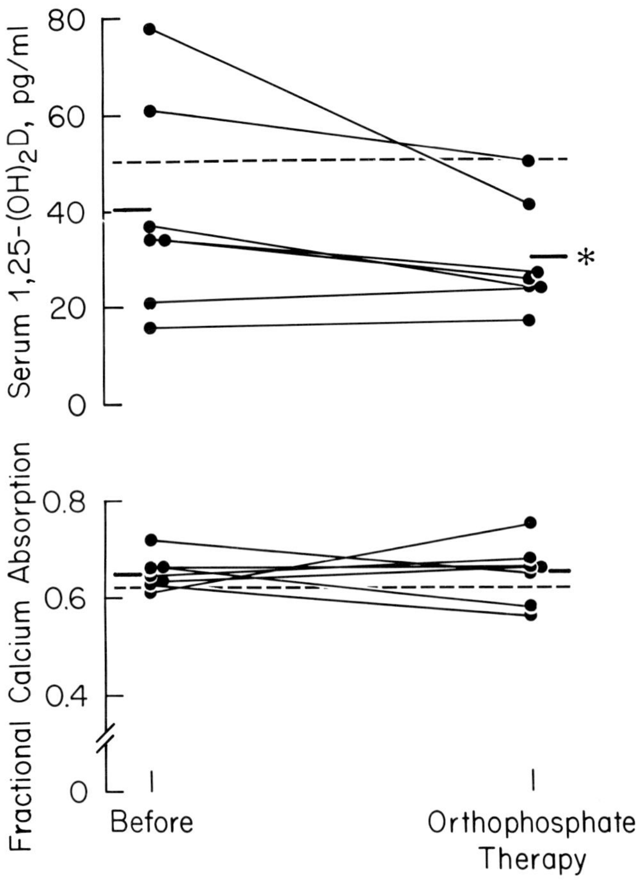

Figure 1. Effect of orthophosphate therapy (1.5 g P/day) on serum 1,25-$(OH)_2D$ and fractional (intestinal) calcium absorption in 7 patients with absorptive hypercalciuria. Bars indicate mean values. Horizontal lines represent upper limits of normal. Significant difference from pre-treatment (before) value is indicated by * for $p<0.05$.

absorption. In absorptive hypercalciuria Type I, however, the serum concentration of 1,25-$(OH)_2D$ remains unchanged and the intestinal hyperabsorption of Ca persists despite a reduction in urinary Ca. Bone density of the distal third of the radius increases during treatment in absorptive hypercalciuria though not in renal hypercalciuria.

The results suggest that thiazide is ideally indicated in renal hypercalciuria but not in absorptive hypercalciuria.

Sodium cellulose phosphate (SCP).[3] According to the unifying scheme for the hypercalciuria, which implicates stimulated 1,25-$(OH)_2D$ synthesis for the high intestinal Ca absorption, an inadequate Ca conservation might be expected because of the excessive skeletal mobilization of Ca from hypophosphatemia and/or high serum 1,25-$(OH)_2D$.

However, patients with absorptive hypercalciuria Type I apparently possess an intact Ca conservation, since (a) inhibition of intestinal Ca absorption by treatment with SCP does not alter Ca balance, (b) the decrement in urinary Ca produced by SCP is proportional to the degree of intestinal Ca absorption, and is higher in patients with absorptive hypercalciuria than in control subjects, (c) although the final urinary Ca during SCP treatment is higher in patients with absorptive hypercalciuria than in control subjects, it is still less than the absorbed Ca, (d) treatment with SCP, at a dose sufficient to restore normal intestinal absorption and urinary excretion of Ca, does not significantly alter or raise above normal serum alkaline phosphatase or urinary hydroxyproline, or decrease significantly bone density.

In contrast, patients with renal hypercalciuria show a less prominent decline in urinary Ca and an exaggeration of secondary hyperparathyroidism during SCP treatment.

These varying responses to treatment suggest separate etiologies for the hypercalciuria, and emphasize the need for differential diagnosis and selective treatment.

REFERENCES

1. Pak, C.Y.C., F. Britton, R. Peterson, D. Ward, C. Northcutt, N.A. Breslau, J. McGuire, K. Sakhaee, S. Bush, M. Nicar, D. Norman, and P. Peters. 1980. Ambulatory evaluation of nephrolithiasis: Classification, clinical presentation and diagnostic criteria. Am. J. Med. 69:19-30.
2. Pak, C.Y.C. 1979. Physiological basis for absorptive and renal hypercalciurias. Am. J. Physiol. 237:F415-F423.
3. Pak, C.Y.C. 1979. Clinical pharmacology of sodium cellulose phosphate. J. Clin. Pharmacol. 19:451-457.

THE ROLE OF SERUM 1,25-$(OH)_2$-VITAMIN D CONCENTRATIONS IN DETERMINING URINARY CALCIUM EXCRETION

Jacob Lemann, Jr., Richard W. Gray and William J. Maierhofer

Departments of Medicine and Biochemistry, Medical College of Wisconsin, Milwaukee, WI, USA

Hypercalciuria is one of the well known risk factors for the formation of calcium oxalate/apatite kidney stones. Increased intestinal absorption of dietary calcium (Ca) has long been known to be present among patients with nephrolithiasis and hypercalciuria (1,2). Since these patients, as a group, do not have clinically significant bone diseae, the additional calcium appearing in the urine, must represent this increase in the intestinal absorption of dietary Ca (3). More recent studies have demonstrated that many of these hypercalciuric stone formers exhibit elevated serum concentration of the renal hormone, 1,25-dihydroxyvitamin D [1,25-$(OH)_2$-D] (4,5,6). This steroid is the most potent form of vitamin D in terms of its capacity to stimulate intestinal Ca absorption (7). Intestinal Ca absorption in humans has been shown to be exquisitely sensitive to prevailing serum 1,25-$(OH)_2$-D concentrations (8). Moreover, elevated serum 1,25-$(OH)_2$-D concentations have been shown to stimulate net bone resorption among humans eating low Ca diets (9,10). In view of these observations, the present studies were undertaken to review the quantitative relationships between daily urine Ca excretion rates or fasting urinary Ca/creatinine concentrations and serum 1,25-$(OH)_2$-D concentrations.

METHODS

We studied 25 healthy men in the Medical College of Wisconsin Clinical Research Center with the permission of the subjects using protocols approved by the Medical College of Wisconsin Human Research Review Committee. Eighteen subjects were studied while they ate constant diets providing an average of 20.1 ± 1.4 SD mmol Ca/day. All 18 were studied on this diet alone and 11 were also studied after 7 to 22 days of ongoing administration of oral 1,25-$(OH)_2$-D_3 (calcitriol) every 6 hours (1 μg/day in 2 subjects, 2 μg/day in 3 subjects and 3 μg/day in 6 subjects). Sixteen subjects were studied while they ate constant diets providing only 4.2 ± 0.6 mmol Ca/day both before and during oral calcitriol (1 μg/day in 2, 2 μg/day in 6 and 3 μg/day in 8 subjects). Serum 1,25-$(OH)_2$-D levels were measured on 3 to 10 occasions during each phase of each study (9). Urinary Ca and creatinine were measured by previously described methods (9).

RESULTS

As shown in Fig. 1 daily urinary Ca excretion rates were directly and significantly correlated to average serum 1,25-$(OH)_2$-D levels for the subjects eating the normal Ca diets and, separately for subjects eating the low Ca diet. The greater increment in urinary Ca excretion for a given increment in serum 1,25-$(OH)_2$-D concentration among subjects eating the normal Ca diet clearly reflects the marked stimulation of intestinal Ca absorption when dietary Ca is available. The progressive increments in urinary Ca as serum 1,25-$(OH)_2$-D levels were experimentally raised among subjects eating the low Ca diet clearly reflects bone resorption since urinary

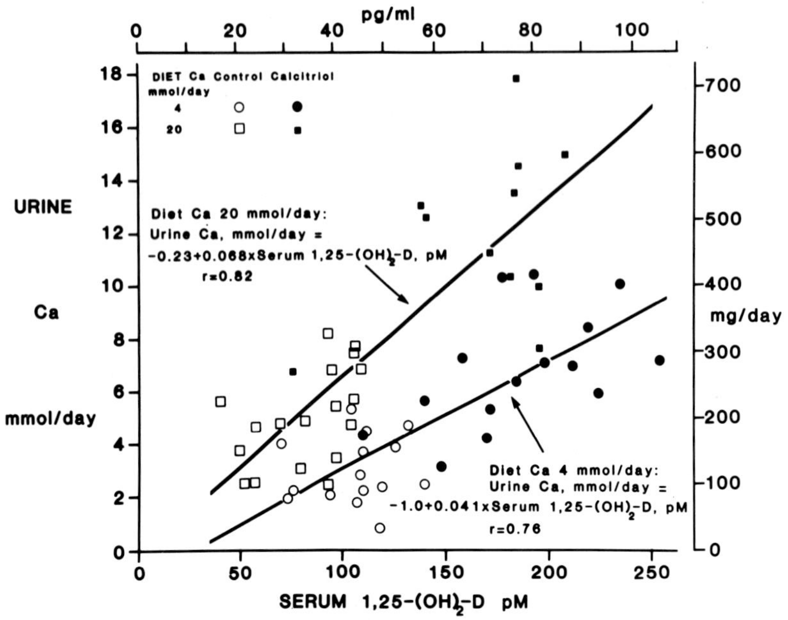

Figure 1

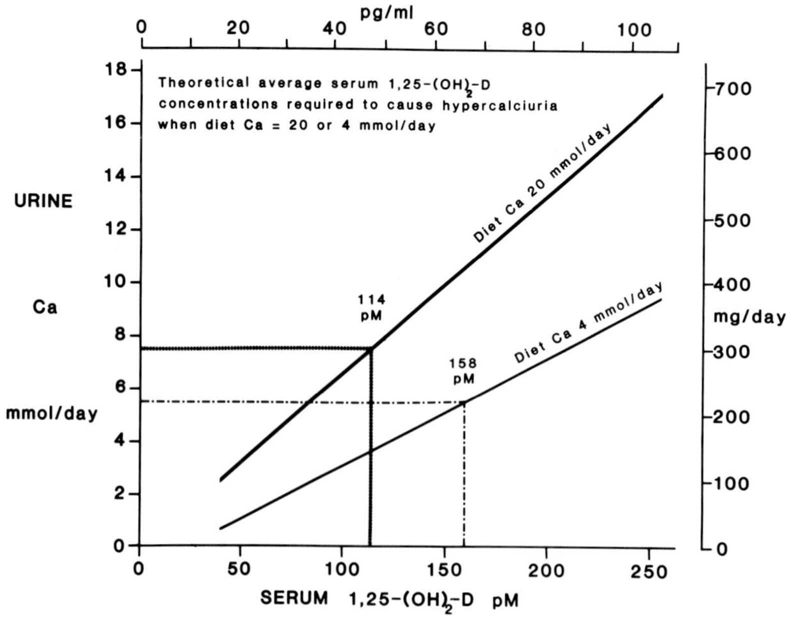

Figure 2

Ca excretion generally exceeded 4 mmol/day, the dietary Ca intake, when serum 1,25 levels exceeded 150 pM.

These data are summarized in Fig. 2. Based on the mean regression line shown in Fig. 1, it is evident that among subjects eating the normal Ca diet that urinary Ca excretion will on the average exceed 7.5 mmol/day (300 μg), the generally accepted upper limit of normal (3), when serum 1,25-$(OH)_2$-D levels average only 114 pM (47 pg/ml). On the other hand among subjects eating low Ca diets an average serum 1,25-$(OH)_2$-D level of 158 pM (66 pg/ml) would be required to cause a daily urine Ca excretion of 5.5 mmol/day (220 mg) an accepted upper limit of normal among subjects eating such diets.

Fig. 3 summarizes the relationship between fasting urinary Ca/creatinine and prevailing serum 1,25-$(OH)_2$-D concentrations. Although the regression relationship was slightly higher for the subjects eating the normal Ca diet than that for subjects eating the low Ca diet, the slopes of the lines were virtually identical and the intercepts were not statistically different. Thus after overnight fasting, the previous level of dietary Ca intake does not significantly influence urinary Ca excretion, consistent with the view that intestinal absorption of the Ca contained in the last meal is no longer occurring. On the other hand the progressive rise in fasting Ca/creatinine as serum 1,25-$(OH)_2$-D levels increase, again must ultimately relfect increased bone resorption (9,10).

These observations are summarized in Fig. 4. Based on the mean regression shown in Fig. 3 for subjects eating the normal Ca diets, fasting urine Ca/creatinine would on the average exceed 0.33 mmol/mmol (0.12 mg/mg), the accepted upper limit of normal (3), only when serum 1,25-$(OH)_2$-D levels exceed 148 pM (62 pg/ml). An average serum 1,25-$(OH)_2$-D level of 178 pM (74 pg/ml) would be required to abnormally elevate fasting urine Ca/creatinine among subjects eating a low Ca diet. Fig. 3 and 4 also emphasize that elevated fasting urinary Ca/creatinine cannot be taken as evidence for a defect in renal tubular Ca reabsorption in the absence of measurement of the prevailing serum 1,25-$(OH)_2$-D concentration. Preferably, evidence for a renal Ca leak would include hypocalcemia and secondary hyperparathyroidism in addition to hypercalciuria.

Presumably these observations are relevant to the evaluation of patients with hypercalciuria and and nephrolithiasis. Additional studies are clearly needed to determine why serum 1,25-$(OH)_2$-D levels may be elevated among these patients and to determine whether either augmented intestinal Ca absorption and/or hypercalciuria occurs in the absence of increased serum 1,25-$(OH)_2$-D levels.

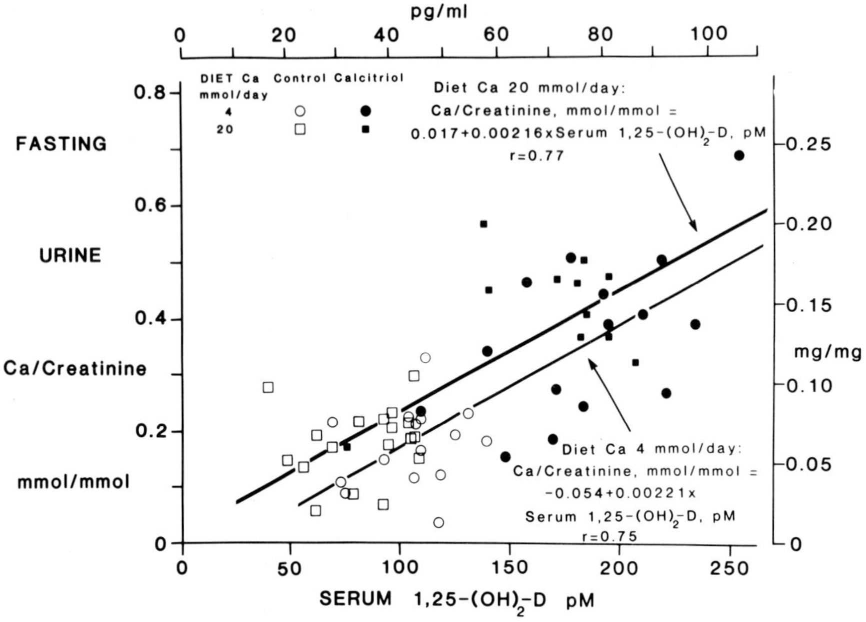

Figure 3

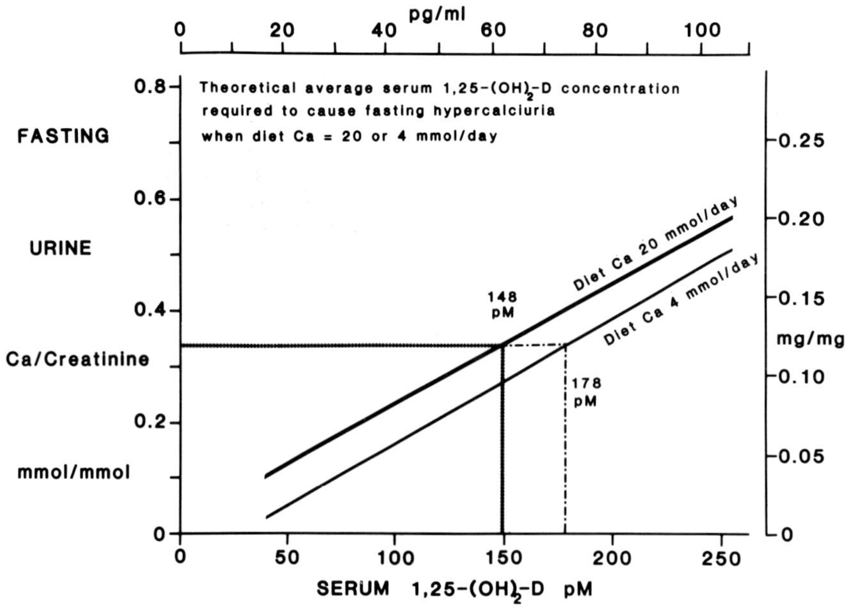

Figure 4

ACKNOWLEDGEMENTS

Supported by USPHS RR00058, AM15089 and AM22014. The authors gratefully acknowledge the assistance of the staff of the Medical College of Wisconsin Clinical Research Center and Core Laboratory.

REFERENCES

1. Edwards, N.A. and Hodgkinson, A. (1965): Clinical Science 29, 143.
2. Pak, C.Y.C., Ohata, M., Lawrence, E.C. and Snyder, W. (1974): J. Clin. Invest. 54, 387.
3. Lemann, J. Jr. (1980): In: Nephrolithiasis, p. 86. Editors: F.L. Coe, B.M. Brenner and J.H. Stein. Churchill Livingstone, New York, Edinburgh and London.
4. Kaplan, R.A., Haussler, M.R., Deftos, L.J., Bone, H. and Pak, C.Y.C. (1977): J. Clin. Invest. 59, 756.
5. Shen, F.H., Baylink, D.J., Nielsen, R.L., Sherrard, D.J., Ivey, J.L. and Haussler, M.R. (1977): J. Lab. Clin. Med. 90, 955.
6. Gray, R.W., Caldas, A.E., Wilz, D.R., Lemann, J. Jr., Smith, G.A. and DeLuca, H.F. (1978): J. Clin. Endocrinol. Metab. 45, 299.
7. DeLuca, H.F. (1981): Annu. Rev. Physiol. 43, 199.
8. Lemann, J. Jr., Adams, N.D. and Gray, R.W. (1983): Mineral Electrolyte Metab. 9, 55.
9. Adams, N.D., Gray, R.W. and Lemann, J. Jr. (1982): Kid. Intl. 21, 90.
10. Maierhofer, W.J., Gray, R.W., Cheung, H.S. and Lemann, J. Jr. (1983): Kid. Intl. (in press).

Discussion of Papers on Idiopathic Hypercalciuria

Moderator: Dr. Frederic Coe

J. TUCCI: Does spironolactone or triamterene interfere with the action of thiazides?

F. COE: I know of no published data concerning the incremental effect of spironolactone or triamterene on urinary calcium excretion in patients taking thiazide. My impression is that Amiloride may further lower urinary calcium.

F. LAFFERTY: Dr. Coe, what percentage of your patients on long-term thiazides develop hypercalcemia?

F. COE: A sustained elevation above two or three standard deviations from the mean is uncommon, perhaps less than 1% per year. That may be because we use thiazide at one third of the normal full dose. I suspect with higher doses of the thiazide we would find it more often.

F. LAFFERTY: What dose are you using?

F. COE: We use about 1/3 of the full dose of whichever drug is being used. In the case of Chlorthalidone, that would be 25-33 mg. a day; in the case of Trichlormethiazide 4 mg. per day; in the case of Hydrochlorothiazide on the order of 25 or at most 50 mg. per day.

J. COBURN: It is clear that the effect of thiazides can be offset if the sodium intake is high; so part of the effect relates to volume depletion.

G. PALMIERI: Occasionally with the use of thiazides, some degree of hypokalemia is observed. The correction of hypokalemia with potassium chloride creates problems with an overload of chloride that indirectly may induce hypercalciuria. We have found that Amiloride will prevent the hypokalemia of thiazides. Do you have any experience with the combination of thiazides and amiloride?

F. COE: There is one study in which a combination of thiazide and a potassium-sparing agent was described. The results were excellent.

J. LEMANN: With these low doses of diuretics that Dr. Coe mentioned hypokalemia is seldom, at least in my experience, a clinical problem, unless of course the patient has another illness that might make even subtle degrees of hypokalemia an unacceptable risk.

H. MALLUCHE: Dr. Coe, you have put forth the hypothesis that there is no longer a separate category of absorptive hypercalciuria or renal hypercalciuria. Let me play the devil's advocate. If that is the case, and the common denominator is just a disturbed interaction between kidney, bone and gut, why do then some patients have a decrease in their urinary calcium if you place them on a very low-calcium diet, while others do not. Another question to Dr. Favus, can you rule out what part of the effects you have observed with thiazides on the gut is due to the changed extracellular fluid volume, and have you seen an effect of thiazides on bone?

J. LEMANN: Let us look back on studies done before the availability of $1,25(OH)_2D$ and PTH assays on the responses of stone formers with hypercalciuria. When these patients are changed from a normal calcium to a low-calcium diet, indeed the urinary calcium falls, but not on the average to levels as low as you see in normal subjects. That is just what you would predict from the data that I showed you when you compare urinary calcium excretion after raising the $1,25(OH)_2D$ levels during normal and low-calcium diets. Urine calcium doesn't fall. Since in Dr. Pak's experience, most of his patients have absorptive hypercalciuria, I can't imagine that most of the earlier reported studies didn't for the most part include patients with absorptive hypercalciuria. I think it is an effect of $1,25(OH)_2D$ on the skeleton that you continue to see; and that doesn't mean it's a renal leak. You have to have other information such as hypocalcemia, secondary hyperparathyroidism with high PTH and urinary cyclic AMP, to substantiate the notion that the residual hypercalciuria on a low-calcium diet is due to a renal leak.

F. COE: I would like to emphasize a point that Dr. Lemann made. Levels of $1,25(OH)_2D$ that can increase 24-hour urinary calcium excretion may not be high enough to raise the fasting urinary calcium level in all cases.

M. FAVUS: Time didn't permit me to discuss the effect of thiazide on bone, but there is a published study indicating thiazides may cause bone resorption. With regard to the effect of volume depletion on calcium absorption, I know of no specific studies that have addressed this point. I would predict that volume depletion would favor decreased calcium excretion and increased net calcium absorption.

M. NORMAN: Dr. Lemann, in normal individuals who are given $1,25(OH)_2D$ and develop hypercalciuria, can you override that hypercalciuria with the thiazide dose that Dr. Coe has suggested while still dosing with $1,25(OH)_2D$. If so, that would make the model very relevant to the underlying disease that we are discussing.

J. LEMANN: As we speak those experiments are in progress.

C. NORDIN: Dr. Coe and Dr. Lemann, you gave fine presentations but there is some confusion on my part. The situation with regards to idiopathic hypercalciuria and the relationship between the 24-hour and the fasting urine calcium in relation to calcium absorption, was reasonably clear until you two got to grips with it. It has now been reduced to a state when it is almost uninterpretable to me. You may not understand what I meant when I described the fasting calcium-creatinine ratio. The fasting calcium-creatinine ratio after a 12 or 14 hour fast represents the minimal obligatory calcium loss of that individual. It is true that occasionally if the absorption of calcium is very high or the intake is very high the previous day, and certainly if you are vitamin D poisoned, then some of that fasting urinary calcium is still an overspill from the previous day. If you are in doubt about that, you can extend the fast for a few hours. You showed some high fasting calcium-creatinine ratios after several days of a low-calcium diet, and you then proceeded to attribute this to disordered $1,25(OH)_2D$ homeostasis. Now there is no way in which $1,25(OH)_2D$ can increase the fasting urinary calcium if the fast is adequate except by attacking bone. You are then seriously suggesting that a significant proportion of idiopathic hypercalciuric stone formers are suffering from an excessive attack of $1,25(OH)_2D$ on bone, though between all of us we have surely collected thousands of cases of idiopathic hypercalciuria without any clinical evidence of bone disease at all, even over many years. Now, when you get an anomalous result like that, it is often wise to put things on their head and see if the relation of X to Y is actually relation of Y to X. There is no way in which a high $1,25(OH)_2D$ level can give you a high fasting urine calcium, but there is a very good way in which a high fasting urinary calcium can give you a high $1,25(OH)_2D$ level. I am quite prepared to believe that among your stone formers are a limited number in whom the minimal obligatory fasting calcium loss is on the high side, probably I think due to increased sodium through-put that is switching on $1,25(OH)_2D$ and causing hyperabsorption of calcium and that is then giving you the high 24-hour urine calcium.

F. COE: Dr. Nordin, thank you for your comments. The administration of $1,25(OH)_2D$ raises fasting urine calcium or causes flagrant negative calcium balance, depending on where you set the dietary intake. What actually happens, as we showed, is that with low calcium diet, bone mineral is lost in the urine.

Now we apologize for that fact, but it nevertheless occurs. I doubt strongly that calcium loss is causing high 1,25$(OH)_2$D levels because, in those patients who were losing bone mineral in the urine, the serum PTH levels were subnormal, urinary cyclic AMP was subnormal, and the serum calcium level was higher than in normal individuals. Renal calcium loss could not have simultaneously raised serum 1,25$(OH)_2$D, lowered PTH, raised the serum calcium, and at the same time, accounted for excessive urine calcium losses. Now Dr. Lemann did the 1,25$(OH)_2$D studies in humans and he may want to comment.

J. LEMANN: Let me say the patients did eat a low-calcium diet. We analyzed them. They did take their 1,25$(OH)_2$D and I do believe Dr. Gray knows how to measure 1,25$(OH)_2$D. We are in the process of doing balance studies on more normal calcium intakes. It turns out that if the dietary calcium intake is normal, even though you have fasting hypercalciuria, as I showed you, the skeleton appears to be protected. That is, calcium balance does not become negative. I suspect that most stone formers on the average do not eat the kinds of very low calcium diets that we artificially produced for these low-calcium diet studies. Therefore, over the long haul their skeleton must be protected. Now the mechanism of the skeletal protection is not clear. Whether it is because of a greater degree of PTH suppression because of the ready availability of dietary calcium for absorption or something else related to calcium intake, I cannot explain. I would welcome any suggestion that you might have to clarify that problem.

A. WASSERSTEIN: Dr. Coe, we have done some studies that are similar to those that you reported today. In the same way, we placed patients on very low calcium diet and found a urinary calcium excretion that was higher than the intake. The majority of patients with idiopathic hypercalciuria have normal parathyroid function so we also came to the conclusion that a low-calcium diet or cellulose phosphate could be dangerous to these patients over a long period because of damage to the skeleton. However, in reviewing the literature, I can't find any evidence that cellulose phosphate results in a negative calcium balance. Do you have any information regarding this?

F. COE: I am not familiar with any precise balance studies using that agent, so I cannot comment.

XVI CALCIUM DISORDERS IN CHILDHOOD

CALCIUM DISORDERS IN CHILDHOOD - OVERVIEW

John G. Haddad

Department of Medicine, University of Pennsylvania School of Medicine, Philadelphia, PA, U.S.A.

Our general focus in this session was to highlight the very interesting time of life when development, rapid growth and skeletal modeling occur. Interest in mineral homeostasis during this period has grown as exponentially as the rate of bone growth itself, but time constraints permitted only a representative sampling of work in the field. Organ development and growth are intimately linked with the ontogenesis of hormone biosynthesis, transport and response machinery. Since the neonatologists are doing such a wonderful job in sustaining very premature infants, there's a whole new group of little folks getting a shaky start in attempting to make the transition from the placental guarantee of minerals in utero to the post-natal uncertainty of diets, infusions and environments.

Dr. Hillman provided some of the important areas to be considered in assessing the difficulties of mineral and skeletal homeostasis during the neonatal period. The availability of minerals and sterols must be taken into account, and sorting out the appropriateness of their disposition in infants represents huge challenges to investigators.

Drs. Anast and Marx addressed the very interesting issue of hypercalcemia in infancy, and the importance of extending observations to renal handling of calcium and studies of family members. Although the basic defect(s) are not characterized in familial hypocalciuric hypercalcemia, the clinical studies now available instruct us to be vigilant concerning this diagnosis.

Although firmly entrenched in the literature, the concept of "vitamin D resistance" is currently undergoing a badly-needed overhaul with newly available methodology. Drs. Glorieux and Liberman discussed new findings and therapeutic approaches in this area. With the recently available techniques in assay of hormones, receptors, hormone effects and histomorphometry, a more rational classification of apparent vitamin D resistance seems likely. Conversely, improved understanding of human diseases of vitamin D metabolism and action should provide clues to and probes for unraveling the mechanisms of vitamin D bioactivity.

These presentations were well-received and the discussions were lively in spite of a late afternoon scheduling on the fourth Symposium day. In addition to the attractiveness of the presented topics and speakers, the session's allure must, in part, be attributable to its concentration on bone and mineral metabolism during the fascinating period of growth and development. It seems very safe to predict a continuing period of growth and development for the field of mineral investigation during childhood.

NEONATAL DISORDERS OF MINERAL HOMEOSTASIS

Constantine S. Anast

Department of Pediatrics, Harvard Medical School and Children's Hospital, Boston, MA, U.S.A.

Calcium homeostasis in the rapidly growing fetus and newborn infant is of great interest but not well understood. Calcium accretion by the fetus during the last trimester of pregnancy approximates 150gm/kg/day which is obtained from the mother through the placenta. At birth the homeostatic mechanisms of the infant must adjust to the abrupt cessation of calcium infusion from the mother. Recent studies have provided insight into the calcium-regulating hormone events that take place during the neonatal period and have provided information regarding abnormalities in calcium metabolism that occur during this period of life. In this discussion an attempt will be made to briefly review the highlights of recent observations in normal and abnormal neonatal calcium metabolism.

CALCIUM METABOLISM IN NORMAL FULL TERM INFANTS

The total, ultrafilterable, ionized calcium and inorganic phosphate levels are higher in cord than in maternal plasma. This indicates that calcium and phosphate are transferred from mother to fetus against concentration gradients. There is no evidence that parathyroid hormone (PTH) and calcitonin (CT) cross the placenta. In normal newborns the plasma calcium decreases progressively after birth so that by the second or third day of life the level is often lower than that found in older infants and children. The plasma calcium usually returns to normal by five to ten days of age in normal full term infants. The serum PTH levels tend to be low in cord blood while the CT levels are normal or somewhat elevated. As the serum Ca normally decreases in the first 48 hours of life, the serum PTH increases to the normal range and the serum CT increases sharply to a peak at 13 to 24 hours of age. After 36 hours of age, there is a progressive decrease in serum CT but the level remains relatively high and above normal at the end of the first week of life. The high serum CT in the neonatal period is consistent with the high C-cell population and CT concentration in the thyroid gland of the newborn infant. It is possible that the elevated levels of CT in the neonatal period play a contributory role in the early fall in serum calcium and that the serum PTH increases as an appropriate physiologic response to the fall in serum calcium. The full term infant appears to be able to convert vitamin D to 25-hydroxyvitamin D (25-OHD) and to 1,25-dihydroxyvitamin D [1,25(OH)$_2$D] in a normal fashion. The plasma levels of 25-OHD in term infants correlate with the maternal values and increase after birth in infants receiving an oral vitamin D supplement of 400 I.U./day.

NEONATAL HYPOCALCEMIA

Early neonatal hypocalcemia occurs during the first 24 to 48 hours of life and is most frequently observed in premature infants. The total serum calcium level often declines to below 7.0mg/dl in premature infants. The pathogenesis of early neonatal hypocalcemia is uncertain. The finding of elevated circulating PTH levels is consistent with an appropriate physiologic response to hypocalcemia in premature infants. This suggests that factors other than parathyroid insufficiency play a pathogenetic role in early neonatal hypocalcemia. One contributing factor may be hypercalcitonemia since premature infants demonstrate a marked increase in serum CT during the first 24 hours of life and an inverse correlation between serum CT and serum calcium has been observed (1). The finding of reduced phosphaturic and renal cyclic AMP responses to parathyroid extract in premature infants suggests that refractoriness to parathyroid hormone may play a pathogenetic role in early neonatal hypocalcemia(2). However, this point remains unresolved. Studies of vitamin D metabolism have been performed on premature infants greater than 31 weeks gestation. Current evidence indicates that these infants have the ability to normally synthesize $1,25(OH)_2D$ (3). However, it is unclear as to whether the premature infant has impaired ability to convert vitamin D to 25-OHD (3,4). Further studies are needed to determine whether impaired vitamin D metabolism plays a role in the pathogenesis of early hypocalcemia.

Late neonatal hypocalcemia occurs at the end of the first week of life commonly in full term infants receiving cow's milk or proprietary milk formulas with relatively high phosphate loads. In contrast to early neonatal hypocalcemia, hyperphosphatemia is a characteristic finding in late neonatal hypocalcemia. In further contrast to early neonatal hypocalcemia, inappropriately low rather than elevated serum PTH levels are frequently observed in infants with late neonatal hypocalcemia. The disorder is self-limited and after several days to weeks the serum calcium returns to normal. The reason for the apparent transient hypoparathyroidism in these infants is unknown.

NEONATAL HYPERCALCEMIA

Hypercalcemia is less common than hypocalcemia in the neonatal period. It is found in association with a number of clinical entities and, if severe, presents as a medical emergency. Some of these disorders, with emphasis on recent observations, will be discussed briefly.

Neonatal Primary Hyperparathyroidism

Neonatal primary hyperparathyroidism is an uncommon but frequently life-threatening disorder. Symptoms of hypercalcemia develop during the early days of life and include hypotonia, constipation and respiratory distress. Serum calcium levels frequently range between 15 and 30mg/dl while the serum inorganic phosphate concentration is frequently less than 3.5mg/dl. However, there are exceptions with serum calcium levels in the range of 11 to 13mg/dl and normal serum inorganic phosphate concentrations. Abnormal skeletal radiographic findings include demineralization, subperiosteal resorption, pathologic fractures, and periodontal osteoporosis. The characteristic pathologic finding in the parathyroid gland is clear cell hyperplasia.

In some cases of neonatal primary hyperparathyroidism there has been no evidence of familial disease although there have been few details concerning family screening. In other cases, consanguinity in normocalcemic parents and/or hypercalcemia in siblings suggests autosomal recessive transmission. In still others, the presence of hypercalcemia in one parent as well as in one or more siblings suggests autosomal dominant transmission. Of great interest is the recent observation of an association between neonatal severe primary hyperparathyroidism and familial hypocalciuric hypercalcemia (FHH)(5). FHH is an autosomal dominant trait, with high penetrance in childhood, in which family members have modest and usually asymptomatic hypercalcemia. The reason for the occurrence of severe neonatal hyperparathyroidism in kindreds with FHH is unknown. Relative hypocalciuria has been observed in several infants with severe neonatal hyperparathyroidism. However, it is uncertain whether relative hypocalciuria is a unique feature of afflicted infants who are members of an FHH kindred or whether most, if not all, infants with neonatal primary hyperparathyroidism have a biochemical phenotype related to FHH.

Neonatal primary hyperparathyroidism is usually, but not always, considered a surgical emergency. If untreated, severely affected infants die between two and seven months of age. Total parathyroidectomy has been advocated because of the high recurrence rate that occurs following subtotal parathyroidectomy. Infants subjected to total parathyroidectomy require life-long treatment for hypoparathyroidism.

Recently we treated a neonate with severe primary hyperparathyroidism with total parathyroidectomy and autotransplantation of 1/3 of one parathyroid gland to the muscle of the forearm. Preoperatively the bones of the infant were severely demineralized, the serum calcium ranged between 20 and 30mg/dl, and the serum parathyroid hormone level was 10 x greater than normal. Postoperatively, serum calcium fell to a range of 11 to 12mg/dl, the serum PTH progressively declined to low levels, and there was marked improvement in bone mineralization. The infant is asymptomatic and at 2 years of age is growing and developing well. Further observations are necessary to determine the long-term effects of the autotransplantation and to determine whether this mode of therapy is superior to total parathyroidectomy. The infant in this study is of interest in that both his mother and father had asymptomatic hypercalcemia and upper normal to elevated serum PTH levels. Relative hypocalciuria (calcium clearance/creatinine clearance less than 0.0125) was present in the infant and mother but not the father who was hypercalciuric. It is possible that in this family there is a genetic abnormality in calcium metabolism resulting in autosomal dominant transmission of mild hypercalcemia and that the infant with severe primary hyperparathyroidism is homozygous for this genetic abnormality in calcium metabolism. The possibility that other infants with severe neonatal hyperparathyroidism are homozygous for an autosomal dominant mild abnormality in calcium metabolism is worthy of consideration. Recent reports indicate that not all infants with neonatal primary hyperparathyroidism require surgical intervention since the disorder may be relatively mild and the infants asymptomatic.

Neonatal Hyperparathyroidism Associated with Maternal Hypoparathyroidism

Congenital hyperparathyroidism may occur in infants born to mothers with poorly treated idiopathic or surgical hypoparathyroidism. The birth weight of these infants is frequently less than 2500gms. The infants usually appear normal at birth although there is one report of a baby with deformity of the skull and chest. Roentgenograms in the neonatal period demonstrate changes consistent with hyperparathyroidism including generalized skeletal demineralization and subperiosteal resorption. In cases where it was measured, the serum parathyroid hormone levels were elevated. In contrast to infants with neonatal primary hyperparathyroidism, these infants frequently have low birth weights, their serum calcium levels are frequently depressed or normal rather than elevated, and the serum inorganic phosphate levels tend to be normal to somewhat elevated rather than depressed. The reason for the differences in biochemical findings in the two groups is uncertain but conceivably could be related to (a) a state of secondary hyperparathyroidism in infants born of hypoparathyroid mothers in contrast to a state of primary hyperparathyroidism in neonatal primary hyperparathyroidism or (b) differences in vitamin D and/or vitamin D metabolite stores since circulating levels of $1,25(OH)_2D$ would be expected to be low in the hypoparathyroid mothers. The mortality rate in infants born of poorly or untreated hypoparathyroid mothers is high, especially in infants with birth weights less than 2000gms. In the infants who survive, the osseous abnormalities regress spontaneously and roentgenograms are normal by 4 to 7 months of age.

The findings in these infants demonstrate the effects of maternal parathyroid deficiency on the offspring. It is postulated that when hypocalcemia secondary to hypoparathyroidism is present in the mother, there is a decrease in calcium transport from mother to fetus. As a result, the fetus is exposed to hypocalcemia *in utero*, leading to hyperplasia of the fetal parathyroid glands. The increased secretion of fetal parathyroid hormone mobilizes calcium from the fetal skeleton. Following birth, the infant's skeleton avidly takes up calcium and with time the parathyroid hyperplasia subsides and bone lesions heal spontaneously. Correction of hypocalcemia in hypoparathyroid women during pregnancy will prevent the development of hyperparathyroidism in the fetus. Transient neonatal hyperparathyroidism secondary to untreated maternal pseudohypoparathyroidism has also been observed.

Idiopathic Infantile Hypercalcemia

Idiopathic infantile hypercalcemia is a disorder of unknown etiology in which hypercalcemia is associated with failure to thrive. A wide spectrum of clinical findings is observed in this syndrome and it is uncertain as to whether this reflects different manifestations of the same underlying metabolic defect on the one hand or different underlying disease processes on the other.

Idiopathic infantile hypercalcemia is frequently found in association with a number of the phenotypic features of the Williams "elfin facies" syndrome which include depressed nasal bones, short and turned up nose, hyperteliorism, receding mandible, prominent maxilla with full pouting cheeks, prominent upper lip shaped in a cupid's bow, low-set prominent ears, epicanthic folds, and strabismus. Cardiovascular disturbances are common in the Williams "elfin facies" syndrome and include supravalvular aortic stenosis and peripheral pulmonic artery stenosis. The serum calcium levels frequently range between 12 and 19mg/dl. The serum phosphorus level is usually normal but may be elevated during periods of azotemia.

The pathogenesis of idiopathic infantile hypercalcemia is uncertain. There is no evidence of abnormal parathyroid function. Excessive vitamin D intake has received attention as a possible etiologic factor especially in Britain shortly after World War II. However, idiopathic infantile hypercalcemia is observed in the absence of excessive vitamin D intake in either the mother or the infant. The possibility of increased sensitivity to vitamin D has been considered. This possibility is consistent with the recent observation of an exaggerated increase in serum 25-OHD following the administration of a vitamin D load to children with Williams syndrome (6). On the other hand, evidence for increased intestinal calcium absorption was reported in one hypercalcemic patient with this disorder in whom serum 25-OHD was normal and serum $1,25(OH)_2D$ was low (7). On the basis of this observation it was postulated that the hypercalcemia in idiopathic infantile hypercalcemia may be due to the transient production of an unknown substance that promotes calcium absorption. In this regard it is of interest that the serum calcium level usually returns to normal by 4 years of age.

Subcutaneous Fat Necrosis

Infantile hypercalcemia occurs in association with subcutaneous fat necrosis. In the afflicted infants, indurated subcutaneous masses with bluish-red discoloration of the overlying skin develop in the early weeks of life. The serum phosphate level and the alkaline phosphatase activity are normal. The reason for the hypercalcemia in these infants is unknown. In one study serum parathyroid hormone levels were low, serum 25-OHD and $1,25(OH)_2D$ levels were normal, and urinary prostaglandin E elevated (8). In this case corticosteroid therapy alleviated the hypercalcemia. It is known that prostaglandins have potent bone resorption actions and thereby can induce hypercalcemia; it is also known that corticosteroids inhibit prostaglandin synthesis. It is uncertain as to whether fat necrosis may either follow or elicit prostaglandin release. In contrast to the elevated urinary prostaglandin observed in the above patient, normal plasma levels of prostaglandin E^2 and E^3 were reported in another infant with subcutaneous fat necrosis (9). The hypercalcemia associated with subcutaneous fat necrosis may persist for several days or weeks and has primarily been treated with glucocorticoids and low calcium diet. If further studies confirm that prostaglandin production is a pathogenic factor in this disorder, then inhibitors of prostaglandin synthetase, such as aspirin or indomethacin, may be effective therapeutic agents.

Blue Diaper Syndrome

This is a rare familial disease in which hypercalcemia and nephrocalcinosis are associated with a defect in the intestinal transport of tryptophane.[10] Bacterial degradation of the tryptophane in the intestine leads to excessive indole production, which is converted to indican in the liver. The oxidative conjugation of two molecules of indican following elimination from the body forms the water insoluble dye indigotin (indigo-blue) which results in blue discoloration of the diaper. The mechanism of the hypercalcemia is uncertain, although oral tryptophane loading in both humans and experimental animals produces an increase in serum calcium.

REFERENCES

1. David, L., Salle, B.L., Putet, G., and Grafmeyer, D. (1981): Pediatr. Res., 15, 803.
2. Kodama, S., Sakurai, T., Seki, A., Morishita, Y., and Matsuo, T. (1975): Kobe Journal of Medical Science, 21, 69.
3. Glorieux, F., Salle, B.L., Delvin, E., and David, L. (1981): J. Pediatr., 99, 640.
4. Hillman, L., and Haddad, J.G. (1975): J. Pediatr., 86, 928.
5. Marx, S.J., Attie, M.F., Spiegel, A.M., Levine, M.A., Lasker, R.D., and Fox, M. (1982): N. Engl. J. Med., 306, 257.
6. Taylor, A.B., Stern, P.H., and Bell, N.H. (1982): N. Engl. J. Med., 306, 972.
7. Gertner, J.M. (1982): Abstracts of 4th Annual Meeting of American Society for Bone and Mineral Research, San Francisco, S22.
8. Veldhuis, J.D., Kulin, H.E., Demers, C.M., and Lambert, P.W. (1979): J. Pediatr., 95, 460.
9. Metz, S.A., and Hassal, E. (1980): J. Pediatr., 97, 336.
10. Drummond, K.N., Michael, A.F., Ulstrom, R.A., and Good, R.A. (1964): Am. J. Med., 37, 928.

NEONATAL OSTEOPENIA - DIAGNOSIS AND MANAGEMENT

Laura S. Hillman, M.D.

Department of Pediatrics, Washington University School of Medicine, St. Louis Children's Hospital, St. Louis, MO U.S.A.

Neonatal osteopenia is usually the result of a combination of adverse factors and treatment depends on defining the key components.

The degree of mineralization accomplished prior to birth is a key beginning point. Calcium and phosphorus are actively transported across the placenta so that maternal deficiencies of calcium and phosphorus are usually compensated for. 25-Hydroxyvitamin D (25-OHD) in the infant is, however, a direct reflection of maternal 25-OHD and mothers with low 25-OHD deliver infants with low 25-OHD. Congenital rickets due to vitamin D deficiency, documented by low infant serum 25-OHD, has been reported primarily among D-deficient Asians residing in Great Britain (1). The key factor prenatally is the length of gestation since bone mineralization occurs during the third trimester and the more premature the infant the less mineralization which has occurred. For most of this paper we will be concentrating on the premature infant who is at greatest risk.

We must first then define the capabilities of the infant, especially the premature, postnatally. Serum vitamin D and 25-OHD was measured in infants who were unsupplemented with vitamin D, during a treatment trial of 25-OHD_3 supplementation, and infants supplemented with 400 IU and 800 IU vitamin D. The vitamin D contained in formula (100-150 IU) was inadequate for the generation of normal vitamin D levels, and significant vitamin D from maternal sources or photoproduction are absent. Infants on 400 and 800 IU have elevated vitamin D, however, not as elevated as might be expected in adults so that vitamin D absorption may be still decreased. Adults can maintain a normal 25-OHD level on even undetectable levels of vitamin D, however infant 25-OHD was normal or low at even very elevated vitamin D levels, suggesting that liver 25-hydroxylation is decreased (2). This would be consistent with a delay in full production of many liver synthesized proteins or compounds.

On the other hand, $1,25(OH)_2D$ production appears normal and elevated levels are seen by 1-2 weeks and progressively increase over the first 12 weeks (3). Delays in renal functions in premature infants in general are far less common than delays in liver function. Whether in premature infants intestine and/or bone is able to respond to the elevated $1,25(OH)_2D$ in adult fashion is unclear.

Maintenance of serum calcium and phosphorus is a more difficult task for infants <1000 grams than those 1000-1240 grams than those 1250-1600 grams. However, at postconceptual maturity (40 weeks gestation), a marked improvement in both calcium and phosphorus occurs and these differences decrease (4). In contrast, serum magnesium is similar between birth weight groups and shows no further increase at postconceptual maturity. The degree of mineralization evaluated by either radiographs or absorption photometry shows a similar pattern with less mature and smaller infants having worse mineralization but all groups showed significant improvement or normalization at postconceptual maturity. The percentage of 72 infants whose x-rays were read as moderate or severe was 77% at 3 weeks, 50% at 6 weeks, 51% at 9 weeks, and 13% at 12 weeks. These data emphasized the problems of the very low birth weight infant and are suggestive of a developmental delay in vitamin D responsiveness in the intestine and possibly the bone.

On top of in utero starting points and development capacities, is superimposed nutrient intake. The two most obvious components are minerals and vitamin D. Seventy-two premature infants previously broken down by birth weight were also broken into infants whose daily calcium intake prior to 3 weeks was >80 mg/kg/day, and those $\leq$80 mg/kg/day. Infants with higher intakes had both higher serum calcium (and phosphorus) and better mineralization although the same pattern of improvement with postconceptual maturity was seen in both groups (4).

Fifty-five infants who had known 25-OHD values out to at least six or nine weeks were divided into infants who could maintain normal 25-OHD levels and correct low 25-OHD levels and infants who had falling 25-OHD levels or failed to correct low 25-OHD levels. Again, the infants with better 25-OHD status had better serum calcium and better mineralization but the pattern with age was similar in both groups (4). Whether 25-OHD is the active substance or whether 25-OHD is a reflection of vitamin D sufficiency with vitamin D or another metabolite the key factor is unclear.

The type of feeding regimen which the infant is electively placed on or is only able to tolerate, in large part determines the type of deficiency which one sees. More often than not, infants who present with severe osteopenia have both a mineral deficiency and a 25-OHD deficiency. Evaluation of nine premature infants who presented with frank rickets and seven infants with severe osteopenia and fractures, showed the majority to be eating a soy formula, elemental formula or a formula designed to mimic mother´s milk (5). Low birth weight (<1000 gm) and low gestation ($\leq$28 weeks) were common features, as is the time of presentation, usually about three months. Low serum calcium, low serum phosphorus, and high alkaline phosphatase are general markers of mineralization problems. Elevated PTH and urine aminoaciduria and low serum 25-OHD confirm that vitamin D deficiency is a major part of the problem. However, poor phosphorus absorption from soy formulae, urine losses on elemental formulae, and decreased content in breast milk-like formulae, undoubtedly adds to the problem.

Premature infants, especially those <1200 grams, who are fed exclusively human milk, develop what is primarily a phosphorus deficiency demineralization. However, infants with low serum 25-OHD get in worse trouble sooner than those with normal serum 25-OHD (6). Serum phosphorus is almost always low, however, a fall below 4.0 mg/dl is usually associated with problems. Urine phosphorus is almost always undetectable and does not help define which infant is in trouble. However, the sudden, marked increase in urine calcium is very helpful in identifying the point when mineralization is in serious jeopardy. Elevation of alkaline phosphatase above 400-500 IU is also worrisome. PTH is usually undetectable and no aminoaciduria is present. Phosphorus supplementation rapidly reverses these findings. We would recommend that all infants <1200 grams fed breast milk be followed with serum and urine calcium and phosphorus to determine the need for phosphorus supplementation. Use of routine phosphorus supplementation is common in Europe and new mineral fortifiers will be commercially available soon.

Infants on TPN develop bone disease very rapidly (7). The key factor is just the inability to deliver adequate calcium and phosphorus intravenously due to precipitation. Inability to deliver adequate vitamin D may also play a role and loss of trace elements in the urine may complicate the picture. Infants fed special formulas, usually because of the inability to tolerate the lactose present in regular cow's milk based formulas, also have increased problems. The poor phosphorus absorption of soy formula is now well established (8). However, problems of calcium and vitamin D absorption are less clear. Casein hydrolasate formulae also have problems, however, mechanisms are unclear. With soy formula, only a third to a half of infants developed significant mineralization problems. Winter-born black infants were at greatest risk suggesting that serum 25-OHD insufficiency may have been the differentiating factor.

Vitamin D deficiency primarily must be considered when the infant is on regular formula or a formula designed for premature infants. VonSydow showed an effect of vitamin D even when whole cow's milk was fed (9). Infants are most often winter or spring-born and black, conditions predisposing to low maternal, and therefore low infant 25-OHD. Infant stores may also be low. Poor maternal diet and lack of skin exposure are often key factors. If the mother is nursing, a low maternal vitamin D may result in low milk vitamin D metabolites. A low serum calcium, moderately low serum phosphorus, elevated alkaline phosphatase, and elevated PTH or generalized aminoaciduria are highly suggestive that a vitamin D deficiency is involved and treatment can be begun on that basis. However, a 25-OHD should be drawn prior to treatment to confirm the diagnosis and can now be run by many commercial laboratories.

Treatment is obviously dependent on the problem which, as noted, is often multiple. Premature infants with phosphorus deficiency due to human milk feedings can be successfully treated by supplementing with 20-25 mg/kg phosphorus as Na or K phosphate and monitoring serum and urine calcium and phosphorus. Infants on TPN whose IV mineral intakes have been maximized can be supplemented with oral vitamin D if tolerated, but need to be begun on enteral feedings and eventual high mineral formula as soon as possible. Premature infants who are on soy formula or elemental formula should be changed to a high mineral (or at least standard) formula if this will be tolerated. If improvement does not occur, an additional vitamin D deficiency must be considered. If possible, a 25-OHD should be checked in all of these cases. Premature infants with suspected or confirmed 25-OHD deficiency have been successfully treated by us using 4,000 IU/day po for two weeks (5). Serum phosphorus usually increases within the first week and x-ray improvement is seen after two weeks. 25-OHD should be rechecked but unless liver disease is present has usually been normal after this course. Once bones have been successfully mineralized, recurrence of problems is rare.

Especially in premature infants, the focus is increasingly on prevention rather than treatment and thus prophylaxis has been focused in two areas: increasing mineral availability and assuring vitamin D sufficiency. Over the last three years three new premature formulas have been released with higher concentrations of calcium and phosphorus but all three have a 2:1 calcium phosphorus ratio based on breast milk. In all three serum calcium is increased, phosphorus retention is maximized, and bone mineralization appears improved. Balance data when compared to in utero accretion data shows comparable calcium "accretion" but low phosphorus accretion (10) and bone density data shows a following of in utero mineralization curves in two-thirds of infants, but not in a third (11). Although the results are promising, this is not the solution for all infants and more work is required to establish optimal mineral contents and ratios.

Establishing the optimal dose of vitamin D to be used for supplementation is complicated. In infants on human milk, standard formula, and standard formula with medium chain triglycerides, calcium absorption increased with doses up to 2000 IU of vitamin D (12). Our data has confirmed an improvement in serum calcium and phosphorus and mineralization in infants fed 800 IU vitamin D over infants fed 400 IU vitamin D. However, we were unable to show an improvement when serum 25-OHD was normalized using supplements of 2 μg/kg birth weight of 25-hydroxycholecalciferol (13). Balance studies using 25-hydroxycholecalciferol have not been done. The difference in findings remains to be explained. At present, 800-1000 IU is a safe recommendation.

In summary, neonatal demineralization, especially in the premature, is a combination of: 1) the developmental limitations of the infant himself, and 2) our knowledge limitations of required feeding needs and availability of those feeds. We are slowly improving our methods, however, it is unlikely that we will ever be able to replace the placenta for nutrient supply and the maternal womb for growing infants with fully mineralized bones.

REFERENCES

1. Ford, J., Davidson, D., McIntosh, W., Fyfe, W. and Dunnigan, (1973): Neonatal Rickets in Asian Immigrant Population. Brit. Med. J. 3, 211.
2. Hillman, L. and Hollis, B. (1983): Serum Vitamin D (D) in Premature Infants. Evidence for decreased conversion to 25-hydroxyvitamin D (25-OHD). Pediatr. Res. 17, 290A.
3. Hillman, L., Salmons, S., Haussler, M., and Dokoh, S. (1983): Serial 1,25 Dihydroxyvitamin D ($1,25(OH)_2D$) serum concentrations in premature infants on varying feeding regimens. Pediatr. Res. 17, 290A.
4. Hillman, L. and Haddad, J. (1982): In: Calcium Disorder. Editors: David Heath and Stephen Marx, Butterworth, London, p. 248, 1982.
5. Hoff, N., Haddad, J., Teitelbaum, S., McAlister, W. and Hillman, L. (1979): Serum concentrations of 25-hydroxyvitamin D in rickets of extremely premature infants. J. Pediatr. 94, 460.
6. Hillman, L., Salmons, S., and Fiore, B. (1982): Phosphorus deficiency in infants less than 1,200 gms fed human milk, relationship to 25-hydroxyvitamin D. Pediatr. Res. 16:166A.
7. Binstadt, D. and L'Heurerex. (1978): Rickets as a complication of intravenous hyperalimentation in infants. Pediatr. Radiol., 7, 211.
8. Shenai, J., Jhaveri, B., Renolds, J., Huston, R. and Babson, S. (1981): Nutritional balance studies in very low-birthweight infants: role of soy formula. Pediatrics, 67, 631.
9. Von Sydow, G. (1946): A study of the development of rickets in premature infants. Acta Pediatr. Scand. 33, Suppl. 2.
10. Shenai, J., Reynolds, J. and Babson, S. (1980): Nutritional balance studies in very low-birthweight infants: enhanced nutrient retention rates by an experimental formula. Pediatrics 66, 233.
11. Green, F., Steichen, J. and Tsang, R. (1982): Effects of increased calcium, phosphorus and vitamin D intake on bone mineralization in very low-birthweight infants fed formulas with polycose and medium chain triglycerides. J. Pediatr. 100, 951.
12. Senterre, J. and Salle, B. (1982): Calcium and phosphorus economy of the preterm infant and its interaction with vitamin D and its metabolites. Acta. Pediatr. Scand. Suppl. 296, 85.
13. Hillman, L., Salmons, S. and Fiore, B. (1982): In: Vitamin D, Chemical, Biochemical, and Clinical Endocrinology of Calcium Metabolism, p. 781. Editors: A. Normal, K.V. Schaefer, D. Herrath, and Gregoliet, Walter De Gruyter, Berlin.

FAMILIAL HYPOCALCIURIC HYPERCALCEMIA: IMPLICATIONS AND QUESTIONS FROM A BROAD SPECTRUM OF CLINICAL FEATURES

Stephen J. Marx, Allen M. Spiegel, Robert W. Downs jr, Roz D. Lasker, and Arthur C. Santora jr

Metabolic Diseases Branch, National Institute of Arthritis, Diabetes, and Digestive and Kidney Diseases, Bethesda, Md, U.S.A.

GENERAL FEATURES OF FAMILIAL HYPOCALCIURIC HYPERCALCEMIA

Familial hypocalciuric hypercalcemia (FHH) or familial benign hypercalcemia has been characterized by the study of kindreds with large numbers of affected members (1). Typically serum calcium concentrations in affected members are 0.5-1.5 mEq/L above the upper limit of the normal range. The pattern of hypercalcemia within each kindred suggests autosomal dominant transmission of the gene, with almost 100% penetrance for expression of hypercalcemia at all ages (Figure 1A).

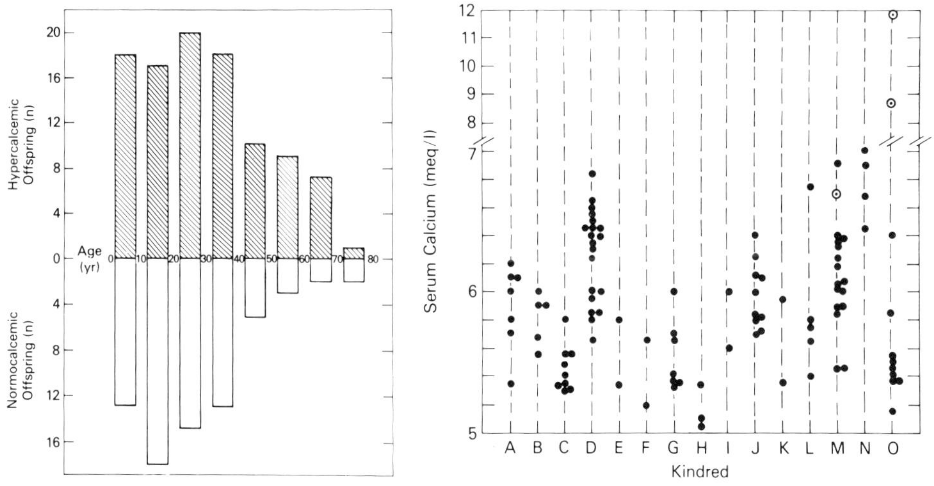

Figure 1A (left panel). Serum calcium in offspring of affected members in fifteen kindreds. Each offspring was classified at the age of first available determination of serum calcium (1).

Figure 1B (right panel). Serum calcium concentrations in hypercalcemic members (prior to any parathyroid surgery) from fifteen kindreds. Each symbol represents one patient; (◎) denotes patient with neonatal severe primary hyperparathyroidism (1).

Approximately one third of affected members have no symptoms attributable to hypercalcemia, but the remainder show a significantly increased prevalence of fatigue, weakness, forgetfulness, polydipsia, arthralgia, and/or headache (1); symptoms are usually mild and rarely cause the person to consult with a physician. Signs attributable to hypercalcemia are uncommon in FHH. In particular, the incidence of nephrolithiasis or of peptic ulcer disease is identical in hypercalcemic and normocalcemic members of these kindreds (1). Severe primary hyperparathyroidism has been recognized among neonates in several kindreds (2). Among adult members recurrent pancreatitis is a definite, though infrequent, association.

In addition to hypercalcemia, mild hypermagnesemia is common, having been identifiable in 50% of our cases evaluated on a metabolic ward (1). The distribution of urinary calcium excretion rates is similar to that in normals or in normocalcemic family members. However, since the mean urinary calcium in FHH is one third of that in typical primary hyperparathyroidism (1) and since urinary calcium excretion is even higher in hypercalcemia with parathyroid suppression than in typical primary hyperparathyroidism, these values are low relative to the levels of calcium in serum. This relative hypocalciuria is useful in diagnosis. Circulating concentrations of parathyroid hormone (PTH) by RIA are usually normal but occasionally elevated; the same is true for urinary excretion of cyclic AMP (3). At surgery the parathyroid glands usually appear grossly normal but are sometimes mildly enlarged. Quantitative analysis of parathyroid histology showed mild hyperplasia in specimens from most operations (4). The outcome of subtotal parathyroidectomy is generally disappointing; almost all patients show a rapid recurrence of hypercalcemia after surgery (1).

VARIATION OF FEATURES BETWEEN KINDREDS

The distribution of serum calcium values is non-uniform from one kindred to another (Figure 1B). In one (kindred N in Figure 1B) all four affected members show serum calcium concentrations above 6.4 mEq/L; in most other kindreds the mean calcium value is between 5.5 and 6.2 mEq/L (see kindred H in Figure 1B for an example of borderline hypercalcemia in affected members). This suggests that there is more than one mutation that can cause FHH.

VARIATION OF FEATURES WITHIN KINDREDS

The heterogeneity between kindreds is difficult to recognize, in part, because of the variability of features within kindreds. Kindred O (Figure 1B - same as Kindred B (2)) illustrates this within-kindred heterogeneity. At least 20 members have shown hypercalcemia (much of this information has been assembled by Drs. Maurice Attie and William M. Law jr). Severe disease was found in the first member to be treated; he had received a diagnosis of neonatal primary hyperparathyroidism in 1959. At age three months, he showed respiratory distress due to hypotonia and an undermineralized, deformed rib cage; serum calcium concentration was 8 mEq/L. He died of respiratory insufficiency 8 days after subtotal parathyroidectomy. A sibling had serum calcium concentrations in the range of 12 mEq/L at two weeks of age. Severe hypercalcemia recurred rapidly after resection of three hyperplastic parathyroid glands. After removal of the fourth parathyroid gland the patient developed normally, requiring therapy for chronic hypoparathyroidism. Subsequent evaluation showed hypocalciuric hypercalcemia in the father and apparently normal mineral homeostasis in the mother. The paternal grandfather of these siblings with neonatal severe primary hyperparathyroidism was last evaluated at age 73. Hypercalcemia had been recognized during family screening; also two of his elderly siblings were found to be hypercalcemic. Extensive questioning revealed only mild arthralgias. He has suffered no serious illnesses. Serum calcium concentration was 5.4 mEq/L. We presume that he has had mild hypercalcemia since birth.

SOME UNANSWERED QUESTIONS

Does FHH have a single etiology? This question must be addressed at several levels. We have already noted that biochemical differences between families suggest different underlying mutations; these could all be alleles at a single locus. More important is the question of whether mutations at distinct loci could cause similar biochemical features; could distinct lesions in one or more pathways cause the same result? And lastly, can the disorder be mimicked at the level of clinical and laboratory features by other types of disturbances? Ionized calcium has been elevated in proportion to total calcium in all kindreds where examined, but the possibility remains of a similar picture (i.e. hypercalcemia without increase in ionized calcium) due to an abnormality in albumin or another divalent cation-binder in plasma.

Is there an absolute diagnostic criterion in the isolated patient? In the absence of knowledge of the underlying molecular disorder(s), a secure diagnosis cannot be made without demonstrating a pattern of disease in multiple members of a kindred; the larger the number of affected members in a kindred, the more secure the diagnosis becomes. Features most helpful in diagnosis are hypercalcemia recognized before age 10, hypercalcemia with relative hypocalciuria (a practical criterion for hypocalciuric hypercalcemia is hypercalcemia with a ratio of calcium clearance over creatinine clearance below 0.01), and absence of features of multiple endocrine neoplasia type 1.

Is primary hyperparathyroidism an integral component of the disorder? We believe it is because we have found the following: PTH concentrations are occasionally high by RIA (3), hyperplasia of the parathyroid glands is often present (4), and neonatal severe primary hyperparathyroidism occurs in multiple FHH kindreds (2). We believe that the FHH trait disturbs calcium metabolism in both the kidney (5). and the parathyroid gland. However, with some large kindreds, PTH concentrations by RIA have been normal; based upon this, FHH has been interpreted by others as a primary disturbance localized to the kidney or to the kidney plus other target tissues for PTH.

What accounts for the association of FHH and neonatal severe primary hyperparathyroidism? Since neonatal severe primary hyperparathyroidism is a rare disorder, its recognition in more than three FHH kindreds (2) cannot be attributed to chance. Equally important is the absence of reports of neonatal primary hyperparathyroidism (of severe or even of mild degree) in any kindred with multiple endocrine neoplasia type 1, type 2, or type 3. In one kindred non-consanguineous parents of a neonate with severe primary hyperparathyroidism both show FHH (2); in another the parents of a severely affected child are consanguineous for FHH (personal communication from Dr. Sara Arnaud (2)). Severity of and transmission patterns of hypercalcemia in these two kindreds suggest that homozygosity for the FHH gene is one cause for this life-threatening manifestation. In most other cases, the homozygous state seems unlikely. Studies of some severely affected neonates have shown hypercalcemia (of mild degree) in only one parent; it seems likely that some factor from the normocalcemic parent modulates expression of the FHH gene from the hypercalcemic parent. This factor might be an otherwise silent gene. There might be a spectrum of genetic lesions because different kindreds with FHH express variable grades of hypercalcemia (see above). Relevant to the mechanism of transmission of severe disease is the observation that among five reported neonates with severe primary hyperparathyroidism and with only one hypercalcemic parent, the normocalcemic parent has been the mother in each case (supplementary table and references supplied on request). The mother might contribute a critical uterine environment. The nature of the possible contribution by uterine environment is undocumented; an influence of maternal serum calcium on the affected fetus seems possible. An affected fetus gestating in a normocalcemic mother may develop secondary hyperparathyroidism in a manner analogous to that of a normal fetus gestating in a hypocalcemic mother. Thus severe primary hyperparathyroidism in the neonate could be a manifestation of FHH and secondary hyperparathyroidism, the latter component being potentially reversible. In support of the uterine environment mechanism and its potential reversibility in the neonate, Eftekhari recently described the offspring of a normocalcemic mother in a kindred with familial hypercalcemia (6) (urine calcium excretion rates have not been reported for this kindred). The newborn showed a serum calcium of 5.8 mEq/L with osteopenia, subperiosteal resorption, and multiple pathologic rib fractures; surgery was deferred, and the neonate then developed asymptomatic hypercalcemia with remineralization of bones by age two months.

What is the optimal management? The answer to this depends upon knowledge of which symptoms and signs can be attributed to the disease. Life-threatening primary hyperparathyroidism in the neonate warrants immediate intervention; recurrent pancreatitis might also improve with measures to lower the serum calcium concentration. Only total parathyroidectomy followed by therapy for hypoparathyroidism has been clearly successful in normalizing serum calcium. Controlled near-total parathyroidectomy (accomplished by total parathyroidectomy and parathyroid autografting) is an experimental approach that has not yet received definitive evaluation. For the majority of cases, our present policy is not to intervene.

CLINICAL IMPLICATIONS

1. FHH is a distinct diagnostic category. Regardless of how it is labeled or how the status of the parathyroid glands is interpreted, clinical features differ from those in familial multiple endocrine neoplasia type 1 or in typical primary hyperparathyroidism. Suspicion of FHH should lead to appropriate family testing. Diagnosis cannot be established without demonstration of characteristic features in other family members.

2. Chronic hypercalcemia can be well tolerated. The near 100% penetrance of hypercalcemia in all decades suggests that hypercalcemia lasts throughout life in FHH. At least one affected patient has survived into his eighties. Relative hypocalciuria and generally normal PTH concentrations probably account for the mild prognosis. Similar features in certain patients with sporadic primary hyperparathyroidism may help define a subset that can be satisfactorily managed without parathyroidectomy.

3. Variability of clinical features is greatest in the neonatal period. Offspring of affected mothers with unaffected mates should be monitored for two reasons: unaffected neonates may exhibit transient neonatal hypoparathyroidism, and hypercalcemic neonates should be properly diagnosed for future counseling. Unaffected mothers with affected spouses should also be monitored; their affected offspring may have increased risk of neonatal severe primary hyperparathyroidism.

4. Many children with FHH remain undiagnosed. Multiphasic screening in adults has uncovered substantial numbers of probands for kindreds with this disorder. When children have been screened in these kindreds, half the offspring of affected members have shown hypercalcemia. Since typical primary hyperparathyroidism is much less common in children than in adults and since typical primary hyperparathyroidism constitutes the majority of cases of asymptomatic hypercalcemia in adults, FHH must constitute a much larger fraction of cases of asymptomatic hypercalcemia in children than in adults.

REFERENCES

1. Marx, S.J., Attie, M.F., Levine, M.A., Spiegel, A.M., Downs, R.W. jr, and Lasker, R.D. (1981): Medicine (Baltimore), 60, 397.

2. Marx, S.J., Attie, M.F., Spiegel, A.M., Levine, M.A., Lasker, R.D., and Fox, M. (1982): N. Eng. J. Med., 306, 257.

3. Marx, S.J., Spiegel, A.M., Brown, E.M., Windeck, R., Gardner, D.G., Downs, R.W. jr, Attie, M., and Aurbach, G.D. (1978): J. Clin. Endocrinol. Metab., 47, 1190.

4. Thorgiersson, U., Costa, J., and Marx, S.J. (1982): Hum. Pathol., 12, 229.

5. Attie, M.F., Gill, J.R. jr, Stock, J.L., Spiegel, A.M., Downs, R.W. jr, Levine, M.A., and Marx, S.J. (1980): Clin. Res., 28, 384 (Abstract).

6. Eftekhari, F. and Yousefzadeh, D.K. (1982): Skel. Radiol., 8, 201.

Discussion of papers of C. Anast, L. Hillman, and S. Marx

D. SLOVIK: Do you have any information about the vitamin D metabolites in patients with familial hypocalciuric hypercalcemia?

S. MARX: Drs. O'Riordan and Bijvoet have studied a large kindred comparing hypercalcemic and normocalcemic members. The serum levels of 1,25 $(OH)_2D$ in those two groups were indistinguishable. This supports the notion that the levels of 1,25$(OH)_2D$ are proportional to the PTH levels in these kindreds. I don't think 25 hydroxy D or 1,25$(OH)_2D$ have very much to do with the etiology of the syndrome.

E. DELVIN: I would like to pose a question to Dr. Hillman regarding the 25 hydroxy D levels that you observed in your premature infants. You came to the conclusion that there might be a liver impairment of 25 hydroxylation of vitamin D. Now, I would suggest that maybe there is another way of explaining these values that you observed. Is it possible that there could be an impairment of the enterohepatic circulation, so that if bile salt synthesis is not mature, you may actually have an impairment of the enterohepatic cycle which would lower the 25 hydroxy vitamin D level in the serum of these preemies?

L. HILLMAN: That is a possibility, although the importance of the enterophepatic circulation regarding 25 hydroxy is still somewhat in doubt. I think our best data suggests that probably it is a 25 hydroxylation defect in the liver but , this is circumstantial in terms of when you look at the premature infant's ability to synthesize a variety of proteins or to conjugate drugs, you see this very similar pattern of relatively low levels until postconceptual maturity is reached, and then there is a sudden increase in 25 hydroxy vitamin D. We see it with D binding protein, ceruloplasm, somatomedin, and a number of other peptides. But that's guilt by association and we can't rule out an increased degradation.

O. MEHLS: I would like to make two comments. One is for Dr. Anast. We recently had the opportunity to follow a patient with hypercalcemia and subcutaneous fat necrosis. Dr. Seibert in our department measured the prostaglandins, which were high. Prostaglandins and hypercalcemia responded well to treatment with aspirin and corticosteroids. It is still undecided as to whether the elevation of prostaglandins are of primary or secondary origin.

I would like to make a second comment regarding the paper of Dr. Hillman. When we talk about vitamin D levels in newborns or premature infants, I think we have to be aware of the paper of Bouillon and associates who showed that we can't interpret these levels without precise knowledge about the D-binding proteins. Pregnancy is the only situation where the D-binding protein is different in the mother and fetus. Therefore, when we measure low levels of either 25 or 1,25 D metabolites, we have to consider the ratio of these levels to the D-binding protein. This will give an idea of the unbound metabolite, which is responsible for the activity of 25(OH)D and 1,25$(OH)_2D$.

L. HILLMAN: The D-binding protein in the preemies follows the same pattern as the 25 hyrdoxy D. It stays low for about the first nine or ten weeks of life and then as postconceptual maturity is reached and the liver "turns on", both the D-binding protein and the 25(OH)D increases; and, indeed, at that point in time there is even a direct correlation of the two. Prior to that time, you know there isn't. We have interpreted this as concurrent liver maturation phenomena. You are right, however, if you think in terms of free 25-hydroxy D, then possibly these low levels of total 25-hydroxy D could mean perfectly normal levels of free 25-hydroxy D. When you are thinking in terms of vitamin D or 1,25$(OH)_2D$, the low DBP makes these levels probably higher and more pharmacologic.

R. SCHILLING: Two questions to Dr. Hillman. If calcium and phosphorus content in human milk is insufficient for premature infants, how do you explain the biochemical signs of phosphorus depletion, but not of calcium? The second question is, if you recommend phosphorus supplementation to human milk, are you not afraid of producing hypocalcemia and secondary hyperparathyroidism by inducing mineralization and increased calcium utilization?

L. HILLMAN: Human milk is indeed low in both calcium and phosphorus, but it's relatively lower in phosphorus than it is in calcium. The calcium absorption from human milk is so good that, although it's lower than you would like for matching in utero skeletal accretion rates, it usually is associated with normal serum calcium levels. The problem is really the phosphorus. The phosphorus demands of the growing preemie are astronomical, not only for the huge mineralization of bone that is required, but also for soft tissue demands; so that it is really the phosphorus deficiency that is of concern. Even though the calcium has been absorbed from the diet, there isn't any phosphorus to move into bone with it and you then see the calcium excreted in the urine. When you restore the phosphorus, the phosphorus and the calcium will again enter into bone formation.

We have this huge sink of bone just waiting to be mineralized so that there is a risk of developing hypocalcemia. But, if we do it slowly enough, we usually don't see significant hypocalcemia. Occasionally, you have to give calcium supplementation. I feel that the best thing to do is prevent the whole process by giving adequate phosphorus from the very beginning so that you don't have to go through these big calcium and phosphorus swings in the blood.

M. WHYTE: Dr. Marx, I'm curious to know whether your FHA kindred members were aware of their biochemical status when you questioned them about symptomatology.

S. MARX: Yes, they were. Unfortunately, that study was done after the diagnosis had been made and neither the interviewers nor the subjects were "blinded." This weakness of the study is much less important in analyzing the data on signs than on symptoms.

A. HODSMAN: Premature infants may be critically ill and in an intensive care unit for some weeks. In view of your data on the possible liver abnormalities of 25 hydroxylation, do you think it would be logical to switch vitamin D supplementation to 25 hydroxy D directly, both parenterally and enterally; and, if so, would you expect the dose requirements to be the same as for vitamin D itself.

L. HILLMAN: We had the theory that if you could bypass both potential decreased vitamin D absorption in the gut and 25 hydroxylation in the liver and give 25 hydroxy D directly, maybe you would have a better or more even effect. We have established that the dose of 2 mcg. per kg. per day of 25-hydroxy D normalizes 25-hydroxy D levels within a week. The problem is it doesn't work in terms of correcting the problem. By increasing the dose of vitamin D from 400 to 800 units, we see better serum calcium levels, lower alkaline phosphatase and better mineralization of bone. When we feed 25-hydroxy D and get even better 25-hydroxy D levels, the serum calcium, if anything falls and the phosphorus increases. The magnesium falls, the PTH decreases, and the bones do not improve. I can't really explain this very well. I think you may need to postulate an effect of vitamin D itself, which is somewhat heretical. The other question is whether the $1,25(OH)_2D$ receptors in these infants are deficient.

G. KLEIN: This is a question for Dr. Hillamn. In light of the fact that a standard pediatric multivitamin infusion is probably going to be developed in the near future, I'd like to know how much intravenous vitamin D_2 you are currently infusing in neonates? The second part of the question is are you currently infusing calcium and phosphorus together in your intravenous solutions for these infants and, if so, how much can you give without precipitation?

L. HILLMAN: As you know, I try and avoid hyperalimentation in these infants. I think we need separate studies to determine what dosages are going to be needed for IV infusion. I think that enterally we're talking about dosages of 100 units/day. I don't think we have anyway of going from our oral data to the IV data. I think someone is going to have to do the IV studies.

There is calcium and phosphorus in the solutions, but unfortunately there is no way to infuse high enough amounts of either mineral to match the *in utero* accretion rates without observing precipitation.

R. CHESNEY: I want to ask Steve Marx if he has any data from either cord blood or from the placenta itself with regards to the serum calcium levels? If you have some anticipated pregnancies, it would be nice if you could get some placenta tissue to try to answer some of these questions.

S. MARX: I don't have this data.

R. CHESNEY: Regarding Dr. Klein's question about intravenous vitamin D, probably a third of the vitamin will stick to the tubing.

DIAGNOSIS AND MANAGEMENT OF HYPOPHOSPHATEMIC DISORDERS

Francis H. Glorieux

Genetics Unit, Shriners Hospital and Departments of Surgery and Pediatrics, McGill University, Montreal, Que. Canada

Chronic hypophosphatemia is one major cause of rickets and osteomalacia in growing children. It may have various causes, either acquired or congenital (Table 1). In most instances, the acquired forms can be controlled by acting on the underlying cause. The inherited syndromes present a challenge however, sometimes for diagnosis and always for management. The most common of the hypophosphatemic disorders is transmitted as a sex-linked dominant trait. Reported sporadic forms may represent new mutations. Affected individuals are diagnosed early in life (hypophosphatemia can be detected at birth in the families at risk) by progressive deformities of the lower limbs (more frequently in varum than in valgum) and stunted growth. Proximal myopathy is absent, as opposed to what is seen in tumor induced hypophosphatemia. Tooth enamel hypoplasia consecutive to long lasting hypocalcemia is also absent, unlike what is observed in vitamin D dependency (VDD). It is important to know that the latter condition when treated with insufficient amounts of vitamin D may mimic vitamin D resistant rickets (VDRR). Differential diagnosis will be based on high PTH and low $1,25(OH)_2D$ circulating levels as well as a rapid and complete response to replacement therapy with $1,25(OH)_2D_3$ in VDD.

In VDRR, rickets is clinically and radiologically evident by age 2. Low plasma phosphate, elevated alkaline phosphatase and decreased renal tubular reabsorption of phosphate are the biochemical markers in the untreated state. Serum calcium and PTH levels are normal and so is $1,25(OH)_2D_3$ concentration in the untreated state (1). A defective regulation of $1,25(OH)_2D$ synthesis has been suggested but would only be an ancillary abnormality (2). Although the basic defect in VDRR has yet to be identified, hypophosphatemia has been shown to be the result of a primary defect in renal phosphate transport (3). Bone histology reveals a moderate to severe osteomalacia (increased osteoid seam thickness, decreased calcification rate) with low turnover and

TABLE 1. Hypophosphatemic disorders in children

Aquired	- Decreased intake	- Prematurity		
		- Phosphate binders		
		- Total parenteral nutrition		
	- Increased loss	- Tumor induced		
		- "Juvenile onset"		
		- Acquired Fanconi	- Heavy metals	
			- "Old" tetracycline	
Congenital	- Increased loss	- Vit. D resistance	- sex linked	
			- sporadic	
			- autosomal dominant	
		- Distal tubular acidosis		
		- Fanconi syndrome	e.g.	- cystinosis
				- tyrosinemia

Supported by the Shriners of North America

normal to increased trabecular bone volume. There is also a peculiar periosteocytic lesion which is not found in other forms of osteomalacia where hypophosphatemia prevails (e.g. tumor induced rickets or florid vitamin D dependency) (4).

"Classic" approach to treatment was based on large amounts of vitamin D (> 50,000 U/d). Although it may improve the rickets, the effective dose was usually close to the toxic range. With long-term administration, the risks of hypercalcemia and renal damage were high. Furthermore, the dwarfism was seldom corrected by vitamin D treatment alone. Since renal phosphate waste is one major expression of the abnormal phenotype, emphasis was placed in the last 15 years, on a treatment regimen based on frequent phosphate supplementation (5). One to 3 grams of elemental phosphorus is administered daily, in 5 divided doses, with no more than a 6-hour interval between doses, all around the clock. Because of the hypocalcemic effect of phosphate loading that could induce secondary hyperparathyroidism, vitamin D_2 was administered concomittantly in doses up to 25,000 IU/d. This treatment will heal the rickets (calcification of the epiphyseal cartilage) but not the osteomalacia (calcification process at the trabecular bone surface) (6,7). Growthrate is also accelerated, with frequent observation of catch-up growth, i.e. passage from a lower to a higher percentile line on the growth chart. If treatment is started before age 5 a spontaneous correction of lower limb deformities can be obtained. Despite these positive effects, control of secondary hyperparathyroidism was difficult. Indeed we were forced in two instances to undertake subtotal parathyroidectomy for correction of "tertiary" hyperparathyroidism. Furthermore, serum levels of alkaline phosphatase seldom returned to normal range, despite healing of rickets on x-rays. This was related to the non-correction of the osteomalacic process at the trabecular bone surface.

When $1,25(OH)_2D_3$ was substituted for vitamin D at the dose of 0.5-1 µg/d in the combined therapy (6), several improvements over the previous regimen were noted. Intestinal phosphate absorption was enhanced allowing a decrease in the daily dose of phosphate. We found that an adequate dose would increase serum phosphate by 1.5 mg/dl 45 minutes after administration in liquid form (Joulie solution) and 60 minutes after administration in tablets (K Phos no. 2, Beach Pharmaceuticals). With the latter an increase of more than 1 mg/dl is still observed 5 hours after the dose. Although this may allow a decrease in the frequency of phosphate dosage, we prefer to maintain the 5-dose schedule, taking in account that full compliance is not always obtained. The control of the phosphate induced hyperparathyroidism was also improved (7). We have not seen any case of "tertiary" hyperparathyroidism since 1977, when the change to $1,25(OH)_2D_3$ was initiated. This observation was corroborated by histologic studies of iliac crest biopsies (6) showing that the parameters of bone resorption (active resorption surface and osteoclast number) that had increased under phosphate therapy (with or without vitamin D_2) decreased significantly. At the same time both static (extent of the mineralization front, thickness of the osteoid) and dynamic (calcification rate, mineralization lagtime) parameters of bone formation were greatly improved, albeit not always fully normalized. Whether this positive effect on bone formation is secondary to an increased availability of phosphate or represents a direct effect of $1,25(OH)_2D_3$ on the mineralization process is not clear. We observed however that for eliciting this response, it was necessary to maintain supraphysiological circulating levels of $1,25(OH)_2D_3$ (6).

The comparison of the growth process under various treatments in VDRR (see abstract on Growth and Skeletal maturation in treated VDRR by G. Chabot and F.H. Glorieux at this meeting) indicate that normalization of the growthrate is primarily a consequence of phosphate supplementation. The change from vitamin D_2 to $1,25(OH)_2D_3$ had no significant effect. It is northworthy that treatment did not accelerate the bone maturation rate, even when catch-up growth occurred. The overall growth period was therefore not shortened and adolescent growth spurt was of normal magnitude and duration.

In contrast with the very good response of the epiphyseal plate but in keeping with the imperfect correction of the mineralization process at the trabecular bone surface, the frequency of the hypomineralized periosteocytic lesions was decreased by the combined phosphate and $1,25(OH)_2D$ therapy but not fully eliminated. Even after 26 months of therapy, the lesions continued to appear in growing osteons indicating that an abnormal osteocytic function may be part of the VDRR phenotype (4).

When bone lesions are reasonably under control, as indicated by a normal growthrate, normal serum alkaline phosphatase concentrations and radiologic healing of rickets , it may be necessary to decrease the dose of $1,25(OH)_2D_3$ from 1 to 0.5 µg/d. This should be done before occurence of hypercalcemia, as soon as the urinary calcium exceeds the normal limit (calcium/creatinine ratio < 0.3, on a random morning urine sample). As said earlier, lower limb deformities will improve under therapy, sometimes correcting completely without orthopedic intervention. If the deformities are severe enough that joint damage may ensue, corrective osteotomies can be considered during the growing period when the above mentioned control conditions are met. Because of the short half-life of $1,25(OH)_2D_3$ it is not necessary to interrupt treatment prior to surgery. The combined [phosphate + $1,25(OH)_2D_3$] regimen can be maintained all throughout the hospitalization period. It is mandatory to monitor the urinary calcium excretion and if the urinary Ca/cr becomes greater than 0.3, $1,25(OH)_2D_3$ should be stopped for a few days. Phosphate supplements are continued and probably help preventing the hypercalcemic episodes often reported to occur in the post-operative state in VDRR. With close follow-up, through bi-monthly visits, of the serum and urinary calcium and phosphate, this treatment approach is efficient and safe. No change in particular were noted in the creatinine renal clearance rate.

Once epiphyses are closed and growth has ceased, one can rightly question the importance of maintaining such a demanding treatment regimen. With the "old" high vitamin D treatment, it was the rule to stop it at the end of the growth period. We know however that at that time and during subsequent years the osteomalacic process is still active (8) even in the absence of any symptoms. It will probably not be the case in our patients treated with phosphate and $1,25(OH)_2D_3$. Whether this will place them in a better position later in life and prevent symptoms to reappear, remains to be established.

REFERENCES

1. Delvin, E.E. and Glorieux, F.H. (1981): Calcif. Tissue Int., 33, 173.
2. Lyles, K.W. and Drezner, M.K. (1982): J. Clin. Endocrinol. Metab., 54, 638.
3. Glorieux, F.H. and Scriver, C.R. (1972): Science, 175, 997.
4. Marie, P.J. and Glorieux, F.H. (1983): Calcif. Tissue Int., In press.
5. Glorieux, F.H., Scriver, C.R., Reade, T.M., Goldman, H. and Roseborough, A. (1972): N. Engl. J. Med. 287, 481.
6. Glorieux, F.H., Marie, P.J., Pettifor, J.M. and Delvin, E.E. (1980): N. Engl. J. Med., 303, 1023.
7. Chesney, R.W., Mazess, R.B., Rose, P., Hamstra, A.J., DeLuca, H.F. and Breed, A.L. (1983): Pediatrics, 71, 559.
8. Marie, P.J. and Glorieux, F.H. (1982): Metab. Bone Dis. Rel. Res., 4, 249.

HEREDITARY HYPOCALCEMIC VITAMIN D RESISTANT RICKETS (HHDR)

Uri A. Liberman, Charles Eil, and Stephen J. Marx

Metabolic Diseases, Beilinson Medical Center, Tel-Aviv, Israel. Endocrinology Branch, National Naval Medical Center, Bethesda, Md, U.S.A., and Metabolic Diseases Branch, NIADDK, Bethesda, Md, U.S.A.

We define rickets as defective mineralization in preosseous cartilage of growth plates and in the organic matrix of growing bone. Osteomalacia, the adult counterpart of rickets, refers to a similar process in bone matrix during endosteal remodeling. Rickets or osteomalacia represent a stereotypic response of skeletal tissue to a variety of hereditary or acquired disturbances not all of which involve defects in calciferol metabolism.

We define resistance to vitamin D as a state where normal levels of the vitamin are associated with subnormal bioeffect; the bioeffect relevant to this chapter is its calcemic effect. Resistance is a broad term that encompasses deficiencies in sensitivity, and/or responsiveness (Fig. 1). Deficient

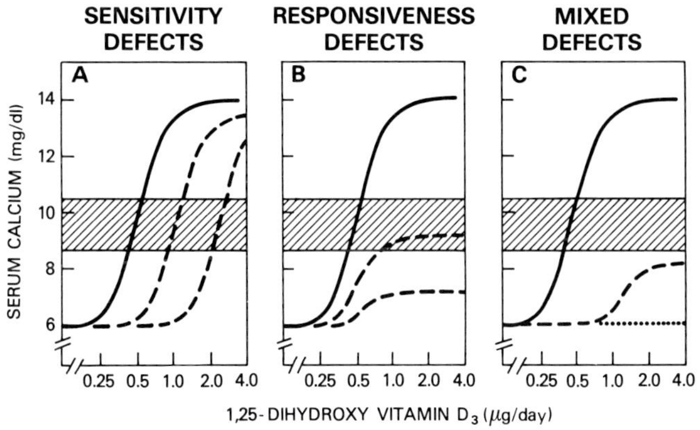

Figure 1. Quantitative and qualitative consequences of resistance (decreased sensitivity, and/or decreased responsiveness) to the calcemic action of $1,25\text{-}(OH)_2D_3$ on a background of vitamin D deficiency and constant calcium intake. Normal response is presented by the solid line in all panels. Panel A: Two grades of decreased sensitivity (dashed lines). Panel B: Two grades of decreased responsiveness (dashed lines). Panel C: Combination of decreased sensitivity and responsiveness (dashed line). Undetectable response (dotted line) (1).

sensitivity is defined as a state where the level of a factor to evoke a half maximal bioeffect is increased. Deficient responsiveness is defined as a state where the maximal bioeffect attainable in normals is not attainable with any level of the factor. We use the term hereditary hypocalcemic vitamin D resistant rickets (HHDR), to describe a primary deficiency in action of vitamin D. As in other hypocalcemic states with normal secretion and action of PTH, secondary hyperparathyroidism with hypophosphatemia develops. The main biochemical differences between hypocalcemic and hypophosphatemic (ex: x-linked hypophosphatemia) rickets are in the serum concentrations of calcium and PTH, both being normal in the latter disturbance.

Vitamin D may be considered as a prohormone whose action requires two distinct processes: hydroxylation to active forms and signalling by active metabolites in target tissues through a steroidal type receptor mechanism. Vitamin D resistance can reflect defects either in biosynthetic transformation (HHDR with low circulating levels of 1,25-$(OH)_2$D) or in target tissue signalling (HHDR with elevated or normal 1,25-$(OH)_2$D concentrations).

HEREDITARY HYPOCALCEMIC VITAMIN D RESISTANT RICKETS TYPE I (HHDR-I)
SYNONYMS: PSEUDOVITAMIN D DEFICIENT RICKETS TYPE I; VITAMIN D DEPENDENT RICKETS TYPE I

HHDR-I describes patients with probable defects in 1-alpha hydroxylation of vitamin D. The clinical and biochemical features of HHDR-I seem to be homogenous among reported cases. Several family studies have revealed a pattern suggestive of autosomal recessive inheritance. Rickets manifests itself before 2 years of age and often during the first year of life. Clinical, radiological, and biochemical features of these patients mimic those in vitamin D deficient rickets but with no direct evidence for nutritional deficiency of vitamin D or any other vitamin. Serum levels of 25-hydroxyvitamin D (25-(OH)D) are normal (or elevated in appropriate proportion to the prior exposure to calciferols). 1,25-dihydroxyvitamin D (1,25-$(OH)_2$D) concentrations in blood are low and remain so even during successful therapy with vitamin D or 25-$(OH)D_3$ (2). Complete remission in patients with HHDR-I can be achieved with high doses of vitamin D preparations lacking a 1-alpha hydroxy configuration or with "physiological" doses of calciferols containing this configuration, i.e., 1,25-$(OH)_2D_3$ or 1-alpha-hydroxy vitamin D_3 (1α-$(OH)D_3$) (Table 1). Due to the basic hereditary defect, remission is dependent on continuous treatment. In HHDR-I, resistance to vitamin D results from impairment in sensitivity without impairment in responsiveness; there is no resistance to 1,25$(OH)_2$D.

TABLE 1. Effective maintenance doses of calciferol analogs in patients with hereditary hypocalcemic vitamin D resistant rickets (HHDR) type I and II.

	Maintenance Dose Of Calciferol Analog			
Disorder	D_2 (μg/day)	25-$(OH)D_3$ (μg/day)	1α-$(OH)D_3$ (μg/day)	1,25-$(OH)_2D_3$ (μg/day)
HHDR I	200-1500	100-400	1-3	0.5-2.0
HHDR II*	1000-150,000	500-5000	10-100	8-50

*Some patients are resistant even to doses higher than these.

HEREDITARY HYPOCALCEMIC VITAMIN D RESISTANT RICKETS TYPE II (HHDR-II).
SYNONYMS: PSEUDOVITAMIN D DEFICIENT RICKETS TYPE II; VITAMIN D DEPENDENT RICKETS TYPE II.

HHDR-II describes a small number of patients with resistance to 1,25-$(OH)_2$D. These patients do not respond to physiological doses of bioactive calciferol analogs, and serum levels of 1,25-$(OH)_2$D are high before and/or during treatment with high doses of calciferol analogs. There are only about 13 kindreds or patients with HHDR-II in the literature (1). The syndrome seems to be hetrogeneous in its clinical and biochemical presentation (Table 2). The unique features in some of these subgroups are reviewed below.

TABLE 2. Clinical and biochemical features of hereditary hypocalcemic vitamin D resistant rickets type II.

Number of Kindreds	Ectodermal Anomalies	Age of Onset	Remission on High Calciferols	Serum Concentration Phosphate	Serum Concentration $24,25-(OH)_2D$
3	No	Late	Yes	Low	NL
2	No	Early	Yes	Low	NL
3	Yes	Early	Yes	Low	NL
4	Yes	Early	No	Low	NL
1	Yes	Early	No*	High	Low

NL - normal; *No response to vitamin D or 1-alpha hydroxylated calciferol metabolites but normocalcemia achieved on $24,25-(OH)_2D_3$ treatment (3).

Late onset of metabolic bone disease with no ectodermal anomalies was reported in three sporadic cases, two with onset of osteomalacia after 10 years of age, and one with onset in adulthood. Complete remission in these patients was achieved with moderate to high doses of bioactive calciferol analogs.

Early onset rickets with no ectodermal anomalies is typified by a brother and sister who presented with hypocalcemic rickets prior to 2 years of age (4). Both exhibited clinical and biochemical remission with large doses of calciferol analogs during a follow-up of more than 10 years. One additional patient with similar features has been reported.

Early onset of hypocalcemic rickets and total alopecia has been reported in at least 7 kindreds. In all patients, rickets was recognizable prior to 2 years of age and alopecia was present prior to age 1 (5). In most of these reports, parental consanguinity and additional affected siblings were noted as well. In 3 kindreds, remission of hypocalcemia and rickets was achieved with high doses of calciferol analogs (Table 2). In 2 patients treated with high doses of vitamin D, 25-(OH)D, $1\alpha-(OH)D_3$ and $1,25-(OH)_2D$ (up to 50-100 times the mean normal levels), no calcemic response was detected. Two additional cases were not responsive to calciferol analogs, but neither received high enough doses and for sufficient periods of time to confirm this.

Early onset of hypocalcemic rickets, hyperphosphatemia, total alopecia and oligodentia was described in one affected member of a kindred (3). Serum levels of $24,25-(OH)_2D$ were below the lower limit of the assay (less than 0.39 ng/ml versus normal 1.5-2.5). On a short course of $24,25-(OH)_2D_3$, hypocalcemia and hyperphosphatemia improved for approximately 3 years; $1,25-(OH)_2D$ levels remained elevated but to a lesser degree.

CELLULAR BASIS FOR HHDR-II

Fibroblasts cultured from normal human skin exhibit high affinity nuclear uptake of $1,25-(OH)_2D_3$ with affinity, capacity and specificity suggestive of mediation by receptors; soluble extracts (cytosol) from these cells demonstrate binding of $1,25-(OH)_2D_3$ with analogous receptor-like properties (5). Evaluations of cultured skin fibroblasts from affected members of 9 kindreds with early onset HHDR-II have been reported. Table 3 summarizes the results of such studies carried by us in members of 6 kindreds (5). Four distinct patterns have been observed *in vitro*: I) Normal capacity and affinity of cytosol binding but unmeasurable whole cell nuclear uptake (kindred A and B, Table 3); II) Whole cell nuclear uptake and cytosol binding-unmeasurable (kindreds C and D in Table 3); III) Decreased capacity and normal affinity of both parameters (kindred E Table 3); IV) Normal capacity and affinity of both measurements (kindred F, Table 3). Pattern III (receptors that are qualitatively normal but quantitatively deficient) may cause impairment in maximal calcemic effect of 1,25$(OH)_2$D (6), (i.e., deficient responsiveness) while pattern I typically is associated with deficient sensitivity to 1,25$(OH)_2$D (4). The recent observations of a biochemical response in cultured fibroblasts to the addition in vitro of 1,25-$(OH)_2D_3$ (stimulation of 25-hydroxyvitamin D 24-hydroxylase activity and inhibition of cell growth) may allow development of in vitro methods for predicting more details of potential for response to calciferol treatment in vivo.

TABLE 3. 1,25-$(OH)_2D_3$ interaction in vitro and in vivo in six kindreds with hereditary hypocalcemic vitamin D resistant rickets type II.

Kindred	1,25-$(OH)_2D_3$ Receptor Analysis in Cultured Cells		Remission of Hypocalcemia on High Doses of Calciferol Analogs
	Cytosol Binding	Nuclear Uptake	
A	Normal	UD*	Yes
B	Normal	UD	Yes
C	UD	UD	Yes
D	UD	UD	No
E	10% capacity	10% capacity	No
F	Normal	Normal	No

*UD - undetectable

THERAPY FOR HHDR-II

A therapeutic trial with doses of calciferol analogs (Table 1) sufficient to maintain serum 1,25-$(OH)_2$D levels 50-100 times the mean normal concentration for several months is essential before deciding if a calciferol lacks detectable bioeffect in vivo. In patients in whom no remission on calciferol is achieved, supplementation with high doses of elemental calcium (2-4 gm/day) could theoretically improve serum calcium and bone mineralization (3). Calcium supplementation could raise serum phosphorus by suppressing secondary hyperparathyroidism. Efforts to treat the hypophosphatemia directly with phosphorous supplements might exacerbate secondary hyperparathyroidism.

REFERENCES

1. Marx, S.J. (1983): In: Vitamin D Metabolism: Basic and Clinical Aspects. Editor: R. Kumar. Martinus Nijhof, Boston. In Press.
2. Scriver, C.R., Reade, T.M., DeLuca, W.F., and Hamstra, A.J. (1978): N. Engl. J. Med. 299, 976.
3. Liberman, U.A., Samuel, R., Halabe, A., et al. (1980). Lancet. 1, 504.
4. Marx, S.J., Spiegel, A.M., Brown, E.M., et al. (1978): J. Clin. Endocrinol. Metab. 47, 1303.
5. Liberman, U.A., Eil, C., and Marx, S.J. (1983): J. Clin. Invest. 71, 192.
6. Liberman, U.A., Balsan, S., Marx, S.J. (1982): Abstracts of 64th Annual Meeting of Endocrine Society, p. 214.

Discussion following papers by Dr. Liberman and Dr. Glorieux

D. SHERRARD: Dr. Liberman, I am interested in the patients who responded to 24,25$(OH)_2D$. Did you look at the bone histology pre and post treatment, and did you look at the 1,25$(OH)_2D$ receptors when you gave the 24,25$(OH)_2D$?

U. LIBERMAN: We don't have bone histology. I didn't give the entire history of the patient. The patient "cured" her rickets without any vitamin D treatment. We believe this happened because of the hyperphosphatemia, though she was still hypocalcemic. She is one of the patients that had a normal cytosol receptor and a normal nuclear uptake of 1,25$(OH)_2D$.

F. GLORIEUX: I was able to look at the bone histology in one of these patients. The bone was sent to us by Dr. Korkor. It showed osteomalacia with high bone turnover and increased resorption as observed in vitamin D dependency type I.

R. JOSSE: What is the explanation for the weakness that occurs in the vitamin D dependent rickets as opposed to the robust infants with equivalent rickets of the hypophosphatemic vitamin D resistant variety?

F. GLORIEUX: I think this is related to the 1,25$(OH)_2D$ deficiency. Work done in St. Louis has shown that vitamin D metabolites are important for normal muscle function. It is striking that after initiation of 1,25$(OH)_2D$, muscle weakness disappears in the vitamin D dependent patients. I think this is one more argument against a state of 1,25$(OH)_2D$ deficiency in the x-linked hypophosphatemic form of rickets.

K. LYLES: For a number of years, I have worked with Drezner in Durham and observed that VDRR patients improve their TMP/GFR with treatment on phosphate and 1,25$(OH)_2D$. They normalize it and they also heal their bones, which you have also shown. Our patients were adolescents, ages 13 and 16, and then adults, while you were taking care of young children. Have you seen any adolescent or young adults with improvement in TMP/GFR after treatment? I think in our older patients we can normalize the TMP/GFR. What has been your experience?

F. GLORIEUX: Over the years, we have not seen any of our older patients show an improvement in the TMP/GFR after treatment. We measure the TMP/GFR in the morning after the phosphate load has been stopped for at least 12 hours to make sure that there is no interference with whatever phosphate might have accumulated in the bladder. The difference may be in methodology. It may also be a question of the dose of 1,25$(OH)_2D$ since we use lower doses than you. I have discussed this issue with you a number of times in an attempt to reconcile our data without success.

R. SCHILLING: Dr. Glorieux, have you ever seen any adverse effects from supraphysiologic 1,25$(OH)_2D$ levels that relate to bone histology? Also, tell us how long you treat your patients?

F. GLORIEUX: With regard to the first question, I think that if there is an adequate balance between the dose of 1,25$(OH)_2D$, which in our hands is about 1 microgram per day, and that of phosphate, we do not see any increased bone resorption from secondary hyperparathyroidism. This is in contrast to our past experience when we saw secondary hyperparathyroidism induced by treatment with phosphate and vitamin D. With regard to the length of therapy, I don't think there is a clear answer. There is no question that we should continue treating until the epiphysis are fused. What should be done afterwards is a question that some of the patients will answer for you. They will stop treatment altogether. In those who will accept continuing treatment and have been treated satisfactorily, I would be tempted to continue therapy.

F. LAFFERTY: Dr. Glorieux, is it possible that your superior results with 1,25$(OH)_2D$ simply reflect the fact that you are pushing the serum calcium and phosphorus to a higher level than you did with ordinary vitamin D?

F. GLORIEUX: Yes, that is one explanation. Although the level that we have achieved when we do titration curves are not much different from one metabolite to another. In fact, we reduce the amount of phosphate we give compared to what we used to give in combination with ordinary vitamin D. This is of benefit to the patient because the intestinal tract does not tolerate a heavy load of phosphate.

R. CHESNEY: We found absolutely no difference in serum phosphorus switching from vitamin D to 1,25(OH)$_2$D. I had a question for Dr. Liberman. Were the patients with alopecia - consanguinous?

U. LIBERMAN: Yes, all the patients with alopecia were consanguinous.

S. POSEN: Dr. Glorieux, would you make some brief comment concerning the gastrointestinal handling of phosphate in hypophosphatemic rickets.

F. GLORIEUX: There has been some controversy about the presence of a decreased intestinal phosphate abosrption. We never found this to be very impressive with loading tests. We did some experiments using jejunal biopsies taken from these patients and then looked at the uptake of radiophosphorus. We could not differentiate the patients from our controls. What is certain is that the intestine will react very postively to the 1,25(OH)$_2$D with an increase in phosphate absorption.

S. AHMED: How old was the patient with total alopecia when you first saw her and how long did you treat her?

U. LIBERMAN: Alopecia usually appears during the first year of life. We try to treat them as soon as possible, as the disease may be fatal. In one of our kindreds four out of eight siblings had the disease. Three died during early childhood. Only after the condition was recognized, high doses of 1,25 (OH)$_2$D were employed and the patient is doing fine. Not all of them responded, however.

A. KORKOR: I would like to make a comment regarding alopecia. The patient that I have with the syndrome had a biopsy of her scalp. On study under electronmicroscopy, there was absolutely no evidence of hair formation. That seems interesting because we can see 1,25(OH)$_2$D receptors in fibroblasts which are precursors of cells that make hair. One wonders whether 1,25(OH)$_2$D receptors and 1,25(OH)$_2$D response is essential during early childhood for the differentiation of the cells that are responsible for making hair.

U. LIBERMAN: This is of course one of the possibilites. In autoradiographic studies 1,25(OH)$_2$D is concentrated in the hair follicles. In most children with the disorder, some hair exists at birth, but it is lost during the first few months of life.

XVII PSEUDOHYPOPARATHYROIDISM (PHP) AND RELATED DISORDERS

PSEUDOHYPOPARATHYROIDISM: AN OVERVIEW

G. D. Aurbach

Metabolic Diseases Branch, NIADDK, NIH, Bethesda, Md. 20205, USA.

In 1942, Albright and his associates (1)described for the first time a syndrome of true hormone resistance which they called pseudohypoparathyroidism or Sebright Bantam syndrome*. The classical syndrome of pseudohypoparathyroidism type I encompasses not only clinical hypoparathyroidism with hypocalcemia and hyperphosphatemia but also certain associated constitutional features including short stature, round facies, obesity, tendency to mental retardation, shortening of the metacarpal and metatarsal bones and subcutaneous calcifications. The associated constitutional features have also been designated Albright's hereditary osteodystrophy (AHO). The original authors found that the subjects were resistant to exogenous parathyroid hormone when tested by the phosphaturic response. This test has been replaced by determining the urinary cyclic AMP response to exogenous parathyroid hormone. The latter test segregates, in a much more efficient manner, subjects with classical pseudohypoparathyroidism from normal subjects and from those with other forms of hypoparathyroidism. Albright and his associates, and many others through the years since their original report, proposed a number of hypotheses in efforts to explain the biochemical abnormality and mode of inheritance of pseudohypoparathyroidism. Among the hypotheses considered by Albright were end organ resistance to normally secreted parathyroid hormone, antibodies to parathyroid hormone, and secretion by parathyroid glands of an abnormal peptide capable of blocking the actions of parathyroid hormone.

The findings of Chase et al (2) of defective production of cyclic AMP in response to PTH redirected attention to the concept of end organ resistance and led to the hypothesis that pseudohypoparathyroidism represented a defect in the parathyroid hormone receptor - adenylate cyclase system accounting for end organ resistance. Subsequent investigations have led to the discovery that the cell membrane content of the guanyl nucleotide regulatory protein (G-unit, which couples receptor activity to adenylate cyclase activity) is deficient in most cases of classical pseudohypoparathyroidism with AHO (3,4). Many of the other hypotheses, including antibody to hormone, have been excluded but recently the concept of an endogenous inhibitor, presumably an abnormal hormone secreted by the parathyroid gland capable of blocking receptors, has once again come under consideration. Dr. Fisher (6 and this volume) presents data that he has obtained with Dr. Chayen indicating that in pseudohypoparathyroidism there is an abnormally high ratio of radioimmunoassayable parathyroid hormone relative to bioassayable parathyroid

---

* After the Sebright Bantam cock which he thought was resistant to androgens. Recently, it has been proved that the female tail-feathering pattern in this variant is not due to resistance to androgens, but rather to an abnormally increased rate of conversion of androgens to estrogens by the skin of these birds (5).

hormone in the plasma of patients with pseudohypoparathyroidism. Moreover, they have found evidence for inhibitory activity in the plasma of patients with pseudohypoparathyroidism (7). This they have determined by adding parathyroid hormone to plasma and carrying out bioassays utilizing the *in vitro* cytochemical bioassay (CBA) for parathyroid hormone developed by the Chayen group (8). Nevertheless considerable amounts of bioactive parathyroid hormone have been detected by two groups, Fisher et al and O'Riordan et al (both reporting in this volume) applying the CBA assay in pseudohypoparathyroidism and the amounts found overlap the normal and hyperparathyroid ranges.

Another point to consider in pseudohypoparathyroidism is that in any condition of excess hormone secretion (primary or secondary hyperparathyroidism) there is development of resistance by the kidney to the effects of parathyroid hormone. This effect, discussed by Dr. O'Riordan, might be attributable to "down regulation" of parathyroid hormone receptors induced by high concentrations of circulating hormone. One could postulate that part of the hormone resistance in pseudohypoparathyroidism is due to this down regulation phenomenon. On the other hand, against this concept is that subjects with pseudohypoparathyroidism adequately treated with vitamin D or infused with calcium (to suppress PTH secretion) continue to express the resistance to exogenous parathyroid hormone as determined by urinary cyclic AMP excretion (2). Moreover, one totally parathyroidectomized patient with the disorder persistently displays the urinary cAMP response defect (2). Patients with hormone resistance in vitamin D deficiency show a correction of this defect after treatment (O'Riordan et al, this volume).

Genetics of Pseudohypoparathyroidism

It has, in the past, been considered that pseudohypoparathyroidism represents a sex-linked disorder in that there are few documented cases of male to male transmission, that the female:male sex ratio in the disorder is approximately 2:1, and that pedigrees of families reported appear compatible with the sex-linked transmission mode. On the other hand, a few families do not fit this pattern; some pedigrees seem compatible with autosomal dominant inheritance, others with autosomal recessive transmission (Drs. Van Dop and Bourne). Part of the confusion concerning heredity in this disorder is due to: 1) too few families with multiple affected members to allow conclusive analysis of inheritance patterns; 2) utilization by different investigators of differing perameters to examine patterns of heredity. Parameters evaluated vary from phosphaturia, physiognomy, blood calcium analyses, urinary cyclic AMP responses, and assays for guanylnucleotide (G-unit) regulatory component. 3)errors in measured parameters have not uniformly been analyzed statistically. One may arrive at a different conclusion concerning genetics using the urinary cyclic AMP response on the one hand vs. G-unit analyses on the other. Utilizing G-unit analyses, Van Dop and Bourne (this volume) find evidence that some families with the disorder may represent recessive or dominant autosomal patterns of inheritance. They readily admit, however, that pedigree analyses reported so far, do not rule out x-linked inheritance. Since the G-unit is composed of two subunits there is the possibility that the gene controlling one subunit is on the sex chromosome and the other subunit could be represented on an autosomal chromosome. Such a mechanism might account for apparent diversity in inheritance. Other possible mechanisms are presented below. Another puzzling feature of the inheritance pattern in pseudohypoparathyroidism is the fact that deficiency of the G-unit averages approximately 50% and never approaches, as found in the cyc^- lymphoma cell mutant, total deficiency, which in the human organism might be incompatible with life.

What can one surmise about the biochemical nature of the disorder--deficiency of G-unit or production of abnormal form of hormone? It is difficult to postulate two distinct genetic defects to account for the same abnormality in any given subject. Moreover, production of a defective hormone seems unlikely to account for the generalized defect in hormone responsiveness described by Levine et al (this volume). Perhaps deficiency of the G-unit, a protein controlling adenylate cyclase in all tissues, can also influence the nature of the product secreted by the parathyroid cell, a process also regulated in part by cyclic AMP. Goltzman (9) has recently described phosphorylated forms of parathyroid hormone. Phospho-proteins are regulated by protein kinases, some of which also are controlled by cyclic AMP. If there be an abnormal distribution of phospho-forms elaborated in pseudohypoparathyroidism due to diminished production of cyclic AMP in the parathyroid cell, one might be able to explain a link between G-unit deficiency and production of parathyroid hormone forms with varying immuno- to bio-activity. Since cyclic AMP has been implicated in control of chondrocyte function (10), it is also possible that brachydactyly in pseudohypoparathyroidism is another consequence of deficiency of the G-unit in the adenylate cyclase complex.

Classically, autosomal dominant gene defects produce in heterozygotes, 50% reductions in enzyme activity since loss of one of a gene pair yields one-half of the normal complement of protein. Fifty percent loss of function in genes carried on the X chromosome might occur in females due to mosaicism, but in affected males the loss of function would be total. This is one of the problems that make the postulate of sex-linkage in pseudohypoparathyroidism difficult: how would one explain thereby male subjects showing 50% of normal complement of the G-unit? Lessons learned in the study of thalassemia may be instructive. In certain forms of $beta^+$ thalassemia (11) the genomic information is normal, but a mutation in an intron causes a splicing defect with consequent abnormal processing of pre-mRNA. The net result is production of significant, but reduced amounts of normal beta hemoglobin chains. Such a splicing defect in biosynthesis of G-unit mRNA in pseudohypoparathyroidism, if localized on the X chromosome, could account for 50% or greater reduction in complement of the protein and be compatible with sex-linked inheritance. Studies in thalassemia (11) are further instructive in proving that similar phenotypic expressions of disease can be caused by many different types of mutations in the genes responsible for hemoglobin synthesis. Like the G-unit, hemoglobin is composed of two different, alpha and beta, protein subunits. Different genes control, normally, synthesis of each subunit (there are still other genes controlling synthesis of gamma and delta chains which normally do not operate post-natally). Mutations in either of the genes for alpha or beta chains can cause thalassemia, which can vary in severity from no discernible clinical effect to life-impairing disease. Moreover, compensatory synthesis of fetal hemoglobins, not normally synthesized in the adult, can occur yielding partially effective proteins. Perhaps in pseudohypoparathyroidism there will be discovered a similarly rermarkable diversity of genetic defects accounting for phenotypic expression of the disorder which also seems to vary in severity.

Currently, the best single unifying hypothesis to account for the genetic defect of pseudohypoparathyroidism with AHO is a deficiency of production of the G-unit. One must recognize moreover that there may well be more than one type of inheritance pattern and gene defect accounting for the phenotype of this syndrome. Ultimate resolution of these problems depend upon structural determination of the G-unit protein and/or application of recombinant DNA technology to elucidate the defect at the polynucleotide level.

REFERENCES

1. Albright, F., Burnett, C.H., Smith, P.H. and Parson, W. (1942): Endocrinology 30, 922.
2. Chase, L.R., Melson, G.L. and Aurbach, G.D. (1969): J. Clin. Invest., 48,1822.
3. Levine, M.A., Downs, R.W., Jr., Singer, M.J., Marx, S.J., Aurbach, G.D. and Spiegel, A.M. (1980): Biochem. Biophys. Res. Commun., 94:1319.
4. Farfel, Z., Brickman, A.S., Kaslow, H.R., Brothers, V.M. and Bourne, H.R. (1980): N. Engl. J. Med., 303:237.
5. George, F.W., Noble, J.F. and Wilson, J.D. (1981): Science, 213,557.
6. Nagant de Deuxchaisnes, C., Fischer, J.A., Dambacher, M.A., Devogelaer, J.-P., Arber, C.E., Zanelli, J.M., Parsons, J.A., Loveridge, N., Bitensky, L. and Chayen, J. (1981): J Clin. Endocrinol. Metab., 53,1105.
7. Loveridge, N., Fischer, J.A., Nagant de Deuxchaisnes, C., Dambacher, M.A., Tschopp, F., Werder, W., Devogelaer, J.-P. De Meyer, R., Bitensky, L., and Chayen, J. (1982): J.Clin. Endocrinol. Metab., 54, 1274.
8. Chambers, D.J., Dunham, J., Zanelli, J.M., Parsons, J.A., Bitensky, L. and Chayen, J. (1978): Clin. Endocrinol 9,375.
9. Goltzman, D., Rabbani, S., Kremer, R. and Bennett, H.P.J. (1983): Program of the Fifth Annual Meeting, Am. Soc. Bone and Mineral Res. A34.
10. Burch, W.M. and Lebovitz, H.B. (1981): J. Clin. Invest. 68,1496.
11. Kan, Y.W. (1983): In: The Metabolic Basis of Inherited Disease, p. 1711. Editors: J.B. Stanbury, J.B. Wyngaarden, D.S. Fredrickson, J.L.

MOLECULAR BASIS OF PSEUDOHYPOPARATHYROIDISM

Cornelis Van Dop and Henry R. Bourne

Departments of Pharmacology, Medicine, Pediatrics and Cardiovascular Research Institute, University of California, San Francisco, CA 94143 U.S.A.

Despite impressive recent progress toward understanding the molecular defects leading to pseudohypoparathyroidism (PHP), major gaps remain. We shall outline advances that led to present concepts regarding the pathogenesis of PHP, and then address possible molecular defects that could underlie the PHP phenotype.

N-PROTEIN

Hormone-sensitive adenylate cyclase consists of three separate protein components: Specific hormone receptor (R), GTP-binding coupling protein (N[1]), and catalytic adenylate cyclase (C). When hormone (H) binds to its specific receptor, the HR complex interacts with N to effect exchange of GTP for bound GDP. The activated N-GTP complex then stimulates C. C activity "turns off" when the N protein's GTPase activity hydrolyzes the bound GTP to GDP (for references see (1)).

Discovery of N resulted from studies of a mutant cell, designated <u>cyc</u>$^-$, which was derived from a S49 mouse lymphoma cell line. <u>Cyc</u>$^-$ cells and membranes, unlike normal (<u>cyc</u>$^+$) cells and membranes, cannot make cyclic AMP (cAMP) in response to stimulation by β-adrenergic agents, choleragen or fluoride ion. However, Ross and Gilman (2) showed that detergent extracts of <u>cyc</u>$^+$ membranes can correct or complement the biochemical defect of <u>cyc</u>$^-$ membranes and restore hormone sensitivity to the adenylate cyclase. This in vitro complementation assay led to discovery of the N protein and allowed its characterization and purification. Plasma membranes from most vertebrate cells contain an N protein activity that can complement the defect of mouse <u>cyc</u>$^-$ membranes in vitro.

N is an intrinsic membrane protein consisting of two dissimilar subunits, designated alpha (42,000 or 52,000 MW) and beta (35,000 MW). The alpha subunit (N_α) contains both the GTP-binding site and (probably) the GTPase enzymatic activity, interacts with fluoride ion to allow activation of adenylate cyclase, and is ADP-ribosylated by choleragen with resulting inhibition of GTPase activity. Hormone receptor-induced exchange of GTP for GDP bound to N dissociates the alpha and beta subunits and the N_α-GTP complex then activates C. <u>Cyc</u>$^-$ cells lack a functional alpha subunit; thus the complementation assay measures detergent-extractable N_α bioactivity.

[1]Also designated G or G/F.

Human erythrocytes lack C, but contain functional N. Because the amount of N activity decreases with erythrocyte ageing, the interpretation of erythrocyte N activity measurements can be misleading in some hematologic conditions.

PHP-I AND N PROTEIN

In 1942 Albright described PHP as a syndrome of resistance to parathormone (PTH) with a characteristic associated morphologic phenotype (for references see (3)). The next major advance toward biochemical understanding of the disorder was the demonstration (4) that exogenous PTH did not raise urinary excretion of cAMP in PHP patients, in contrast to normal and hypoparathyroid subjects. The subsequent finding (5) that a synthetic cAMP analog increases urinary phosphate excretion and raises serum calcium in PHP patients, as in normal subjects, indicated that the PHP defect is not due to resistance to cAMP but rather involves inadequate stimulation of cAMP synthesis by PTH. These patients are now classified as Type I because several "PHP, Type II" patients have been described in whom PTH does not effect phosphaturia while urinary cAMP excretion is normal or elevated.

Subsequently, several reports indicated that many PHP-I patients showed resistance (usually subclinical) to several other peptide hormones--including thyrotropin, vasopressin, glucagon, and gonadotropins. These endocrine abnormalities do not result from hypocalcemia or reduced PTH effect, since correction of hypocalcemia does not correct them. There is considerable evidence that cAMP is the intracellular second messenger for these hormones and PTH. Thus each of the multiple endocrine abnormalities seen in PHP-I, including hypocalcemia, can be indirectly attributed to deficient cAMP synthesis. Because these hormones act via unique receptors, PHP must involve a defect in a cellular component at a site distal to hormone receptor.

Drezner and Burch (6) demonstrated that PTH-sensitive adenylate cyclase in the renal biopsy from a patient with PHP required additional GTP for maximal activation. This suggested that the PHP defect might involve the N protein. Two laboratories then showed (7,8) that erythrocytes from most PHP-I patients had only 50% of the N protein activity found in erythrocytes of normal subjects. Later studies in our laboratory demonstrated deficient N protein activity in platelets, cultured fibroblasts, and virus-transformed lymphoblasts from these same PHP-I patients. This persistence of decreased N protein activity in cells cultured in vitro indicates that decreased N protein activity is encoded in the genome of individual cells and is not due to the abnormal hormonal milieu or metabolic imbalance of PHP-I patients. Reduced N protein has recently also been demonstrated (9) in kidney biopsy material of the PHP-I patient previously described by Drezner and Burch (6).

Erythrocytes from some PHP-I patients contain normal N protein activity. These patients are now classified as PHP-Ib, to distinguish them from PHP-Ia patients in whom N protein activity is reduced. PHP-Ib clearly differs from PHP-Ia. The molecular defect in PHP-Ib remains undefined and the disorder is probably heterogeneous.

INHERITANCE PATTERNS

Before N protein assays were available to differentiate PHP-Ia from PHP-Ib, an X-linked dominant mode of inheritance was postulated for PHP. This was based on the female predominance (~2:1) and the lack of documented male-to-male transmission of the disease in affected pedigrees. The wide range of clinical severity seen in affected patients and the lack of a reliable biochemical marker for the disease left some doubt regarding these conclusions. Using N protein deficiency as a marker for PHP-Ia, we found families with recessive and dominant patterns of inheritance (10). Although pedigrees analyzed thus far do not rule out X-linked inheritance, we think that autosomal dominant inheritance is most likely.

MOLECULAR PATHOPHYSIOLOGY OF PHP-Ia

There is substantial evidence that N_α exists as several distinct forms in hormone-responsive cells. Thus, single cells can contain N_α polypeptides with varying molecular weight and charge, and changes in N activity occur in association with heterologous desensitization of adenylate cyclase.

Johnson et al. (11) found that choleragen catalyzed [^{32}P]-ADP-ribosylation of two proteins (42,000 and 52,000 MW) in S49 mouse lymphoma cells. Subsequently, these two forms of N_α have been found in varying proportions in different tissues and copurified in preparations of N isolated from rabbit liver (1). Proteolytic digestion maps of these two forms are nearly identical (12). Furthermore, N_α mutations in S49 mouse lymphoma cells that affect pI or abundance of the protein alter both the 52,000 and 42,000 MW forms. Thus, one gene probably codes for the two forms of N_α. The two forms probably result either from post-transcriptional modification (resulting in deletion of an intron during mRNA processing), or from post-translational modification of the protein. Gilman et al. (1), comparing the two isolated molecular forms of N_α in reconstitution experiments using <u>cyc</u>$^-$ membranes, found only minor functional differences. Despite these findings, it is possible that the two forms perform unique coupling functions in native membranes.

In addition, two-dimensional gel electrophoresis of choleragen-treated N_α from wild type S49 lymphoma cells has demonstrated several forms with different isoelectric points but the same molecular weights. Our studies of retinal transducin, a protein from the retina which is homologous to N, showed that choleragen specifically attaches only one ADP-ribose at a unique site on the protein. Thus, if the N protein is also ADP-ribosylated at only one site, the multiple forms with different isoelectric points probably result from a post-translational modification of N_α.

Finally, heterologous desensitization of adenylate cyclase in fibroblasts by prostaglandin E_1 results from an uncharacterized alteration of N which reduces the coupling efficiency of N to C (13). In this case the desensitization-induced reduction of N activity in the cyc$^-$ complementation was not associated with changes in choleragen-catalyzed ADP-ribosylation of N_α (13). Heterologous desensitization in rat liver, however, did decrease choleragen-catalyzed radiolabeling.[2]

In summary, several lines of evidence suggest that post-translational modifications of N protein occur, but the nature of these changes and their effects on hormone receptor-adenylate cyclase coupling are not well-characterized. Aberrations in one or more of these pathways could lead to the PHP phenotype by reducing N activity.

The S49 mouse lymphoma cell line, which dies upon exposure to cAMP and hormones that stimulate cAMP synthesis, has been useful for characterizing normal N protein function by providing clonal populations of mutant cells resistant to these hormonal effects. $\overline{\text{Cyc}^-}$, the mutant described above, completely lacks N activity. Several other mutants with structurally and functionally altered N_α have been characterized (for references see (15)). One of these, H21a, interacts normally with HR complex, as demonstrated by an N-induced decrease in affinity of R for H. However, the N protein in H21a membranes is incapable of stimulating adenylate cyclase with fluoride or guanine nucleotides. A second mutant, unc, contains a mutant N protein which activates C in the presence of fluoride or guanosine triphosphates but cannot alter the affinity of R for H or interact with the HR complex to effect exchange of GTP for bound GDP. In addition, two-dimensional gel electrophoresis of the ADP-ribosylated N_α from unc demonstrates a change in its isoelectric point without a change in molecular weight. Other mutants exhibit partially reduced N protein activity, as measured by hormone stimulation of adenylate cyclase in membranes, complementation of cyc⁻ membranes, and choleragen-catalyzed ADP-ribosylation. Similar mutations of the human N_α protein could result in the PHP-I phenotype.

In conclusion, the demonstrated decrease in N protein activity in cells from PHP-Ia patients can account for their resistance to the effects of multiple hormones that act via cAMP. Several different molecular defects could result in this decreased N activity. At present, further studies of PHP are hampered by the low cellular concentrations of N. To characterize more fully the N protein defect in PHP-Ia, it will be necessary to devise both immunologic assays for N protein that do not depend on its biologic activity, and recombinant DNA techniques for isolating and characterizing the N_α structural gene and its expression.

Finally, although not discussed here, PHP-Ib probably represents a group of disorders which may affect several gene products, including N protein, cyclic nucleotide phosphodiesterases or anion membrane transport proteins.

REFERENCES

1. Gilman, A.G., Sternweis, P.C., Northup, J.K., Hanski, E., Smigel, M.D. and Kahn, R.A. (1982): Adv. Pharmacol. Therapeut., 4, 79.
2. Ross, E.M. and Gilman, A.G. (1977): Proc. Natl. Acad. Sci. (U.S.A.), 74, 3715.
3. Van Dop, C. and Bourne, H.R. (1983): Ann. Rev. Med., 34, 259.
4. Chase, L.R., Melson, G.L. and Aurbach, G.D. (1969): J. Clin.

[2] R.P. Robertson, personal communication.

Invest., 48, 1832.
5. Bell, N.H., Avery, S., Sinha, T., Clark, C.M., Jr., Allen, D.O. and Johnson, C., Jr. (1972): J. Clin. Invest., 51, 816.
6. Drezner, M.K. and Burch, W.M., Jr. (1978) J. Clin. Invest., 62, 1222.
7. Farfel, Z., Brickman, A.S., Kaslow, H.R., Brothers, V.M. and Bourne, H.R. (1980) New Engl. J. Med., 303, 237.
8. Levine, M.A., Downs, R.W., Jr., Singer, M., Marx, S.J., Aurbach, G.D. and Spiegel, A.M. (1980) Biochem. Biophys. Res. Commun., 94, 1319.
9. Downs, R.W., Jr., Levine, M.A., Drezner, M.K., Burch, W.M., Jr. and Spiegel, A.M. (1983): J. Clin. Invest., 71, 231.
10. Farfel, Z., Brothers, V.M., Brickman, A.S., Conte, F., Neer, R. and Bourne, H.R. (1981): Proc. Natl. Acad. Sci. (U.S.A.), 78, 3098.
11. Johnson, G.L., Kaslow, H.R. and Bourne, H.R. (1978): J. Biol. Chem., 253, 7120.
12. Hudson, T.H. and Johnson, G.L. (1980): J. Biol. Chem., 255, 7480.
13. Kassis, S. and Fishman, P.H. (1982): J. Biol. Chem., 257, 5312.
14. Farfel, Z., Salomon, M.R. and Bourne, H.R. (1981): Ann. Rev. Pharmacol. Toxicol., 21, 251.

Discussion following paper by C. Van Dop

J. POTTS: Can you use any of the assays such as the CYC-complementation or the ADP-ribosylation assay to support your thought that in the one case, the dominant form, there is a reduced amount of protein and in the other there might be a translational defect causing the functional differences?

C. VAN DOP: Well, the major problem relates to the complementation assay which is not very sensitive so that we have not been able to obtain adequate kinetic data on adenylate cyclase upon addition of detergent extracts to the membranes.

Secondly, in the model of protein deficiency in the S-49 lymphoma cells it has been documented that there are protein abnormalities that result in altered isoelectric points, but we've not been able to find this in patients with pseudohypoparathyroidism.

R. NEER: Is it possible to evaluate the presence of the N inhibitory protein in patients with pseudohypoparathyroidism type 1-B?

C. VAN DOP: You mean the inhibitory N?

R. NEER: Yes.

C. VAN DOP: We have not measured those yet, mainly because there is not a facile assay available for measuring that inhibitory N (which is different from the stimulatory N protein which I am discussing). We will be studying that, but as of now, I do not have any data.

G. AURBACH: Dr. Van Dop, you mentioned that the G unit is composed of at least two separate protein subunits. Could this conceivably allow for genetic abnormalities in more than one gene that could have something to do with influencing G unit concentration?

For example, if there were subnormal amounts of the 35-K subunits, could that possibly influence the final result in complementation assays?

C. VAN DOP: It could, however, on the basis of Gilman's studies with the 35-K or beta subunits, when increased it seems to inhibit adenylate cyclase activation whereas deficiencies of that protein in contrast would be expected to increase the sensitivity of the cyclase system to stimulatory hormones. He has done these experiments by isolating the alpha and beta subunits and then re-adding each to a defined system.

PARATHYROID HORMONE BIOACTIVITY IN FAMILIAL PSEUDOHYPOPARATHYROIDISM TYPE I

J.A. Fischer, C. Nagant de Deuxchaisnes, N. Loveridge, M.A. Dambacher, F. Tschopp, E. Werder, L. Bitensky and J. Chayen

Research Laboratory for Calcium Metabolism, Departments of Orthopedic Surgery and Medicine, and Pediatrics, University of Zurich, Zurich, Switzerland; Department of Rheumatology, St. Luc Hospital, Louvain University in Brussels, Brussels, Belgium; Division of Cellular Biology, Kennedy Institute of Rheumatology, London, U.K.

Pseudohypoparathyroidism is defined as a form of clinical hypoparathyroidism in which the end-organs of parathyroid hormone (PTH) do not respond to the administration of the hormone (1-3). The fact that the urinary cAMP responses to exogenous PTH are low or absent (2) in pseudohypoparathyroidism type I (PSPI), led to the hypothesis that the metabolic abnormality might be a defect of PTH renal receptors. This view was supported by the observation that a receptor-cyclase coupling protein (N protein) was found to be deficient in renal membranes of a patient with PSPI (4) whose PTH-dependent adenylate cyclase required greater than normal concentrations of GTP for activation (5). Moreover, erythrocyte N protein activity was deficient in many but not all PSPI patients (6,7).

The levels of bioactive PTH (bioPTH) have been found to be normal or close to the normal range in the face of markedly raised levels of presumably intact immunoreactive PTH-(1-84) (iPTH) (8). One explanation is that receptors of PTH are blocked by the presence in the circulation of a factor which interferes with the biological response of the hormone. We have demonstrated that plasma of PSPI patients blocked the activity of exogenously added PTH on guinea-pig kidney used in the cytochemical bioassay (9).

In the present report, we investigated the inhibition of PTH bioactivity by plasma of PSPI patients and of their siblings with normal urinary cAMP response to PTH. PSPI patients in five families (A, B, C, D and E) and their mothers in four families (A, B, D and E) had characteristic signs which included short stature, brachymetacarpia and/or brachymetatarsia, subcutaneous ossifications, a round face and mental retardation (Table 1, Fig. 1) (1-3). All the other relatives examined and a sixth family (F) lacked the signs of Albright's osteodystrophy. The urinary cAMP response to PTH, as evaluated according to a slightly modified protocol of Chase et al. (2,3), was reduced or absent in the 17 PSPI patients. 10 relatives responded normally to the administration of PTH. 12 PSPI patients of 5 families (A, B, C, D and E) exhibited partial deficiency of N protein activity (6) in red blood cells ($53\pm3\%$, SE; normal $102\pm3\%$) ($P<0.001$) (10). In one father and six mothers deficient N protein activity ($63\pm4\%$) was associated with normal urinary cAMP response to PTH. In one sister N protein activity was 99% and she responded normally to PTH. In a sixth family (F) N protein deficiency did not correlate with urinary cAMP responsiveness to PTH. N protein activity was similarly deficient in PSPI patients and in some of their siblings with normal urinary cAMP responsiveness to PTH.

Mean levels of bioPTH of 9.8 ± 3.8 pg/ml in 15 PSPI patients (4.7 ± 1.7 pg/ml in 6 untreated PSPI patients) and of 6.8 ± 1.7 pg/ml in 9 relatives with normal urinary cAMP response to PTH were similar to those of normal subjects (5.7 ± 0.5 pg/ml) (8,9). But, iPTH levels (8) were raised above normal values in 15 of 17 PSPI patients and in 3 of 10 relatives examined. The elevated levels of

Correspondence: Dr. J.A. Fischer, Klinik Balgrist, Forchstrasse 340, 8008 Zurich, Switzerland

Table 1. Clinical and laboratory data (for pedigrees see Fig. 1)

Position in pedigree	Age, sex	BioPTH (pg/ml)	iPTH (pg/ml)	Recovery (%)	Urinary cAMP ($nmol/min/m^2$) Basal	Maximal	N protein (%)	Treatment (µg/day)
A family								
A-1	44 F	3.4	220	28	1.5	57.4	60	-
A-2	16 F	<0.1	1840	<1	1.1	11.6	-	0.5 1,25-D_3
A-3	13 M	0.2	341	19	2.7	6.0	50	0.5 1,25-D_3
A-4	12 M	51	390	14	0.2	5.1	47	0.5 1,25-D_3
A-5	8 F	-	480	-	3.1	9.4	-	0.5 1,25-D_3
A-6	42 F	<1.0	890	52	2.2	87.8	55	-
A-7	11 F	0.4	390	1	3.8	1.4	39	0.5 1,25-D_3
A-8	7 F	-	270	-	4.7	11.0	51	-
B family								
father	40 M	11.6	390	70	-	-	96	
mother	38 F	12.0	160	130	1.3	50.4	58	-
daughter	10 F	36	900	<1	12.5	15.5	45	330 DHT
daughter	6 F	18	680	23	5.0	6.4	56	280 DHT
son	14 M	7.1	260	78	-	-	99	-
C family								
father	39 M	11.2	85	70	2.0	52.0	75	-
mother	40 F	0.8	240	86	2.0	100	77	-
son	12 M	1.1	510	1	3.3	3.9	51	530 DHT
son	8 M	6.0	890	6	5.7	6.7	56	300 DHT
daughter	8 F	13.0	220	4	4.0	246	99	-
D family								
mother	48 F	8.6	380	3	2.6	48.0	50	-
son	17 M	6.0	69	3	1.1	1.7	69	1750 D_3
son	11 M	<1.0	560	<1	1.1	11.1	76	-
E family								
mother	32 F	-	100	-	1.3	63.1	68	-
daughter	10 F	4.7	780	17	1.3	1.5	52	-
son	7 M	2.9	760	9	2.7	10.0	48	-
F family								
F-1	81 F	10.1	360	<1	2.0	50.0	67	-
F-2	59 F	5.3	300	60	-	-	120	-
F-3	14 F	4.2	200	105	-	-	107	-
F-4	52 F	5.7	250	98	-	-	91	-
F-5	20 F	3.1	210	<1	-	-	101	-
F-6	50 F	3.0	340	7	-	-	95	-
F-7	27 M	0.7	210	20	1.0	39.0	70	-
F-8	48 F	10.4	640	<1	2.0	7.0	104	-
F-9	17 M	9.1	1380	<1	2.0	3.0	78	-
F-10	38 F	0.1	890	6	4.0	9.0	99	-
Normal range		1-26	<300	49-90	<6	16.8-268	91-113	-

1,25-D_3, 1,25-dihydroxyvitamin D_3; DHT, dihydrotachysterol

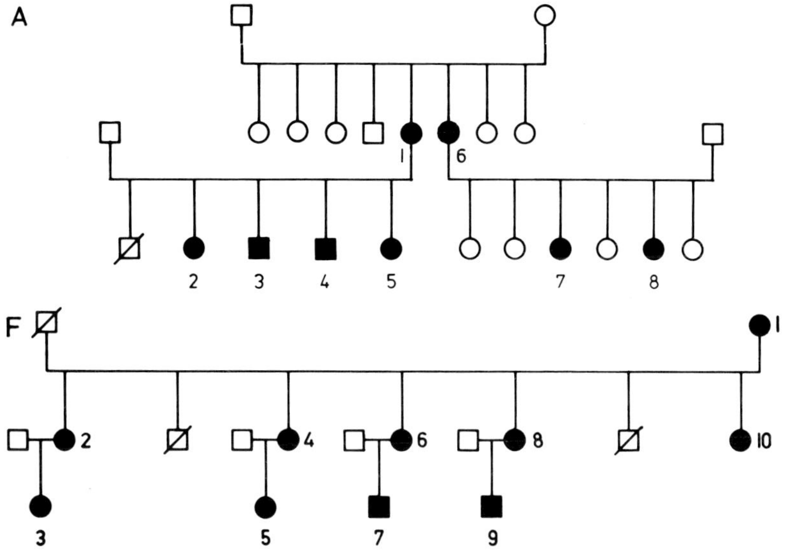

Figure 1. Pedigree of the A and F families. Empty symbols, not examined; Ø, deceased. Quadrangles are male and circles female subjects.

iPTH represent predominantly a peak co-eluting with intact PTH on gel permeation chromatography (not shown). One explanation is that receptors of PTH are blocked by the presence in the circulation of a factor which interferes with the biological response of the hormone. In accord with this possibility, the recovery of cytochemical bioactivity of exogenously added bovine PTH (100 pg/ml) to the plasma of PSPI patients was below 1% in 5 and ranged from 1% to 23% in 10 patients (mean $7 \pm 2\%$) as compared to 49% to 90% (mean $69 \pm 4\%$) in normal subjects ($P<0.001$) (9). In 9 relatives with normal urinary cAMP response to PTH the recovery of exogenously added PTH ranged from <1% to 130% (mean $44 \pm 15\%$); however, PSPI patients had lower recovery values than their siblings ($P<0.025$).

Thus we have demonstrated the presence, in the plasma from PSPI patients and some of their relatives, of a factor which partially inhibits the biological action of PTH on guinea-pig kidney. This factor was not present in the plasma of a patient who had undergone total parathyroidectomy (84% recovery), and the factor therefore might originate from the removed parathyroid glands (9). Nevertheless, the N protein activity was low in this patient (11) and the urinary cAMP excretion did not respond to PTH in a normal manner (2), even though he had normal phosphaturic and hypercalcemic responses after, but not before parathyroidectomy (12). In some patients with PSPI, the decreased or absent phosphaturic and hypercalcemic responses to PTH can be restored by treatment with vitamin D and normalisation of raised endogenous iPTH levels (see reference 13). Stimulation of renal adenylate cyclase activity is not necessarily linked to the phosphaturic effect of PTH. In agreement with this view is the finding that the PTH fragment-(3-34) inhibited the stimulation of renal adenylate cyclase by the biologically active fragment-(1-34) in vitro, but had no agonist or antagonistic effects on renal phosphate transport in vivo (14). PTH-(3-34), moreover, caused dissociation of cAMP production and calcium release in cultured bone explants (15). Also, in the cytochemical bioassay system, the effect of intact PTH-(1-84) is blocked by the 3-34 peptide (16). The possibility raised by our studies is that even if PTH receptors were intact, they might be partially blocked by the presence, in the circulation of PSPI patients and some of their relatives, of a factor the nature of which remains to be elucidated.

1. Albright, F., Burnett, C., Smith, P.H. and Parson, W. (1942): Endocrinology, 30, 922.
2. Chase, L.R., Melson, G.L. and Aurbach G.D. (1969): J. Clin. Invest., 48, 1832.
3. Werder, E.A., Fischer, J.A., Illig, R., Kind, H.P., Bernasconi, S., Fanconi, A. and Prader, A. (1978): J. Clin. Endocrinol. Metab., 46, 872.
4. Downs, Jr., R.W., Levine, M.A., Drezner, M.K., Burch, Jr., W.M. and Spiegel, A.M. (1983): J. Clin. Invest., 71, 231.
5. Drezner, M.K. and Burch, Jr., W.M. (1978): J. Clin. Invest., 62, 1222.
6. Farfel, Z., Brickman, A.S., Kaslow, H.R., Brothers, V.M. and Bourne, H.R. (1980): N. Engl. J. Med., 303, 237.
7. Levine, M.A., Downs, Jr., R.W., Singer, M., Marx, S.J., Aurbach, G.D. and Spiegel, A.M. (1980): Biochem. Biophys. Res. Commun., 94, 1319.
8. Nagant de Deuxchaisnes, C., Fischer, J.A., Dambacher, M.A., Devogelaer, J.-P., Arber, C.E., Zanelli, J.M., Parsons, J.A., Loveridge, N., Bitensky, L. and Chayen, J. (1981): J. Clin. Endocrinol. Metab., 53, 1105.
9. Loveridge, N., Fischer, J.A., Nagant de Deuxchaisnes, C., Dambacher, M.A., Tschopp, F., Werder, E., Devogelaer, J.-P., De Meyer, R., Bitensky, L. and Chayen, J. (1982): J. Clin. Endocrinol. Metab., 54, 1274.
10. Fischer, J.A., Nagant de Deuxchaisnes, C., Dambacher, M.A., Werder, E., De Meyer, R., Devogelaer, J.-P. and Bourne, H.R. (1982): Calcif. Tiss. Intl., 34, S39 (abstract).
11. Farfel, Z., Brothers, V.M., Brickman, A.S., Conte, F., Neer, R. and Bourne, H.R. (1981): Proc. Natl. Acad. Sci. USA, 78, 3098.
12. Nagant de Deuxchaisnes, C. and Krane, S.M. (1978): In: Metabolic Bone Disease, vol. 2, p. 217. Editors: L.V. Avioli and S.M. Krane, Academic Press, New York.
13. Stögmann, W. and Fischer, J.A. (1975): Am. J. Med. 59, 140.
14. McGowan, J.A., Chen, T.C., Fragola, J., Puschett, J.B. and Rosenblatt, M. (1983): Science, 219, 67.
15. Herrmann-Erlee, M.P.M., Nijweide, P.J., van der Meer, J.M. and Ooms, M.A.C. (1983): Calcif. Tiss. Intl., 35, 70.
16. Loveridge, N., Kent, G.N. and Heath, D.A. (1982): Clin. Sci., 63, 75P (abstract).

Supported by Swiss National Science Foundation Grant 3.813-0.81 and the Arthritis and Rheumatism Council for Research.

Discussion following paper by J. Fischer

G. AURBACH: This observation about the abnormal ratio of immunoreactive over bioactive hormone in the plasma of these subjects is certainly interesting.

J. O'RIORDAN: Could I have my first slide just to express our experience with the cytochemical bioassay. The patients that we have studied with untreated pseudohypoparathyroidism have invariably showed in the cytochemical bioassay elevated concentrations of bioactive hormone, and they have been similar to the concentrations of biologically active hormone found in patients with vitamin D deficiency.

When these patients are treated, the bioactive hormone concentration decreases in the pseudohypoparathyroid patients as well as in the patients with vitamin D deficiency. So at least in this group (and the hormone measurements were made by the same observer), the hormone seems to be biologically active, and the glands seem to respond appropriately. We would agree that there is a disassociation, however, in response of the immunologically-active hormone.

F. BRINGHURST: With regard to the inhibitory effect which you see in the cytochemical bioassay, has it been possible to inhibit the effect, i.e. the standard response to PTH by prior incubation of the tissue with diluted plasma from these patients, or are all these simultaneous additions?

J. FISCHER: These have been simultaneous additions. In response to Dr. O'Riordan, I might add that there are discrepancies concerning normal ranges. I fully agree that some of the patients with pseudohypoparathyroidism present measurable bioactive PTH values, however, plasma values of bioactive PTH measured by several groups of investigators have been from 0.2 to 33 pg/ml in normal subjects. It would therefore seem that the majority of patients reported by Dr. O'Riordan, with vitamin D deficiency as well as with pseudohypoparathyroidism display bioactive PTH concentrations which are not elevated.

J. RAY: I am a litte confused about the special case you showed with the normal ratio and wondered if you were suggesting that the inhibitor you are discussing is coming from the parathyroid gland?

J. FISCHER: We have indeed found that the recovery of exogenously added PTH was normal in a patient following parathyroidectomy. The inhibitory factor may therefore originate from the parathyroid glands.

F. KOLB: In 1960, we described four patients evidencing osteitis fibrosa which was reversible when we normalized serum calcium. This is the best bioassay of parathyroid hormone. Therefore, I think the hormone is biologically active, at least in some patients.

J. FISCHER: Thank you, but the point is how much, especially in the context of our own findings.

RESISTANCE TO MULTIPLE HORMONES IN PSEUDOHYPOPARATHYROIDISM: ASSOCIATION WITH DEFICIENT ACTIVITY OF GUANINE NUCLEOTIDE REGULATORY PROTEIN

Michael A. Levine, Robert W. Downs, Jr., and Allen M. Spiegel

Department of Medicine, Johns Hopkins University School of Medicine, Baltimore, Md., U.S.A., and Metabolic Diseases Branch, NIADDK, NIH, Bethesda, Md., U.S.A.

Pseudohypoparathyroidism (PHP) is an heritable metabolic disorder characterized by the biochemical features of hypoparathyroidism (hypocalcemia and hyperphosphatemia) with apparently normal parathyroid hormone (PTH) secretion. The hallmark of this disorder as originally described by Albright is resistance of the target organs, bone and kidney, to the action of PTH (1). In addition to the biochemical abnormalities, many but not all patients exhibit a unique somatic appearance (subsequently referred to as Albright's hereditary osteodystrophy) encompassing multiple developmental dejects: (1) round face and stocky build; (2) brachydactyly; and (3) heterotopic ossification. Characterization of the molecular basis for PHP commenced when Chase and Aurbach showed that the action of PTH on target tissues, bone and kidney, is mediated by cyclic AMP, and found that patients with PHP lack the normal brisk rise in urinary cyclic AMP after infusion of PTH (2). Their studies indicated that in PHP type I there is a defect in the target organ PTH receptor-adenylate cyclase system, proximal to the generation of cyclic AMP. Although hypoparathyroidism is the most commonly recognized endocrine deficiency in PHP, the presence of other clinical abnormalites in patients with PHP, such as hypothyroidism and hypogonadism, suggested that hormone resistance in the syndrome may be more generalized than heretofore appreciated. This led us to speculate that a defect in a component of the adenylate cyclase complex common to all tissues, such as the guanine nucleotide regulatory protein (G unit), might account for hormone resistance in PHP. Recent studies from this laboratory (3) as well as by Bourne and co-workers (4) have demonstrated a deficiency of G unit activity in erythrocytes from many patients with PHP. We report here biochemical and clinical studies which suggest that PHP patients with deficient erythrocyte G unit activity have a disorder which is generalized to cyclase-dependent tissues. Moreover, it appears that PHP patients with normal erythrocyte G unit activity may have a defect limited to PTH target tissues.

PATIENTS AND METHODS

Subjects

Twenty-nine patients were studied. The diagnosis of PHP type I was confirmed by documentation of a markedly blunted urinary cyclic AMP response to a standard intravenous infusion of PTH. Patients were characterized as to the presence (+ AHO) or absence (- AHO) of Albright's hereditary osteodystrophy based on the finding of brachydactyly. Palpable or radio-opaque heterotopic ossifications were considered confirmatory of AHO. Patients showing neither brachydactyly nor subcutaneous ossifications were considered to represent the (-) AHO variant of PHP.

Methods

Assays of G unit activity were performed as previously described (3), and were based on activation of adenylate cyclase in detergent-solubilized turkey erythrocyte membranes by G units in detergent (Lubrol PX) extracts of human erythrocyte membranes. Cyclic AMP production in this system was proportional to added human erythrocyte G units. Results of assays are expressed as a percentage of the activity of a standard membrane preparation consisting of pooled erythrocytes from 5 normal individuals, and represent the mean of at least three determinations.

The presence of target organ specific hormone resistance was evaluated by determining the responsiveness of diverse cyclase-dependent tissues to their respective tropic peptides. Data were analyzed with students' t-test for unpaired samples. The 95% confidence interval was used for testing significance. Unless otherwise stated, results are expressed as mean ± 1S.D.

Results and Discussion

Fifteen of our patients (13 females) showed features of AHO and 14 patients (12 females) had normal somatic phenotypes. Serum calcium was similarly reduced in (+)AHO and (-) AHO groups (4.10 ± 0.36 vs 3.97 ± 0.48 mEq/l) and plasma PTH was elevated in each member of both groups. Erthyrocyte G unit activity was determined in all subjects (Figure 1). Patients who lacked features of Albright's hereditary osteodystrophy showed normal G unit activity, whereas in 13 of 15 (+) AHO patients there was approximately a 50% reduction in G unit activity [.92 ± .08 vs .43 ± .03, ($p<0.001$)] (Figure 1). There was no significant difference between the G unit activity of (-) AHO patients and controls including normal volunteers, hyperparathyroid and hypoparathyroid patients.

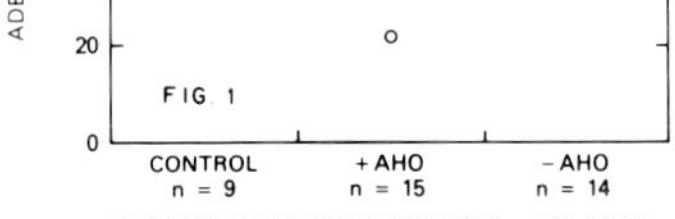

*SIGNIFICANTLY DIFFERENT FROM CONTROL, AHO P<0.001

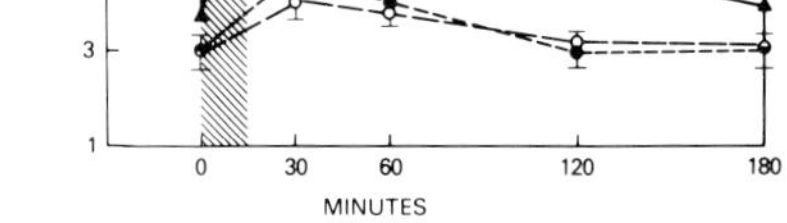

Based on the results of the G unit assay, patients with PHP were divided into two groups, one showing normal erythrocyte G unit activity (NGU), and the other showing deficient erythrocyte G unit acvtivity (DGU). Sixteen patients were thus classified as NGU (12 females, 4 males), 14 of whom were (-) AHO, and 2 of whom were (+)AHO. The DGU group comprised 13 PHP females, all of whom satisifed the criteria for (+)AHO. Despite markedly different values for erythrocyte G unit activity, the time course and magnitude of the changes in urinary cyclic AMP following PTH infusion (250 U, PTE, Lilly, given i.v. time 0-15 m) were similar in both DGU (●) and NGU (O) groups. Normal individuals (▲), by comparison, showed a brisk urinary cyclic AMP response, with peak values 40 to 50 times basal (Figure 2).

Abnormal thyroid function was found in virtually all patients with deficient G unit activity. Basal thyroid hormone (thyroxine and triiodothyronine) concentrations in serum were often slightly reduced and even when normal were accompanied by elevations in basal thyrotropin (TSH). Peak TSH responses to thyrotropin-releasing factor (500 mcg, i.v.) were characteristic of primary hypothyroidism. Moreover, despite greater elevations in TSH, DGU patients showed lesser increases in triiodothyronine 180 minutes following TRH than NGU patients (Table I). In the absence of goiter or antithyroid antibodies, the data are compatible with resistance of the thyroid to TSH. By contrast, NGU patients with PHP generally showed normal basal and stimulated TSH (Table 1), and normal serum thyroid hormone concentrations.

Table 1. Endocrine Studies

Group	Basal TSH (μU/ml)	Peak TSH (μU/ml)	T_3 (ng/ml)	Plasma cAMP (μM x min)
DGU	15.0 ± 6.5	54.3 ± 22.7	27.5 ± 26	5.1 ± 2.2
NGU	4.5 ± 2.0	19.5 ± 6.6	45.0 ± 16.8	8.6 ± 3.4
Control	2.0 ± 1.1	16.5 ± 6.7	53.6 ± 23.6	8.6 ± 3.6
Control v DGU	$p<.001$	$p<.001$	$p<.001$	$p<.01$

Hepatic responsiveness to hormone stimulation was assessed by measuring the rise in blood glucose and plasma cyclic AMP following a bolus injection of 0.5 mg of glucagon. The rise in plasma cyclic AMP was significantly reduced in the DGU group of patients (Table 1). The distal effect of hepatic cyclic AMP generation, glucose release, was normal in both groups, and indicates that despite the presumably reduced adenylate cyclase activity in DGU patients, sufficient intracellular cyclic AMP does accumulate to transduce the hormone signal and express the distal physiologic effect (i.e., hyperglycemia). Adrenocortical responsiveness to ACTH (250 mcg, cosyntropin) was assessed only by measuring the distal physiologic response, rise in serum cortisol, and was normal in all patients.

Gonadal dysfunction was common in DGU patients. Ten of 11

females showed either primary or secondary amenorrhea. In the majority of the patients we studied basal gonadotropins were not elevated nor was there an exaggerated gonadotropin response to luteinizing hormone-releasing factor.

Our studies clearly show that PHP type I is a heterogeneous disorder composed of at least 2 groups of individuals: patients who show NGU and those who show DGU. Deficient erythrocyte G unit activity correlates well with the apparent presence of hormone resistance in diverse adenylate cyclase-dependent tissues, and implicates this defect as the cause of a generalized disorder of adenylate cyclase. The limited nature of the endocrine perturbation in patients with NGU implicates abnormal PTH or altered PTH-receptor interactions as the basis for hormone resistance in these patients, but at present there is no direct evidence to support this hypothesis. It also remains possible that some PHP patients with NGU will be found to have multiple hormone resistance, and will prove to have another defect in the adenylate cyclase system (e.g. increased phosphodiesterase activity) that leads to generalized hormone resistance. Further support for the hypothesis that a deficiency of G unit activity could account for generalized hormone resistance in PHP comes from studies of other accessible tissues. We have recently found that cultured fibroblasts from DGU patients with PHP (who show resistance to multiple hormones) accumulate significantly less cyclic AMP in response to hormone stimulation than do control fibroblasts (5). This observation is consistent with the premise that a reduction in functional G units may impair the ability of various tissues to respond to a variety of agents whose mechanism of action involves activation of adenylate cyclase. Finally, the relationship between AHO and G unit activity is unclear. Although in our experience (-) AHO patients show normal G unit activity, the reverse is not true. We and others have observed (+) AHO patients who show normal G unit activity. Thus it is unlikely that a deficiency of G units per se leads to the AHO phenotype.

In summary, we have shown that many PHP patients manifest deficient erythrocyte G unit activity and are resistant to multiple hormones. We believe that this relationship is not coincidental, but rather that the defect reflects a generalized disorder of adenylate cyclase.

References

1. Albright, F., Burnett, C.H., Smith, P.H. (1942): Endocrinology, 30:922.
2. Chase, L.R., Melson, G.L., Aurbach, G.D. (1969): J.Clin.Invest., 48:1822.
3. Levine, M.A., Downs, R.W., Jr., Singer, M.J., Marx, S.J., Aurbach, G.D., Spiegel, A.M. (1980): Biochem. Biophys.Res.Commun., 94:1319.
4. Farfel, Z., Brickman, A.S., Kaslow, H.R., Brothers, V.M., Bourne, H.R. (1980): N.Engl.J.Med., 303:237.
5. Levine, M.A., Eil, C., Downs, R.W., Jr., Spiegel, A.M. (1983): J.Clin.Invest., in press.

Discussion following paper by M. Levine

T. FEIGELMAN: The incidence of the dysmorphic feature, namely AHO, with the short metacarpals and metatarsals and short stature along with multiple hormone resistance is most interesting. What I find challenging is the associated incidence of mental deficiency that goes along with this syndrome. I've reviewed a large number of mentally retarded individuals, and we have found that the incidence of short stature and short metacarpals in almost 4% of these patients. This 4% seems to run across the lines of various mental deficiency syndromes. About 1/3 of the patients have Down's syndrome. Sporadically, these people have hypothyroidism, primary or secondary, some have hypogonadism, hypoadrenalism, and a few even diabetes insipidus. Very few, if any, have hypocalcemia or hyperphosphatemia, and none really seem to require vitamin D. In view of what may be a high incidence of this dysmorphic feature in the mentally retarded population and the assocation of the G unit deficiency with this dysmorphic feature, I wonder whether or not we have an assocation with mental development.

M. LEVINE: This brings up an interesting point. I will say that two of the patients that we saw who had AHO, and more have been seen subsequently, did not have decreased G unit activity. It is possible that the G unit activity deficiency is somehow related to the expression of AHO. How it's related is unknown at the present time. I would also point out that many of the components of the phenotype of AHO are suggestive of a widespread developmental defect in tubular bone or other mesenchymal bone structures. This may not be unique to pseudohypoparathyroidism and may occur in other syndromes in which development defects occur. Archibald studied the incidence of metacarpal bone shortening and about 10% of the population will have modest shortening of a third or fourth metacarpal. The brachydactyly seen in pseudohypoparathyroidism can be distinguished from that in other syndromes, however.

Addressing the point of mental retardation and G unit deficiency, one certainly finds it reasonable to suggest that there may be an influence of adenylate cyclase (G unit activity), in development of the brain. It's known, for example, that the retina has a protein which is a GTP substrate, and there probably are other elements of the CNS system in which G protein or adenylate cyclase is important for proper development.

M. KLEEREKOPER: If this G-protein deficiency is ubiquitous, why is the clinical expression so predominantly a hypoparathyroid state? Are there some patients with say primary hypothyroidism where there is a deficiency and the hypoparathyroidism is very minimal?

M. LEVINE: Yes, as Dr. Van Dop has alluded, the vitamin D status of the patient is extremely important in determing whether or not a defect in adenylate cyclase per se, or the G unit will be manifested as hypocalcemia. We have seen two patients in whom clinical hypothyroidism has been the presenting complaint. Hypocalcemia in one has never been documented, and in the other, has been transient. Neither patient has required treatment with calcium or vitamin D. Their response to PTH is deficient and the urinary cyclic AMP response cannot be distinguished from patients who clearly have hypocalcemia. But these patients required treatment with physiologic replacement of thyroxine; so it's clear that the stoichiometry of the G unit with other components of adenylate cyclase and phosphodiesterase from tissue to tissue as well as other factors such as vitamin D status, can be important in determing the clinical expression of the genetic defect.

M. PARFITT: Are there cases of AHO, as you have defined it in whom all endocrine and molecular studies are normal?

M. LEVINE: No, I have not seen that. At the very least they have had an abnormal response to PTH.

INHERENT AND ACQUIRED RESISTANCE TO PARATHYROID HORMONE IN MAN

J.L.H. O'Riordan, G.N. Hendy and I.G. Lewin

Department of Medicine, The Middlesex Hospital, London W1N 8AA, U.K.

Resistance to the action of parathyroid hormone (PTH) can be inherent, as in pseudohypoparathyroidism, but it can also be acquired as in primary and secondary hyperparathyroidism and it can be induced in normal subjects. Responsiveness can conveniently be examined by following the changes in the concentration of circulating cyclic AMP that follow injection of 200 units of bovine parathyroid hormone intravenously. Normally this causes a brisk rise in plasma cyclic AMP, as well as an increase in the urinary excretion of cyclic AMP and the phosphaturic response to the hormone. This response can be blocked by prior infusion of 1,000 units of bovine parathyroid hormone over the preceding two hours (figure 1), resistance to the hormone being produced without any change in serum calcium. (4). The response recovers completely, within 12-18 hours. Infusion of the biologically active N-terminal 1-34 fragment of parathyroid hormone can also impair the response to intact parathyroid hormone so that inactive C-terminal fragments are not involved in the genesis of this resistant state. However, infusion with a biologically inactive fragment (3-34) of the N-terminus does not block the response to intact hormone so that biologically inactive fragments of the N-terminus, certainly those lacking the first 2 residues, are also not responsible for the refractory state.

The changes in plasma cyclic AMP after administration of parathyroid hormone are largely due to effects on the renal adenyl cyclase so that the

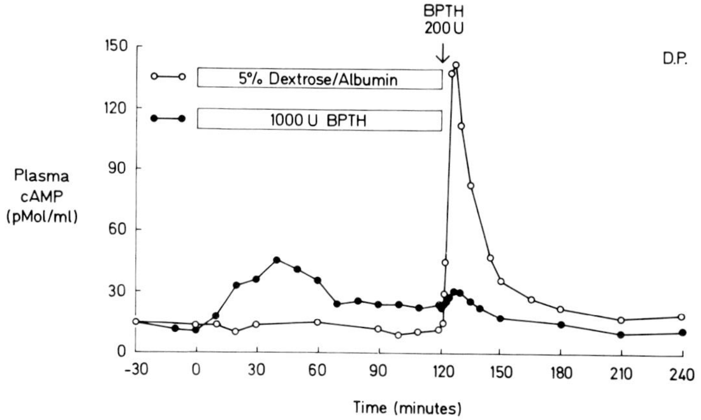

Fig. 1: During a 2 hour infusion, into a normal subject, of 1,000 units of BPTH, the plasma cyclic AMP concentration initially increased and then declined during the latter part of the infusion. At the termination of the infusion an injection of 200 units of hormone resulted in a markedly impaired response as compared to the response after a control infusion of dextrose/albumin.

response is greater when measured in renal effluent than it is in peripheral venous blood and is dependent on renal function. (3). Even moderate impairment of renal function is associated with marked reduction in responsiveness to parathyroid hormone (figure 2). The greater the degree of renal failure, the greater the impairment in the response to injected bovine parathyroid hormone. The resistance is correlated with serum creatinine and with concentration of endogenous parathyroid hormone and in severe chronic renal failure there is no significant increase in plasma cyclic AMP after the administration of bovine parathyroid hormone. This impairment in response can be reversed by successful renal transplantation.

In primary hyperparathyroidism the response to exogenous hormone can also be blunted. It increases, however, albeit not to normal, after removal of a parathyroid adenoma, when the concentration of endogenous hormone is normal (figure 3). This recovery of responsiveness occurs more gradually, over a period of months. In some patients with mild primary hyperparathyroidism the response may be within the normal range, but increases after removal of the parathyroid adenoma. In some patients with primary hyperparathyroidism the resistance can in part be attributed to mild impairment of renal function but resistance can also occur when renal function is entirely normal. Since recovery of responsiveness occurs much more slowly after removal of a parathyroid adenoma, than it does after infusion of hormone into normal subjects, it is unlikely that the same mechanisms are involved. Resistance to the action of parathyroid hormone occurs in subjects with vitamin D deficiency who are hypocalcaemic and have secondary hyperparathyroidism with normal renal function. When the deficiency is corrected by treatment with vitamin D, responsiveness to parathyroid hormone increases to normal (1). This is associated with a reduction of the concentration of endogenous hormone to normal. (figure 4).

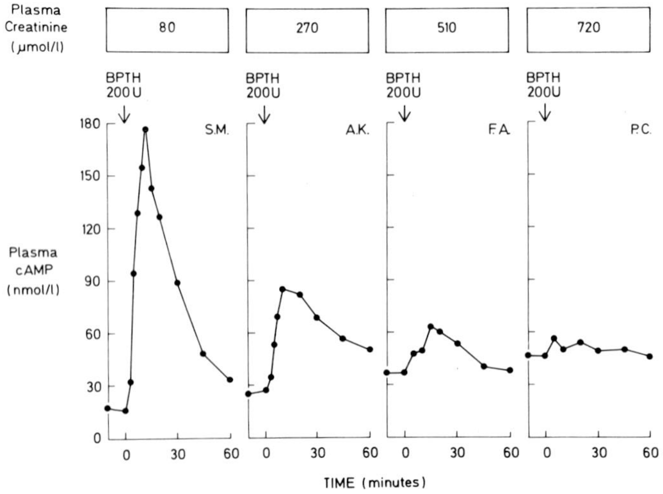

Fig. 2: Shows the increasingly marked impairment in plasma cyclic AMP response to an injection of 200 units BPTH in 3 patients with varying degrees of decreased renal function as compared to the response in a normal subject (S.M.).

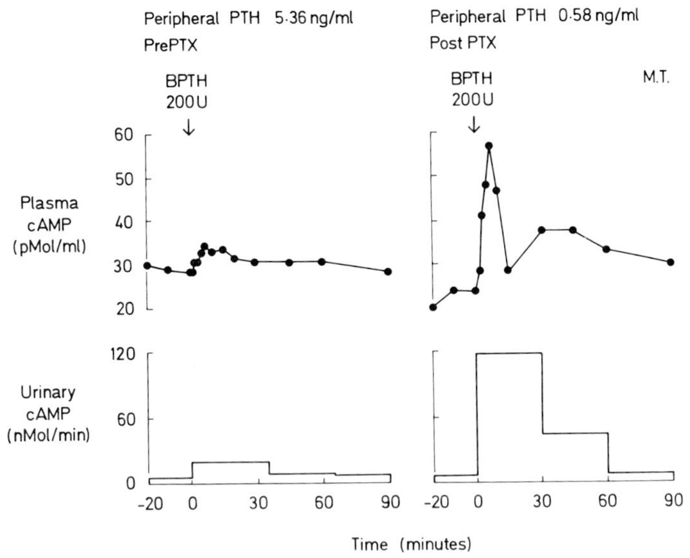

Fig. 3: Shows the effect of parathyroidectomy on the plasma cyclic AMP response to an injection of 200 units of BPTH in a patient with primary hyperparathyroidism and normal renal function.

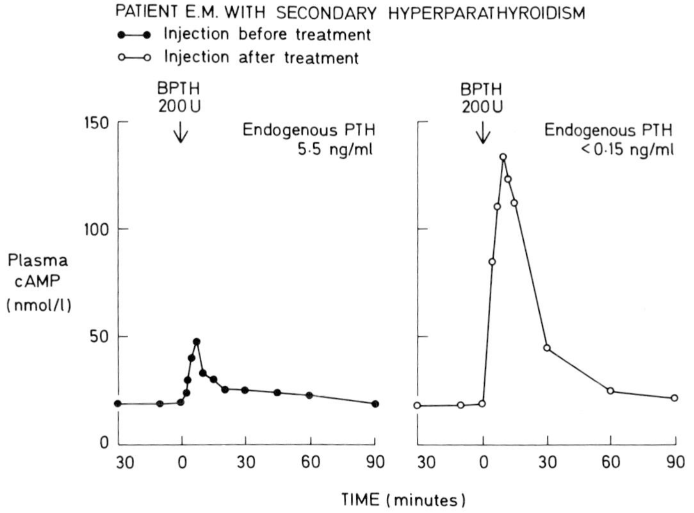

Fig. 4: Shows the effect of vitamin D therapy on the plasma cyclic AMP response to an injection of 200 units of BPTH in a patient with the secondary hyperparathyroidism of vitamin deficiency.

In some patients with vitamin D deficiency raised plasma phosphate may be associated with hypocalcaemia and secondary hyperparathyroidism (2). The hyperphosphataemia might be taken to indicate that there was resistance to the phosphaturic action of the hormone; the cyclic AMP response is, however, normal, so that this situation mimicks that in so called "pseudohypoparathyroidism type 2".

Resistance to parathyroid hormone can be associated thus with hypercalcaemia or hypocalcaemia and can be induced without there being any change in serum calcium. It seems that high concentrations of parathyroid hormone in each of these situations is associated with the development of resistance. A variety of mechanisms may be involved in reduction of reduced responsiveness, such as changes in occupancy of receptors or alteration in their affinity or number and there may be uncoupling of the receptor and cyclase, at the level of the G subunit.

REFERENCES

1. Lewin, I.G., Papapoulos, S.E., Hendy, G.N., Tomlinson, S. and O'Riordan, J.L.H. (1982): Clin. Sci. 62, 381.
2. Lewin, I.G., Papapoulos, S.E., Tomlinson, S., Hendy, G.N., and O'Riordan, J.L.H. (1978): Quart, J., Med. 188, 533.
3. Tomlinson, S., Barling, P.M., Albano, J.D.M., Brown, B.L., and O'Riordan, J.L.H. (1974): Clin. Sci. Molec. Med. 47, 481.
4. Tomlinson, S., Hendy, G.N., Pemberton, D., and O'Riordan, J.L.H. (1976): Clin. Sci. Molec. Med. 51, 59.

Discussion following paper of G. O'Riordan

G. AURBACH: Dr. A. Spiegel has been studying a very similar protocol to the one just shown by Dr. O'Riordan, infusing exogenous parathyroid hormone, measuring plasma cyclic AMP, but at the same time sampling plasma from the patients and carrying out highly sensitive adenylate cyclase assay. He finds recovery of injected hormone to be the same in normal subjects as in those with pseudohypoparathyroidism. These tests give no evidence for the possibility of an endogenous inhibitor.

C. NORDIN: Your examples of resistance to PTH in renal failure and in osteomalacia with secondary hyperparathyroidism could, of course, be due as you imply to the high PTH levels. It is conceivable that vitamin D itself plays some part? In two of the examples you gave, there was deficiency of $1,25(OH)_2D$ and when you gave the vitamin D the PTH decreased. Now, I know the obvious implication is of what you said, but could it be that $1,25(OH)_2D$ is required to express the action of PTH in that situation?

J. O'RIORDAN: Anything is possible, but I would point out that in the normal subjects you see a similar phenomenon and I don't believe that over that time period significant changes in $1,25(OH)_2D$ would have occurred.

J. POTTS: Dr. O'Riordan's observations are quite intriguing with regard to Dr. Fischer's findings, i.e., that high PTH levels can modify response to exogenously-administered hormone with the response measured in vivo. Now, what do you think about the situation with regards findings in the cytochemical bioassay, particularly since the patient who had been parathyroidectomized did not show any trouble with recovery or inhibitory action?

J. FISCHER: That brings up the issue also that he did not exhibit a urinary cyclic AMP response, I would like to ask a question, especially to Dr. O'Riordan. How far do these patients respond with a phosphaturic or perhaps a hypercalcemic response which are more truly biological effects than involvement of the second messenger?

J. O'RIORDAN: We have not really focused so much on the phosphaturic response. It might be of interest to consider phenomena that occur in some patients with vitamin D deficiency who occasionally have hyperphosphatemia. Those patients with high PTH and low serum calcium might be regarded as having Type II pseudohypoparathyroidism despite the fact that the cyclic AMP response can be normal. There is no evidence in this particular group of PTH resistance. The abnormal situation is corrected with treatment by physiological amounts of vitamin D.

D. RAO: Dr. O'Riordan, we have found the same dissociation of cyclic AMP and phosphaturic responses to PTH infusion in vitamin D deficiency. In response partly to Dr.Nordin's question, I must cite one patient in whom TMP/GFR was initially high, but decreased after treatment with a gluten-free diet without vitamin D and thus, indicating that it probably is PTH rather than vitamin D mediated.

M. KLEEREKOPER: Dr. O'Riordan is it really fair to give the same amount of PTH, irrespective of the pool of PTH of the patient in which you are injecting? Have you tried different doses of parathyroid hormone in somebody with primary or secondary hyperparathyroidism to see whether you can get a better response?

J. O'RIORDAN: Yes, we have given larger doses, and we have not seen a difference in response. I might say that in normal subjects you can show the plasma cyclic AMP response is dose dependent. For simplicity and practical reasons we have confined the study to an effective single dose in our various groups.

H. WRAY: I'm interested in the statements that have been made about vitamin D status and the responsiveness in the pseudohypoparathyroid patients. How does this relate to the phosphaturic response which we find is the least variable. Sometimes patients with an absent cyclic AMP response have an entirely normal phosphaturic response. Is there any connection with the vitamin D status in these patients?

J. FISCHER: In a patient we reported some years ago, we normalized serum calcium and iPTH with vitamin D. He responded with a normal phosphaturic response.

S. KRANE: It's interesting that the studies of Dr. O'Riordan mimic those that were reported by Dr. Goldring several years ago, testing parathyroid hormone responses of cultured human cells such as foreskin fibroblasts and giant cell turmos. Exposure to PTH blocks the subsequent cyclic AMP response from re-exposure to PTH. If you incubate with 3-34, 8-18 norleucine inhibitor analog this does not desensitize, but blocks the simultaneous response. So what you observed in vivo was what was observed in vitro several years ago using human cells. As far as $1,25(OH)_2D$ is concerned, Dr. Goldring also described the fact that $1,25(OH)_2D$ actually suppresses the cyclic AMP response to PTH in these cultured cells. Using one of the fibroblasts from one of the Japanese patients with $1,25(OH)_2D$ receptor deficiency, this suppression of the PTH response was not seen, whereas in the other cells from the same patient, that had receptors, there was a suppressed response to PTH. So what has been discussed here is all consistent with what's been observed and described in vitro.

J. O'RIORDAN: I think it's interesting to speculate as to what changes one is producing. It is easy to talk about down regulation, change in numbers of receptors, or affinity of receptors and to speculate about the role of coupling through the G protein in vivo. One can only observe, however, the phenomenon at this state and wonder what changes one is producing at the receptor level.

M. EPSTEIN: In light of these abnormalities in nonaffected sibs, what advice should be given a nonaffected sib when she wants to have children?

M. LEVINE: This is a difficult question, and I think it falls back on analysis of the mode of inheritance in any one kindred. I think there is sufficient evidence that genetic heterogeneity is present in this disorder and it is difficult to give good risk values. In an unaffected sib, if one could detect in the family that there were a G unit defect and the sib who was preparing to have a family did not show the G unit defect, one would feel comfortable in saying that at least the somatic cells had escaped the genetic defect. However, one doesn't know what's happening in the germ line, and in fact that sort of problem can explain some families where in the first and second generation appear to be autosomal recessive, but subsequent generations appear to express dominant type of inheritance. I would say there is a 50% chance in patients who are affected, probably very low in those who are not.

J. O'RIORDAN: Could I make one point about the pattern of the pseudohypoparathyroidism certainly as I see it in England, namely, that we very rarely see patients with the beautiful family trees that you have studied. They are mostly sporadic cases so that the genetics in that situation are difficult to discern.

G. AURBACH: This is one of the key problems in the disorder. There are too few families with multiple affected members to make much sense of the genetics.

R. NEER: The inhibitor that Dr.Fischer describes appears to derive from the parathyroid glands. If that be true, one might expect the inhibitor could be removed by antibodies to parathyroid hormone or by an affinity column to which these antibodies were coupled. Have you had an opportunity to explore that possibility?

J. FISCHER: No, but I would say this would not necessarily follow because we don't know what is being recognized by the antibodies. Your proposal is certainly worthy of further consideration.

XVIII SCIENTIFIC POSTER SESSIONS

FIRST SCIENTIFIC POSTER SESSION - ASSAYS FOR PTH AND VITAMIN D, BONE HISTOMORPHOMETRY, EVALUATION OF SKELETAL MASS, MISCELLANEOUS LABORATORY STUDIES

MODERATORS: L. AVIOLI, H. DUNCAN

1. "Lack of Effect of 1,25(OH_2D_3) and 24,25$(OH)_2D_3$ on parathyroid hormone Secretion in Human Parathyroid Cells in Vitro." G. Akerstrom, C. Rudberg, S. Ljunghall, L. Wide

2. "Studies on Vitamin D in Internal Medicine" Ph. Arlet, C. Gaillemin, Y. Botreau, M. Fuffaut, Y. LeTallec

3. "Post-Menopausal Osteoporosis Screening from Phalangeal Mineral Density by Radiographic Absorptiometry" R.S. Bachtell, C. Colbert, R. Coleman

4. "In Vivo Estimation of Total Body Bone Mineral (TBBM) Using Dual Photon Absorptiometry" J. Borg, A. Gotfredsen, C. Christiansen

5. "Clinical Application of In Vivo Estimation of Total Body Bone Mineral (TBBM) by Dual Photon Absorptiometry" A. Gotfredsen, J. Borg, L. Tjellesen, L. Nilas, O. Als, C. Christiansen

6. "A Probable Mechanism of In Vivo Resorption of Apatite from Bone" S. Chatterji

7. "Bone Loss in Osteoporosis as Quantified by Computed Tomography" M.A. Dambacher P. Ruegsegger, J.A. Fischer, M. Anliker

8. "Comparison of Histomorphometry and Computed Tomography in Quantitating Trabecular Bone" A.J. Olah, P. Ruegsegger, M.A. Dambacher

9. "The Hepatic Osteodystrophy: Evaluation of the Plasma Levels of 25$(OH)D_3$ in Subjects with Cirrhosis of the Liver" M.D'Amore, F.P. Cantatore, A.C. Amoruso, G. Santoro, M. Carrozzo

10. "A Comparison of Salivary 25 Hydroxy Vitamin D with Free 25 Hydroxy Vitamin D in Serum" A. Fairney, P. Saphier

11. Effects of Intracerebroventricular PTH Peptides in Pain Threshold and on Brain Prostaglandins Level in the Rat" C.E. Fiore, G. Clementi, A. Prato, D. Grimaldi, L. Malatino

12. "Effect of Section Thickness on Analysis of Mineralization Dynamics in Tetracycline-labelled Bone Biopsies" J.M. Harrelson, B. Lobuagh, K.W. Lyles, M.K. Drezner

13. "Femoral Bone Densitometry and Vertebral Dual Photon Absorptiometry" J.F. Heron, J.P. Sabatier, J. Dallet, J. Lefevre

14. "The Evaluation of Rates of Bone Loss by Serial Densitiometry. Correlation with Metabolic Calcium Balances in Osteoporosis" R. Hesp, U. Elsasser, J. Reeve

15. "Complementary Determination of 25 Hours Whole Body Retention of Methylendiphosphonate. A Simple Index of Bone Metabolism" L. Hyldstrup, N.B. Morgensen, G.F. Jensen, P. McNair, I. Transbøl

16. "Differences Between Vertebral Crush Fracture and Hip Fracture Syndromes" C. Johnston, Jr., P.J. Meunier

17. "Evaluation of Mid-C-Regional PTH (MID-C-PTH) As A Co-marker for Bone Turnover in Uremic Patients" H. Juppner, R. Baethke, R.D. Hesch

18. "Radioimmunoassay of Intact Human PTH Using Synthetic hPTH (28-48) As Immunogen and Ligand" M.J. Atkinson, T. Schettler, R.D. Hesch

19. "Three-Dimensional Shape and Thickness of Trabecular Bone Osteons" J. Kragstrup, F. Melsen, H.J.G. Gundersen, L. Mosekilde, T.Karring

20. "Thickness of Lamellae in Normal Human Iliac Trabecular Bone" J. Kragstrup, F. Melsen, L. Mosekilde

21. "Computerized Simulation of Bone Remodeling-Graphic Demonstration of Dynamic Processes" H. Krumme, G. Delling

22. "Effects of Nifedipine on Serum Calcium and Parathyroid Hormone in Man" S.C. Kukreja, P.C. Deedwania, L.T. Mann, G.A. Williams

23. "Ionized Calcium as Hypercalcemia Indicator" L. Larsson, G. Toss

24. "Cultured Bovine Parathyroid Cells Display Generalized Resistance to Extracellular Calcium" M.S. LeBoff, D. Beaudoin, E.M. Brown

25. "Discriminant Analysis of Serum Glycoproteins: A Method to Differentiate Causes of Hypercalcemia" A.A. Licata, C. Hawker

26. "Bone Mineral Density of the Lumbar Spine by Dual Photon Absorptiometry: In Vivo and In Vitro Studies" L. Markhard, R. Lindsay, D.W. Dempster, N. Pushparaj, D.W. King, G. Valiquette, W. Hawkins

27. "Total Body and Spinal Bone Mineral in Normal Women" R.B. Mazess

28. "Correlation Between Spinal and Peripheral Bone Mineralization Measured by Localized Neutron Activation Analysis" B. Maziere, D. Kuntz, C. Sejourne, B. Naveau, D. Comar

29. "Inhibitory Effect of Follicle Stimulating Hormone on Parathormone in Rat Calvaria In Vitro" M.S. Meyer, T.M. Chalmers, J.J. Reynolds

30. "Metabolic Bone Disease in Adults: The Value of Bone Histology" P.D. Miller, W.E. Huffer, R.A. Krebs, B.J. Neal, D.O. McIntyre

31. "The Use of CT Scanning for the Diagnosis of Osteoporosis" B.E.C. Nordin, A. Robertson, A. Crowe, C.E. Cann

32. "Vitamin D and its Metabolites are Essential to Normal Insulin Secretion" S. Kadowaki, A. Norman

33. "Bone Mineral Density Quantitation In Vivo. A Comparison of Three Methods" D. O'Keeffe, D. Powell, D.J. Dowesett, J.T. Ennis

34. "Effects of Ranitidine on Serum Parathyroid Hormone Levels in Normal Subjects" E. Palummeri, M. Passeri, M. Marchesi, M. Pedazzoni, A.M. Malagnino

35. "Bone Turnover Evaluated by A New Simple Model of 99mTc-Methylen Diphosphonate Kinetic" M. Passeri, M. Bernini, R. DiRuvo, E. Palummeri, C. Gennari

36. "Dual Photon Absorptiometry of the Lumbar Spine: Normal Spine Mineral Ranges" M.R. Powell, F.O. Kolb, J.J. Prendergast

37. "Effects of EDTA and Hypercalcemia on Plasma Prolactin, Parathyroid Hormone and Calcitonin in Normal and Parathyroidectomized Individuals" J.P. Raymond, R. Merceron, R. Issac, F. Wahbe

38. "Axial and Peripheral Skeletal Mineral Status by Dual Photon Absorptiometry of 153-GD in Prednisone Treatment" O. Schaadt, H. Bohr

39. "Clinical Aspects of Trabecular and Cortical Bone Mineral Scanning by Dual Photon Absorptiometry of 153-GD" O. Schaadt, H. Bohr

40. "Extracellular Calcium Potentiates the Magnesium-induced Inhibition of PTH Release and Elevation in Cytosolic Calcium Concentration in Dispersed Bovine Parathyroid Cells" D. Sholback, E. Brown

41. "Renal 1,25$(OH)_2$D Response to Intravenous hPTH-(1-34) in Normal Subjects" D.M. Slovik, M.A. Daly, J.T. Potts, Jr., R.M. Neer

42. "Single Photon Densitometry in Women: Comparison of Intercollegiate Swimmers, Tennis Players and Age Matched Controls" P. Jacobson, W. Beaver, S. Grubb, T. Taft, R. Talmage

43. "Distribution and Metabolism of Some Alkaline-Earth Elements in Bone with Respect to Reference Japanese Man" G. Tanaka, H. Kawamura, K. Shiraishi

44. "Skeletal Blood Flow in Metabolic Bone Disease" M. Tellez, J. Reeve, K. Walton, P.J. Meunier, R. Wootton

45. "Changes of Trabecular Bone Mass (TBM) Assessed by Computerized Tomography (CT) During Chronic Hemodialysis (CHD) and After Transplantation (Tx)" A. Torres, M.L. Mendez, M. Losada, J. Garcia, B. Maceira, S. Suria, V. Lorenzo

46. "An Ionized Calcium Regulated Calcium Clamp Technique in Man" O. Torring, H.E. Sjoberg

47. "Plasma Concentrations of Vitamin D Metabolites in Patients with Primary Billiary Cirrhosis" Z. Varghese, E. Keck, O. Epstein, K. Farrington, S. Sherlock, J.F. Moorhead

48. "Direct and Indirect Measurements of Osteoid Seam Width in Human Iliac Crest Biopsies" S. Vedi, J.E. Compston

49. "Age Related Changes in Bone Formation in Normal British Subjects" S. Vedi, J.E. Compston

50. "Measurement of Total Resorption Surface in Human Iliac Crest Biopsies" S. Vedi, A. Webb, J.E. Compston

51. "Decreased Serum Ionized Calcium and Normal Vitamin D Metabolite Levels with Antioconvulsant Drugs" R.S. Weinstein, G.F. Bryce, B.B. Gallagher

52. "Bone Necrosis and Metabolic Bone Disease" S.Y.P. Wong, C.R. Dunstan, E. Hills, C. Needs, J. Garvan, R.A. Evans

53. "Effect of Calcium and Some Calciotrophic Drugs on Hormonal Homeostasis" I. Zofkova

OVERVIEW OF FIRST POSTER SESSION

L.V. Avioli and H. Duncan

School of Medicine, Washington University, St. Louis, MO 63110; Dept. of Medicine, Division of Rheumatology, Henry Ford Hospital, Detroit, MI 48202, U.S.A.

There are increasing numbers of observations which suggest that measurements of bone mass or mineral density in an arm or leg do not necessarily have a correlation with the vertebral bone mass. Despite these observations, the accumulated data have prompted investigations of: (1) the precision and accuracy of the methods; (2) the appropriateness of comparing one skeletal site with another; (3) the relevance of cortical bone and trabecular bone mass and volume to each other; and (4) the clinical syndromes associated with bone loss, particularly related to the specific age, sex and reproductive status of the normal and target populations. Consequently a number of papers and posters focused on different aspects of these situations.

The introduction of the dual photon absorptiometric method of bone mass assessment has permitted an accurate measurement of vertebral bone mass and total body bone mineral (i.e., calcium). Borg, Gotfredsen, Christiansen, et al. compared the mineral content of the distal forearm with total body mineral. In healthy subjects, age and sex matched, there was no significant difference between the two methods. The reproducibility of the results of the dual photon method showed a co-efficient of variation at an acceptable value of 2 to 3 percent. Similar figures were reported by other authors (Heron, et al., Markhard et al., Powell et al., Schaadt and Bohr). Both methods documented a reduction of mineral mass at the time of the menopause. In men, there was a diversion of observations with respect to the radial mass measurements and the total bone mineral, the latter revealing no decline with age. Some limitations of methods which assessed vertebral bone mass were recognized in a paper of Marcod et al. (and voiced by Nordin) wherein the *in vivo* mineral mass of individual vertebrae was determined and then the *in vitro* estimate of the same vertebrae was determined both with and without the transverse and spinous processes. It is alleged that the appendages of the vertebrae are metabolically unlike trabecular bone. After the menopause, spinal bone mineral content was 8 to 9% lower than before, for a given radial bone mineral content, while the relationship between total body bone mineral and the radial mineral content was not altered by the menopause (Markhard et al.). These relationships were examined also in osteoporotic patients and in patients receiving glucocorticoid therapy (Gotfredsen et al., Markhard et al., Mazess and Schaadt and Bohr). Studies on the osteoporotic group showed uniform bone loss. The best discriminant between osteoporotics (symptomatic) and normals was the central density assessment for the vertebrae (Markhard et al.), which again excluded appendages of the vertebrae and avoided the error associated with edge location; this latter, is particularly troublesome in assessment of densitometric values in the severely osteoporotic patients (Markhard et al. and Powell).

In patients with rheumatoid arthritis, bone mineral was significantly lower than that observed in normals. This was further decreased when these arthritic patients were treated with glucocorticoids (Gotfredsen). However, Schaadt and Bohr reported that whereas the bone mineral content was significantly reduced in the axial skeleton by the use of glucocorticoid therapy, there was no significant change in the femoral cortical bone mass in the same patients. It may be of note that in Schaadt's group of 64 glucocorticoid treated subjects, 13 had chronic liver disease which may have altered slightly the nature of the metabolic bone status. In this regard, D'Amore et al. and Atkinson et al. demonstrated that approximately 55% of their patients with chronic liver disease had 25 hydroxy vitamin D levels below the normal range, and a high frequency of this low plasma level was also reported in primary biliary cirrhosis by Varghese et al. and in alcoholic cirrhosis by Arlet et al.

New quantitative methods and more refined approaches to the measurement of mineral content and structure of the vertebral body have been introduced by modifications of computerized tomography techniques. Five presentations were directed both towards the accuracy of the method (Dambacher et al., Olah, Rüegsegger, Nordin et al., O'Keeffe et al., Torres et al.), as well as to comparison with other methods. Dambacher et al. observed considerable variations in the rate of trabecular bone loss in osteoporotic postmenopausal females. As a group, they lost 2.7% of bone per year. Three of 12 had no bone loss in a 3 year observation, whereas the remaining 9 showed losses between 2 and 20% over the same period. Interestingly, most of these patients lost bone in a step-wise fashion; phases of relative stability were followed by brief phases of acute bone loss. Preliminary studies using fluoride (80 mg. per day) in osteoporotic females revealed that only 1 in 3 subjects responded with an increase in trabecular bone during the two year treatment period. Cortical bone showed no differences between the treated and the nontreated group. There was also a report describing a good coorelation between the estimates of trabecular bone density measured by histomorphometry and that determined by the non-invasive computerized tomography (Ohal, Rüegsegger and Dambacher).

Neutron activation of both total and regional body estimates of mineral content apparently fails to differentiate between the extraosseous mineral and bone (Mazier et al.). This report showed that postmenopausal bone loss from the 7th thoracic vertebra correlated poorly with the mineral content of bone loss in the hand. In another study trabecular bone mass of the 4th lumbar vertebra was determined by computed tomography in 17 patients treated with hemodialysis for 1 to 4 years, and in 6 patients who received a renal transplant. This paper of Torres et al. reported a mean increase in trabecular bone mass of 10.5% in the dialyzed patients and this change correlated closely with the quantitation of radiological subperiosteal resorption of the cortex, as well as the serum alkaline phosphatase levels, thus suggesting influence of parathyroid hormones. Although the 6 renal transplant subjects showed a decrease of 13.73% of total bone mass at 3 months after transplantation, at 12 months the mean trabecular bone mass had shown an increase of 7.34%. As with many studies of patients with renal osteodystrophy, there are regional peculiarities and further investigation by this method at different centers is necessary.

Reeve and coworkers correlated bone mass measured in calcium balances over an 18 day period with serial densitometric studies and photon absorptiometry; they conceded that the computed tomography studies would be more precise. Further attempts at measuring bone turnover in different metabolic diseases and in normals was made by the use of labelled and unlabelled diphosphonate compounds (Hyldstrup et al. and Passeri et al.) with analysis of blood dilution curves and urinary excretion; correlation between both methods was high ($r = 0.93$).

Qualitative and quantitative histological studies (Miller et al., Vedi, Kompston and Webb, Wong et al.) emphasized that degrees of histological osteomalacia may be overlooked. It is evident again that careful definition and attention to methods involved have to be clearly understood when references to clinical and histological osteomalacia are made. Detailed studies of the construction of trabeculae (Kragstrup, Melsen et al.) focussed attention upon the lamellar orientation and the lamellar thickness. These observers noted that lamellar thickness in males was unchanged throughout life, while a slight but significant increase in thickness was noted in females. There was no specific change in the pattern at the time of the menopause. They felt that the lamellar thickness was a standardized pattern and that attention to its variation in metabolic bone disease and bone stability might be as important as the bone mineral content itself. A unique computerized model identifying the bone remodelling unit was presented by Demling et al.

Harrelson et al. suggested that some histomorphometric studies of tetracycline labelling might be different in different laboratories if sections of variable thickness were used for these histological calculations. This group observed that there was a gross discrepancy between their estimate of the "mineralization front" dimensions (tetracycline labelling length) when a 5 micron thick section was compared with a section 10 microns thick, each obtained from the same block. They suggested that differences as great as 30% increase were noted in the length of the tetracycline label on the thicker slide, whereas the observations on successive sections at 20 and 40 microns in thickness, there was an increase of tetracycline labelling length of 10% and 28% respectively above that seen on the 10 micron thick slide. Frost suggested that in thicker slides the depth of "optical sectioning" is considerably thinner than the section itself and "racking up and down" the microscope objective to view the full thickness would increase the distribution and number of optical sections, hence giving rise to altered measurements. There are also other reasons to compare inter-laboratory values, since the methods of fixing, embedding, staining and cutting techniques as well as duration of exposure to the ultra violet light all need standardization.

Increasing emphasis was placed upon the importance of recognizing separate clinical fracture syndromes; vertebral compression fractures occurred a decade earlier than the mean age for long-bone fractures in postmenopausal women (Johnston and Meunier). These authors reported observations on iliac bone biopsies from approximately 30 individuals of each group. In those who sustained vertebral fractures, the serum PTH level was significantly higher and the radial bone mass was significantly lower than normal. Those with femoral fractures had PTH levels which were also higher than normal, but the radial mineral mass was normal. They recognized that these were deviations from the expected results when PTH, calcium, trabecular and cortical bone masses were measured in all subjects. Jacobson et al. reported on a population of normal college women subjected to single photon absorptiometry studies and included tennis players (10), swimmers (17) and age matched controls (34). All but one had normal monthly menstrual cycles, but the use of birth control pills was not identified. The tennis players' non-dominant radial photon absorptiometric readings were not different from those of the controls. However, the radial bone width and bone mineral content of the dominant hand of the tennis players and the swimmers were increased above normal. Speculations on the amount of activity needed to maintain this mineral advantage were numerous. Utilizing single and dual photon absorptiometry at the radial and lumbar sites respectively, these authors also examined groups of premenopausal and postmenopausal female tennis athletes. The results indicated that these groups as a whole showed wider radii and more bone mineral per unit volume than their non-athletic age-matched controls. It is evident that longitudinal studies are imperative in followup of this interesting study.

In the assessment of patients with hypercalcemia, Licata and Hawker, indicated that there was a simultaneous alteration of serum glycoproteins in patients with malignancies. Consequently, analysis of the glycoproteins and sialic acid could help differentiate malignant from benign hypercalcemia. Larson and Toss emphasized that ionized calcium ("the active calcium fraction") correlates better with abnormal metabolic clinical states than the total or corrected serum calcium levels. This factor was utilized by Weinstein et al. in a series of 109 patients receiving anti-convulsant drugs. These workers observed that serum ionized calcium levels increased after therapy with calcium and vitamin D, and there was a simultaneous decrease in seizure frequency. The bone mineral content in these subjects was 89.8 $\pm$ 0.6% of normal values and the bone histology showed features of high turnover bone rather than osteomalacia.

By using a radioactive fluoride and blood flow study, Tellez et al. showed that the skeletal blood flow in osteomalacia was increased and that the blood flow through bone in osteopenia was reduced proportional to the reduction of the bone mass. However their observation that a considerable amount of bone is supplied by blood from the portal system of the bone marrow reinforces the necessity to study the endosteal and trabecular bone surfaces and their interrelationship with the bone marrow. It is at these sites where the dominant changes in osteopenic states occur. In the past it has been suggested provocatively that osteoporosis is a "disease of the expanding bone marrow."

SECOND SCIENTIFIC POSTER SESSION - BONE PHYSIOLOGY, HYPERCALCEMIA PARATHYROID DISORDERS - PRIMARY AND SECONDARY, OSTEOMALACIA AND RENAL OSTEODYSTROPHY

MODERATORS: C. ARNAUD, A. NORMAN

1. "Bone Mineral Density and Surgery for Primary Hyperparathyroidism" E.M. Alhava, P. Karjalainen

2. "Pathophysiology of Osteoporosis After Kidney Transplantation" D. Babarykin, R. Rosental

3. "Aluminum (AL) Accumulation in Nondialyzed (ND) Azotemic Children Due to Oral Aluminum Hydroxide (AH)" S.P. Andreoli, J.M. Bergstein, D. J. Sherrard

4. "Chromosome 20 Deletion in Multiple Endocrine Neoplasia Syndrome Types 2A and 2B" V.R. Babu, D.L. VanDyke, C.E. Jackson

5. "Hypercalcemia Due to Renal Carcinoma Producing 25(OH)D_3? G. Beccari, E. Grossi, A. Del Noce

6. "Can Adrenergic Stimulation Tests Be Used in the Diagnosis of Hyperparathyroidism?" L. Benson, S. Ljunghall, C. Rudberg, L. Wide, G. Akerstrom

7. "No Effects of Secretin Infusion on PTH in Normal Subjects or Patients with HPT" L. Benson. S. Ljunghall, L. Wide, G. Akerstrom, K. Oberg

8. "Treatment of Osteoposoris and Similar Diseases with Ipriflavone" A. Bossanyi, L. Feuer

9. "Preliminary Investigation into the Metabolic Fate of (10S(19)^{3}H)-Dihydrotachysterol - 2(^{3}H-DHT_2) in Rats" R. Bosch, W.J. Visser, J.M.M. Roelofs, S.A. Duursma

10. "Renal Osteodystrophy Progress despite Parathyroid Hormone Loss in Peritoneal Dialysate" G. Buccianti, M.L. Bianchi, G. Valenti, E. Corghi M. Cecchettin, E.E. Polli

11. "The Influence of Sucralfate Ingestion on Aluminum (Al) Metabolism in Normal Rats" M.A. Burnatowska-Hledin, G.H. Mayor

12. "Oncogenic Hypophosphatemic Osteomalacia with Low Serum 1,25$(OH)_2$D Unresponsive to Parathyroid Extract" L. Checchio, H. Linto Wray

13. "Vitamin D Deficiency and Osteomalacia in Patients with Hip Fractures - An Unrecognized Epidemic" S.H. Doppelt, R.M. Neer, M. Daly, L. Bourret, A. Schiller, M. Holick, H.J. Mankin

14. "Effects of Primary Oxalosis on Bone Structure and Metabolism" F. Christ, H.U. Klehr, G. Anders

15. "The Cellular Basis of Metastatic Bone Disease in Patients with Breast Cancer" S.F. Cramer, W.R. Rader

16. "Subtotal Parathyroidectomy for Hyperparathyroidism Associated with Renal Failure" F.L. Delmonico, A.B. Cosimi, N.T. Rubin, C.A. Wang

17. "Osteomalacia in Dialyzed Patients: A Role for Vitamin Therapy?" M.C. de Vernejoul, H. Halkidou, R. Berlénguer, M. Bussine, L. Miravet

18. "Respective Role of Desferrioxamine and of Osmosedwater Dialysis in Arresting Progression of Aluminum-induced Osteomalacia" M.D. de Vernejoul A. Meyrier, H. Halkidou, L. Miravet

19. "Bone Disease During Long-term Parenteral Nutrition" M.D. de Vernejoul, B. Messing, M. Bussine, J. Bielakoff, L. Miravet

20. "Primary Hyperparathyroidism: Persistent Autonomy During 4-8 Year Post-Surgical Follow-up" B. Duarte, R.J. Santen, L.M. Demers, R.E. Reitz, T.S. Harrison

21. "PTH, Vitamin D, Aluminum and Bone in Chronic Renal Failure" C.R. Dunstan, R.A. Evans, S.Y.P. Wong, E. Hills, A.W. Norman, G.F. Bryce

22. "The Effect of 1,25 DHCC and 24,25 DHCC Alone and in Combination in Chronic Renal Failure" C.R. Dunstan, R.A. Evans, S.Y.P. Wong, E. Hills, A.W. Norman, A. Alfrey, G.F. Bryce

23. "Bone Mineral Content (BMC) in Diabetic and Nondiabetic Hemodialysis Patients" R. Estes, G. Willie, C. Cruz, G. Zasuwa, N.W. Levin, A. M. Parfitt, M. Kleerekoper

24. "Iatrogenic Bone Aluminum Intoxication in Patients with Mild to Moderate Renal Failrue" M.C. Faugere, K. Abreo, A. Smith, R.M. Friedler, H.H. Malluche

25. "Pharmacologic Doses of 24,25-Dihydroxycholecalciferol (24,25-D_3) Do Not Produce 'Medical Parathyroidectomy' in Hypercalcemic Kidney Transplant Recipients" M. Friedlander, R. Horst, C. Hawker

26. "Bone Lesions and Dental Caries After Gastrectomy" M. Fukuda, M. Hirota, Y. Yamagishi, S. Sato

27. "The Morphometry of Hepatic Osteodystrophy in Primary Biliary Cirrhosis: Relationship to the Liver Disease" C.N. Ghent, A.B. Hodsman, C. Anderson

28. "Parathyroid and Vitamin D Response to Parenteral Aluminum Administration" W.G. Goodman, D.A. Henry, R. Horst, R.K. Nudelman, E. Slatopolsky, J.W. Coburn

29. "Dynamic Testing, Using a New Radioimmunoassay for NH_2- Terminal PTH - Improves Discrimination Between Normal and Abnormal Parathyroid Function" S.T. Harris, R.M. Neer, G.V. Segre, J.T. Potts, Jr.

30. "Carbamazepine and Bone Mineral Metabolism" V. Hoikka, E.M. Alhava, P. Karjalainen, T. Keranen, K. Savolainen

31. "Serum Aluminum in Hemodialyzed Patients with Renal Osteodystrophy" S. Hosokawa, S. Kohira, T. Tomoyoshi

32. "The Relationship Between Mild Renal Osteodystrophy (ROD) and Severe ROD Group in the Value of Serum Immunoreactive Parathyroid Hormone (iPTH) and Serum Immunoreactive Calcitonin (iCT) of Chronic Hemodialyzed Patients" S. Hosokawa, S. Kohira, T. Tomoyoshi

33. "Bone 'Buffering' Capacity in Aluminum Associated Bone Disease (AABD)" B.U. Ihle, M. Cochran, G. Becker, D. Campbell, P. Kincaid-Smith

34. "Functional Evaluation of Parathyroid Adenomas and Hyperplasia by Immunoperoxidase Staining" W.W. Johnson, R.E. Lewis, Jr., B. Allen, N.C. Nelson, J.M. Cruse

35. "Histological Methods of Assessing Bone Resorption in Uremia" J.A. Kanis, T. Cundy, M. Beneton, C.G. Woods, M. Earnshaw, R. Smith

36. "Fanconi Syndrome - Osteomalacia and Hypoparathyroidism" S. Khoury, J.R. Tucci

37. "Evidence for A Generalized Derangement in the Regulation of Renal 25-OH-D-1α-Hydroxylase (1-OHase) in X-Linked Hypophosphatemic Rickets (XLH)" B. Lobuagh, M.K. Drezner

38. "Sodium Etidronate Alters Vitamin D Metabolism in Man" P.J. Lawson-Matthew, D.F. Guilland-Cumming, A.J.P. Yates, R.G.D. Russell, J.A. Kanis

39. "Assessment of an Oral Calcium Tolerance Test in the Diagnosis of Primary Hyperparathyroidism (HPT)" P. Madvig, R. Marcus

40. "Acute Mid-day Changes in Serum Ionized Calcium and Parathyroid Hormone Mid-region Immunoreactivity: Accentuated Diurnal Fall in Calcium During Lactation" L. Mallette, J. Kirkland

41. "Various Types of Skeletal Remodeling in Three Patients with Osteosclerosis" E. Manzke, D. Leupold, H. Gruber, D. Baylink

42. "Reversible and Irreversible Skeletal Disease in Celiac Enteropathy (Non-tropical sprue)" G. Marel, D.S. Rao, M. Kleerekoper, M. Mathews, B. Frame, A.M. Parfitt

43. "Blood Pressure Response to Changes in Serum Calcium During Hemodialysis" J.C. Maynard, C. Cruz, G. Zasuwa, J. Meister, D. Kaufman, D. Valade, M. Kleerekoper, N.W. Levin

44. "The Periosteal and Juxtaperiosteal Components of Hyperparathyroid Bone Resorption in Chronic Renal Failure" H.E. Meema, D.G. Oreopoulos

45. "Osteomalacia in Adults: Clinical and Biochemical Features" P.D. Miller, W.E. Huffer, R.A. Krebs, B.J. Neal, D.O. McIntyre

46. "Response to Desferrioxamine Infusion in Patients with Dialysis Osteomalacia" D.S. Milliner, A.C. Alfrey, D.J. Sherrard, S.M. Ott, J.H. Shinaberger, A.R. Nissenson, J.W. Coburn

47. "Comparison of 1α(OH) Vitamin D3 and Calcium Carbonate for the Control of Hyperparathyroidism and Hyperaluminemia in Patients on Chronic Hemodialysis" Ph. Moriniere, I. Gregoire, M.A. Herve, J. Gueris, Y. Tahiri, J.L. Sebert, A. Fournier

48. "Aluminum (Al) Intoxication Hypercalcemia and Osteomalacia in Hemodialysis Patients: Treatment with Desferrioxamine" A.H. Mudde, A. P. Roodvoets

49. "Collagen Markers in Cancer" G.M.A. Palmieri, H.B. Niell, J. Seyer, C.L. Neely, M.S. Soloway, A.B. Hinton

50. "Bone Aluminum in a Liver Transplant Patient" J.A. Pitcock, G.M.A. Palmieri, J.W. Williams, T.G. Peters, S. Vera, S.R. Acchiardo

51. "Mangement of Tumor-Induced Hypercalcemia with Amino-Hydroxypropylidene Biphosphonate (APD)" L. Portmann, J.M. Haefliger, G. Bill, P. Burckhardt

52. "Ultrasonic Guidance of Fine Needle Biopsies of Parathyroid Adenomas" J. Rastad, P.G. Lindgren, L. Grimelius, S. Ljunghall, B. Stenkvist, H. Johnansson, G. Akerstrom

53. "Pathogenesis of Aluminum-Associated Osteomalacia in Hemodialysis Patients" E.S. Ricanati, S.M. Ott, K.L. Klein, M. Lamm, N.L. Miller, D.J. Sherrard, A.C. Alfrey, E. Slatopolsky, J.W. Coburn

54. "Effects of Thyroid Hormone Excess on Mineral and Bone Metabolism" J.D. Lalau, J.L. Sebert, A. Marie, A. Smadja, A. Fournier, J. Quichaud

55. "Adenyl Cyclase Bioassay for PTH- Some Clinical Experiences" M.S. Seshadri, Y.L. Chan, M. Wilkinson, S. Posen

56. "The Use of Cimetidine in the Preoperative Preparation of the Primary Hyperparathyroid Patient" J.K. Sherwood, F.W. Ackroyd, M. Garcia

57. "Cimetidine for the Preoperative Preparation of the Patient with Primary Hyperparathyroidism" J.K. Sherwood, F.W. Ackroyd, M. Garcia

58. "Cimetidine in the Diagnosis of Parathyroid Disease" J.K. Sherwood, F.W. Ackroyd, M. Garcia

59. "Familial Adult-Onset Hypophosphataemic Osteomalacia with Fanconi Syndrome. Studies of Myopathy" R. Smith, R.J. Newman, G.K. Radda, M. Stokes, A. Young

60. "The Relevance of Routine Skeletal Surveys of Patients on Maintenance Hemodialysis" M. Sundaram, M.K. Wolverson, E. Heiberg, J.B. Shields

61. "Oncogenic Osteomalacia and Siadh Due to Oat Cell Carcinoma" M. Fallon, H.C. Taylor, M.E. Velasco

62. "Recurrent Hyperparathyroidism in Chronic Renal Failure" H. Takagi, Y. Tominaga, K. Uchida, N. Yamada, M. Kawai, T. Morimoto, H. Suzuki

63. "Polymorphism of Parathyroid Glands of Secondary Hyperparathyroidism in Patients with Chronic Renal Failure" H. Takagi, Y. Tominaga, K. Uchida, N. Yamada, K. Kawahara, T. Kano, H. Suzuki

64. "'Osteoporosis' and Non-Secretory Myeloma" E.J. VanSlyck, M. Kleerekoper, J.P. Abraham, M.J. Deegan

65. "Does Calcium Mediate High Renin Renal Hypertension?" E.T. Zawada, Jr., M. Johnson

OVERVIEW OF SECOND POSTER SESSION

Claude D. Arnaud, M.D. and Anthony W. Norman, Ph.D.*

Endocrine Unit, V.A. Medical Center and Departments of Medicine and Physiology, University of California, San Francisco, CA, U.S.A.

*Department of Biochemistry, University of California, Riverside, CA, U.S.A.

Twelve posters were selected from the Tuesday, May 10, 1983, poster session for 5 minute presentations before a general meeting of the participants; six concerning parathyroid disorders, and six related to clinical problems of vitamin D metabolism. Each of these was followed by a lively 10-15 minute discussion period which brought out important details of individual studies and related information obtained in similar investigations performed by discussants.

Harris et al. used a new, extremely sensitive radioimmunoassay (RIA) of the biologically active region of parathyroid hormone (PTH) to perform dynamic testing of parathyroid function in normal subjects and patients with surgically confirmed primary hyperparathyroidism (1°HPT). Calcium infusions in normal subjects regularly decreased serum immunoreactive PTH (iPTH) to undetectable values (<5 pg/ml). In sharp contrast, increasing serum ionized calcium (Ca^{++}) by 1.9 mM did not decrease serum iPTH below 8 pg/ml in 1° HPT patients. Further studies using EDTA infusions to lower serum Ca^{++} permitted these investigators to develop a family of "log dose" curves describing the relationship of serum Ca^{++} to iPTH. These curves revealed a higher serum Ca^{++} "set point" for serum iPTH suppression in 1° HPT patients than in normals, clearly demonstrating the "semi-autonomous" nature of abnormal parathyroid gland tissue. Perhaps the most important practical clinical consequence of this work is that dynamic testing of the type described showed abnormalities of iPTH responses to Ca^{++} infusions in patients with mild hypercalcemia and normal basal values for serum iPTH. More discouraging, however, was the investigators' confirmation of previous studies showing that dynamic testing fails to discriminate between patients with "hyperplasia" and "adenoma."

Madvig et al. evaluated the oral calcium tolerance test (previously described by Broadus et al. to distinguish normal subjects from patients with 1°HPT) in age matched older normals (mean age = 63) and patients with 1°HPT (mean age = 60). They were able to validate the test in younger subjects based on increases in urine and serum calcium and decreases in urine cyclic AMP. However, they found that the differences in calcium excretion, serum calcium, and urine cyclic AMP between older aged matched normal and 1°HPT patients were minimal and that such testing failed to distinguish between these two groups. Although it will be interesting to see if future evaluation of the calcium tolerance test in older subjects will show similar results, the present study is extremely important because the majority of patients with 1°HPT are over 50 years old. The test generates a number of somewhat costly laboratory measurements and it probably should not be used to evaluate older patients until it is investigated further.

One of the most important current questions in the management of older patients with mild or "asymptomatic" 1°HPT is whether surgical cure of 1°HPT will result in an improvement in the frequently observed decreased bone mineral density. Alhava et al. provided a preliminary answer in his interesting presentation. He measured distal radial bone mineral density in 30 older patients with 1°HPT (26 women, 4 men) before and after parathyroidectomy. Before surgery, there was an 11% decrease in this index compared to controls. After surgery, bone mineral density progressively increased until it was only 2% lower than controls at 48 months. Further studies of this type, using multiple methods and sites of bone mineral density measurement are clearly indicated; but for the moment, the results of Alhava's simple but important study suggests that, 1) the diagnosis of 1°HPT should be intensively sought in all patients with diminished bone mineral density and, 2) parathyroidectomy should be performed in such patients if 1°HPT is identified and the patient is a reasonable surgical risk.

The localization of parathyroid tumors, so that they can be easily removed at surgery, is one of the most formidable problems in the treatment of 1°HPT. Recent non-invasive techniques, such as ultrasound of the neck and computerized tomography of the neck and mediastinum have provided a reliable means of localizing lesions which might be parathyroid in origin. Rastad et al. have gone one step further and performed fine needle biopsies of tumors in patients with suspected 1°HPT under ultrasonic guidance to histologically identify such lesions. Their report suggests the possibility of a simple, rapid means of histologically proving the diagnosis of 1°HPT in hypercalcemic patients, thus circumventing more costly and classical metabolic investigations. We (CDA) have used a similar approach, supplemented with PTH bioassay or RIA of extracts of biopsy obtained tissue, with considerable success except that our investigations have been confined to patients with recurrent or persistent 1°HPT.

The advisability of continued medical treatment, as opposed to surgical extirpation of hyperplastic parathyroid glands in patients with chronic renal failure, remains a difficult clinical decision. Delmonico et al. reported their experience with the results of subtotal parathyoidectomy (3 glands and all but 50-75 mg of a remaining gland) in 38 such patients with bone pain. Hyperparathyroidism of clinical significance occured in only 2 patients, 5 and 8 years after parathyroidectomy and resection of the residual parathyroid tissue in these patients restored eucalcemia. With the gradual appearance of greater surgical sophistication in parathryoid surgery and the major advances in non-invasive localization techniques, I (CDA) expect that the frequency of surgical therapy for secondary hyperparathyroidism will increase and the sequellae of hyperparathyroidism during the post-transplant period will diminish.

The chronic treatment of malignancy associated hypercalcemia (MAH) remains one of the most challenging and difficult problems in clinical medicine. Although Bijvoet et al. have demonstrated the usefulness of the drug, Amino-hydroxypropylidene biphosphonate (APD), in this syndrome, Portman et al. reported their experience with it in 14 patients with MAH. In confirmation of the Bijvoet group, serum calcium decreased towards normal within 4 days of the initiation of APD treatment, and tended to remain in the normal range for as long as 4 weeks. Relapses occured within several weeks in 4 patients and 2 of these responded to retreatment. Few adverse effects were observed; one patient developed hypocalcemia and another, fever. Unfortunately, APD is not available in North America and there seems to be some question as to whether it will ever undergo extensive, multicenter evaluation. Based on the studies available, however, it represents a very appealing approach to the management of a vexing therapeutic problem.

Of particular note were the studies of Lobaugh and Drezner, who reported on the regulation of the renal 25-hydroxyvitamin D-1α-hydroxylase (1α-hydroxylase) in X-linked hypophosphatemic rickets (XLH). Their studies were carried out in Hyp mice and examined whether the renal 1α-hydroxylase activity in the Hyp mouse responds to known modulators of enzyme activity in comparison to the 1α-hydroxylase of the normal mouse kidney. Neither phosphate depletion, nor high levels of PTH, nor low levels of serum calcium significantly elevated the measurable 1α-hydroxylase enzyme activity of the Hyp mouse. Thus, their evidence suggests that the renal 1α-hydroxylase of the Hyp mouse is not stimulated above basal levels by any of the generally acknowledged modulators of the 1α-hydroxylase activity; this in turn suggests that there may be a ubiquitous defect of regulation. It is intriguing to speculate that this may also be the case in the human form of XLH.

Checchio et al. determined whether subjects with oncogenic hypophosphatemic osteomalacia are capable of elevating their serum level of $1,25(OH)_2D$ in response to the administration of exogenous parathyroid hormone extract. Hypophosphatemic osteomalacia is known to be associated with benign mesenchymal tumors and such subjects characteristically have inappropriately low circulating levels of $1,25(OH)_2D_3$. These workers noted an absence of a detectable increase in serum $1,25(OH)_2D$ after infusion of PTH in spite of a normal urine cyclic - AMP response. This suggests that the defect in oncogenic hypophosphatemic osteomalacia is an inability to respond to the changes in renal tubular cyclic AMP.

Freidlander et al. reported the results of administration of phamacological doses of 24R-25-dihydroxyvitamin D_3 in three hypercalcemic adults with 1°HPT and normal kidney function. They were provided 60 µg/day of $24,25(OH)_2D_3$ for a period of three months. In spite of reports that the parathyroid gland has receptors for $24,25(OH)_2D_3$, these authors noted no changes in serum iPTH at any time. Consequently, the authors concluded that $24,25(OH)_2D_3$ did not suppress parathyroid hormone secretion in the clinical setting of persistent hyperparathyroidism.

Two papers presented results which bear on the very topical problem of aluminum intoxication in patients with end-stage renal failure. Aluminum accumulation in bone may reduce bone formation and cause osteomalacia in dialysis patients as well as in patients treated with total parenteral nutrition. The mechanisms of the bone toxicity remain undefined and yet present the clinician with challenging problems of management. Goodman et al. developed an animal model of this disease wherein six dogs received parenteral aluminum (1 mg/kg/day for 3-5 weeks). Serum immunoreactive PTH (iPTH) and vitamin D levels were measured as well as serum calcium and other blood parameters. The maximum serum iPTH response to EDTA induced hypocalcemia was the same before (510% versus 476%) as after 10 days of aluminum loading, serum ionized calcium also did not change. Intriguingly, the serum levels of $1,25(OH)_2D$ fell from 27 to 12 pg/ml and in four dogs serum $1,25(OH)_2D$ was undetectable by day 17. These results indicate that the short term administration of aluminum neither reduces basal iPTH levels nor impairs the PTH response to acute hypocalcemia in vivo. However, it does mediate, by unknown mechanisms, a reduction in the serum level of $1,25(OH)_2D$. These data are consistent with the suggestion that aluminum intoxication may result in the impaired renal synthesis of $1,25(OH)_2D_3$.

Milliner et al. studied the responses to infusion of desferrioxamine in patients maintained on dialysis who have detectable osteomalacia as a consequence of possible aluminum intoxication. The basis of the study is that desferrioximine (DFO) is capable of chelating aluminum. The objective was to determine whether prolonged treatment with DFO might reduce the body burden of aluminum. The authors evaluated the serum and bone content of aluminum and the changes in serum aluminum after the infusion of desferrioxamine (DFO) in 9 hemodialysis patients with bone biopsy proved osteomalacia. Following the IV infusion of DFO (either 40 mg/kg or 80 mg/kg), serum aluminum rose to 408% and 583%, respectively, of the baseline value. Furthermore, there was an associated removal of aluminum during hemodialysis with dialyzer clearances of 34 ml/min with cuprophane membranes. These studies dramatically indicate that infusion of DFO can mediate a substantial increment in serum aluminum in dialysis patients and suggest that further trials with DFO are warranted to identify whether it is possible, with prolonged treatment, to significantly reduce the body burden of aluminum.

Doppelt et al. evaluated the incidence of vitamin D deficiency and osteomalacia in patients with hip fractures in the Boston, Massachusetts, area. Of 142 patients with hip fractures admitted to the Masschusetts General Hospital, 22% had serum 25(OH)D levels below normal (normal = 8-55 ng/ml). Thirty percent of the patients had biopsy proved osteomalacia. These results suggest that a surprisingly high percentage of patients with hip fractures are vitamin D deficient and have consequent osteomalacia. The important questions regarding this study are whether the patient population studied were in some way selected and whether future studies in other geographic areas will be confirmatory.

THIRD SCIENTIFIC POSTER SESSION - OSTEOPOROSIS, PAGET'S, CALCITONIN HYPERCALCIURIA, PEDIATRIC BONE DISEASES

MODERATORS: R. LINDSAY, D. FRASER, A TASHIJIAN

1. "Bone Loss in Osteoporosis: Reduced Bone Formation and Increased Resorption Indices both Correlate with Negative Calcium Balance M. Arlot, J. Reeve, D. Slovik, J. Vismans, J.C. Renier, P.J. Meunier

2. "Effect of Parity on the Age-related Bone Loss in Control and Thyrotóxic Women" A. Argyropoulos, K. Alevizaki, D. Ikkos, K. Ntalles, P. Singhellakis, H. Vassilopoulos

3. "Lack of Hypercalcemia in Immobilized Children" S. Bachrach, T. Sterner

4. "Pathogenesis of Postmenopausal Osteoporosis" J.R. Buchanan

5. "Renal Resistance to PTH with Osteitis Fibrosa Cystica" M. Burnstein, S. Kottamasu, B. Frame

6. "Growth and Skeletal Maturation in Vitamin D Resistant Rickets (VDRR) Treated with Oral Phosphate Salts and Vitamin D_2 or $1,25(OH)_2D$" G. Chabot, F.H. Glorieux

7. "Hypercalcitonemia in Toxic-Shock Syndrome (TSS)" R. Chapman, C. Lauter, L. Ospina, J. Colville, D. Batts

8. "Renal Tubular Calcium (Ca) Reabsorption (TRCa) in Idiopathic Hypercalciuria (IH)" G. Colussi, M. Surian, G. Pontoriero, G. Rombola, M.E. DeFerrari, F. Malberti, P. Cosci, A. Marni, L. Minetti

9. "Reduced Bone Mineral Mass in Secondary Amenorrhea" E. Corghi, M.P. Caraceni, T. Motta, M.L. Bianchi, L. Soldati, E.E. Polli

10. "Calcium Absorption in Corticosteroid Treated Subjects With and Without Osteoporosis" R.G. Crilly, B.E.C. Nordin, D.H. Marshall

11. "Effect of Carbohydrate Content of Low Calorie Liquid Diets on Calcium Balance During Dieting for Obesity" M. Davie

12. "Bone Matrix Protein Profile in Femoral Head Specimens from Osteoporosis and Osteoarthrosis Cases" J.M. Mbuyi, J. Dequeker

13. "Reflex Sympathetic Dystrophy and Vertebral Crush Fracture Syndrome" J. Dequeker, P. Geusens, A. Verstraeten

14. "The Prophylaxis of Nutritional Rickets: The Lessons of the Glasgow Prevention of Asian Rickets Campaign" M.G. Dunnigan, J.B. Henderson, B.M. Glekin, W.B. McIntosh

15. "Vitamin D Deficiency in Saudi Arabia Inspite of the Sunshine" A.T.H. Elidrissy, S.H. Sedrani, K. Arabi

16. "The Treatment of Paget's Disease of Bone" R.A. Evans

17. "Calcitriol Replacement Therapy During Pregnancy and Lactation in a Vitamin D Dependency Type I Patient (VDD-I)" E.E. Delvin, F.H. Glorieux, G. Chabot

18. "Calcitonin Secretion in Glucocorticoid-Treated Patients" C. Gennari, M. Bernini, P. Nardi, L. Fusi, F. Zacchei

19. "Mineral Content of Forearms of Babies Born to Asian and Caucasian Women" D. Gillies, P. Congdon, A. Horsman, J. Dibble

20. "Semi-Quantitative Determiniation of Chronic Osteoporosis from Radiographs of Long Bones" C.S. Revak, T. Gillespy,III

21. "Flouride and Subclinical Rickets Among Immigrant Children in Glasgow" K.M. Goel, R.W. Logan, E.M. Sweet, R.A. Shanks

22. "Reduced Prevalence of Rickets in Asian Children in Glasgow" K.M. Goel, S. Campbell, R.W. Logan, E.M. Sweet, G.C. Arneil

23. "Familial Hypercalcemia: Hypercalciuria and Hypocalciuria in A Small Kindred" D.A. Hanley

24. "Changes in Bone Mass During 1½ Years (3-Amino-1-Hydroxypylidene)-1-1-Biophosphonate (APD) Treatment of Generalized, Osteolytic Multicystic Paget's Disease" L. Hyldstrup, J. Karlsen, G.F. Jensen, P. McNair, I. Transbol

25. "Identification of Subpopulations in Postmenopausal Osteoporotics by Cluster Analysis" J.L. Ivey, H.E. Gruber, D.J. Baylink, C.H. Chesnut

26. "Smokers Bones Revisited by Epidemiological Approach" G.F. Jensen, L. Hyldstrup

27. "Paget's Disease Mimicking Metastasis" S. Kattapuram, W. Phillips

28. "Vitamin D Metabolism and Prophylaxis in the Preterm Infant" I. Kovar, P. Mayne, J. James, I. Barnes, U. Hennes

29. "Hypocalcemia in Patients with Carcinoma of Prostate" S.C. Kukreja, A. Shanmugam, J.H. Shah, G.A. Williams

30. "Assessment of the Efficacy of Fluoride Associated With 25 OH Cholecalciferol in the Treatment of Primary Osteoporosis" D. Kuntz, P. Marie, B. Naveau, B. Maziere

31. "Long Term Phosphate Supplementation: Clinical and Metabolic Effects in Renal Stone Formers" B. Wikstrom, U. Backman, B.G. Danielson, B. Fellstrom, G. Johnansson, S. Ljunghall, L. Wide

32. "Postpregnancy Osteoporosis and 1,25 Dihydroxyvitamin D_3 Deficiency" R.A. Mackin, O. Gluck

33. "Bone Histomorphometry (BH) and Glomerular Filtration Rate (GFR) in Children with Renal Osteodystrophy (ROD) Due to Chronic Renal Failure (CRF)" A.T. Mazur, R. Baron, M. Norman

34. "Determinats of Trabecular Bone Volume in Corticosteroid Treated and Hyperthyroid Patients" B.E.C. Nordin, J. Aaron, R.G. Crilly, R. Francis, M. Peacock

35. "Determinats of Trabecular Bone Volume in Osteoporotic Men" J. Aaron, B.E.C. Nordin, K. Sagreiya

36. "Trabecular and Cortical Bone Studies in Femoral Neck Fractures" J. Aaron, A. Horsman, B.E.C. Nordin

37. "Histological and Compositional Changes of Bone in Disease Osteoporosis in Monkeys" W.J. Niklowitz, T.E. Bunch, W.S.S. Jee, D.R. Young

38. "Bone Histomorphometric Analysis on Osteogenesis Imperfecta" H. Norimatsu, O. Inoue, K. Ibaraki, H. Takahashi

39. "Post-Traumatic Osteopenia: A Morphological Study in Man" K. Obrant

40. "Bone Metabolism in Homozygous Beta-Thalassemia" S. Ortolani, M. Cecchettin, J. Duriez, P. Favini, P. Massaro, F.M. Ulivieri, E.E. Polli

41. "Polyostotic 'Fibrous Dysplasia'" P. Osterberg, B. Magee, D.R. Hadden

42. "Age Related Changes in Gastrin-Calcitonin Relationship as a Pathogenic Factor of Senile Osteoporosis" M. Passeri, E. Palummeri, L. Cella, G. Cervellin, D. Provvedini

43. "Osteolytic Paget's Disease, Generalized Osteopenia and Otosclerosis in a Missouri Kindred" H.M. Perry,III, M.D. Fallon, W.A. Murphy, L.V. Avioli, M.P. Whyte

44. "Diffuse Non-secretory Osteosclerotic Myeloma with Extensive Erythrophagocytosis" S. Raman, B. Frame, S.M. Saeed, K. Tolia, U. Raju, S. Kottamasu

45. "In Vitro Secretion of Calcitonin and Carcinoembryonic Antigen by C-Cell-Carcinoma" F. Raue, G. Boller, E. Rix, H. Schmidt-Gayk, R. Ziegler

46. "Pathophysiology of Neurologic Dysfunction in Vertebral Paget's Disease" L. Reinstein, D. Seibert, K. Hladik, G.E. Reahl,Jr.

47. "Composition, Structure and Ultrastructure of Urinary and Other Calculi As A Key to Aetiology" A.L. Rodgers

48. "Spongiosasklerose bei systemischer Mastozytose" V. Rosinus

49. "Occurrence of Hypercalcemia in Gaucher Disease: Evidence of Altered Vitamin D Metabolism" R.H. Roswell, S. S. Bottomley

50. "Hypercalcemic Infantile Renal Tumors Heterotransplantation to Nude Mice" M.F. Rousseau-Merck, A. Bourdeau, F. Russo-Marie, M. Garabedian, C.Nezelof

51. "Abnormalities of Collagen Synthesis in Osteogenesis Imperfecta" D. Rowe, J. Shapiro, M. Poirier, S. Schlesinger

52. "Management of Bone Disease in Children Undergoing Continuous Ambulatory Peritoneal Dialysis (CAPD): Value of High-Dose Calcitriol" I.B. Salusky, L. Paunier, H. Kangarloo, E. Slatopolsky, J.W. Coburn, R.N. Fine

53. "Very Low Birth Weight Infants Develop Nutritional Phosphorus Depletion Syndrome" R. Schilling, F. Haschke, J. Kovarik

54. "Unusual Clinical Presentation of Osteogenic Sarcoma" F. Shai, A.G. Smith, J. Abouzeid, F. DeSoto-La Paix, F. Fani

55. "Critical Evaluation of Therapeutic Exercise Programs in Postmenopausal Spinal Osteoporosis" M. Siniki, B. Mikkelsen

56. "Hyperphosphatemic Tumoral Calcinosis with Bone Involvement: A Case Report" T. Sugimoto, T. Fujita, Y. Imai, T. Fukami, K. Ohbayashi, M. Tsutsumi, K. Sakaguchi, H. Baba, R. Hishikawa, M. Fukase, Y. Yoshimoto K. Mizuno, H. Takedaya

57. "Observations on Fluoride Action on Bone Matrix" A.K. Susheela, J. Kochar, M. Jha

58. "Histomorphometry of Ilium in Glucocorticoid-Induced Osteoporosis" H. Takahashi, T. Tanizawa, T. Konno, J. Inoue, T. Haba

59. "Migratory Regional Osteoporosis of the Lower Extremities with Veterbral Osteoporosis" R.A.L. Sutton, N.J. Robert

60. "Histological Heterogeneity of Osteoporosis" R.S. Weinstein

61. "Lumbar Canal Stenosis in Paget's Disease: Staging the Clinical Syndrome and Its Treatment" G.M. Weisz, R. Sekel

62. "Variable Radiographic Response of Osteolytic Paget's Bone Disease to Ethane-1-Hydroxy-1, 1-Diphosphonate (EHDP) Therapy" M.P. Whyte, W.A. Murphy, F.R. Singer, J.G. Haddad, Jr.

63. "Disorders of CA-Phosphate-Metabolism in Normocalcaemic Individuals With Basal Ganglia Calcifications" R. Windeck, D. Strauss, N. Graben, G. Benker, D. Reinwein

64. "Optimizing Treatment of Paget's Disease with EHDP" A.J.P. Yates, C.J. Preston, K.I. Mundy, D.J. Beard, A.D. Paterson, J.A. Kanis, R.G.G. Russell

65. "Effect of Elcalcitonin in Osteoporosis" S. Yoshikawa, N. Tsuyama, M. Shiba, M. Igarashi, H. Orimo

66. "Dynamic Bone Histomorphology in 17 Hydroxylase Deficiency" Y. Yoshimoto, Y. Imai, T. Sugimoto, T. Fukami, H. Baba, M. Tsutsumi, K. Sakaguchi, R. Hishikawa, T. Fujita

67. "Calcium Glycerophosphate as a Source of Calcium and Phosphorus in Total Parenteral Nutrition of Baby Pigs" D.E. Yuen, R.K. Whyte, H.H. Draper

68. "Paget's Disease in Germany: Aspects of Incidence, Distribution and Treatment" R. Ziegler, H. Minne, G. Holz

69. "Hypophosphatemic Rickets with Hypocalciuria and Elevated Serum Levels of $1,25(OH)_2D$" M. Tieder, R. Samuel, A. Halabe, R. Arie, D. Modai, D. Gabison, U.A. Lieberman

70. "Hereditary Familia Renal Phosphate Leak with Bone Lesion, Hypercalciuria and Nephrolithiasis" R. Arie, R. Samuel, A. Halabe, U.A. Lieberman

71. "Stipled Epiphysis - Periarticular Calcifications and Cyst-Like Bone Destructions in Hypophosphatemic Bone Disease" O. Schaadt, J. Sylvest, E. Rostgaard Christensen, I. Goldmann

72. "Benign Giant Cell Tumor Complication Extensive Paget's Disease" M.R. Clements, E.B. Varley, T.M. Chalmers

73. "Homocysteinuria and Osteoporosis" T. Feigelman

OVERVIEW OF THIRD POSTER SESSION

Donald Fraser, M.D., Armen Tashjian, M.D., Robert Lindsay, M.D.

Seventy three scientific posters were presented during the Third Poster Session. Twelve were chosen for further oral presentation, four were studies of childhood disorders, three localized bone pathology and five involving osteoporosis. The presentations of these twelve studies were succinct and surprisingly informative, while generating many questions and much healthy discussion.

CHILDHOOD DISORDERS

Children with chronic renal failure are prone to develop osteodystrophy at an early stage. However, the histological response of bone to vitamin D metabolites while the kidneys gradually deteriorate is unclear. Mazur et al carried out sequential bone histomorphometry in 28 undialyzed patients, treated for 1-2 years with vitamin D compounds, usually 25-OHD_3, 1-2 μg/d. Before starting therapy all had GFR $<$75 ml/min/1.73m^2 and all had bone lesions (either predominantly osteomalacia, predominantly osteitis fibrosa, or OM +OF). As expected, GFR decreased during the two-year study; approximately half the patients were dropped because end-stage failure supervened. Bone histomorphometry became normal in one-third of patients during therapy, but only (with two exceptions) if GFR was $>$ 25 ml/min/1.73 m^2. The results support the use of vitamin D therapy early in the course of chronic renal failure before GFR falls below 25 ml/min/1.73 m^2. In answer to a question whether 1,25$(OH)_2$ D_3 was recommended as treatment, the authors stated they had observed healing with this sterol, but had insufficient data to recommend it over 25-OHD_3.

Children with chronic renal failure developed secondary hyperparathyroidism and renal osteodystrophy while undergoing continuous ambulatory peritoneal dialysis (CAPD). Salusky et al studied 21 uremic children who had substantial degrees of secondary hyperparathyroidism during CAPD despite customary doses of calcitriol or DHT, and normal levels of serum Ca and P_i. By slowly increasing the dose of calcitriol to 26$\pm$ 4 ng/kg/d, until plasma Ca was between 11.0 and 11.5 mg/dl, skeletal radiographs became nearly normal or improved in 19 of the 21 patients, serum alkaline phosphatase decreased in two-thirds and iPTH decreased significantly in half. Serum phosphate did not increase significantly. The authors believe that aggressive calcitriol dosing in renal failure children on CAPD has a beneficial effect on the skeletal lesions. When questioned whether another approach to treatment of the skeletal lesions might have been to increase the concentration of the dialysate calcium, the authors pointed out that the dialysate in use already contained a calcium concentration of 1.75 mmol/L (6 mg/100 ml), well above the upper normal range of ionized calcium.

Of the several forms of heritable rickets, familial hypophosphatemic vitamin D resistant rickets (VDRR) has proved to be one of the most difficult to treat. Hypophosphatemia is clearly the cardinal biochemical abnormality, and in recent years combined treatment with phosphate salts and large doses of vitamin D metabolites has been advocated. At this symposium, Chabot and Glorieux have provided data on linear growth and skeletal maturation. Eight girls and two boys were treated for 3-10 years on a schedule that provided 1-3 g phosphorus in 5 divided doses daily, and vitamin D_2, 25-50,000 IU/day or, since 1977, 1,25$(OH)_2D_3$, 0.5-1.0 μg/d.

Irrespective of whether children were normal or short in stature on entry into the study, prepubertal growth velocity during therapy was 6.3 cm/yr and during puberty maximum growth velocity, assessed in girls, was 9.8 cm/yr, both satisfactory responses. Treatment did not increase the rate of bone maturation above normal nor was the time of epiphyseal fusion accelerated at puberty. Thus, the improvement in statural growth achieved by treatment was not offset by increased skeletal maturation, and the individual's growth potential was not adversely affected by treatment. Although 1,25$(OH)_2D_3$ provided better control of osteomalacia and phosphate-induced secondary hyperparthyroidism, vitamin D_2 therapy had an equally satisfactory effect on growth.

Although biochemical abnormalities of collagen have been reported in isolated cases of osteogenesis imperfecta (OI), no systematic pattern of pathology has emerged in this genetically heterogeneous disease. At this symposium, Rowe et al report studies of collagen synthesis in cultured skin fibroblasts of 36 patients. They first classified the patients into OI forms I, III, IV according to a minor modification of the clinical criteria of Sillence et al (J. Med. Genetics 16:101, 1979). Results were not reported for OI Type II (congenital lethal recessive). When fibroblast cultures were classified according to their synthesis or types I and III collagen and their constituent α- chains, each of the three forms of OI manifested a distinctive biochemical pattern. Collagen synthesis in OI III did not differ from that of 29 control subjects, whereas abnormalities were observed in the other forms - defective type I collagen synthesis in OI I, and defective synthesis of α-2(I) chain in OI IV. This important research provides a biochemical basis for the varied genetic expression of OI, and will help in diagnosis.

BONE PATHOLOGY

Toshitsugu Sugimoto and colleagues from Kobe, Japan described a 19 year old man with periarticular calcinosis surrounding many joints, calcification of the aortic wall, and areas of both increased and decreased skeletal density by x-ray. The disorder began in childhood. The laboratory findings included hyperphosphatemia with an elevated Tm PO_4/GFR in the presence of normal renal function, delayed plasma clearance of an oral phosphate load, and normal plasma calcium concentration. Plasma PTH was normal, and exogenous PTH elicited enhanced phosphaturia and urinary cAMP excretion. Plasma $1,25(OH)_2D_3$ was low (18 pg/ml). Double tetracycline labeling studies were interpreted as showing a normal mineral appositional rate and accelerated periosteal resorption. The authors concluded that soft tissue calcification was probably due to an increased Ca X P product secondary to an undefined renal tubular defect in the handling of phosphate. The mechanisms underlying the bone changes were unknown.

H.M.Perry III, et al of St. Louis, presented their findings on a kindred with Paget's disease of bone. Members of three generations were affected with appendicular lesions of Paget's disease, as well as generalized osteopenia and otosclerosis. The bone disease of some members responded to treatment with human calcitonin. Male to male transmission was demonstrated. Otosclerosis affected 70% of the family members and segregated as an autosomal dominant trait which appeared to be inherited independently of Paget's disease.

Friedhelm Raue and co-workers described studies of the in vitro secretion of calcitonin (CT) and carcinoembryonic antigen (CEA) by primary cultures of several human medullary thyroid carcinomas. Spontaneous release of CT and CEA was observed for up to 55 days in culture. Calcium, pentagastrin, glucagon, and cimetidine added to the culture medium enhanced modestly CT secretion but had no effect on the accumulation of CEA in the medium. Immunoperoxidase staining revealed CT and CEA in the same cells. The authors concluded that classical stimuli for CT secretion do not release CEA from malignant C-cells in vitro.

Seizo Yoshikawa et al presented the results of their investigations on the effects of eel calcitonin in patients with osteoporosis. They divided 130 cases of post menopausal and senile osteoporosis into 4 groups: no treatment controls; eel CT group; dietary calcium supplementation alone(700mg/day); and eel CT plus calcium supplementation. Results were evaluated after 6 months by metacarpal densitometry. Patients treated with eel CT plus calcium had a significant increase in bone density as compared to the control group. CT or calcium alone had no effect. They found no increase in serum, PTH or antibiodies to eel CT in treated patients. The authors concluded that eel CT plus calcium supplementation may be beneficial in the treatment of osteoporosis, although because of the short duration of their studies additional trials will be necessary.

OSTEOPOROSIS

Of the five abstracts selected in this section, two dealt with glucocorticoid induced osteoporosis, perhaps evidence not only of the importance of the disorder but also the problems which clinicians are faced in dealing with treatment or prevention of this side-effect of steroid therapy. In Takahashi's study the histomorphometric changes were greatest with highest dose and longest administration, although there was some doubt about the influence of the underlying disease, particularly in relationship to the reduction in mineral apposition rate found in female patients on high dose steroid treatment for more than 4-5 months. This paper also presented evidence that mean well thickness is reduced in steroid osteoporosis, in agreement with other published data.

In a somewhat similar study, reduction in forming surfaces was found only in those steroid treated patients who had developed osteoporosis and not in those whose trabecular bone volume was normal. This suggests, assuming other conditions were similar, that some individuals may have some resistance to the effect of steroids in bone, the reasons for which are not clear. In another study from the same laboratory, Crilly contended that only those individuals who showed malabsorption of calcium developed steroid osteoporosis. Curiously, in the discussion, it was suggested that the trabecular bone was the same in both the crush fracture group and those with normal spines. Clearly the inconsistencies between patients and studies require more detailed investigation. Crilly's paper did suggest that the use of calcium supplements by themselves may not be an efficient method of prevention for steroid osteoporosis. Takahashi, in a very small group of patients with steroid osteoporosis, found little effect in treatment with a cyclical regime of 1α-hydroxycholecalciferol and eel calcitonin.

In an abstract examining calcitonin secretion during glucocorticoid treatment, Gennari et al showed a significantly reduced calcitonin response to calcium infusion. The patients were used as their own controls during a pre-treatment phase. This study provides a possible link between steroid osteoporosis and postmenopausal osteoporosis where the reduced calcitonin response to calcium infusion in women and with increasing age has been suggested as a factor of possible pathogenetic importance. The importance of the calcitonin in senile osteoporosis is also suggested by the study by Passeri and associates who observed that the calcitonin response to a protein load was lacking in this disorder. In view of this, perhaps more detailed therapeutic studies of the type performed by Takahashi may be important.

In an abstract examining the role of the vitamin D metabolites, Buchanan suggested that the prime defect in the pathogenesis of postmenopausal osteoporosis was also malabsorption of calcium. He showed reduced levels at 24,25 dihydroxyvitamin D and a reduced ratio of 24,25 dihydroxyvitamin D to 1,25 dihydroxyvitamin D in patients with established disease. These abnormalities were partially corrected by simulation of calcium absorption, including the use of 1,25 dihydroxyvitamin D as therapy. The authors suggest that this supports the theory that calcium malabsorption is the prime defect. However, to establish this, more detailed studies of D metabolites and the relationship of such changes as documented here would be required at a stage in the disorder when rapid bone loss was progressing.

XIX ORAL SESSIONS

ORAL SESSION A - SELECTED TOPICS

MODERATORS: H. DUNCAN, J. POTTS, JR.

1. "*In Vitro* Studies of Parathyroid Hormone Regulation" G. Akerstrom, C. Rudberg, L. Grimelius, H. Johansson, S. Ljunghall, J. Pertoft, L. Wide

2. "The Effect of Cimetidine on PTH Levels" J.K. Sherwood, F.W. Ackroyd, M. Garcia

3. "Parathyroid Suppressibility During Calcium Infusion As Evaluated by Neprogenous cAMP (NcAMP) in Man" P. Singhellakis, A. Nikou, Ch. Nicolou, K. Alevizaki, D. Ikkos

4. "Parathyroid Hormone Metabolism In Primary Biliary Cirrhosis: A Possible Defect In Hormone Metabolism" M.J. Atkinson, T. Schettler, E. Keck, I. Vido, R.D. Hesch

5. "Changes in Bone Metabolism Related to Age and Sex. Determination of 24 Hours Whole Body Retention of MDP in 125 Normal Persons" L. Hyldstrup, N.B. Mogensen, P. McNair, G.F. Jensen, I. Transbol

6. "Function of Cryopreserved Human Parathyroid Tissue" J. Norton, A. Spiegel, G. Aurbach, P. Schneider, M. Brennan

7. "Impaired Renal Production of 1α,25-Dihydroxyvitamin D in Nephrotic Syndrome" M. Kubota, M. Ito, K. Hirano, H. Koide, J. Ohno

8. "Bone Mineral Content of Femoral Bone and Lumbar Spine in Women with Fracture of the Femoral Neck" H. Bohr, O. Schaadt

9. "Age-Related Loss of Trabecular Bone in Pre-menopausal Women: A Biopsy Study" R. Marcus, J. Kosek, A. Pfefferbaum, S. Horning

10. "Microradioscopic Assessment of Bone Resorption: Preliminary Findings Using Zeiss MOP-3 Image Analyzing System" H.E. Meema, D.G. Oreopoulos, T.M. Murray

11. "Post-Traumatic Osteopenia: An Electron Probe Analysis with Special Reference to the Calcium Concentration in Different Parts of Trabeculae" K.J. Obrant, R. Odselius

12. "Measurement of Human 25 OHD_3 1α-Hydroxylase in Renal Specimen" Y. Seino, K. Satomura, K. Yamaoka, M. Ishida, H. Yabuuchi, Y. Tanaka, H.F. DeLuca

13. "Hydroxylysine Glycosides: A New Assay Method and Its Application to Assess Collagen Turnover in Spinal Cord Injury Patients" G. Rodriguez, J. Claus-Walker

14. "Mineralization of Trabecular Osteoid in Osteoporosis: A Comparison Between Sr-85 and Tetracycline Kinetics" J. Reeve, M. Arolt, R. Hesp, C. Edouard, P.J. Meunier

15. "How Useful is Osteocalcin as an Index of Bone Metabolism in Man?" R.G.G. Russell, J. Beresford, J. Poser, L. Coulton, M. Sharrard, A.J.P. Yates, J.A. Kanis

ORAL SESSION A: SELECTED TOPICS

Moderators: Howard Duncan and John T. Potts, Jr.

Henry Ford Hospital, Detroit, MI, U.S.A.; Department of Medicine, Harvard Medical School and Massachusetts General Hospital, Boston, MA, U.S.A.

Akerstrom and colleagues reported results of their studies to examine secretory responsiveness of adenomatous parathyroid glands (primary hyperparathyroidism) and hyperplastic glands (secondary hyperparathyroidism). They used dispersed cells prepared for excised tissue, maintained as primary cultures. Variations in calcium content of the media induced changes in rate of release of parathyroid hormone measured by immunoassay. Responses among the glands regarding degree of suppressibility of hormone secretion differed greatly. No significant differences could be assigned, however, between the adenomatous glands, as a group, and the hyperplastic glands. These results were felt to be similar to the findings of Brown and others. Questions were raised, without obvious answers, concerning the differences in tecnniques (gland slices versus dispersed cells) and responses *in vivo* to calcium suppression to results seen *in vitro*.

Extensive studies previously reported in part were reviewed by Sherwood and associates concerning suppression of hormone secretion by cimetidine. The interesting and provocative results were discussed extensively by the audience, some of whom had not been able to confirm the findings of Sherwood et al. In discussion, the possible effects of varying bioavailability and blood levels of the drug and the timing of sampling for hormone measurements, as well as methodological variations, were raised as possible explanations for the discordant results, but no conclusions could be reached.

Evaluation of the usefulness of suppression of levels of nephrogenous cyclic AMP during intravenous calcium infusion as a means of distinguishing among normal subjects and patients with primary hyperparathyroidism, and individuals with secondary hyperparathyroidism were reported by Singhellakis and his collaborators. Studies were performed in 89 controls, 16 patients with secondary, and 19 patients with primary hyperparathyroidism. Patients with secondary hyperparathyroidism lowered cyclic AMP levels as briskly as normals; reduced suppressibility and even paradoxical rises were seen in the primary group. The results led the authors to propose the utility of the test as an adjunct in differential diagnosis (Editor's note: The similar degrees of suppressibility of glands *in vitro*, whether from primary or secondary hyperparathyroidism, contrast sharply with the results of these *in vivo* studies - the explanation being unclear).

A report from the Hesch laboratory concerned investigations in 14 subjects with primary biliary cirrhosis aimed at evaluating the possible influence of altered Kupffer cell function on hormone metabolism and, consequently, bone turnover. Attention was called to the observations of the St. Louis group that peripheral metabolism may be required to generate an amino-terminal fragment that acts on bone. The group used three different radioimmunoassays to assess hormone metabolism by comparison of ratios of hormone content measured by each assay, one assay being felt to measure intact hormone, one the middle of the molecule, and one predominantly the carboxyl region. Jueppner interpreted the results to show reduced hormone metabolism in patients with more severe degrees of biliary cirrhosis. The speculation was offered that osteopenia in this disease might reflect reduced production of an amino-terminal fragment (which was not itself measurable directly). Discussants pointed out the multiplicity of changes in metabolism generally in patients with severe cirrhosis which made difficult any firm conclusions regarding a cause and effect relation between metabolism of parathyroid hormone and the status of the skeleton.

By using whole body retention of technicium-labeled diphosphonate, Hyldstrup and his colleagues indicated that the retention of diphosphonate represented a measure of bone turnover and correlated to some extent with the level of serum alkaline phosphatase, which itself was felt to represent bone formation. The changes of the order of 7% were felt to be reliable and significant, and at high turnover states there was an increased retention of two to threefold. This form of balance study has, so far, been confined to short-term studies. Repeated observations showed a three to six month delay in returning to normal following parathyroidectomy. These figures match well with the predicted "sigma" equilibration time following stimulus.

The NIH group concerned with studies in patients with hyperparathyroidism reported their results in patients requiring re-exploration of the neck who had gland tissue cryopreserved. Dr. Norton summarized results in 17 patients who had reimplantation into the forearm of 1 mm minced sections of cryopreserved parathyroid tissue. The tissue had been preserved for periods of 6 months to as long as 48 months. Autotransplantation featured 25-30 separate forearm implants. All patients had been rendered hyperparathyroid and were maintained on supplemental calcium and vitamin D. In 7 patients, previously without detectable parathyroid hormone levels post-surgically, successful autotransplantation was accomplished, as assessed by detection of higher levels of immunoassayable hormone in the forearm view on the side of the transplant. These patients became normocalcemic without supplemental treatment and had restoration of normal systemic parathryoid hormone levels. Some inadequate restoration of autotransplant function was noted in 3 additional patients; no function at all could be detected in the other seven of the total of 17 patients. After a two-year post-transplant evaluation, no evidence of hyperfunction was detected even though some of the transplanted tissue came from adenomas. Causes of failure were discussed, as well as a note of caution concerning possible hyperfunction if the period of evaluation of the results of transplant is extended by several years. Hopeful directions for improvement in functional preservation of tissue were also commented on, particularly variation in induction of cryopreservation.

Kubota and associates evaluated the question of the cause of the low levels of vitamin D metabolites seen in the nephrotic syndrome. Reasoning that if the sole defect is excessive renal loss of vitamin D binding protein with its metabolites (as part of the renal protein wasting of the syndrome) then correlations should be found between serum protein concentration and vitamin D metabolites before, during, and after treatment with prednisone to reduce proteinuria. With successful treatment and clinical remission, 25-OH-D and $24,25(OH)_2D$ levels rose promptly; good correlation existed with serum protein concentration. $1,25(OH)_2D$ levels were 17.1, 28.4, and 15.8 pg/ml initially, during treatment, and after remission, respectively; no correlation was seen with serum protein. Occasionally, $1,25(OH)_2D$ levels rose later as clinical remission continued. One interpretation offered was that impaired renal synthesis of $1,25(OH)_2D$ is involved in the pathophysiology, not merely renal loss of the metabolite. Discussion centered on the significance of the low levels of $1,25(OH)_2D$ throughout the study and whether firm conclusions could be drawn (without other tests, such as stimulation of $1,25(OH)_2D$ production) concerning impaired renal synthesis of $1,25(OH)_2D$.

Two papers also addressed the issue of variation of bone mass with age. It was noted that different sampling sites do not necessarily parallel each other, even in the same person. Bohr and Schaadt used a dual photon absorptiometry to show that there was a lineal loss of bone in the femoral neck in subjects varying in age from 20 years onwards, whereas the femoral shaft mineral content fell more rapidly after 60 years. Their subjects were all women, of whom 47 had had recent femoral neck fracture and 38 were healthy matched controls. The bone mineral content of the femoral shaft in the fracture group was significantly reduced. Among other factors, influencing the propensity to fracture were muscle mass, eye sight, dizziness, and, in addition, abnormal crystal structure in bone at specific sites of the femoral neck fracture to which Reeve referred in his studies.

The volume of trabecular bone in iliac crest biopsies was determined histomorphometrically by Marcus and his associates. Their biopsies were unique in that they were taken from females, ages 15 to 56, who had no metabolic bone disease, who were all premenopausal, but diagnosed as lymphoma with no disease below the diaphragm. All were biopsied before systemic therapy for their primary disease. These studies agreed with Riggs's observations on iliac bone, with those of Arnold on the study of vertebrae, and with those of Frost in the study of rib cortex, in that bone volume decreased steadily during the reproductive years from the age of 25 onwards. However, other studies have suggested that this diminution of bone volume does not begin until the middle or late thirties. Marked variations of bone volume were noted within each age group, and it is conceivable that the site of onset of demineralizing process could have some relationship to the physical activity of the individual concerned, as represented in studies of Talmadge et al and of Frost elsewhere at this meeting. Eighty-two men, ages 16 to 64, were similarly evaluated and showed that during this aging process they lost approximately half of the bone volume per year that was lost by women (the figure for women was in the range of 0.7 bone volume per year). These figures agreed fairly well with the dual photon absorptiometry methods. It is recognized in this study that it is a cross-sectional assessment and lacks the predictability that any one individual with better bone at any time will be at an advantage, 10, 20, or 30 years further along. Again, longitudinal studies are exceedingly important.

A different approach to trabecular size, volume, and structural detail was demonstrated by Meema and associates, using microradiographic methods. By using magnifying systems and fine grain x-ray plates, clear definitions of the longitudinal tunneling of bone cortices in high turnover metabolic states were identified and measured. Meema felt that the individual bone metabolic unit resorption sites on trabeculae could be identified and the volume calculated as approximately 0.0012 cmm. (Editor's note: These studies, of course, are singularly effective in evaluating changes in hand x-rays, for such detail of larger bones at greater distances from the x-ray plate do not lend themselves to developing this fine detail.)

Obrant and Odseline presented some histological evidence that there was a mineralization defect of trabeculae which occurred at some distance from the site of injury of the same bone. He studied trephine biopsies taken approximately 7 to 13 months after the distal injury to the tibia. The trephine itself was taken some 15 to 18 cm distant, usually at the proximal end of the tibia in the region of the proximal diaphysis. Trephine specimens were not demineralized, but were imbedded in methyl methacrylate, and sections were cut and stained using Von Kossa stain, Goldner stain, and a separate section was mounted unstained. Obrant described areas of buried osteoid, alternate layers of mineralization occurring next to incompletely mineralized osteoid, particularly seen on Goldner stain, and some trabeculae which were completely unmineralized. On the unstained section, an electron probe analysis of mineral content of the osteoid was performed by adaptation of the scanning electron microscope, whereby an adjacent section to that which demonstrated alternate layers of different mineralization in the Goldner stain, revealed the same alternation of mineral content by the electron probe.

Speakers from the audience noted that such phenomena were also seen in cases of renal osteodystrophy and that the Von Kossa stain was not the best to demonstrate the presence of calcium due to its low pH and demineralizing capacity, and its greater specificity for phosphate than for calcium. It was also noted that high turnover bone states produce a relative hyperosteoidosis and that this relatively localized phenomenon in the region of the injured site would be recognized as a "regional acceleratory phenomenon," whereby any mild or major noxious stimulus generates a local high turnover state in an attempt to repair. This reaction involves the majority of tissues in the region, including bone. The authors had not reported any information on other metabolic bone states using these methods.

A group of Japanese workers reported on a new micro-assay for renal 25-hydroxyl -hydroxylase in human kidney biopsy specimens. Advantage was taken of the screening program for renal disease in Japanese schoolchildren. Seven children had renal biopsies performed after persistent hematuria and proteinuria. Seino and his co-workers adapted the Tanaka and DeLuca tissue assay to micro-methodology suitable for work with the small amounts of renal tissue remaining after diagnostic histological studies. The assay was validated on specimens of rat kidneys using rats who were made D-deficient versus normal rats. The assay used 1 microgram of 25-OH D/mg tissue. Examination of linearity studies, varying substrate, tissue mass, and incubation time established conditions for a suitable assay at 20 minutes.

By comparison with the rat data and assumption about the normality of D metabolism in these minimally affected children, the work provides a normal range for human renal 1 -hydroxylase as 28.8-117 pg/mg tissue/20 minutes incubation and may prove useful in future studies with clearly diseased kidneys that are biopsied.

Rodriguez and Claus-Walker discussed a method of studying the catabolism of collagen derived from bone and from skin, as applied to spinal injury patients in whom disturbances of both these tissues and of metabolism is evident. These workers exploited the observation that metabolic products of bone collagen produced a hydroxylysine derivative, galactosyl hydrolysine, while the comparable derivative from skin collagen is identified as the glucosyl-galactosyl hydroxylysine. It is recalled that both types of collagen are Type 2. Whereas both these values tend to return towards normal values after the first six months of immobilization, it was felt that the presence of a more-than-average rapid deterioration of one of the collagen types, i.e., glucosyl-galactosyl hydroxylsine, may permit prognostications regarding the development of skin ulcers.

A combined histomorphometric and kinetic study by Reeve and a group of international colleagues examined the interrelationship of measurements of osteoid surface, osteoid volume, and tetracycline labeling, with bone formation and bone resorption as assessed by kinetic data derived from the turnover of SR-85. In the trabecular bone of these osteoporotic patients, it was noted that not all osteoid seams accepted a double label of tetracycline when the patient had been appropriately exposed. This included not only early and late developing osteons, bone remodelling units, but those which were in "the middle" of their normal development. (These features had originally been described by Frost in bone cortex in 1964). The lack of double labeling represented either a temporary arrest or a greatly extended mineralization lag time, that is, a dissociation between the different stages of activity of the basic metabolic unit (BMU). Only when the measurement of the surface of osteoid adjacent to double labels was used in calculation for new bone formation, did the correlation with kinetic data (using SR-85) become significant. It was evident that rates of osteoblast function as measured by tetracycline labelling were not necessarily always proportional to the osteoid production and that the flat osteoblast may not perform in the same manner as the cuboidal or plumb osteoblast. (Editor's Note: These observations are in accord with those of others who have studied individual cellular performance of osteoblasts in osteon development of dogs). It was suggested by Reeve that closer attention be paid to the pattern and the extent of single and double tetracycline labelling, as it is observed in different metabolic disturbances and that calculations be appropriate to the double and single tetracycline surfaces involved. (Editor's Note: The functions of the osteoblast may be better understood with respect to its size, age, and whether it arises in the normal BMU sequence, or under the influence of flourides on a previously quiescent surface, at which site osteoblasts are fewer and labeling of the osteoid less complete and apparently less subject to other standard hormonal influences).

Russell and co-workers reported that osteocalcin, the major non-collagen protein in human bone, is <u>not</u> a reliable measure of osteoblastic activity. In high bone turnover states, i.e.,

Paget's disease, there was generally an increase in serum level of osteocalcin, but as with alkaline phosphatase, the levels are crude measures of bone cell activity. In a bone cell culture, it was shown that alkaline phosphatase and osteocalcin production may respond in a different manner to the same stimulus. For these reasons, the limitations of predictability of bone cell population behavior *in vivo*, from observations made on bone cell responses *in vitro*, were strongly re-emphasized.

ORAL SESSION B - SELECTED POSTERS

MODERATORS: J. COBURN, B. FRAME

1. "Bone Changes AFter Billroth I and II Gastric Resections" E.M. Alhava, M. Paakkonen, P. Karjalainen

2. "Hyperparathyroidism in MEN-1, Natural Course and Effects of Parathyroid Surgery" L. Benson, K. Oberg, S. Ljunghall, J. Malmaeus, G. Akerstrom

3. "Vitamin D Status and Bone Histomorphometry After Billiopancreatic Bypass for Obesity" J.E. Compston, S. Vedi, G.J. Watson, L. Pitton, N. Scopinaro

4. "Bone Disease Associated with Total Parenteral Nutrition" K.N. Jeejeebhoy, C.S. Tam, W.C. Sturtridge, M. Shike, J.E. Harrison

5. "The Relationship of Hepatic Osteodystrophy (OD) to Calcium and Vitamin D Metabolism in Early Primary Biliary Cirrhosis (PBC)" A.B. Hodsman, C. Anderson, G. Jones, C.N. Ghent

6. "Mortality and Morbidity in Untreated Hypercalcemia: A Cohort Study with 12 Years of Follow-up" S. Ljunghall, H.O. Adami, S. Jakobsson, M. Palmer, G. Akerstrom

7. "Neuromuscular Involvement in Primary Hyperparathyroidism" S. Ljunghall, G. Johansson, Y. Olsson, E. Stalber, G. Akerstrom

8. "Disodium EDTA Infusions for the Differentiation of Primary Hyperparathyroidism with Normal Basal Immunoreactive Parathyroid Hormone Values from Non-parathyroid Hypercalcemia" L. Mallette, R. Berger

9. "Asymptomatic Celiac Disease Presenting as Osteomalacia" P.D. Miller, W.E. Huffer, R.A. Krebs, B.J. Neal, D.O. McIntyre

10. "Localization of Hyperfunctioning Parathyroid Adenoma" R. Morita, C. Shigeno, M. Hino, M. Fukunaga, K. Yamamoto, K. Nakajima, N. Hayashi, T. Harioka, Y. Dodo, Y. Nakano, T. Odori, K. Torizuka

11. "Exogenous Hyperthyroidism with Osteoporosis" H.M. Perry, III, M.D. Fallon, D.D. Droke, M. Bergfeld, S.L. Teitelbaum, L.V. Avioli

12. "Oral Therapy of Aluminum-Hydroxide ($Al(OH)_3$) in Long Term Treated Patients (LTTR.P.) on Hemodialysis (HD) with Special Regard to the Effect on Renal Osteopathy (RO)" W. Schulz, F. Weidig, G. Popperl, J.J. Deuber

13. "Medical Treatment of Primary Hyperparathyroidism with Diphosphonates" A.J.P. Yates, A.D. Paterson, D.L. Douglas, C.J. Preston, D.J. Beard, E.C. Cameron, S. Woodhead, R.G.G. Russell, J.A. Kanis

14. "Are Vitamin D Metabolites Other Than 1,25$(OH)_2D_3$ Physiologically Important in Man?" J.A. Kanis, J. Clayton, D. Guilland-Cumming, S.K. Johnson, P. Lawson-Matthew, R. Vaishnav, R.G.G. Russell

ORAL SESSION B, SELECTED TOPICS

Jack W. Coburn and Boy Frame (Moderators)

Medical and Research Services, V.A. Wadsworth Medical Center and Dept. of Med., U.C.L.A. Sch. Med., Los Angeles, CA; Univ. Mich. Sch. Med., Ann Arbor, MI & Henry Ford Hosp., Detroit, MI, U.S.A.

Dr. Alhava of Kuopio, Finland, presented data on the bone findings in patients who had undergone Billroth gastrectomy I compared to those with a Billroth II gastrectomy. Bone mineral content and biochemical parameters were studied 21-27 years after gastrectomy in 19 patients with a Billroth I procedure, in 19 patients with a Billroth II gastrectomy, and also in age and sex-matched controls. There were no differences in the bone mineral content by photon absorptiometry nor in serum biochemical findings between the two gastrectomy groups, except that the mean serum alkaline phosphatase levels were slightly higher in the Billroth II than Billroth I group. In both groups, bone mineral content was slightly lower than in age-matched controls. No patient had clinical evidence of osteomalacia and none had evidence for vitamin D deficiency. Thus, clinically significant bone diseases are rare after the use of these surgical techniques and with diets that were ingested by these patients, observations different from those in England during World War II.

Dr. Benson, et al., of Uppsala, Sweden, reported the clinical findings in 10 kindreds with multiple endocrine neoplasia, type I. In these families, 36 patients had hyperparathyroidism, usually the first manifestation, 9 had pituitary tumors, and 19 had various types of pancreatic tumors; only 5 displayed all 3 features of the syndrome. On follow-up evaluation, the best surgical procedure for the parathyroid hyperplasia in the syndrome was total parathyroidectomy with autotransplantation in the forearm. In patients treated in this manner, serum calcium could be normalized, while recurrence of hyperparathyroidism was common after sub-total parathyroidectomy. From questions during the discussion, it is apparent that there is no method to identify the presence of this syndrome when hyperparathyroidism is seen in the first case encountered in a kindred, i.e., there was nothing distinctive about the hyperparathyroidism.

Dr. Compston, et al., of London, England, reported the results of a study, including bone biopsy data, in 41 patients evaluated 12-61 months after biliopancreatic bypass surgery for obesity. There was biopsy evidence of metabolic bone disease in nearly 70% of patients, plasma phosphate levels were slightly lower in those with bone disease, while the levels of plasma 25-hydroxyvitamin D and other biochemical features were normal. Thus, evidence for metabolic bone disease was common, but the pathogenesis of this bone disease was unclear and simple vitamin D deficiency was not likely to be responsible.

Dr. Harrison of Toronto presented data on bone disease in patients treated with long-term total parenteral nutrition. She showed evidence for a significant improvement in bone disease, characterized by hyper-osteoidosis, occurring in association with the withdrawal of vitamin D from the TPN solution. Also, an increased fraction of the mineralization front was covered with tetracycline. One case showed the reappearance of wide osteoid when the patient was later treated with $1,25(OH)_2D_3$. In the discussion, the potential significance of aluminum loading in the Toronto patients with severe osteomalacia was raised, since Sherrard et al had found positive aluminum stains in the Toronto patients who had osteomalacia. However, the patient with recurrence of osteomalacia after $1,25(OH)_2D_3$ apparently did not exhibit aluminum. The puzzling mechanism whereby normal quantities of vitamin D can apparently produce an osteomalacia-like bone disease were discussed without any clear-cut answers.

Dr. Hodsman, et al., of London, Ontario, reported studies of bone and mineral metabolism in 14 consecutive patients with early primary biliary cirrhosis without skeletal symptoms. Four showed biopsy evidence of osteomalacia and 3 showed osteoporosis; the bone biopsies in the remainder showed mild abnormalities but were non-diagnostic. The levels of $24,25(OH)_2D_3$ were lower in the patients with "hepatic osteodystrophy." Alterations of serum levels of other vitamin D metabolites, 25(OH)D and $1,25(OH)_2D$ were not present; a surprising finding was increased urinary calcium in those with nutritional osteomalacia. No explanation for the abnormalities was apparent; there were no measures of calcium absorption.

Dr. Ljunghall, et al., of Uppsala, Sweden, presented interesting long-term follow-up observations of patients with asymptomatic and untreated hypercalcemia, presumed to be due to hyperparathyroidism. The course of the hypercalcemic individuals were compared to that of age and sex-matched cohorts. There was slightly higher mortality in the hypercalcemic group compared to the normocalcemic controls ($p<.05$), although this was not explained by any specific cause of mortality. However, death rates due to malignancy tended to be higher although not statistically different in the hypercalcemic group. These observations, if they continue to hold with further follow-up, supports the indications for parathyroid surgery in patients with asymptomatic hyperparathyroidism and mild hypercalcemia.

Dr. Ljunghall, et al., of Uppsala, Sweden, also reported a study of muscle function with electrophysiological measurements in patients with primary hyperparathyroidism; muscle biopsies were done in a substantial number of patients. The electrophysiological data showed very slight and often non-specific abnormalities in a small fraction of patients; moreover, it was thought unlikely that these changes were responsible for vague symptoms of muscle weakness or fatiguability. The authors concluded that symptomatic muscle disease was uncommon in hyperparathyroidism, except in rare patients with gross and severe hypercalcemia. In the discussion others, including Dr. Mallette, concurred with this view.

Dr. Mallete, et al., of Houston, Texas, reported studies utilizing EDTA infusions for the study of iPTH response to hypocalcemia in patients with primary hyperparathyroidism, particularly those with normal basal serum levels of iPTH. They noted very rapid and supranormal increment of serum iPTH levels as the serum ionized Ca fell, observations compatible with a rightward shift of the "set point" for PTH release. These observations indicate the presence of abnormal parathyroid hormone release in almost all patients with hyperparathyroidism.

Dr. Miller, et al., of Denver, Colorado, evaluated 187 patients referred because of axial osteopenia and compression fractures. Fifty-nine patients had bone biopsy evidence of osteomalacia, i.e., wide osteoid seams. In the subgroup of patients with osteomalacia but with no apparent cause of the osteomalacia, 50% had intestinal biopsies; and celiac disease was discovered in 70% of this latter group. Biochemical studies revealed minor biochemical abnormalities in some but not all of the patients; these alterations included an increase in serum alkaline phosphatase, increased serum iPTH levels, and low levels of 25-hydroxyvitamin D. Of interest, there were no symptoms of malabsorption in the patients with celiac disease, indicating that this diagnosis would not have been made without the bone biopsy. These results indicate that celiac disease may be common in elderly patients presenting with axial skeletal loss. Verification of these interesting observations is clearly needed.

Dr. Morita, et al., of Kyoto, Japan, reported their experience with various methods for the pre-operative localization of parathyroid adenoma. As the first choice, they recommended the used of ^{201}Tl-chloride for scintiscan with subtraction of the ^{123}I-images of the thyroid gland, with a sensitivity of this procedure of 57%. Ultrasonography had a sensitivity of 75%, but this procedure required a highly skilled ultrasonographer; also, parathyroid and thyroid tumors could not be differentiated. The most accurate method was the CT scan after injection of contrast media; the sensitivity was nearly 90%; again, thyroid and parathyroid tumors were not separated. In a few patients venous samples for iPTH measurements were obtained using catheterization of the veins draining the parathyroid glands. The sensitivity of this last procedure was high, but it has the greatest morbidity of any of the procedures. This represented an interesting study comparing various methods for parathyroid gland localization.

Dr. Perry, et al., of St. Louis, Missouri, described 3 post-menopausal women with osteopenia and vertebral crush fractures who gave a history of ingesting excessive doses of exogenous thyroid hormone. There was mild hypercalcemia, hyperphosphatemia, and increased serum alkaline phosphatase. Bone biopsies, evaluated by tetracycline labelling, showed increased turnover with increased osteoclastic and osteoblastic activity. These features may separate these patients from the usual patient with post-menopausal osteoporosis.

Dr. Schulz, et al., of Bamburg, West Germany, reported the relationship between oral therapy with aluminum-hydroxide gels, plasma aluminum levels and other features of renal osteodystrophy in 126 hemodialysis patients in whom reverse osmosis had been utilized for water purification. The results showed that oral aluminum hydroxide was the major factor associated with increased plasma aluminum levels in these dialysis patients. Serum Al levels correlated with the dosage of PO_4-binders and the duration of dialysis. Serum iPTH levels were inversely related to the plasma aluminum levels, evidence which may support experimental studies in animals that aluminum can cause suppression of PTH release. Patients with high serum Al levels also had stainable Al along the the mineralization front bone biopsy specimens. He suggested that oral Al loading, although not a common cause of encephelopathy, can lead to skeletal pathology in dialysis patients.

The effects of two diphosphates, clodronate (Cl_2MDP) and etidronate (EHDP), were studied in patients with hypercalcemia due to primary hyperparathyroidism by Yates, et al., of Sheffield, England. From the reduction in fasting urinary calcium excretion and urinary hydroxyproline excretion noted during treatment, they suggested that there was decreased bone resorption during clodronate therapy. Serum calcium decreased in all but did not fall to normal. Moreover, Cl_2MDP was far more potent than EHDP in this effect, and serum P and $TmPO_4$/GFR rose in those given EHDP. The effect on lowering serum calcium was not sustained with long-term administration; none-the-less, the results suggest that Cl_2MDP might be useful in the management of patients who are poor surgical risks.

Dr. Kanis, et al., of Sheffield, England, reviewed evidence which suggests that vitamin D sterols other than 1,25-dihydroxy-vitamin D_3 may play a physiological role in calcium regulation. Indirect evidence is based on the seasonal variations in plasma levels of 24,25-dihydroxyvitamin D; these correlated with changes in bone mineral content while the latter were not related to the plasma levels of 1,25$(OH)_2$D. He suggested that 24,25$(OH)_2D_3$ may lead to enhanced bone mineralization compared to the effects of 1,25$(OH)_2$D. Data showing greater body retention of Ca after 24,25$(OH)_2$D treatment than with 25$(OH)_2$D above were reviewed. This area of investigation continuses to be puzzling. However, a physiological role for 24,25$(OH)_2$D cannot be confirmed until more data are available.

ORAL SESSION C - SELECTED POSTERS

MODERATORS: C. JOHNSTON, S. KRANE

1. "Osteoporosis of Pregnancy: Comparison with Juvenile Osteoporosis" R. Smith, J.C. Stevenson, C.G. Winearls, C.G. Woods

2. "Excessive Ingestion of Fluoride and Bone Pathophysiology" A.K. Susheela, M. Jha

3. "Plasma 25-OHD Levels in Femoral Neck Fracture Cases in South Australia" G. Morrison, M. Hone, D. Sharpe, H. Morris, B.E.C. Nordin

4. "Bone Fractures in Patients with Paget's Disease. Results of Treatment with Calcitonin" C. Mautalen, G. Ghiringhelli, Z. Rubin, C. Massironi

5. "The Prevention of Osteoporosis by Postmenopausal Estrogen Replacement" F.W. Lafferty, D.O. Helmuth

6. "Value of the Calcitonin Test in Symptomatic Postmenopausal Osteoporosis" P. Geusens, J. Dequeker, A. Verstraeten

7. "Osteoporosis and Immune Function" T. Fujita, Y. Yoshimoto, Y. Nakao, T. Matsui, Y. Imai, T. Fukami, T. Sugimoto

8. "Osteosclerosis and Hypoplastic Anemia (Acquired 'Osteopetrosis')" E. Hills, W.G. Hughes, R.A. Evans, C.R. Dunstan, S.Y.P. Wong

9. "Severe Osteoporosis Associated with High Alcohol and Tobacco Consumption in Man" M.C. de Vernejoul, J. Biekaloff, J. Gueris, L. Miravet, A. Ryckewaert

10. "Treatment of Post-Menopausal Osteoporosis with 1,25-Dihydroxyvitamin D_3" A. Caniggia, R. Nuti, F. Lore, A. Vattimo

11. "Fluoride and Calcium Interactions: Syndromes of Bone Disease and Deformities (Human Studies)" S.P.S. Teotia, M. Teotia, D.P. Singh

12. "Clinical Aspects of Trabecular and Cortical Bone Mineral Scanning by Dual Photon Absorptiometry of 153-Gd" O. Schaadt, H. Bohr

13. "Erosive Spondylarthropathy in Hemodialyzed Patients - A New Syndrome?" D. Kuntz, B. Naveau, T. Drueke, A. Dryll

14. "Bone Gla-Protein - A Marker for Osteoblastic Activity" H.H. Malluche, M.C. Faugere, P. Fanti, P.A. Price

Simultaneous Oral Session (C)

SELECTED TOPICS IN METABOLIC BONE DISEASE

Moderators: C.C. Johnston, Jr., M.D. and Stephen M. Krane, M.D.

R. Smith and associates, from Oxford and the Royal Postgraduate Medical School, London, presented 7 patients who developed spinal osteoporosis in relationship to pregnancy. In 6 of these patients, the disease improved; and in fact, 2 went through subsequent pregnancies without recurrence. In 1 patient, the disease was progressive. Routine biochemical measurements were normal and transiliac bone biopsies showed osteoporotic bone with no increase in osteoid or cellular activity. In some of these patients, $1,25(OH)_2D_3$ values were low; and in fact, may have been low in most in relationship to their pregnancies. These findings are quite similar to those found in 10 patients who were studied presenting with juvenile osteoporosis. Among this group, 5 spontaneously improved when growth ceased. These two syndromes may represent the same underlying disease process.

F.W. Lafferty from University Hospital, Cleveland, Ohio, discussed long-term effects of estrogen replacement therapy in 61 treated, postmenopausal women, compared to 63 control subjects followed for 3-16 years, with a mean follow-up of 8.6 years. The estrogen replacement consisted of conjugated estrogen, 0.625 mg daily for three out of four weeks. A loss of height of 1.5 inches or more had an incidence of 33.1 per 1,000 patient-years among estrogen-replaced subjects, and 66.9 among the controls--a significant difference, with the major effect occurring after age 65. It was noted that the loss of height occurred in an irregular, step-wise pattern in both groups and, in 95% of the cases, was unassociated with pain. Abnormal electrocardiograms and diabetes mellitus developed in significantly fewer estrogen-treated patients than controls, and there was no significant increase in carcinoma of the endometrium or breast. These data suggest that estrogen replacement is safe and will reduce the incidence of compression fractures in postmenopausal women.

M.C. de Vernejoul and associates from Paris reported on 11 men between the ages of 30 and 50 (mean age 44) with idiopathic osteoporosis. Eight of the 11 had greater than normal alcohol consumption (180 gr vs 44 gr of alcohol per day for controls), and five had elevated levels of γ-glutamyl transferase. In addition, 10 of the 11 were heavy smokers (400 gr vs 16 gr per day of tobacco). Serum calcium, phosphorus, and immunoreactive parathyroid hormone were all normal. In patients studied, trabecular bone volume was lower than normal, as was mean wall thickness and the mean trabecular thickness. There was a significant correlation between trabecular bone volume and mean trabecular thickness, but not between trabecular bone volume and mean wall thickness. Bone formation rate at tissue level was decreased. The mean interstitial bone thickness, which is inversely related to resorption, was not different from controls. It was concluded that osteoporosis in this population resulted from decreased bone formation and no change in bone resorption, and that high alcohol and tobacco consumption was a risk factor for osteoporosis in Man.

Fujita and associates from the Department of Medicine, Kobe University, studied immune function in osteoporotics. Tuberculin intracutaneous tests were performed in 240 subjects above the age of 55. Negative reactors increased with advance in age, from 15% below 65 to 95% above 90. Significant association was found between bone mineral content below 0.4 gr/cm^2, indicating definite osteoporosis and negative tuberculin reaction. Above the age of 76, negative reactors showed significantly lower BMC than positive reactors. Among subjects without spinal compression fracture, 48% were negative reactors and 74% of those with fractures gave negative reaction. Administration of levamisole for two months changed the negative reaction to positive in 50% of the osteoporotics, and $1\alpha(OH)D_3$ induced similar changes in 80%, suggesting a stimulation of immune function. Osteoporotics had increase in $OK^{T}4/^{T}8$ helper/suppressor ratios. It was concluded that aging is generally accompanied by a decrease in cell-mediated immune function, but such decreases were apparently more pronounced in osteoporotics, and that such defects seem to be influenced favorably by $1\alpha(OH)D_3$.

P. Geusens and associates, Leuven, Belgium, reported on the value of calcitonin tests in symptomatic postmenopausal osteoporotics. Salmon calcitonin was injected intramuscularly and blood and urine samples were collected at regular intervals up to 24 hours in 46 patients. Serum calcium decreased and urinary calcium increased early after injection. Urinary hydroxyproline increased slightly, immediately after injection; however, there was considerable individual variation. In general, patients with increased bone resorption (as evidenced by increased hydroxyprolinuria before calcitonin), had a more pronounced response to calcitonin; however, this was not found in all cases. It was concluded that the wide variation in changes in serum calcium and hydroxyprolinuria reflects the diversity of bone turnover in patients with symptomatic disease.

Professor Caniggia, Siena, presented data from an open trial of the use of $1,25(OH)_2D_3$ in the treatment of symptomatic osteoporosis. The trial was carried out in 37 women, 25 of whom presented with vertebral fractures. All received 1 μg per day of synthetic $1,25(OH)_2D_3$ for several months after the diagnosis had been confirmed by pretreatment biopsies. There was an improvement in bone pain and increased mobility in the majority of the women, but bone mineral content as assessed by photon absorptiometry did not change significantly. Fractional calcium absorption, which was decreased before treatment, was restored to normal in all patients, and no evidence of hypercalcemia was found. Urinary calcium increased in all cases, but urinary hydroxyproline did not increase, suggesting hypercalciuria was not due to an effect on bone. There was no change in blood urea nitrogen or serum and urine creatinine. The results suggest that $1,25(OH)_2D_3$ may have some value in the treatment of osteoporosis, and additional studies are being undertaken to further evaluate it.

B.E.C. Nordin and associates presented data from 41 female

patients with femoral neck fractures (mean age 73.9 years), and 53 elderly normal women (mean age 71.2 years), studied in Adelaide, South Australia. The mean plasma 25(OH)D level in the fracture cases was 38.4 $\pm$ 3.4 nmol/l, and in controls, 67.6 $\pm$ 4.0 nmol/l. Normal value for 44 laboratory workers in the same area was 75.6 nmol/l. When fracture cases were divided into those from nursing homes vs those admitted straight from their own homes, plasma 25(OH)D was significantly lower in the latter. It was concluded that even in Adelaide, with 2,500 hours of sunshine per annum, low 25(OH)D's are found in females with femoral neck fractures.

Susheela, from the All India Institute of Medical Sciences, reported studies on structural and functional deviations in cortical and cancellous bone produced in rabbits given high doses of fluoride. Morphometric studies revealed increased periosteal thickness and diameter of osteones in the cortical bone, whereas the cancellous bone developed cartilagenous loci. There was noted to be an increase in glycosaminoglycans in the trabecular bone and among the various constituents. Dermatan sulphate was increased in cancellous bone. This appeared to be localized in the cartilagenous foci. Human subjects who had received high fluoride intake had serum glycosaminoglycan content which was similar to that found in the animal model.

Teotia and associates from the Postgraduate Department of Human Metabolism and Endocrinology in Meerut, India, studied the interaction between fluoride and calcium intakes in patients with bone disease and deformities. Groups with high and low fluoride content and adequate and inadequate calcium intakes were contrasted. The incidence and severity of bone disease and bony leg deformities was greater in residents in endemic areas of fluorosis with dietary calcium deficiency. Also, the severity and prevalence of bone disease and deformity was larger in subjects exposed to high intakes of natural fluoride than in subjects residing in non-endemic areas. The bone diseases found included osteoporosis, rickets, osteomalacia, and parathyroid bone disease. Deformities were largely confined to the knees and legs. The presence of high fluoride and low calcium intake appeared to be responsible for the development of the deformities.

Dr. Schaadt, from the University of Copenhagen, reported on his use of the dual photon technique for measurement of bone mass in the lumbar spine, femoral neck, and femoral shaft. The method was quite accurate and had a precision of better than 2% in repeated measurements. His studies demonstrated that bone mineral loss with aging and in patients treated with Prednisone and those with primary osteoporosis were characterized by significantly greater loss from the axial than from the peripheral skeleton. Some patients had reduced axial bone mass with normal peripheral measurements, whereas other patients had decreased bone mass in both areas. It was concluded that it is necessary to make measurements in the clinically-relevant areas for adequate evaluation of bone mass.

Dr. Malluche, from University of Kentucky in Lexington, reported on his evaluation of bone GLA-protein as a marker of osteoblastic activity. Bone biopsies and serum levels of bone BGP were measured in 21 dialyzed patients with renal osteodystrophy. Bone histology showed low-turnover osteomalacia in 5 patients and the BGP was above normal here (71.4 $\pm$ 28.1 ng/ml vs a normal of 6.78 $\pm$ 0.20 ng/ml). Eleven patients had mixed uremic osteodystrophy and clearly elevated BGP (257 $\pm$ 76 ng/ml), and 5 patients had hyperparathyroid bone disease with extreme elevations in BGP (874 $\pm$ 210 ng/ml). There was significant correlation between BGP and the surface of osteoid, bone osteoblastic interface, osteoblastic index, surface and volume of fibrosis, and mineral apposition rate. There was no signficant difference in serum levels of $1,25(OH)_2D_3$, alkaline phosphatase, parathyroid hormone, serum calcium, and phosphorus between the three histologic groups. These data indicate that BGP may be useful in the evaluation of the patient with renal dystrophy.

Mautalen and associates, from Buenos Aires, reported on 10 patients with Paget's disease who had pathological fractures. In 5 cases, the treatment was conservative and calcitonin was given in a daily dose of 50 to 100 units. All healed within 3 to 6 months. Three of these patients had received EHDP therapy during 8 months to four years prior to the fracture. Delayed union was observed in 4 fracture patients treated surgically, and in another patient, severe demineralization precluded ambulation. Calcitonin was subsequently given to these patients, and healing ensued. Of these latter 5 patients, 3 had previously received EHDP during 2 to 12 months after surgery. It is suggested that calcitonin is useful in the treatment of bone fractures of Paget's disease.

Hills and associates, from Sidney, Australia, presented data on an 18-year-old female who had hypoplastic anemia. The hemoglobin was 7.8 gr/dl; the white count and thrombocyte count were normal; calcium, phosphorus, alkaline phosphatase, parathyroid hormone, and calcitonin were also normal. Bone x-rays showed uniform dense osteosclerosis. A bone marrow biopsy showed marked reduction in hemopoietic tissue with focal aggregates of lymphocytes. An iliac crest wedge biopsy was performed after double tetracycline labeling. Bone formation was normal with osteoid surfaces of 11%, osteoblast surfaces 5.1%, and total bone formation rate 344 $um^3/mm^3/day$. Resorption parameters were normal, with an osteoclast count of $1.0/mm^2$. No cartilage remnants were seen. It was speculated that the most probable cause of osteosclerosis and aplastic anemia in this patient is a marrow stem-cell defect leading to defective production of both hemopoietic tissue and osteoclasts.

Kuntz and associates, from Paris, France, described 10 patients aged 46 to 71, who were on chronic hemodialysis, and had x-rays which revealed destruction of the intervertebral disc, with a narrowing of the interspace and a variable degree of bone destruction. In 8 cases, these lesions were present in the cervical spine, and in 2 cases, in the thoracic and lumbar spine. Infection was suspected; however, vertebral pain was absent or minimal, and spine motility was normal. Disc biopsy in 3 cases was bacterialogically negative. This syndrome is called "erosive spondylarthropathy", and appears to be present in some patients on chronic hemodialysis.

ORAL SESSION D - SELECTED TOPICS

MODERATORS: C. ANAST, J. HADDAD

1. "Steroid-Sensitive Hypercalcemia Associated with Common Variable Immunodeficiency: Pseudo-Hypervitaminosis D" J.M. Lemire, L. Paunier, S.C. Jordan, J.W. Coburn, E. Slatopolsky, R.L. Horst, D.J. Sherrard, F.R. Singer, R.N. Fine

2. "Effects of $1,25(OH)_2D_3$ on Renal Phosphorus Threshold in Hypophosphatemic Rickets (XLH)" O. Mehls, F. Manz, K. Kettenmann

3. "Relationships Between Radiological and Biochemical Evidence of Rickets" A.A. Motaal, G. Gettinby, W.B. McIntosh, G.R. Sutherland, B.M. Glekin, M.G. Dunnigan

4. "Effect of Gastric Surgery on Stimulated Calcitonin Secretion" S. Ortolani, P. Salvini, I. Lamarina, E. Corghi, P. Favini, F.M. Ulivieri, E.E. Polli

5. "Mineral Economy in Preterm Infants Fed with Human Milk" B.L. Salle, J. Senterre, G. Putet, E.E. Delvin, F.H. Glorieux

6. "Calcium and Phosphorus Homeostasis in Children with Infantile Spasms During ACTH Therapy" R. Riikonen, O. Simell, J. Jaaskelainen, J. Perheentupa

7. "Rickets in Malnourished Children" N. Raghuramulu, V. Reddy

8. "Osteomalacia in Pseudohypoparathyroidism - The Role of Hypocalcemia and Hyperparathyroidism" J.M. Pettifor, E. Sochett, M. Quirk

9. "Effects of 1,25-Dihydroxycholecalciferol on Skeletal Growth in Osteodystrophic Uremic Children" M.L. Bianchi, E. Aimini, A. Edefonti, S. Ortolani, F. Sereni, E.E. Polli

10. "Low Perinatal Vitamin D Level and Its Relation to Infantile Rickets in Saudi Arabia" A.T.H. Elidrissy, F. Serinius, A. Swailim, P. Dandona

11. "Dietary Advices for Recurrent Stone Formers (RSF): New Developments" Ph. Jaeger, L. Portmann, A.F. Jacquet, P. Burckhardt

12. "Bone 'Buffering' Capacity in Aluminum Associated Bone Disease (AABD)" B.U. Ihle, M. Cochran, G. Becker, D. Campbell, P. Kincaid-Smith

13. "Calcium-Regulating Hormones in Children Receiving Total Parenteral Nutrition" G.L. Klein, R.L. Horst, E. Slatopolsky, L.J. Deftos

14. "Prolonged and Progressive Bone Mineral Loss Following Renal Transplantation in Children" R.W. Chesney, P.G. Rose, R.B. Mazess

15. "Evidence for Primary Parathyroid Gland Hyperfunction in Idiopathic Hypercalciuria" R.A. Evans, E. Hills, S.Y.P. Wong, C.R. Dunstan, Y. Eade. L. Wyndham

ORAL SESSION D - OVERVIEW

Constantine S. Anast

Department of Pediatrics, Harvard Medical School and Children's Hospital, Boston, MA, U.S.A.

Disturbances in mineral and bone metabolism continue to be frustrating problems in patients with chronic renal disorders. Moreover, additional problems have been recognized as experience has been gained with various forms of therapy. Thus, aluminum used in salts to bind phosphate accumulates at the bone-osteoid junction. Such patients may have normal or only slightly elevated levels of circulating parathyroid hormone. Ihle et al demonstrated with calcium infusion studies that patients with aluminum associated bone disease had significantly diminished calcium clearance compared to controls. They concluded that these patients had a diminished buffering capacity to acute changes in serum calcium and that hypercalcemia in chronic renal failure patients may be secondary to aluminum associated bone disease rather than to secondary hyperparathyroidism. In fact, patients with hyperparathyroidism had an increase in buffering capacity to acute changes in circulating calcium. Thus, the added complications produced by aluminum in patients with renal osteodystrophy indicate that aluminum therapy should be used with caution and that other methods should be investigated to help control serum phosphate concentration. Another observation of concern is that of Chesney et al who observed a progressive loss in bone mineral content in the majority of children following renal transplantation. They demonstrated that the bone mineral loss was secondary to a reduced renal function and glucocorticoid administration. They suggest that these children may be at serious risk for bone disabling disease in the future. On a positive note, Bianchi et al report that the administration of $1,25(OH)_2D_3$ to osteodystrophic uremic children over a one-year period resulted in an increase in bone mineral content, an increase in linear growth, and a reduction in circulating parathyroid hormone. Further studies are needed to determine the consistency of this effect as well as to determine whether there will be continued improvement over a longer period of time.

Idiopathic hypercalciuria continues to be an enigma. The possible roles of parathyroid hormone, vitamin D metabolites, hyperabsorption, and primary renal loss of calcium continue to be elusive. In view of these complexities, decisions regarding modes of prevention and therapy remain difficult. On the basis of studies in recurrent stone formers, Jaeger et al offer practical advice that very well may be profitable to follow until the puzzle of idiopathic hypercalciuria is unravelled. They point out the utility of a high fluid intake in the prevention of recurrence of nephrolithiasis. Problems with compliance with a high fluid intake are well recognized and must be dealt with in each individual patient. Jaeger et al also point out that a low calcium diet may lead to an increase in urinary oxalate in calcium hyperabsorbers. The increase in urinary oxalate would counteract the benefits of the decrease in urinary calcium and thereby defeat the purpose of the low calcium diet. Thus, they suggest that if dietary calcium is to be reduced, dietary oxalate should be simultaneously reduced, especially in the calcium hyperabsorbers.

Vitamin D deficiency as a result of poor dietary intake and limited exposure to sunlight remains a problem in various parts of the world. Three separate studies of vitamin D deficiency in this symposium provided new and interesting information. These observations were: (1) Malnutrition *per se* does not appear to affect the metabolism of vitamin D. (2) The serum calcium in cord blood is normal and higher than that in maternal blood in infants and mothers with low vitamin D stores. This suggests that the transplacental calcium transport may not be dependent upon the vitamin D status. (3) The serum alkaline phosphatase activity followed by serum Ca x PO_4 are the most important discriminating variables in predicting radiological evidence of rickets. Circulating 25-OHD levels do not show significant discrimination.

It is of interest that osteomalacia may be observed in patients with pseudohypoparathyroidism. Histomorphometric and biochemical studies by Pettifor et al suggest that the osteomalacia in these patients is secondary to hypocalcemia and that the pathogenesis is similar to that in calcium deficient rickets. Thus, measures to correct the hypocalcemia in these patients is important if osteomalacia is to be prevented.

Total parenteral nutrition is used as a therapeutic adjunct in the treatment of a number of disorders and, indeed, in certain circumstances may be life-saving. However, boney abnormalities of uncertain etiology, including demineralization, osteomalacia, and rickets, have proved to be serious complications. Biochemical abnormalities noted in adults include hypercalciuria, low serum $1,25(OH)_2D$, and hypophosphatemia. However, there is only limited information regarding possible abnormalities in children receiving total parenteral nutrition. Klein et al report normal to high serum $1,25(OH)_2D$ and decreased fractional excretion of calcium after three weeks of total parenteral therapy in children. Rickets was observed in one child and demineralization in another. Although these preliminary observations are of interest, the three-week period of study is relatively short and fails to provide substantive insight into this complex and serious problem. It is apparent that more detailed studies over more prolonged periods of time are needed to gain a better understanding of the pathogenesis of this complication.

Mehls et al demonstrated that the administration of $1,25(OH)_2D_3$ resulted in a significantly higher TmP/GFR in children with X-linked hypophosphatemic rickets. The significance of this finding is uncertain since it was not clear whether the effect on tubular reabsorption of phosphate was a direct one or whether it was possibly mediated through a decrease in circulating parathyroid hormone.

For a variety of reasons, it has become commonplace to feed human milk to low birth weight infants. However, hypophosphatemic rickets has been observed in several low birth weight infants who received human milk and has been attributed to the low phosphate concentration of human milk. Salle et al report that vitamin D does not increase calcium retention in these infants but that calcium retention is significantly increased by supplementation of human milk with phosphorus and vitamin D. Thus, it is possible that the benefits of human milk in premature infants can be achieved without the complications of metabolic bone disease by supplementing human milk with phosphate and 1200 units of vitamin D per day.

Abnormalities in mineral and bone metabolism are observed in patients with immunodeficiency but the underlying mechanism that links these two basic disorders together is unknown. Lemire et al present indirect evidence in support of the possibility of increased sensitivity to $1,25(OH)_2D$ in a patient with immunodeficiency associated with hypercalcemia, increased bone density, and hypercalciuria. The increased sensitivity to $1,25(OH)_2D$ was suggested by probable increased gastrointestinal absorption of calcium in the presence of normal circulating $1,25(OH)_2D$ levels. More direct evidence is needed to support this hypothesis. Detailed studies in patients of this type may provide basic information regarding the interrelationship between the macrophage system and altered calcium metabolism.

XX WORKSHOPS

WORKSHOP ON RADIOLOGY OF METABOLIC BONE DISEASE

S.R. Kottamasu, M.D.,[1] D.S. Rao, M.D.,[2] H.E. Meema, M.D.,[3] and H.K. Genant, M.D.[4]

Departments of Diagnostic Radiology[1] and Internal Medicine,[2] Henry Ford Hospital, Detroit, MI, U.S.A.; Department of Diagnostic Radiology,[3] Toronto General Hospital, Toronto, Ontario, Canada; and Department of Diagnostic Radiology,[4] University of California, San Francisco, San Francisco, CA, U.S.A.

S.R. Kottamasu illustrated an overview of metabolic bone disease with several clinical and radiologic case studies.

Case 1. A 55 year-old male with pain and limitation of motion of the left lower extremity.

Radiographs demonstrate hyperostosis of the left hemipelvis, femur, tibia, and medial rays of the foot. The findings in the hemipélvis resemble Paget's disease, however, wavy and sclerotic bone contour extending along one side of tubular bones, like flowing candle wax, is characteristic of MELORHEOSTOSIS. (Fig. 1,2)

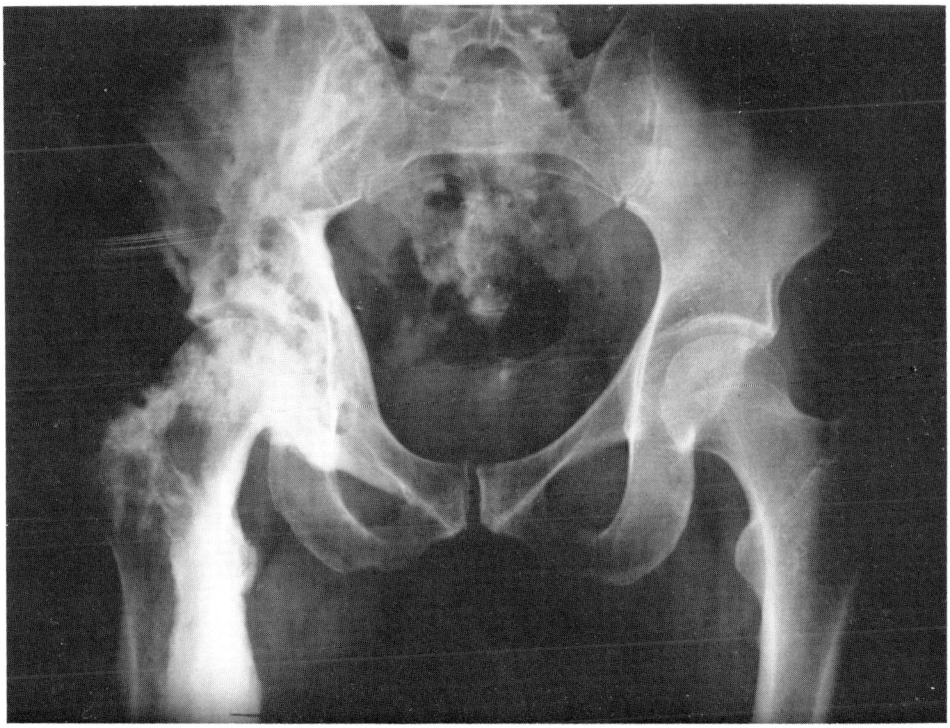

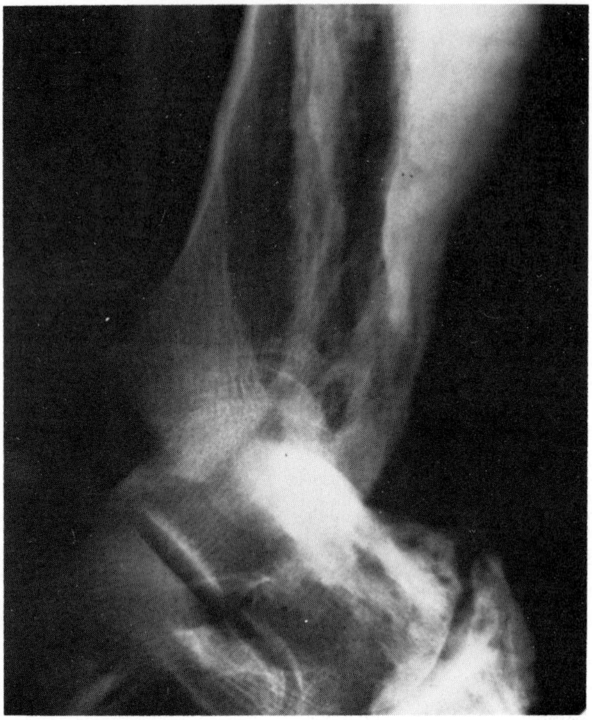

Case 2. A 15 year-old male following blunt trauma to the foot. Radiographs demonstrate numerous, well circumscribed foci of increased density in various bones, an incidental finding, characteristic of OSTEOPOIKILOSIS. (Fig. 3)

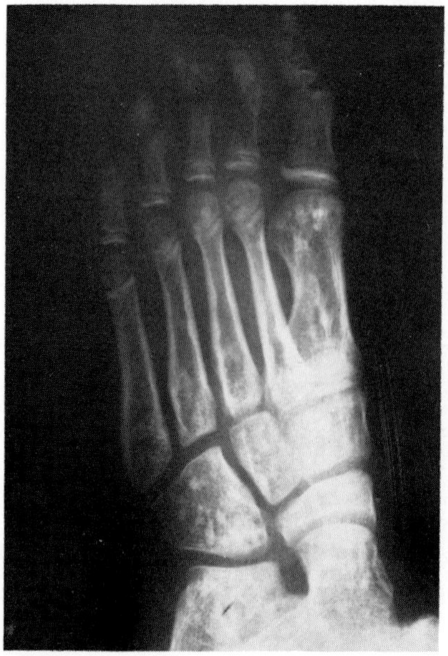

Pathologically, the focal sclerotic areas are foci of compact bone in spongiosa.

Case 3. A 5 year-old boy with waddling gait and muscular weakness.

Radiographs of lower extremities show symmetric cortical thickening involving mid-diaphyses of femur, tibia, and fibula. (Fig. 4)

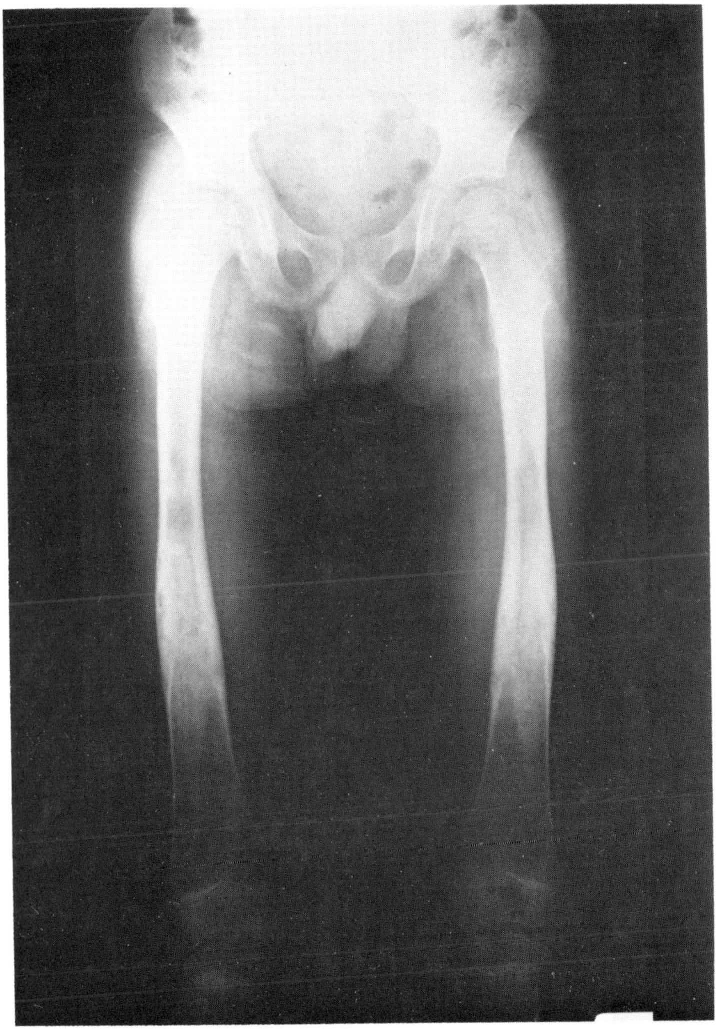

Radiographs of a 40 year-old male, father of Case 3, demonstrate sclerosis and marked cortical thickening with increase in the outer diameter of the bones. Metaphyses and epiphyses are conspicuously unaffected. (Fig. 5)

The findings are characteristic of ENGELMANN'S DISEASE (progressive diaphyseal dysplasia).

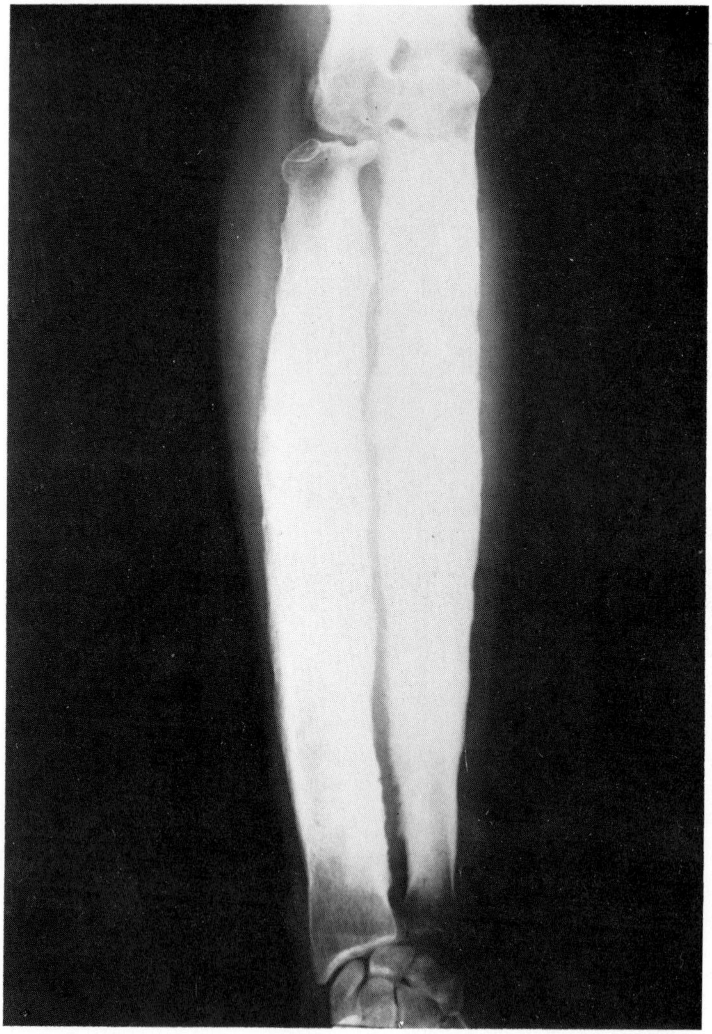

Case 4. Radiographs of the spine in a 45 year-old male show typical "bone-within-bone" appearance. One of the classic conditions in the differential diagnosis of this radiologic finding is OSTEOPETROSIS. Subsequent radiographs demonstrate generalized osteosclerosis, absence of corticomedullary demarcation and pathologic fracture of the proximal femur.

Case 5. Rickets in osteopetrosis.

Some children with congenital form of osteopetrosis develop radiologic changes of rickets and abnormal biochemical changes (low serum calcium, phosphorus, and increased alkaline phosphatase).

Pathogenesis is not well understood and treatment is unsatisfactory.

Case 6. A 55 year-old male with pain in the left lower thigh.

Radiographs of the femur demonstrate multiple lytic lesions involving the distal femur, some of the lesions are intracortical and the lesions extend to the distal articular surface of the femur. The proximal end of the lesion has a "blade of grass" appearance, characteristic of the osteolytic phase of Paget's disease, OSTEOPOROSIS CIRCUMSCRIPTA.

Case 7. A 15 year-old girl with headaches.

Radiographs demonstrate multiple lytic lesions in the fronto-parietal region of the skull. Follow up radiographs show sclerosis and thickening of bone at the sites of previous lytic lesions. (Fig. 6)

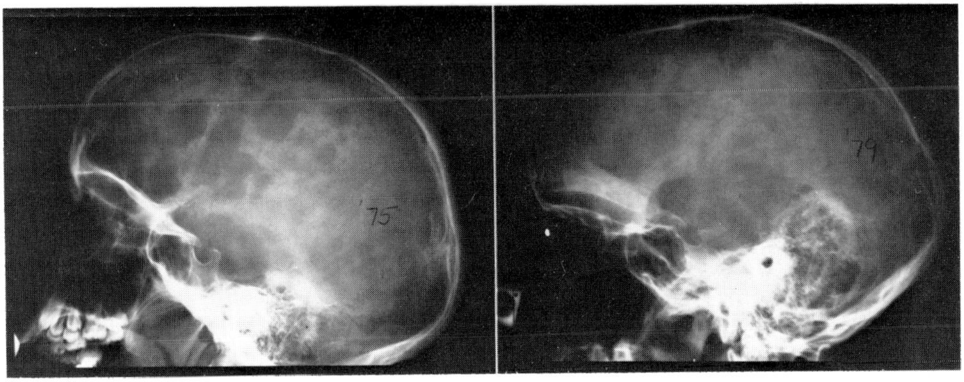

This case demonstrates spontaneous progression of the lytic phase of FIBROUS DYSPLASIA to the more commonly recognized sclerosic phase. This transition is less frequently documented in fibrous dysplasia than in Paget's disease.

Case 8. A 45 year-old woman with skin rash and hepatomegaly.

Skeletal radiographs demonstrate generalized mixed osteosclerotic and lytic pattern. This, associated with a brownish macular skin rash that urticates and hepatosplenomegaly, suggests the possibility of SYSTEMIC MASTOCYTOSIS. (Fig. 7)

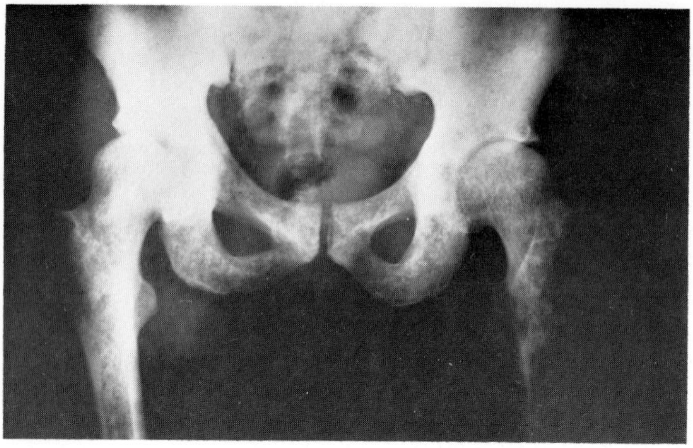

15 to 20% of patients with mastocytosis have detectable bone lesions. Skeletal lesions in mastocytosis may be lytic, sclerotic, or mixed, and may demonstrate focal, multifocal, or diffuse distribution.

Case 9. A 60 year-old male with generalized and progressive, severe skeletal pain and tenderness. Serum chemistries are normal except for a modest elevation of alkaline phosphatase. (Fig. 8)

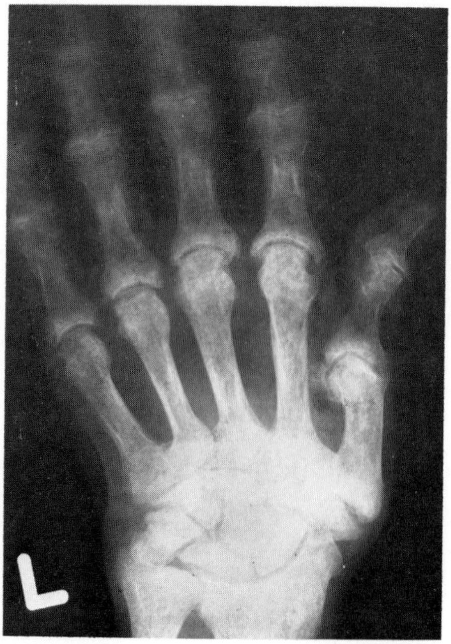

Radiographs demonstrate indistinct cortices, coarse trabecular pattern, and spotty areas of increased bone density. Outer diameters of all the bones of the hands are increased symmetrically, a feature characteristic of FIBROGENESIS IMPERFECTA OSSIUM. There is loss of birefringence of collagen fibers on polarizing microscopy.

Case 10. A 60 year-old with generalized osteosclerosis and lytic lesions involving two ribs.

A bone scan showed only minimal increased uptake in the lytic lesions in the ribs. Serum protein electrophoretic pattern was normal.

Bone biopsy demonstrated an OSTEOSCLEROTIC FORM OF MULTIPLE MYELOMA. The table lists the major causes of generalized osteosclerosis.

DIFERENTIAL DIAGNOSIS OF GENERALIZED OSTEOSCLEROSIS

1. Osteoblastic Metastatic Bone Disease
2. Hyperparathyroidism - primary or secondary
3. Myelosclerosis
4. Osteopetrosis
5. Lymphoma
6. Pyknodysostosis
7. Fluorosis
8. Systemic Mastocytosis
9. Tuberous Sclerosis
10. Van Buchem's Disease
11. Osteosclerotic Multiple Myeloma
12. Fibrogenesis Imperfecta Ossium

Case 11. A 35 year-old man presented with a pathologic fracture through a lytic lesion in the right tibia.

The skeletal survey demonstrated additional lytic lesions involving the left tibia and fibula. Follow-up films in six months showed SPONTANEOUS HEALING OF BROWN TUMORS WITH SCLEROSIS FOLLOWING PARATHYROIDECTOMY.

Case 12. A 14 year-old girl with bilateral slipped capital femoral epiphysis. There is subperiosteal resorption involving the phalanges of the hand. There is a lytic lesion in the left distal clavicle, consistent with a Brown tumor. The lab findings reveal persistent hypocalcemia, elevation of serum phosphorus, alkaline phosphatase and iPTH, and resistance to the administration of exogenous PTH.

This case represents RENAL RESISTANCE TO PARATHYROID HORMONE WITH OSTEITIS FIBROSA (pseudo-hypo-hyperparathyroidism).

H.E. Meema discussed the periosteal and juxtaperiosteal components of hyperparathyroid bone resorption in chronic renal failure.

Subperiosteal resorption in finger phalanges is a pathognomonic sign of hyperparathyroidism. It is generally considered to represent centripetal osteoclastic bone resorption from the periosteal surfaces, i.e. surface erosion. This does not fully explain why in some cases there remains a thin remnant of periosteal bone covering large juxtaperiosteal resorption spaces. A longitudinal microradioscopic study of the evolution of subperiosteal resorption in patient with resorption in patient with chronic renal failure shows increased juxtaperiosteal resorption (a variant of intracortical resorption in many areas where there is subsequent development of subperiosteal resorption. It thus appears that intracortical resorption, which is more a nonspecific manifestation of high bone turnover than a specific sign of hyperparathyroidism, often precedes development of subperiosteal resorption. This explains why both subperiosteal and intracortical resorption correlate significantly with the extent of elevation in iPTH, although the correlation is higher for subperiosteal than for intracortical resorption.

H.K. Genant reviewed the clinical applications of computed tomography of the spine.

The normal ranges of vertebral mineral and age-related bone losses were determined from cross-sectional studies of 120 normal males and 203 normal females, aged 20-80 years. The normal mean value for young males and females was approximately 175 mg/cm. Males, by a linear regression, lost an average of 0.84%/year, and females by a cubic regression, lost an average of 1.2%/year. Correcting for age-related bone marrow fat changes altered the observed rates of loss only by about 10%.

Cross-sectional studies in 80 perimenopausal women showed an average 5.6%/year vertebral cancellous mineral loss by QCT compared with 3%/year peripheral cortical mineral loss by photon absorptiometry and radiogrammetry. Longitudinal studies in 31 women following oophorectomy showed an average 9%/year vertebral cancellous bone loss, and peripheral cortical bone loss was 2 to 3%. Crosssectional studies in 25 young women with various forms of amenorrhea showed an average decrement from normal of 30% in vertebral mineral values and 10% in peripheral cortical values.

Cross-sectional studies in 48 males with idiopathic osteoporosis showed a mean decrement from normal of 48% in vertebral mineral and 15% in peripheral cortex. When expressed as a percent of normal, peripheral measurement correlated (r=0.63) with vertebral measurements but did not provide a reliable individual estimate of vertebral mineral loss or of atraumatic spinal fractures. Vertebral QCT measurement provided an index of fracture risk by revealing a threshold at approximately 110mg/ cm, above which fractures were rare and below which fractures were common.

The greatest advantages of spinal QCT for noninvasive bone mineral measurement lies in the high precision of the technique, the high sensitivity of the vertebral spongiosa measurement site, and the potential for widespread application.

MANAGEMENT OF PRIMARY HYPERPARATHYROIDISM: Report on a workshop discussing a proposed clinical study to prospectively evaluate the benefits and risks of surgical and non-surgical approaches to mild hyperparathyroidism

G.B. Talpos, M.D., M. Kleerekoper, M.D., A. Kambouris, M.D., and D.R. Moore, M.D.

Departments of Surgery and Medicine, Henry Ford Hospital, Detroit, MI U.S.A.

Earlier presentations and discussions at this symposium left many questions unanswered concerning the optimal management of patients with primary hyperparathyroidism (PHPT) in whom the hypercalcemia is minimal and in whom signs and symptoms directly referable to hypercalcemia and/or HPT are lacking. This has often been referred to in the literature as "asymptomatic PHPT" but this term has been deliberately excluded from this paper. Many patients with mild HPT are not truly asymptomatic. They pose a clinical problem in that their symptoms cannot be readily recognized as those of PHPT and the clinician cannot predict which of these many complaints might be alleviated by "corrective" surgery(1).

With this in mind, a workshop was held to discuss a prospective study of the management of PHPT. There was general agreement that the current literature on PHPT does not provide adequate answers concerning optimal management of patients with mild PHPT. Few studies have addressed this issue and only one is randomized and prospective(2,3). Although documentation exists that a skilled surgeon can correct hypercalcemia due to PHPT in more than 95% of patients (4), little evidence exists that this is of short-or long-term benefit in mild diseases. In fact there is a paucity of information concerning the benefits of surgery in patients with any degree of hypercalcemia(5).

Answers to many of these questions could be provided by a well designed properly conducted prospective randomized clinical trial evaluating benefits and risks of surgical and non-surgical management of patients with PHPT. Some of the questions which could be addressed, as generated by the participants of the workshop, are given in Table I.

TABLE I. Questions to be addressed by a prospective clinical trial.

A. Patient's Questions:
- If I feel well now, how will I feel better after surgery?
- How long before complications develop if I don't have surgery?
- What if I don't have surgery at all?

B. Physician's Questions:
- What is the natural history of skeletal complications and how is this effected by surgery?
- What is the cost of surgery versus medical follow-up?
- Are there factors present at the time of diagnosis which can predict the clinical course of the disease in an individual patient?
- Do different forms of PHPT exist and do these relate to the different secretory abnormalities (set point change versus non-set point change) or to different histologic abnormalities?
- What is the success rate of surgery?
- What is the complication rate of non-surgery?
- Are these complications reversible?
- Are these complications avoidable by non-surgical means?
- What constitutes cure?
- Which surgeons should perform the initial parathyroidectomy?
- Which surgeons should perform follow-up explorations?

Serious concerns were raised about the feasability of conducting such a trial. The best recognized published prospective clinical trial of the management of PHPT was conducted at the Mayo Clinic(6). A principal investigator of of that trial, Dr. Donald Scholz, reported to the workshop that the single limiting factor to the conduct of their trial was inadequate funding. Another major difficulty encountered was the waning enthusiasm of the patient's primary care physician through the necessary long follow-up period. These concerns were echoed by many of the participants. Without attempting to minimize these difficulties it was agreed to proceed with a design of a clinical trial in order to better seek funding of such an undertaking.

Discussion then concentrated on establishing a diagnosis of PHPT in a cost effective manner. Table II contains the minimum evaluation required to confirm PHPT. It also contains the parameters utilized to exclude non-parathyroid causes of hypercalcemia such as sarcoidosis, milk-alkali syndrome, and various types of malignancy. Although some investigators had operational definitions which differed, those present agreed to incorporate these guidelines as the minimum for the purposes of the proposed trial. Data which had been collected could always be excluded if not relevant, but data which had not been collected could never be assessed.

TABLE II. Minimal criteria to diagnose PHPT and exclude non-parathyroid causes of hypercalcemia.

History and Physical Examination.

- Serum calcium greater than or equal to two standard deviations above the mean on more than one occasion (calcium measurements can be either ionized or protein-corrected total serum calcium).
- Multi channel biochemical profile
- Complete blood count
- Urinalysis
- Chest radiograph
- Serum and Urine protein electrophoresis
- Immunoreactive PTH
- 24 hour urine for calcium and creatinine
- Intravenous pyelogram
- T4, T3 if age greater than 70

The next issue addressed by the workshop participants was to determine which patients with PHPT could be ethically randomized into different treatment categories. Patients with any of several serious conditions associated with hypercalcemia would be immediately moved into the surgical treatment group. Providing these patients with the usual treatment for hypercalcemia from PHPT - namely surgery - should protect them from possible detrimental effects of the study. A list of the conditions which would mandate surgery is found in Table III.

Although the major categories for randomization of appropriate patients are surgery and non-surgery, interest was expressed in further subdividing the non-surgery category. This would allow inclusion of other treatments which were also discussed at the Symposium such as cimetidine, propanolol, estrogen and diphosphanates in addition to a simple observation group (7,8). The services of a biostatistician would be utilized in constructing the overall experimental design and a determination would be made concerning the practicality of assessing the number of patients necessary to provide statistical significance with this increased number of treatment categories.

The desirability of surgical input and especially standardization of the surgical approach was briefly discussed when it was announced that the American Association of Endocrine Surgeons (AAES) was interested in supporting this study. The concensus of the workshop participants was to leave further deliberations in this area to the AAES. Continued communication with this surgical organization was encouraged.

TABLE III. Conditions which would mandate parathyroidectomy if present at any time.

A. Signs and Symptoms.
- Renal lithiasis
- Clinically evident bone disease
- Pancreatitis
- Recurrent peptic ulcer disease
- Disabling "soft" PHPT-associated symptoms
- Distance from medical care making follow-up unlikely
- Intercurrent thyroid surgery
B. Laboratory Investigation.
- Serum calcium greater than 13 mg/DL on one occasion, greater than 12mg/on two occasions, or greater than 11.5 mg/DL on three occasions.
- Urinary calcium greater than 400 mg/24 hrs. on 750 mg. calcium diet for 48 hours.
- Metabolic bone disease (bone mineral content greater than two standard deviations below the mean)
- Renal insufficiency
- Anemia less than 10 grams hemoglobin/DL

After four hours of discussion the workshop was drawn to a close. Some issues were left untouched due to lack of time. More importantly, however, a strong initiative was begun to evaluate current treatment of PHPT. A committment was made to continue evolving a protocol with which to seek proper funding. Individuals interested in participating in design of this study itself were invited to contact the authors.

REFERENCES

1. Coe, F and Favus, M (1980) Does Mild,Asymptomatic Hyperparathyroidism Require Surgery? New England Journal of Medicine 302: 224-5

2. Neer, R (1983) Natural History of Untreated Hyperparathyroidism. Submitted for Publication.

3. Larsson, L, Toss, G, Lennquist, S, Tegler, L and Tilling (1983) A Preliminary Report from a Prospective Study on Mild Hyperparathyroidism. Submitted for Publication.

4. Wells, S and Leight, G (1983) The Surgical Management of Patients with Primary Hyperparathyroidism. Submitted for Publication

5. Posen, S, Clifton-Bligh, P. Reeve, T. Wagstaffe, C, and Wilkinson, M (1983) Is Parathyroidectomy of Benefit in Primary Hyperparathyroidism. Submitted for Publication.

6. Scholz, D and Purnell, D. (1981) Asymptomatic Primary Hyperparathyroidism: A 10 year prospective study. Mayo Clinic Proc. 56: 473-478.

7. Bilezikian, J (1983) Medical Management of Primary Hyperparathyroidism. Submitted for Publication.

8. Marcus, R, Madvig, P, Crim, M, Kosek, J and Pont, A (1983) Estrogen Therapy for Postmenopausal Women with Primary Hyperparathyroidism. Submitted for Publication

AUTHOR INDEX

SUBJECT INDEX

Prepared by N.C. Netelenbos

University Hospital, Free University, Amsterdam